THE POLITICAL COST OF AIDS IN AFRICA

Evidence from six countries

Published by Idasa, 357 Visagie Street, Pretoria 0001

© Idasa 2008
ISBN 978-1-920118-65-5

First published 2008

Edited by Lois Henderson
Cover by Marco Franzoso
Layout by Bronwen Müller
Production by Idasa Publishing

Bound and printed by Logo Print, Cape Town

THE POLITICAL COST OF AIDS IN AFRICA

Evidence from six countries

Edited by Kondwani Chirambo

*id*asa

2008

Contents   Page

Contributors

Editor and project leader

Kondwani Chirambo

Kondwani Chirambo, the programme manager of IDASA-GAP, conceptualised and initiated the AIDS and Elections Project for IDASA in 2003 and published the first research paper to provide empirical evidence on the impact of HIV/AIDS on the electoral process, focusing on Zambia. Chirambo holds a Master of Arts Degree in Mass Communications from the University of Leicester, United Kingdom; and an Advanced Diploma in Human Rights Law from the Raoul Wallenberg Institute, University of Lund, Sweden. Chirambo is a doctoral candidate in Communication Science with the University of South Africa (UNISA). He has published widely on AIDS and governance including *Democratisation in the Age of HIV/AIDs*; and *HIV/AIDS and Governance in Southern Africa: Emerging Theories and Perspectives* (principal editor and co-author).

Email: kchirambo@idasa.org.za

Researchers

Malawi

Alister Chawundumuka Munthali

Dr Munthali is the Deputy Director of the Centre for Social Research in charge of research and training. He is a medical anthropologist and obtained his PhD in anthropology from Rhodes University, South Africa in 2003 and a Masters of Arts from the University of Amsterdam in 1999. His areas of interest are the social aspects of HIV/AIDS, child labour, disability, occupational health and safety, adolescent sexual and reproductive health and urban health. He has published in internationally refereed journals such as the African Anthropologist, the Nordic Journal of African Studies and the Malawi Medical Journal.

Email: amunthali@csrunima.org

Professor Wiseman Chirwa

Professor Chirwa is a former Director of the Centre for Social Research, University of Malawi. His current research projects include: State of Democracy in Malawi; Civil Society and Poverty Reduction; and Institutions of Democratic Governance in Malawi. He is editor of the Malawi Journal of Social Science and has published widely in journals and edited books.

Email: wisechirwa@yahoo.com

Peter Mvula

Dr Mvula is a socioeconomist and has a Masters of Professional Studies (International Development) and a PhD in Rural Development, concentrating on rural livelihoods from the University of East Anglia (UK), obtained in 2002. He is also a gender analyst and trainer. Dr Mvula has done surveys in the fields of rural livelihoods, the nutritional status of rural communities, food security, safety nets and rural livelihoods, health-related issues, poverty analysis and disaster and relief operations.

Email: Peter_mvula@hotmail.com

Zambia

Derrick Elemu

Derrick Elemu holds a Masters of Arts in Development Studies, specialising in the Politics of Alternative Development Strategies, Gender, Human Rights and Good Governance from the Institute of Social Studies (ISS), The Hague, Netherlands. He is also the current Chairperson for the CODESRIA National Working Group in Zambia. As part of his responsibilities at the university he engages in research, both on behalf of the university and for other organisations. He also undertakes research as a consultant with local and international NGOs and development agencies.

Email: elemud@gmail.com

Elijah Rubvuta

Elijah Rubvuta is the Executive Director of the Foundation for Democratic Process (FODEP). He has over ten years of experience in various capacities with one of Zambia's leading non-partisan election monitoring civic organisations. FODEP has monitored every election in the country since 1992. Rubvuta holds a Masters degree in Development Studies from the Institute of Social Studies in The Netherlands and a Bachelor's degree in Social Work & Public Administration from the University of Zambia. He has participated in a number of social research studies.

Email: rubvuta@gmail.com

Adrian Muunga

Adrian Muunga is a democratic governance consultant and partner of MEG Associates in Zambia. He also conducts political party capacity-building programmes and public opinion research. Muunga is currently the Civil Society APRM Co-ordinator, managing a secretariat that co-ordinates civil society input into the African Peer Review process. He previously served as National Co-ordinator for the Netherlands Institute for Multiparty Democracy (IMD) and has worked for the National Democratic Institute (NDI) in Zambia, Zimbabwe, South Africa, Malawi, Togo and The Gambia. He is a founding member of the Foundation For Democratic Process (FODEP) and a graduate of the University of Zambia.

Namibia

Graham Hopwood

Graham Hopwood is the Manager of the Public Dialogue Centre at the Namibia Institute for Democracy (NID) in Windhoek. He is also a Co-editor of Insight Namibia, Namibia's only current affairs magazine. He holds a BA Hons degree in English Language and Literature from the University of Liverpool, UK. His published work includes Tackling Corruption: Opinions on the Way Forward In Namibia (Editor) published by the Namibia Institute for Democracy (NID) (2007); Guide to Namibian Politics published by NID (2004 and 2006); Regional Councils: At the Crossroads (occasional paper published by NID 2005); The Swapo Extraordinary Congress: Uncharted Territory (research paper published by IPPR 2004); The Men Who Would Be President (research paper published by IPPR 2004); Walvis Bay: South Africa's Hostage (a booklet published by Catholic Institute for International Relations 1991).

Email: graham@nid.org.na

Justine Hunter

Justine Hunter is the Executive Director of the Namibia Institute for Democracy (NID) in Windhoek. She has a Masters degree in Political Science, History and Anthropology from the Rheinische-Friedrich Wilhelm University, Bonn, Germany. She also has a PhD in Political Science from the Albert-Ludwigs-University, Freiburg i.Br. Germany. Her thesis was on The Politics of Memory and Forgetting in Independent Namibia: Dealing with Gross Human Rights Abuses Committed during the Era of Armed Liberation Struggle, 1966-1989 (publication forthcoming). Her publications include Who Should Own the Land? Analyses and Views on Land Reform and The Land Question in Namibia and Southern Africa (Windhoek: NID 2004).

Email: hunter@nid.org.na

Doris Kellner

Doris Kellner is the Programme Manager: Civic Education Programme of the Namibia Institute for Democracy (NID) in Windhoek, where she is responsible for the conceptualisation and execution of numerous traditional and interactive civic and voter education programmes, including multimedia campaigns, publications, national competitions, national and regional workshops and conferences. She has a BA Hons degree in Communication Science from Rand Afrikaans University, Johannesburg and a Masters of Business Leadership from the University of South Africa (Unisa).

Email: kellner@nid.org.na

Tanzania

Flora Kessy

Flora Lucas Kessy is a Senior Social Scientist at the Ifakara Health Research and Development Centre (IHRDC) and holds a PhD in Agricultural and Consumer Economics with a major in Family and Consumer Economics and a minor in Women and Gender in the Global Perspective from the University of Illinois at Urbana Champaign (2001). She also has a Masters degree in Management of Natural Resources and Sustainable Agriculture from the Agricultural University of Norway (1996) and a Bachelor of Science, Food and Technology from Sokoine University of Agriculture, Morogoro,

Tanzania (1991). Kessy has researched and published on issues related to poverty, gender and development, household food security, and reproductive health, in particular family planning and HIV/AIDS.

Email: fkessy@gmail.com

Ernest Mallya

Professor Ernest Mallya is Associate Professor in Public Policy and Administration at the University of Dar es Salaam. He studied in Tanzania for his first two degrees (BA and MA) and earned a PhD from the University of Manchester, England in 1994. He has worked on projects in various domains within the governance field. Included among the research and government institutions in which he has worked are: the former Civil Service Department (Tanzania), the German Technical Cooperation Agency (GTZ), the Economic and Social Research Foundation (ESRF) of Tanzania, The International Health Policy Programme (IHPP), the UNDP/Maastricht School of Management (MsM), the Kvistgaard/Hedeselskabet (Denmark), the Electoral Institute of Southern Africa (EISA) and Idasa.

Email: emallya@hotmail.com

Oswald Mashindano

Dr Oswald Mashindano is a Senior Research Fellow with the Economic and Social Research Foundation (ESRF), where he is Coordinator of Research and Monitoring. For the past 18 years, Mashindano has undertaken research and teaching at the University of Dar es Salaam, Tanzania. He teaches microeconomics, agricultural economics and rural development, and natural resources and environmental economics. He has also lectured in quantitative methods and research methodology. Mashindano is the author of various publications. His most recent published articles include Private Foreign Investment and the Poorest Countries: The Case of Tanzania; and The Agricultural Sector and Poverty in Tanzania: The Impact and Future of the Reform Process. He has also coauthored several books, including Maendeleo Stahimilivu (Sustainable Development); Tourism Growth and Sustainable Development; and Mining for Sustainable Development in Tanzania.

Email: omashindano@hotmail.com

Senegal

Cheikh Ibrahima Niang

Dr Cheikh Ibrahima Niang is a Senior Lecturer at the Institut des Sciences de l'Environnement (Institute for Environmental Sciences) and in the department of sociology of Cheikh Anta Diop University, Dakar, Senegal. His Masters degree in anthropology and his PhD in environmental sciences were cosupervised by the late Dr Anta Diop. Currently, Cheikh I. Niang teaches social anthropology and research methodology. He supervises several masters and doctoral students on the social aspects of the environment, HIV/AIDS and health. He is coeditor of a journal on social aspects of HIV/AIDS in Africa.

Email: ciniang@sentoo.sn

South Africa

Per Strand

Dr Per Strand holds a PhD in political science from Uppsala University, Sweden. His thesis – Decisions on Democracy: The Politics of Constitution-Making in South Africa 1990-1996 – seeks to explain how the compromise on the democratic constitution emerged through negotiations, brinkmanship and the recognition of mutual interests between the key parties. He has extensive lecturing experience in Comparative Politics at the Department of Government at Uppsala University. He is currently a Lecturer in Political Science Theory and Methodology in the Department of Political Studies at the University of Cape Town, South Africa. A permanent resident in South Africa, Strand is affiliated to the Centre for Social Science Research at the University of Cape Town.

Khabele Matlosa

Dr Khabele Matlosa is the Senior Adviser (Director) in the Research Department at the Electoral Institute of Southern Africa (EISA). He holds a PhD in Political Economy from the University of the Western Cape, Cape Town and an MA in Development Studies from the University of Leeds, UK. He has lectured extensively at undergraduate level on political development and governance in Southern Africa at the National University of Lesotho (NUL), the University of the Western Cape and at post-graduate level in the Masters of Policy Studies (MPS) programme of the Southern African Political Economy Series (SAPES) Trust based in Harare, Zimbabwe. Prior to joining EISA, Dr Matlosa was the Director: Research and Policy Studies Faculty at SAPES Trust.

Ann Elaine Strode.

Ann Strode is a Senior Lecturer at the School of Law; University of Natal, Pietermaritzburg. She served as special legal adviser to the National HIV/AIDS and STD Directorate; was the regional director for Lawyers for Human Rights and a member of the University of Natal's HIV/AIDS Vaccine and Ethics Research Group. She has consulted for international and donor agencies in various capacities. Strode recently completed a consultancy for Idasa's Governance and Aids Programme on Institutional Governance of the HIV/AIDS Pandemic in South Africa. She holds an LLM, LLB and BA in Religious Studies and Political Science, from the University of Natal.

Researchers at Idasa-GAP

Josina Machel

Josina Machel is the Coordinator of the Institutional Capacity Building Project (Parliaments and Political Parties) in GAP. She holds a Master of Sciences degree in Sociology, (Gender) from the London School of Economics and Political Science, UK and a Bachelor of Social Science, Sociology and Political Science from the University of Cape Town, South Africa. Previously Machel worked for the Anglo-American Operations Ltd as Human Resources Officer: HIV/AIDS Programmes. She leads Idasa-GAP's work on policy on the African continent and strategic institutional interventions.

Christele Diwouta

Christele Diwouta is a Programme Assistant in Idasa-GAP. She holds an LLM in Human Rights and Democratisation from the University of Pretoria; a Maitrise in Business Law from the University of Dschang, Cameroon and an LLB from the University of Buea, Cameroon. Diwouta worked as research

assistant with the Centre for the Study of AIDS, before joining Idasa-GAP. She has participated in election observation missions to Madagascar organised by the Electoral Institute of Southern Africa (EISA) and in the Idasa observation mission to the Nigerian general elections of 2007. She has also contributed to Idasa publications on child labour and human rights.

Justin Steyn

Justin Steyn is a PhD candidate at Wits University. He is currently a researcher at Idasa. His speciality is political philosophy, with an emphasis on free agency in active social engagement. In his studies he has focused on human rights, democratic theory, moral philosophy, distributive justice, political economy and gender studies.

Acknowledgments

The road leading to this publication has been a long, bumpy one, with new challenges at every turn. We have learned from this exercise some invaluable lessons about the methodologies required to unravel topics of a politically sensitive nature; about the etiquette called for in engaging the various high-level personalities and institutions that contributed to the content of the study and, finally, about the nature of the beast itself – exploratory research.

The exploratory studies conceptualised, undertaken and led by the Governance and AIDS Programme (GAP) of Idasa over the past five years clearly revealed the relationship between AIDS and democratic governance on the one hand, and the capacity deficits of many of our institutions irrespective of the epidemic on the other.

These studies are the culmination of a project that began in 2003 amidst scepticism concerning the subject matter and its relevance to the overall national responses to HIV/AIDS. Yet in many instances, when audiences were faced with speculative theories, the fascination with the outcomes became self-evident. It has taken time to register new waves of acknowledgement about the importance of the work and its relationship to traditional areas such as politics, human development and health.

Over the years, the work has expanded to cover seven countries: Botswana, Namibia, Malawi, Senegal, South Africa, Tanzania and Zambia. In all the countries, Idasa worked with state entities and civil society organisations. I take this opportunity to underline that the work could not have been possible without the involvement and dedication of our local partners; the Center for Social Research (CSR) at the University of Malawi; the Namibia Institute for Democracy (NID); the Economic and Social Research Foundation in Tanzania (ESRF); the Foundation for Democratic Processes (FODEP) in Zambia; and the Institute for Environmental Sciences at the University of Cheik Anta Diop, Dakar, Senegal. The researchers from these partner agencies, all of them senior academics and practitioners, have - apart from undertaking the country-based research - played pivotal roles in mobilising local political figures in the wide-ranging national forums that informed the pre- and post-research phases of the multi-country studies.

Without the involvement of officials from government, political parties, national assemblies, electoral commissions, People Living with HIV/AIDS, election NGOs, research institutions and above all the donor agencies that financed it, this would have been an exercise in futility.

It is hence with immense gratitude that we extend our thanks to the Swedish International Development Cooperation Agency (SIDA), which financed this most comprehensive of all our studies in this area. The multi-country research was a follow-up to a pilot study conducted in Zambia in 2003, which was funded by the Ford Foundation and subsequent research in South Africa undertaken in 2004/5 supported by the Rockefeller Brothers Fund (RBF).

The support of these three donor agencies has placed GAP at the helm of a new body of knowledge that establishes the empirical link between HIV/AIDS and democratic governance, using the electoral process as an entry point. Based on its ground-breaking research, GAP has begun a process of developing strategic approaches for political leaders/policy-makers as a contribution to the effective management of the pandemic.

We may recall that the AIDS and Elections Project was an initiative that emerged out of consultations with political agencies at the highest level, among them: the Electoral Commissions Forum of SADC Countries (SADC-ECF), senior representatives from the United Nations Development Programme (UNDP) and the Joint United Nations Programme on HIV/AIDS (UNAIDS) country offices, the SADC Parliamentary Forum, the SADC Health Sector Coordinating Unit, civil society and donor agencies and the presidency of South Africa represented by Former Deputy President Jacob Zuma.

The second Governance and AIDS Forum was held on 22-24 May 2007 in Cape Town to discuss the findings of the multi-country study and was opened by the then acting Minister of Health, Mr Jeff Radebe (Minister of Transport). It brought together technical experts from the SADC region and francophone West Africa to examine the outcomes and suggest initiatives that might galvanise targeted policy responses. Electoral commission directors from the regions, AIDS experts, finance ministry officials, political party leaders and government department officials from South Africa participated in the deliberations that commanded worldwide media coverage. In short, the contributions to this project have been many and varied.

Finally, let me sincerely thank the staff of Idasa-GAP for their dedication to addressing the deficits in the research through additional work and interviews. In particular, Josina Machel, Christele

Diwouta and Justin Steyn played important roles in delivering a product that was as close to our original vision as possible. Marietjie Myburg lubricated our public communication in several innovative ways. Jennifer Dreyer, and before her Vasanthie Knaicker, managed our administrative processes with great efficiency. Moira Levy and Bronwen Müller of Idasa's Publishing Department spent the second half of 2007 assisting with the onerous task of publishing the book.

Special thanks to AFRIGIS PTY Limited for developing the Geographical Information Systems (GIS) maps and related graphs for this project.

Dr Anne Chikwana, formerly Idasa's Coordinator of the Afrobarometer project, assisted partners with useful directions and insights on the use of public opinion data. Ann Strode of the University of KwaZulu-Natal and Dr Khabele Matlosa of the Electoral Institute of Southern Africa (EISA) continued to play important roles at various stages of the studies. Through all this, Paul Graham, the Chief Executive of Idasa, was always available to us to be consulted and to provide moral support.

If we have failed to acknowledge others whose valuable input we benefited from, we do so with sincere apologies.

Kondwani Chirambo,
Manager Idasa-GAP

Preface

Elections are not enough to establish a democracy. The African Charter on Democracy, Elections and Governance establishes 11 principles of democratic governance, not only "the holding of regular, transparent, free and fair elections" but also those dealing with gender equity, corruption, representation, participation, political parties and transparent state processes.

Nevertheless, without elections and the possibility that these bring for the alternation or renewal of leadership, accountability to citizens by leaders, public choice, and a culture of citizen initiative and ownership of political systems, democracy cannot exist.

Despite encouraging signs of a shift in many countries on our continent to multiparty electoral systems, democracy itself is nowhere guaranteed; fledgling multiparty states have had to contend with endemic poverty, social and political upheaval, assaults on civil liberty and other challenges to the emergent new order.

Idasa's Governance and AIDS Programme (GAP) recognises that HIV/AIDS can destabilise the institutions of democratic governance, especially in countries where they are new and vulnerable.

Idasa established GAP to assist countries affected by the disease to explore its impact on governance and to investigate the best forms of parliamentary representation for managing the disease. It has undertaken public research and engaged in conversations with a range of stakeholders, taking its investigation to the very heart of the problem – the effect of the disease on electoral officials, institutions, voters and elected leaders, in fact on the electoral process itself.

This research has been conducted publicly through a combination of investigative work and engagement with those affected and infected by the disease. It has both immediate policy implications and more general policy lessons. It also considers the general political and social consequences of the disease – for determining budget priorities, allocating resources, shaping economies and communities, and determining the quality of public services, amongst many others. In particular, it looks carefully at the consequences for electoral systems and election management, and for the administrations, contestants and voters without whom our societies degrade their democratic legitimacy and efficacy.

We have to accept for the moment that we cannot cure the disease. And while, with considerable difficulty, we can encourage individuals to protect themselves against infection and prevent others from contracting it, we still have to adapt our societies to deal with the millions of people who are already HIV-positive – through medication, nutrition, daily care, and social and individual wellbeing – and with the consequences of unnatural death rates amongst adults of child-rearing and socially productive ages.

Until we can end HIV/AIDS, and even in the period from a cure to the last infection, we will have to establish AIDS-resilient societies. This book is about what may need to be done in one very important area.

This work would not have been possible without the support of the Swedish International Development Cooperation Agency (SIDA), which financed much of the research in this study. Thanks are also due to the Ford Foundation and the Rockefeller Brothers Fund for their role in financing this work.

Idasa has been privileged to work with five partners in this project: the Center for Social Research at the University of Malawi, the Namibia Institute for Democracy, the Economic and Social Research Foundation in Tanzania, the Foundation for Democratic Processes in Zambia and the Institute for Environmental Sciences at the University of Cheik Anta Diop, Dakar, Senegal. Our heartfelt thanks to them as well.

Paul Graham
Executive Director, Idasa

INTRODUCTION

Kondwani Chirambo

1. Introduction

The Political Cost of AIDS in Africa is an expedition into the unexplored realms of a pandemic that today poses an unprecedented development challenge to a continent seeking revival amidst the rigours of globalisation.

It is a journey that takes us into the inner sanctums of politics and the uneasy environment generated by AIDS therein. It is, in essence, a discussion that unravels the challenges to political participation experienced by ordinary citizens living with HIV/AIDS.

It is a study that quantifies both the political and economic costs associated with the loss of elected representatives and voters to AIDS; one that ultimately illustrates the threat posed by the pandemic to the sustenance of democratic institutions.

In the final analysis, this book presents observations and recommendations for possible reasoned[i] interventions, in the short and long term. It is the fourth and most comprehensive volume produced by Idasa as part of a five-year undertaking to establish the impact of HIV/AIDS on the electoral process within the broader context of democratic governance.

We launched this study with a pilot in Zambia (Chirambo: 2003), following it up with a comprehensive exploration of South Africa (Strand; Matlosa; Strode & Chirambo: 2005) and a preliminary release of our multicountry synthesis report (Chirambo: 2006).

The publication represents the work of African researchers in six countries. It constitutes case studies of Namibia, Malawi, Tanzania, South Africa, Senegal and Zambia, with a comparative section following this chapter. The book will delve into deep-seated national issues, relating not only to the electoral process but also to the political management of the HIV/AIDS epidemic. Its outcomes, we hope, will have broader policy relevance not only to strategies dealing with HIV/AIDS, but also to initiatives on electoral system design.

Followers of our work in the fields of HIV/AIDS and governance will recall that it was slightly over four years ago that senior political leaders, technocrats, academics and policy specialists from 12 countries in southern Africa and intergovernmental organisations converged upon Cape Town to discuss the governance ramifications of the pandemic.

In many ways, the two and a half day conference, organised by the Governance and AIDS Programme (GAP) of Idasa and the United Nations Development Programme (UNDP), was the first serious attempt to move what some might have considered a highly academic subject to the policy arena with a clear intent to demystify the link between two seemingly unrelated fields.

Idasa facilitated a process of dialogue on the implications of AIDS for democratic governance at the conference dubbed the Governance and AIDS Forum (GAF) involving senior representatives of regional bodies such as the Southern African Development Community (SADC) Health Sector Coordinating Unit (SADC-HSCU), the SADC Electoral Commissions Forums (SADC-ECF), the SADC Parliamentary Forum, the UNDP, UNAIDS; the presidency in South Africa, donor agencies and research institutions.[ii] Country-specific stakeholder meetings were held in Namibia, Malawi, Tanzania, South Africa, Senegal and Zambia in 2005/6 that included senior state and non-state actors. These were reference group meetings which served to validate findings and further regional input, leading to the second GAF held in Cape Town on 22-24 May 2007. These participatory processes were meant to engender wider "ownership" of the problem and a shared policy approach based on the outcomes.

The first GAF conference was subsumed by speculative theory issuing from academics and defence analysts from the United States who postulated a complete collapse of state systems in Africa, particularly since many countries on the continent seemed to fit into the World Bank's definition of "fragile states."[iii] With its catastrophic consequences characterised by gradual decimation of the relatively younger, economically productive and often more educated segment of the population, US scholars envisaged AIDS as almost certainly likely to further weaken the pillars of democracy: the economy, political institutions and political culture.[iv] This analysis failed to critically consider the hubs of resilience within African societies such as extended family and kinship systems, all of which, although overwhelmed, continue to be one of the reasons why our societies at the very basic level of human organisation, have held together.[v]

The second GAF was challenged to seek solutions as a demonstration of the resolve of the African states in responding to the threats posed by AIDS to political institutions based on the findings of 2003, 2005 and 2006. Significantly, the second GAF was driven by African scholars who provided much richer understandings of their own contexts and were moved to challenge western experiences and definitions of democratic governance, which will be ably expounded in the chapter on Senegal by Dr Cheikh Ibrahima Niang.

One of the most critical issues to arise from the 2003 GAF, which has eventually led us to this book, was the need to investigate the impact of HIV/AIDS on political stability, particularly relating to the electoral process a key indicator of democratic governance. Raised by the SADC-ECF, this issue was one that had occupied debates in academic circles and within Idasa for some time before that.

2. Policy relevance

There are three main factors that have stimulated interest by political decision-makers and academics in this project:

- Firstly, both topics – HIV/AIDS and electoral reform – are matters of public policy concern. Their interrelationship may begin to catalyse a new form of discourse on electoral engineering and on strategies against HIV/AIDS, particularly in high-prevalence countries. Several of the southern African countries, including Botswana, Namibia, Lesotho, Malawi, Mauritius, South Africa, Zimbabwe and Zambia, have been entertaining the reform of their electoral systems, largely inherited from British colonialism (Matlosa; 2004; EISA 2004).

- From an academic point of view, the research is ground-breaking and has added new knowledge to the understanding of HIV/AIDS and its dynamics and has also, on the other hand, challenged conventional analysis and studies on political processes.

- Finally, experts on democratisation consider the electoral process as a means to improve AIDS policy because leaders with the right credentials could assume power and effectively address the crisis. It has also been assumed that problems of weak mandates of the winners might arise if too few people turn up at the polls due to illness, care-giving and deaths. Mass manipulation of electoral outcomes through ghost voting could also manifest, thus generating tensions and conflict. Concerns around instability therefore remain central to this discussion.

It may be unwise to conclude from this preamble that the interest in the two topics comes from a dis-

cursive culture that continues to embrace a sense of openness on both matters. The reality cannot be further from the truth. On the one hand, electoral reform has been mired in inexplicable self-interest by succeeding generations of politicians in several countries, with a tendency toward lethargy at critical points of constitutional reform. Except for Lesotho, where armed conflict after the highly disputed election results of 1998/9 led to significant reform to the electoral model, the other countries have undergone long, drawn-out and inconclusive constitutional processes.

Ostensibly, the need to reform is an idea born of disgruntlement from opposition parties, trade unions and civil societies seeking greater accountability, gender and ethnic diversity, and transparency in government.

In South Africa, the Congress of South African Trade Unions (Cosatu), a strategic liberation partner of the African National Congress (ANC), has been at the forefront of agitating for a transformation of the country's Proportional Representation (PR) system to a Mixed Member Proportional (MMP) or Parallel system because of concerns around lack of accountability on several fronts including health.[vi] Put more succinctly, electoral processes, as will be argued in the Senegal chapter, can be galvanised by many factors, including fraudulent electoral management systems, corruption, and cultural, economic and political exclusions influenced by electoral systems that serve parochial ethnic/elitist needs. Hence, the incentive to seek reform would have been animated by considerations that have a much longer history than HIV/AIDS.

We cannot, at this juncture, determine whether research initiated by Idasa will catapult HIV/AIDS to the top of the list of priorities that are likely to influence the political trajectory of these debates. We can say, however, that influential regional and national entities, including the SADC-PF's Committee reviewing the Norms and Standards of Election Practice have engaged with these matters in their deliberations with Idasa and appear to take cognisance of the gravity of the situation.

Through these technical committees, we may begin to see a change in the manner in which HIV/AIDS is discussed in political circles despite the now evident denialism that permeates the corridors of power across the continent regarding disclosures.

Historically, official acknowledgement of the disease as a potential political problem rarely manifested even as the AIDS epidemic peaked in the early to mid-1990s. But as the 20th century drew to a close, policy actors began marginally to show a sense of worry about deaths amongst political leaders.

It is worth noting for instance that seven years ago, the UNDP/SADC Human Development Report (2000) warned of "…the slow collapse of the political, social and economic systems in the worst affected countries if measures are not taken to mitigate the impact of AIDS. For example, in some of the worst affected countries, repeated by-elections and delays in court cases attributed to AIDS-related illnesses and deaths is on the increase posing a challenge to the fragile emerging democracies in the (Sub-Saharan African) region" (SADC/UNDP/SAPES, 2000: pp. 150-151).[vii]

Despite this, HIV/AIDS did not still form part of the debate on electoral reform. Policy experts argue that in order to gain the attention of the policy-makers, issues raised for the national agenda need to significantly qualify as public emergencies. Wayne Parsons (2003), in explaining the models in agenda-setting developed by Cobb and Elder, posits that an issue for public discussion is generated by both internal and external "triggers".

Natural catastrophes, unanticipated human events, unfair distribution of resources, among others could constitute an array of "triggering devices." AIDS, we assert, is a catastrophe of scale and has been declared an "emergency" by several African countries requiring a public policy intervention,[viii] therefore any unknown impacts of empirical significance is likely to be of value to the improvement of national responses.

At a global political level, no less an authority than the United Nations (UN) acknowledges that HIV/AIDS presents a governance and security challenge and is therefore likely to affect the manner in which member states manage their political, economic and social affairs at all levels. (Hunter 2003; UNDP 2002; UNDP-HDR 2002; WHO/UNAIDS Global Report on HIV/AIDS; 2006). [ix]

Explaining the complexity of the epidemic in this regard, Peter Piot, Executive Director of UNAIDS, describes AIDS as "a massive attack on global human security" and attributes the failure of governments to recognise this to the timeframe of years and decades that the epidemic takes to manifest. This recognition of AIDS as a security matter is timely as the notion of security has been expanded by UNDP from implying the absence of conflict to meaning all fundamental conditions that are needed for people to live safe, secure, healthy and productive lives.[x]

Similarly, electoral reform is certainly a matter of public or common concern over which governments engage civil society, opposition parties and donor communities. It is also triggered in part by requirements for equal and equitable representation and access to power and resources.[xi] The status of both topics under review in terms of their policy import therefore cannot be in doubt.

For its part, Idasa links its research on AIDS and governance to the disciplines of the intended target groups, by demonstrating how the pandemic affects the decision-makers themselves and their constituencies. This approach underlines Sandra Braman's (2003: p.48) assertion that in order for policy-makers to appreciate the value of social science research, those in the profession must learn to link their work to the disciplines in which the policy-makers are trained or located. Not surprisingly, the choice of elections, the means by which state power is organised, has resonated positively with elected representatives.

We have focused on five key areas: electoral systems, electoral management and administration, parliamentary configuration, political parties and voter participation. The institutions and actors involved in the electoral process all play a significant role in most instances in democratic accountability and the stability of government.

We do not for a moment equate elections with democracy. We do nonetheless underline the centrality of elections to modern democracies and particularly to emergent democracies in Africa. We critically analyse the place of the institution of elections within the concept of governance and its normative cousin, democratic governance. Our initial impression is that AIDS has the potential to unsettle a number of the strategic democratic institutions, thereby also affecting governance: the non-hierarchical manner in which nations are expected to manage their political, economic and social affairs based on a set of values, policies and institutional arrangements that include state and non-state actors.

3. Hypothesis, methodology and impediments

The electoral process as defined in this study is characterised by rules, institutions and a set of political actors. All the key elements under study have a bearing on democratic governance, as will be expounded in this chapter. Our aim therefore is to respond to the question: What is the impact of HIV/AIDS on the electoral process in Africa?

To explore the question, the project has investigated the following areas of the electoral process:

- Electoral systems: Increased deaths amongst elected representatives will be financially demanding on the state as by-elections mount in countries employing Single Member Plurality (SMP) systems and Mixed Member Proportional (MMP) systems.

- Parliamentary configuration: Power shifts arising from AIDS-induced by-elections are being analysed. Weaker parties are likely to lose policy influence as they fail to recapture seats that are declared vacant following deaths amongst their elected representatives.

- Electoral management and administration: Loss of core staff and part-time support personnel may affect efficiency; raise re-training costs and affect institutional memory. The management of the voters' roll will be problematic because of so many dead voters

- Political parties: The potential impact on political leadership and organising capacities of political parties is being studied: succession, financial implications and support bases may all be affected by attrition due to AIDS amongst cadres, leaders and stalwarts.

- Voter and civic participation: Focus Group Discussions (FGDs) investigate the impact of sickness, stigma and discrimination on voter participation from the perspective of PLWHAs. Will people infected and affected by HIV/AIDS withdraw from elections for lack of enthusiasm, or due to a sense of hopelessness? Conversely, will it galvanise PLWHAs and other civil society actors to demand treatment and care as a right?

3.1 Electoral systems: the link to democratic governance and human development

Defined as the mechanisms that translate votes cast into seats and power in parliament and other decision-making mechanisms, electoral systems influence who is elected, how they are elected and therefore who decides on our governance priorities (including AIDS policy). Researchers in this area

(Reynolds et al: 2005; Matlosa et al: 2007) indicate that the electoral systems can influence the quality of governance, the inclusivity of policy decisions and the nature of democratic accountability fostered by the party system.

More recently, the works of Gassner, Onhiveros and Verardi (2005) show strong correlations between the electoral systems and human development based on their effect on social security and welfare spending. The researchers employed simple econometric techniques and used several definitions of human development. The authors reveal that in majoritarian systems such as the First-Past-The-Post (FPTP) system (which is constituency-based) politicians will channel their resources to the districts where they are likely to obtain the most votes. The study further shows that under the majoritarian systems politicians will be more targeted since competition is concentrated in constituencies or geographically determined zones. Conversely, proportional systems, characterised by large voting districts, register higher levels of human development given the ambition by politicians to appease diverse groups nationwide (ibid).

> "We find that countries which have proportional systems enjoy higher levels of human development than those with majoritarian ones, thanks to more redistributive fiscal policies. We also find that when the degree of proportionality, based on electoral size, increases, so does human development" (Gassner, Onhiveros and Verardi; 2005; p. 1 para 1).

Human development relates mainly to widening people's choices regarding the acquisition of knowledge, accessing resources and living long healthy lives.[xii] Human development is closely linked to concepts of governance as articulated in a variety of authoritative works. Governance underlines the importance of transparency, accountability and the participation of all (marginalised) persons in decisions that affect their well-being (SADC/UNDP/SAPES: 2000: DPRU; 2001).

Electoral systems will be one of the institutions in the governance superstructure that link the governed and the governors in respect of how they select their development blueprints through an election.

In theory therefore, electoral models will contribute to enhancing the principles of participation and accountability so citizen choices on education, employment and health, among others, may be expressed through representation in decision-making processes. It may hence be inferred that electoral systems are integral to good or democratic governance frameworks[xiii] and are also relevant to human development.

This obviously implies that the choice of an electoral model has much wider developmental implications than may be normally envisaged. The next few paragraphs explain how each one of the electoral systems works and how they may influence governance.

The four main types of electoral system employed in southern Africa (and Senegal) that have been investigated in terms of their vulnerability to HIV/AIDS by Idasa are as follows:

Table 3.1: Electoral systems	
Countries	Electoral system
Zambia	FPTP
South Africa	PR
Namibia	PR
Malawi	FPTP
Tanzania	FPTP
Senegal	Parallel system
Lesotho	MMP
Idasa 2007	

Single Member Plurality (SMP)

Popularly referred to as First-Past-The-Post (FPTP), this system is considered the simplest. The country is divided into electoral zones and political parties field one candidate each to compete for the constituency seat. Independent candidates in most cases can compete as well. The candidate who receives the most votes is declared victor (even if one does not obtain more votes than all the others combined). One of the key elements of this system is the requirement for a by-election or supplementary election to fill vacancies in the event that the elected representative dies, resigns or crosses the floor. There are seven SADC countries that operate the FPTP electoral system: Botswana, Malawi, Mauritius, Swaziland, Tanzania, Zambia and Zimbabwe, most of which are former British colonies.

In the FPTP system, political parties tend to be personality-based, without clear policy and ideological direction and it's the strongest candidates (representing political parties or standing as independents), in the end, that claim a presence at constituency and national levels. The FPTP or SMP system is relatively stronger on accountability as leaders are directly elected by the voters and may lose power in

succeeding polls if their performance is judged as poor. There is a range of criticisms directed at the SMP which include:

- Wasted votes, as losers' total votes will not translate into any form of representation;
- The translation of votes to seats tends to be disproportional;
- The system may disadvantage ethnic minorities as it's a game of numbers: small parties and women will also find it difficult to win in highly polarised and patriarchal environments;
- It often leads to a de-facto bi-party system;[xiv]
- On the basis of the work of Gassner, Onhiveros and Verardi (2005), we may add the relatively lower human development impacts observed under this system.

It can be argued therefore that the choice of electoral system allows for a particular class or section of society to access power and decide on AIDS priorities. Depending on the choice of system, decisions on AIDS could be representative of wider societal concerns or they could be decided on by a dominant ethnic group to the exclusion of minority considerations on the epidemic.

Single Member Majority (SMM)

The Single Member Majority (SMM) system is similar to the SMP in that the country is divided into electoral constituencies. However, the fundamental characteristic is that candidates will be required to garner an absolute majority of votes (50 + 1 %) in the constituency to be declared winner. Sometimes, where candidates fail to achieve an absolute majority, a run-off is called. The SMM has been used for presidential elections in some countries in the Southern African Development Community (SADC) region, such as Angola.

Proportional Representation (PR)

Global trends suggest that Proportional Representation (PR) systems are gaining in popularity as they contribute to conflict resolution through their inclusive nature, and are therefore being touted as a means for democracy consolidation (Matlosa, et al: 2007). There are various types of PR systems practised worldwide; but the commonly used variant is the closed party list system. Under this system, the entire country is considered a single constituency. Political parties will contest this space and will be allocated seats according to the proportion of votes they obtain nationally. For example, a party that wins 40% of the total votes casts will theoretically secure 40% of the seats in Parliament.

The parties will use the closed lists submitted to the Electoral Management Body (EMB) to assign MPs to seats in hierarchical order. There is no requirement for a by-election when a vacancy occurs. Rather, parties will be allowed to fill the void with the next person on the party list. Angola, Mozambique, Namibia and South Africa are the countries in the SADC that apply the PR model.

Experts posit that PR models often encourage the formation of policy-based political parties. This is because, inevitably, the competing organisations need to appeal to the various interest and ethnic groups within the population to garner a decent percentage of the national vote that could translate into a proportional number of seats in parliament. Some of its strengths include:

• Encouraging gender diversity as women can be deliberately infused on to party lists for parliament;

• Promotes conflict resolution as minority parties will have an opportunity to gain a foothold in Parliament, particularly when there is a low minimum threshold;

• Encourages the formation of parties or like-minded groups of candidates who will inevitably develop strategic visions to secure national appeal;

• Every vote counts; very few are wasted. With low thresholds, nearly every vote contributes to electing a candidate;

• Encourages nation-wide campaigns as opposed to parties restricting themselves to (ethnic or traditional) strongholds;

• Power-sharing between parties is encouraged;

• Tends toward longevity and stability of government as power configurations will not constantly change due to by-election losses, for instance;

• Higher levels of human development have been attributed to the PR system.

The PR system's weaknesses, in the eyes of most of its critics, are its tendency to:

• Build fragmented party systems and coalition governments which in turn lead to legislative "gridlocks" as representatives may not reach common ground on key issues;

• It may facilitate the presence in parliament of extremist parties;

• Voters cannot enforce accountability as the mandate to appoint MPs rests entirely with the elected party. There is no public input into who goes on to the closed party list;

• The PR system uses mathematical formulae which may be too complex for ordinary citizens to understand. The lack of appreciation of electoral systems is itself problematic in terms of the confidence it may generate in the long run (Reynolds et al: 2005; Matlosa et al: 2007).

3.1.1 Mixed systems

Most countries will consider dealing with the short comings of either the FPTP or the PR systems by combining them into a mixed system. The Mixed Member Proportional (MMP) system and the Parallel system are both categorised as "mixed" but they do have their distinct differences, which are explained below.

Mixed Member Proportional (MMP)

It has to be underlined that while South Africa uses the PR system at national level, at local government level it employs the Mixed Member Proportional (MMP) system, which is a combination of the PR and FPTP systems. The system facilitates the election of one stream of Members of Parliament (MPs) or councillors through the FPTP system and the other through the PR system. In the MMP system any disproportionalities manifesting from the FPTP (or other) system is compensated for by the PR element. Only one SADC country, Lesotho, has adopted the MMP system at national level thus far (EISA: 2003).

The Parallel system

The Parallel system is also classified as a mixed system. However, the fundamental difference between it and the MMP system is that while in the latter the PR component compensates for disproportional outcomes from the FPTP (or other) system, in the Parallel model the two systems are independent of each other and are managed separately. In the SADC region Seychelles is the only country to apply the Parallel system.[xv] In this study, Senegal is the only country to employ this model. Senegal changed its electoral system for the national parliament from list PR in 1978 to the current mixed, Parallel model which has been used since 1983 (Reynolds el at: 2005). There have been several modifications to the system which will be presented in the Senegal chapter.

3.2 The political significance of an electoral system

Reynolds *et al* (IDEA: 2005) describes the choice of electoral system as one of the most important institutional decisions for a democracy because it has a significant impact on the political future of any country. It is an undertaking that should involve all stakeholders. And yet, its importance not withstanding, it is rare that electoral systems are in fact deliberately chosen. Influence from colonialism, neighbours or perhaps regional bodies might more often be the reason a particular model is chosen, he asserts. In instances where there is an opportunity for a measured approach to selecting an electoral system International IDEA proposes the following criteria:

- Providing representation: an electoral system must ensure that geographical representation, ideological divisions and party political situations are taken into account;

- Elections must be accessible and meaningful: People's votes must have a bearing on how the country is governed. Thus the choice of electoral system should influence the legitimacy of institutions;

- Facilitating stable and efficient government: The system must avoid discrimination against particular parties and interest groups; voters must perceive the system to be by and large fair;

- Providing incentives for reconciliation: Electoral systems must also serve as tools for conflict resolution within societies allowing for inclusivity of all ethnic and interest groups to the extent possible;

- Holding the government accountable: The system must facilitate accountability;

- Encouraging political parties: The system must be seen to encourage the growth of political parties, a key factor in the consolidation of democracy;

- Promoting legislative opposition and oversight: The electoral system should assist in ushering in a viable opposition which can exercise legislative oversight over government;

- Taking into account international standards: The system must embrace international covenants, instruments and treaties affecting political issues which form the principles of free, fair and periodic elections and which advance the principle of one person, one vote;

- Making the election process sustainable: The resources of a country must be taken into account. The availability of skills and financial resources are both paramount in operating an electoral system (Reynolds, *et al*, 2005).

This last point provides us an entry point into the discussion on AIDS as it relates to the sustainability of electoral models in the age of HIV/AIDS. Some of the countries discussed in the study seem to rely rather heavily on donor support in many sectors, including their electoral processes. Sustainability must almost certainly be one of the key considerations to be made in their electoral engineering undertakings.

3.2.1 Parliaments: power and gender balance

The operationalisation of electoral systems leads to representation and participation of various interests in decision-making mechanisms such as Parliament and local government. Depending on the system employed, there may be diversity or under-representation of certain segments of society. Often the aim of well-meaning nations is to ensure that the electoral system leads to fair outcomes, where the interests of the vast majority and minorities are expressed in the highest policy institutions.

We notice from a casual examination of the status of each Parliament in this study that countries using the PR have generally fared much better in gender balance compared to those employing plural/majority systems such as the SMM and FPTP. For the SADC countries, it was evident that only Angola, Mozambique, Namibia and South Africa attained the minimum threshold of 30% of women in decision-making mechanisms by 2005 a requirement of the SADC Declaration on Gender and Development of 1997.[xvi]

In the case of these four SADC states, women were deliberately infused into parliament, mainly by political parties weighting their lists of candidates toward the women in addition to having a gender quota within the party structures. The FPTP system will often struggle to meet these requirements as there can be no guarantee that a party with a relatively good gender balance will succeed in getting all or some of its female candidates into power through competitive elections. Patriarchal biases creep into both primary processes within party structures and amongst the electorate during campaigns. Maintaining the gender status quo once female candidates are lost to disease or other causes is highly unlikely in these circumstances.

Organised women's groups in some countries have been used to assist female candidates in political parties to assume power. In Zambia, in the 2001 general elections, the Zambia National Women's Lobby Group (ZNWLG) campaigned in favour of women candidates with some measure of success but not enough to infuse any form of gender equity (Chirambo *et al*, 2002). Out of the 198 women nominated by their parties to stand as candidates in the parliamentary elections only 19 won seats in the 158-seat parliament. (The total parliament size is 158 seats: 150 are elective with 8 being non-elective seats.) Compared to 1996 when only 59 women contested parliamentary positions, this was seen as an improvement in women's attempts to claim their place in decision-making processes.[xvii]

In Senegal in 1994, women drawn from politics, trade unions and activist groups banded together to form the Council of Senegalese Women (COSW). In the 1998 legislative elections the COSW launched strong female empowerment campaigns across all political parties and directed at parties, the media and the public. The resultant pressure pushed some political parties to institute 25% to 40% quota systems for women representatives. Although a bill was introduced by government in 2007 to provide for half of all candidates on the party lists presented by political parties to be women, the judiciary declared it unconstitutional. The exclusionary tendencies in the Senegalese system, it is argued in that country's chapter, are latent and inherited from French colonialism.

Tanzania's electoral model, while described as FPTP, has a legislated gender quota which is accessed through the PR model. Because of this, Tanzania has also been able to achieve the 30% threshold. There is, therefore, a need to stress the importance of the electoral system in configuring power in this regard.

Many experts will agree that representation in parliament can influence the way policy matters are prioritised. We noted earlier that vacancies in the FPTP system are filled through new competitive elections or by-elections, regardless of whether they occur as a result of an MP resigning, being dismissed or dying. In this study therefore, we are interested in establishing whether the frequency of by-elections, some of which may be caused by HIV/AIDS, necessarily leads to power shifts in parliament, with weaker parties failing to retain the seats they previously held. Do parties end up losing policy influence? We know of course that in the PR system political parties will fill any vacancy via appointment. We will learn much more in the Senegal chapter about vari-

ations in replacement of MPs in the Parallel model as practiced in Senegal, through the use of substitute MPs.

3.2.2 Electoral management and administration

Legal and constitutional framework

It is a well-documented fact that the overall integrity of any election hinges, to a large extent, on the legal framework and the uprightness of the institutions that conduct the polls. The legal framework consists of constitutional provisions, electoral acts and regulations or statutory instruments constituting such acts. Electoral procedures, the conduct of elections and the institutions that administer them are predetermined within this framework.

Cognisant of this fact, the African Union, in its draft African Charter on Democracy, Elections and Governance, emphasises the need for the continent to develop independent electoral bodies. Chapter 7, Article 17 (1) of the Charter stipulates the requirement for member states to "establish and strengthen independent and impartial national electoral bodies responsible for the management of elections".

Prior to an election, there will often be two important processes that inform the management and administrative mechanisms in planning the poll. These are:

• The national census;

• Delimitation of boundaries.

The census: The national census is a survey of people resident in a country, which provides relevant data from national to community level. This information is essential for government planning, for business and for the community at large. The information establishes the demographic profile of the country, indicating how many people are citizens and how many of these are above or below voting age. Censuses have a long history dating back to ancient Egypt, China and Babylon when governments needed information so they could plan armies, as well as monumental projects such as the building of the pyramids or effect land re-distribution.[xviii]

Delimitation: Knowledge of population size and distribution enables the implementation of the delimitation process or demarcation of constituencies. A delimitation commission will be established to draw the constituencies' boundaries by applying a stipulated formula which defines the average size of the electorate to be assigned to each constituency. The demarcation of constituency boundaries is extremely sensitive and can be a source of post election conflict.

It is possible for governments in countries using the FPTP system for instance to re-engineer the boundaries, that is create more constituencies in areas in which the party in power enjoys majority support, therefore enabling it to get a larger proportion of the parliamentary seats. The SADC Parliamentary Forum (SADC-PF), which has a long history of election observation in Africa and has been used by both the executive arms of the SADC and the AU as a reference point in developing their charters, does take note of this and recommends that the impartiality of delimitation commissions in drawing up boundaries be re-affirmed in the constitutions of SADC countries. A number of key steps are suggested:

- The tenure of office of the commissioners should be guaranteed in the constitution;
- There should be no political interference in the demarcation of boundaries. The exercise should be left to the technical competence of the boundary delimitation commission;
- The commission should consult stakeholders in the process;
- Gerrymandering must be outlawed;
- Recommendations of the boundary delimitation commission should not be altered by any stakeholder.[xix]

3.3 Electoral commissions

The information from the delimitation commission will in turn inform the management and administrative processes of the electoral commission. Electoral commissions lie at the heart of a stable democracy, lending credibility and integrity to the democratic process by ensuring that the rules are applied fairly; and that to the extent possible, the majority of citizens participate in freely making their choice of policy. In practice, electoral commissions are often accused of lacking independence, particularly since the government of the day or the president may have a hand in confirming nominations of commissioners or appointing them. Controversies surrounding electoral outcomes will not usually spare the electoral management body, hence the need to evolve a widely acceptable system of selection and appointment of chief electoral administrators and supervisors.

Recommendations from the SADC and the AU emphasise the need to avoid political interference from the executive in putting electoral commissions in place. Some of the recommendations by the SADC-PF include:

- The complete independence and impartiality of the electoral commission in dealing with all political parties should be re-affirmed in the constitution;
- Selection of commissioners should be done by a panel of judges set up by the Chief Justice or the equivalent "on the basis of the individual's calibre, stature, public respect, competence, impartiality and their knowledge of elections and political development processes";
- Selection of commissioners should be done in consultation with all political parties and stakeholders with final approval coming from parliament;
- The commission should have financial autonomy i.e. with its own budget directly voted for by parliament (and not allocated by the ministry of finance or any government department);
- The electoral law should empower the commission to recruit and dismiss its own staff based on professional considerations, rather than hire public service workers whose loyalty to the commission is not guaranteed;
- Electoral commissioners should have security of tenure entrenched in the constitutions of SADC states.

It is interesting to note that the recommendations imply an electoral process can be undermined by the manner in which a management mechanism is put in place or lack of consultation with other stakeholders or even by lack of financial autonomy, among other things. There is also evidently a move to depart from the use of temporary public workers as election officers because of potential accusations of partiality, depending on which department supplies the workers. If they are drawn from the office of the president, for instance, there are likely to be debates over the fairness of the outcomes.

The reality is that most Electoral Management Bodies (EMBs) do rely on the services of public service workers as support staff during elections anyway. Except for Namibia (among the countries we have studied), these countries from time to time enlist the services of public workers, particularly teachers and municipal workers. The aspirations of new democracies, we would imagine, would be to build the capacity of trained support staff over time to ensure that post-election conflict is minimised through diligent management. However, we do know from other authoritative studies that HIV/AIDS has been a major cause of deaths amongst public service workers, including teachers, and we ask therefore to what extent this form of attrition may undermine the management of elections.

Citizen and voter registration systems

Lastly, the voters' roll is perhaps the most sensitive instrument in any election. It represents the aggregate number of registered voters and will ultimately serve as a key indicator of voter turnout. The representation of marginalised voices can also be extrapolated from voter databases, providing researchers, political parties, election monitors and others an opportunity to determine levels of political enthusiasm or validity of the data and ultimately the credibility of the electoral process.

In order to achieve this level of confidence, EMBs will need to have fairly sophisticated voter registration systems that will enable the removal of dead voters from the registers in good time before major elections. Knowing the size of the voter population before the poll is fundamental to allaying fears of fraud from opposition elements. To lubricate this process, states will need to institute citizen registration systems that are technologically compatible with the voters' rolls so that death certificates can be timeously processed and dead electors eliminated from the registers. The advent of AIDS may increase this work load for both home affairs ministries and EMBs. Worse still, countries without citizen registration systems or with outmoded systems are likely to struggle to cope with the number of deceased.

Political parties

On the advent of independence or liberation most African states experienced the emergence of party systems dominated by the nationalist or liberation

movements that existed at the time of achieving majority rule. With broad-based popular support for nationalist/liberation movements, opposition parties struggled to compete with the relatively more sophisticated rivals. In several of the countries in this study, including Malawi, Tanzania and Zambia, de facto one-party states were declared within ten years of independence from the British in the 1960s. This meant all official opposition was outlawed and the sum effect was that the party system was undermined even further (IDEA; 2000).

It was not until the early 1990s that a new wave of opposition emerged, usually breakaway groups from the founding party, to challenge those in power. Encouraged by relaxed registration rules, political parties began to make considerable contributions to democratic accountability, allowing for diverse interests to emerge. Studies by the United Nations Economic Commission for Africa (UNECA) indicate that in 2005, Chad had 73 political parties, South Africa 140, Mali 91, Ethiopia 79, Burkina Faso 47, Morocco, Nigeria and Botswana each 30, Egypt 17 and Ghana 10 (UNECA, 2005).

While there was a flood of parties, it has to be stated that experts noted the advantages of incumbency which placed ruling parties in a position to accentuate a de facto dominant-party system. This has been the case in Namibia, Botswana, Tanzania, Zimbabwe and South Africa. South Africa, with a PR electoral system at national level and state financing for political parties, has a relatively stable party environment as there seems to be an incentive to exist beyond elections. However, it is also characterised by a dominant party in the form of the ANC.

In most cases, political parties' performances will be determined in part by the nature of the electoral system. PR systems seem to reflect fairer outcomes while the FPTP system is often seen to present obstacles for the opposition, as discussed above. Party performances will also be determined by the amount of resources they have. Without a doubt, all parties would be assisted greatly if state funding was available without overly inhibiting pre-conditions. Malawi, Mozambique, Namibia, Seychelles, South Africa and Zimbabwe are some of the countries with state funding provisions for political parties.

There are however marked differences in the manner in which such funding is made available: in some countries the funding is restricted to election periods, while in others it is provided between and beyond the election period. The requirement in most cases for parties to qualify for funds is that they garner a prescribed number of seats in parliament.

Figure 3.1: Parties per Parliament

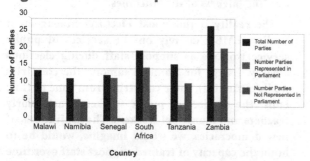

That being the case, it is hardly surprising that only one or two parties will in the end benefit from state resources. The level of funding available to a particular party will assist in levelling the playing field to some extent: they will be able to employ campaign staff, acquire transport to access the remotest parts of a country and deploy advertising in print and electronic media, as well as other communicative technologies (IDEA, 2000).

Because of the preconditions attached to accessing party funding, the reality is that launching a new party often means struggling against existing older parties in nearly all spheres. New parties will not have the organisational skills, finances or administrative systems to survive beyond an election or two. Often, they will also not have an ideology and will be guided simply by the desire to seek high office. While some of the current opposition parties were formally in power at independence, such as the United National Independence Party (UNIP) in Zambia and the Malawi Congress Party (MCP), most of them were formed in the early 1990s and will have narrow political bases (IDEA; 2000; UNECA, 2005). Most opposition political parties are headed by patrons who not only finance the institutions but also provide the leadership and they often have to close down after losing at the polls.

In Malawi for instance, of the nine parties that won parliamentary seats in the 2004 election, only three were more than ten years old. These were the Malawi Congress Party, the Alliance for Democracy and the United Democratic Front. The rest were created within three years of the 2004 election. In Zambia, nearly all the opposition parties that contested the second multi-party election in 1996 had collapsed by the time the country held its third election in 2001, except for UNIP which in fact boycotted the poll. Riddled with a range of institutional inadequacies, political parties may find epidemic such as HIV/AIDS weaken them further. There are three levels at which HIV/AIDS may impact on political party structures:

- Organisational: The loss of cadres and members affects electioneering capacity;

- Financial: Loss of members reduces subscriptions;

- Leadership: The loss of a patron may mean the end of a party or compromise electoral viability and financial status.

Voter participation

Without the support and participation of citizens, the legitimacy of our political systems is to be doubted. Our emphasis on citizen participation in governance processes in this regard was to determine to what extent, if at all, AIDS sickness and care-giving prevents people from adding their voices to the policy arena. Low participation can be problematic for democracies as issues of legitimacy creep in when too few people are involved in electing a government. Political scientists have warned about low participation in elections across the world for decades. Although turn-out as a percentage of registered voters in some cases may appear impressive, it can be disheartening when calculated as a percentage of eligible voters or the Voting Age Population (VAP).

Africa has not been spared this scrutiny and in several instances relatively low participation has been attributed to political disillusionment, poor incentives to vote, lack of service delivery by successive regimes, poverty, lack of transport, inaccessible terrain and the weather. Valid as these might seem, for a long time no consideration was given to AIDS as contributing factor.

If millions of people are ill, or are tending to sick relatives, surely they would be inclined to consider matters of personal survival ahead of attending a rally or standing in a long queue to elect a candidate for parliament unless of course there is a real belief that electing a particular candidate might dramatically usher in an era of better health care, non-discrimination in employment and accessing other economic goods. So there would be two sides of the same coin: either HIV/AIDS drives people underground and causes them to withdraw from the electoral process or it serves as a catalyst for infected and affected peoples to hold their representatives accountable for (lack of) service delivery.

We are supported by the outcomes of the Afrobarometer surveys which provide an analysis of citizen perceptions of state performances, in particular affecting health and AIDS. Through this instrument, we seek to understand whether AIDS is considered a national priority by Africans; the extent to which people experience HIV/AIDS at a personal level and their expectations in terms of government responsibility. While the Afrobarometer experts have done their own analysis of the findings, we attempt to go further in some respects to find other explanatory factors that cause Africans to express certain views. We therefore ask the question: does HIV/AIDS positively or negatively affect voter participation; if so, in what ways?

4. Terminologies

In the course of discussing the spread of AIDS on the African continent, we shall constantly use words such as prevalence or incidence which might, in error, be confused by readers who are unfamiliar with the terminology. Prevalence refers to existing infections in the 15-49 age bands while incidence denotes new infections occurring in the same cohort each year. The 15-49 age cohort is the UNAIDS recommended measure to understand the extent of HIV in a population (or the percentage of persons aged between 15 and 49 who are infected with the virus (NAC, 2004)). This in effect means a 16% prevalence rate translates into 16% of 15-49-year olds being HIV-infected. It would not imply that 16% of the entire population in a country is infected, an error that AIDS experts constantly remind us in communicating HIV/AIDS national status (ibid).

5. Choice of countries

We selected the countries for this study on the basis of their electoral systems which needed to be compared in respect of their vulnerability to HIV/AIDS. In order for us to understand the dynamics of the disease, we needed to see whether countries with lower prevalence rates had a relatively low attrition rate among elected representatives, for instance. Southern African countries have exceedingly high levels of HIV in adult populations. Except for Mauritius, Seychelles and unexplored Angola and DRC, the other ten countries in the region carry a large caseload of HIV/AIDS cases (eight of them have adult prevalence of 15% or more).[xx] The four other countries did not fit the bill for our purposes as the first two were islands and quite removed from mainland Africa. Angola and DRC were post-conflict nations with relatively weak institutions which would render it exceedingly difficult for us to gather information that would be reasonably comparable. We elected to include a West African state with a demonstrable record of early responses, a different history of colonisation and cultural experience, and a radically different religious make-up.

The seven countries eventually selected for this study were therefore Senegal, Botswana, Namibia, Malawi, Tanzania, South Africa and Zambia (The Botswana study was not completed in time to form part of this book.)

6. Methodology

In this study, the AIDS pandemic will be considered the independent variable while the electoral process is the dependent variable (Tredoux & Durrheim, 2002).[xxi]

The research has been structured around a standard methodology: Literature reviews of authoritative journals and studies; interviews with political party leaders, electoral officials, parliamentarians, election-based bodies; statistical analysis of epidemiological data, electoral data and Afrobarometer data; focus group discussions with PLWHAs and care-givers who are mainly registered or eligible voters; stakeholder meetings with cross-sectional participation from state and non-state actors.

Stakeholder meetings were held at the beginning of the research process where methodologies were discussed at national level and contributions made by other actors. These have been followed by post-research dissemination meetings with the same group of senior stakeholders where preliminary findings have been tested to the finalisation process. A number of dissemination/stakeholder meetings have also included official involvement from government ministers or speakers/deputy speakers of national parliaments, directors of electoral management bodies and presidents of leading political parties.

7. Limitations

We must, however, also state the difficulties encountered in pursuing this project. To begin with:

- Records on actual cause of death are not available due to confidentiality considerations. Researchers have had to draw inferences by analysing trends and age cohorts and determine whether they fit the AIDS mortality profiles;

- The available data on mortality among elected representatives is drawn from different periods of time in some respects. In countries such as Namibia and South Africa information prior to 1994 is scanty or non-existent;

- Not all countries have institutionalised citizen and voter registration systems; in cases where these exist, they will not always be directly compatible. This renders it extremely laborious for authorities to capture deaths and purge dead electors from the voters' rolls in time. Because of that, there is a high probability this investigation will not have unravelled the full extent to which voter registration systems have been compromised by AIDS, if at all;

- Some countries have not had a voters' register until recently or have changed the existing roll with every election, rendering longitudinal impact studies almost impossible to achieve as there is no guarantee of the accuracy of previous or current rolls. Also, such information is not directly comparable between countries because of the unique circumstances affecting each of them;

- As with all exploratory research, the project provides answers and also generates a myriad new questions. However, limited resources prevent the investigation of all perspectives that arise from this project.

8. Organisation of chapters and readership

Finally, while our previous publications have tended to be directed more at the academic and policy communities, in this edition we attempt to gravitate toward a general readership. The book is organised into seven chapters; six of these present comprehensive country reports. The overview chapter will provide the background and comparative overview of the outcomes of the multi-country studies. The chapters will discuss at length the following matters:

- The AIDS pandemic, its impact and policy challenges;

- A synthesis of studies attempting to explain the disparities in infection rates between southern and western Africa;

- A brief historical background of the SADC and its collective efforts to fight AIDS (with references to Senegal);

- A definition of the concepts of governance and democratic governance and how they relate to HIV/AIDS;

- A discussion on the electoral processes within the context of democratic governance and its link to HIV/AIDS;

- An overview of the research outcomes and recommendations.

Following the generic framework of AIDS and the electoral process presented in the overview chapter, chapter two will examine the highly uncertain environment in Malawi, particularly controversies around the voter registers and the legitimacy of leadership; chapter three will address the post-liberation scenario in Namibia and the challenge of combating HIV/AIDS for a young nation seeking to consolidate its democratic institutions while chapter four will locate itself in South Africa's politically charged AIDS debate, the electoral reform discourse and the ravages of AIDS amongst registered voters in the nine provinces. In chapter five Tanzania highlights the contradictions of two governments that form a single union: Tanganyika and Zanzibar as the United Republic of Tanzania, and challenge us to understand the disparities in infection between the largely Islamic island and the mainland and also to interrogate the strategic bipartisan political partnership formed by parliamentarians to fight AIDS. Chapter six tackles the case of Zambia where heated debates on compulsory testing for leaders emerged in the wake of a constitutional review effort that seems to ignore the evidence of high attrition amongst parliamentarians from undisclosed illnesses and the impact this might have on the country's political trajectory. Chapter seven on Senegal re-considers the whole notion of democratic governance in highly critical fashion, applying historical and cultural analysis, and speaks to the meaning of democratic governance in Africa within the context of the influences of global capital on both definitions and outcomes of governance.

Endnotes

i   Meehan (1998; p 136, Para 1) asserts that: "what identifies a reasoned choice or action is the element of deliberate weighing or comparing of outcomes, balancing the benefits to humans of selecting each of the alternatives".

ii See Chirambo K & Caesar M (Eds) (2003); AIDS and Governance in Southern Africa: Emerging Theories and Perspective. Cape Town: Idasa.

iii Also known as Low Income Countries Under Stress (LUCUS) that are defined by weak policies, institutions and governance.

iv Youde J. (2001) All the Voters will be Dead: HIV/AIDS and Democratic Legitimacy and Stability in Africa (Iowa).

v   Lately, social researchers in Africa seem to agree that without the extended family and kinship systems, the impact of HIV/AIDS on African societies would have been much worse. Africa hosts 95% of the 13 million so-called AIDS orphans. See Matshalaga N. & Powell G., (2002) Mass Orphanhood in the Era of HIV/AIDS: Bold Support for Alleviation of Poverty and Education may Avoid a Social Disaster. http://www.pubmedcentral.nih.gov/articlerender.fcgi?artid=1122118 & IRIN news report: Malawi: Illegal Orphanages Mushroom: http://www.irinnews.org/report.aspx?reportid=61374

vi   www.cosatu.org.za/congress/conggg/all-res.htm

vii   Author's italicisation.

viii Parsons W. (1995) argues that public policy has to do with those spheres which could be designated as "public"; that are held as common to all; the dimension of human activity which is regarded as requiring governmental or social regulation or intervention or at least common action.

ix   Author's italicisation.

x   Statement by Peter Piot, Director, UNAIDS, UN University, 2 October, 2001. http://www.africaaction.org/docs01/piot0110.htm

xi   For instance the SADC Declaration on Gender and Development of 1997 seeks gender balance, recognising the disadvantaged position in decision-making mechanisms, concerns arising from the Beijing Declaration and Platform for Action. See The SADC MPs Companion on Gender and Development in Southern Africa (2002) SARDC/SADC-PF.

xii   Author's italisation.

xiii In *Deepening Democracy in a Fragmented World. UNDP Human Development Report 2002*. New York, available at www.undp.org p: 51, the UNDP states that "from a human development perspective, good governance is democratic governance".

xiv   See Matlosa K., Chiroro B., Letsholo S., (2007): Politics of Electoral System Reform and Democratisation: Contemporary Trends in Southern Africa. EISA; Johannesburg. Conference paper.

xv   Reynolds et al (2005): Electoral System Design: the International IDEA Handbook: IDEA: Stockholm.

xvi   The SADC MPs Companion on Gender and Development in Southern Africa. Harare (2002): SARDC/SADC Parliamentary Forum.

xvii Zambia National Women's Lobby Group: End of Year Report January-December 2001; Submitted to Netherlands Embassy; p 19.

xviii http://www.statistics.gov.uk/census2001/cb_8.asp. The resolution of Cosatu's 8th National Congress in 2003 sought to introduce a 65% constituency-based system combined with 33% proportional representation.

xix   SADC Parliamentary Forum: (2001) Norms and Standards for Elections in the SADC Region: Windhoek: SADC-PF.

xx   SADC and International Cooperating Partners: Framework on Regional Support to HIV and AIDS in Southern Africa. 2006.

xxi   Tredoux C. & Durrheim explain that "Variables are measured entities (or attributes of entities that can take on different values i.e. as height, weight. Independent variables are variables that are presumed to affect or determine other variables. Dependent variables are affected or determined by independent variables" pp 9-14).

References

Braman S. (2003) Communication Researchers and Policy-making. Massachusetts: Massachusetts Institute of Technology.

Chirambo K., Nel N. and Erasmus C. (2003) Zambia Presidential, Parliamentary and Local Government Elections, 2001; Evaluation of Impact of Donor Investment. Pretoria: Idasa.

DPRU. (2001) Human Development Indicators in the SADC Region.

Development Policy Research Unit, University of Cape Town.

EISA (2003) Principles for Election Management, Monitoring and Observation in the SADC Region. Johannesburg: Electoral Commissions Forum/Electoral Institute of Southern Africa.

Gassner M., Onhiveros U. and Verardi V. (2005) Electoral Systems and Human Development. Journal of Human Development Alternative Economics in Action. Vol 7 No 1, March 2006.

Hunter S. (2003) Who Cares? AIDS in Africa. New York. Palgrave Macmillan.

IDEA. (2000) The Functioning and Funding of Political Parties in the SADC Region: An Overview; Conference on Sustainable Democratic Institutions in Southern Africa. Stockholm: IDEA.

Matlosa K., Chiroro B. & Letsholo S. (2007) Politics of Electoral System Reform and Democratisation: Contemporary Trends in Southern Africa. Johannesburg EISA, conference paper.

NAC. (2004) The HIV/AIDS Epidemic in Zambia: Where are we now? Where are we going? Lusaka: September.

NAC. (2004) HIV/AIDS Communication Strategy. Lusaka: May.

Parsons W. (1995) Public Policy: An Introduction to the Theory and Practice of Policy Analysis. Cheltenham: Edward Edgar Publishing Ltd.

Reynolds A., Reilly B. & Ellis A. (eds) (2005)

Electoral System Design: The International IDEA Handbook. Stockholm: IDEA.

SADC/UNDP/SAPES. (2000) Human Development Report. Challenges, Opportunities for Regional Integration. UNDP/SAPES.

Tredoux C. & Durrheim (eds) (2002) Numbers, Hypotheses & Conclusions: A Course in Statistics for the Social Sciences. Cape Town: UCT Press.

UNECA. (2005) Striving for Good Governance in Africa. Addis Ababa: United Nations Economic Commission for Africa.

UNDP. (2000) Zimbabwe Human Development Report. Governance. UNDP.

UNDP. (2002) Deepening Democracy in a Fragmented World. Human Development Report 2002. New York: United Nations Development Programme. available at www.undp.org

SAPES-UNDP-SADC (2000) Human development Report: Challenges and Opportunities for Regional Integration. SAPES Book No 9.

WHO/UNAIDS. (2006) Global Report 2002-2005.

The political cost of AIDS in Africa

Evidence from six countries

Kondwani Chirambo

1. Making sense of disparities in infection rates

A global epidemic has consumed the world since the early 1980s when the HI virus was discovered, with Africa bearing the heaviest brunt. UNAIDS estimates that by December 2004 the epidemic had killed 20 million people and a total of between 35.9 and 44.3 million people worldwide were living with the virus. Of these 57% (25.4 million) are in Sub-Saharan Africa (UNAIDS/WHO: 2004; 2006).

HIV prevalence in Africa ranges from 0.7-9% in countries such as Senegal in West Africa; 1% in North Africa; to 15-30% in adult populations in most of southern Africa, the region most affected by the epidemic (CHGA; 2004: UNAIDS/WHO: 2005).

Figure 1.1: Population 2005

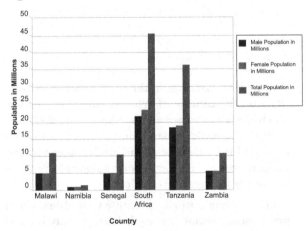

Source: WHO 2006, graph by Idasa

Leading health economists and social scientists have described AIDS as a "long wave" event (Barnett and Whiteside; 2002)[1]; one that will require long-term strategic planning and implementation to address its impact on current and future generations. HIV/AIDS is distinct from other epidemics and indeed other predominantly sexually transmitted diseases for a number of reasons:

- The symptoms are not immediately visible and can remain invisible for up to ten years or more. This facilitates a silent diffusion through society via unprotected sex, poor medical facilities, intravenous drug use and Mother-To-Child Transmission (MTCT);

- Because it is a "catastrophe in slow motion" predominantly transmitted through heterosexual intercourse it comes with stigma and discrimination and therefore generates denialism;

- Unlike other major killers such as tuberculosis, malaria or indeed other sexually transmitted infections (STIs), it has no cure;[2]

- It is unprecedented in terms of the human catastrophe it has caused;

- It is the first disease to be labelled a global security threat by the United Nations Security Council, and the first to command a discussion by the entire Security Council (Hunter: 2003).

Figure 1.2: HIV/AIDS prevalence 2005

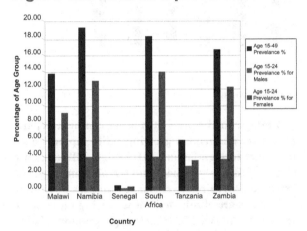

Sources: WHO 2006; graph by Idasa

Since its manifestation, life expectancy in southern Africa has declined from 60 years to below 40 years in the most affected countries, particularly in the sub-region defined by the Southern African Development Community (SADC), which constitutes Angola, Botswana, the Democratic Republic of Congo (DRC), Lesotho, Mauritius, Malawi, Mozambique, Namibia, Seychelles, South Africa, Swaziland, Tanzania, Zambia and Zimbabwe.

Data from 2006 suggest the SADC hosts less than 2% of the global population,[3] but by many accounts has the highest concentration of HIV in the world, with approximately 39% or 14.9 million of the 38.6 million people living with HIV (at the end of 2006). The region carries the additional burden of 41% of children orphaned by AIDS.[4]

Due to the decimation of working age populations, food security and nutrition have been under threat. Agriculture, the mainstay of the majority of the people in the region, is already experiencing the impact of HIV/AIDS. The Food and Agricultural

Organisation (FAO) estimates that more than seven million workers have been lost due to HIV/AIDS in the Sub-Saharan region, with agriculture experiencing the severest impact. The SADC also acknowledges the effect on business in the sub-region as productivity declines due to absenteeism and deaths amongst workers and profit margins are compromised as spending on sickness and death benefits rises (SADC: 2003).

Figure 1.3: Adult mortality per 1 000 (2004)

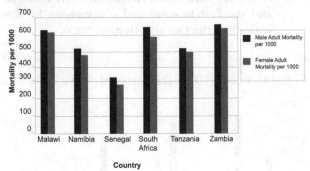

Source: WHO 2006

Strategic institutions such as government departments are enduring a growing skills gap and need to attract foreign labour. AIDS-related illnesses are also affecting recruitment and training amongst the armed forces as relatively large numbers of eligible candidates are eliminated while serving officers are left out of international training programmes due to their HIV status (UNAIDS: 2006).

Despite AIDS, during the mid to late 1990s, population growth rates in the SADC increased, with some countries reporting growth rates of 3.5% per annum. Experts attributed the growth rates to a fall in infant mortality rates and the sustenance of high fertility levels in the SADC which increased from 4.9 in 1990 to 5.1 in 1997. This picture had changed by the dawn of the millennium.

Mortality amongst adults in several countries has since trebled. The trends show increases in

Figure 1.4: Average life expectancy (2004)

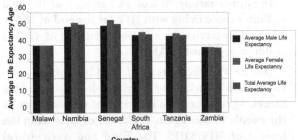

Source: WHO 2006

infant mortality as more children became infected. Generally, mortality profiles in the region, according to some experts, have become reminiscent of the 1950s (SADC: 2003)[5].

The SADC predicts that the unprecedented demographic effects of the HIV epidemic will have dire implications for the social and economic development of the region:

- The overall population growth is predicted to be lower than it would have been without HIV/AIDS;
- Poverty will increase amongst the populations of the region unless significant response mechanism are deployed;
- The ILO predicts that by 2010 the labour force in countries with the highest rates will have labour forces 20% smaller than they would have had under conditions of no-AIDS (ibid).

2. Why is the SADC most affected by HIV/AIDS?

Why is the SADC region the most affected by HIV/AIDS on the continent? Why are infection levels so much lower in western and northern Africa? While a detailed scientific explanation of these phenomena is beyond the expertise of this study, we can briefly examine some of the key reasons advanced over time by experts from various disciplines.

The reasons posited constitute a combination of pre-existing social, cultural, legal, economic and political conditions which were thought to have provided fertile ground for the spread of HIV.[6] Initial arguments attempting to explain the severity of the SADC AIDS epidemic were at best speculative. Some of the inter-linking factors that are today discussed are as follows:[7]

- High levels of gender-based violence and particularly sexual violence and rape of women and children;
- Low HIV risk perception;
- Pervasiveness of transactional and transgenerational sex among young people, especially young women;[8]
- The HI Virus (type 1) found in the SADC region is more virulent than the type 2 found in West Africa;[9]

- Social, cultural and legal practices that place women in an unequal position in society and thus increases their exposure to HIV/AIDS;[10]

- High mobility and varied patterns of migration, some of which is specifically linked to employment and was particularly central to the economic and political history of the region;

- High levels of politically-motivated conflict and violence for at least the last 20 years in individual countries within the region, including internal displacements;[11]

- High levels of multiple and concurrent sexual partnerships by men and women with insufficient consistent, correct condom use, combined with low levels of male circumcision are the key drivers of the epidemic in the sub-region.[12]

Some of the arguments may not have general validity and will therefore not explain the disparities in infection rates between southern and western Africa, mainly because the studies appear to be concentrated in the SADC region.

In relation to human mobility, Crush *et al* (2006) explain that the incidence of HIV in Sub-Saharan Africa has been found to be higher near roads where people profess to have personal migration experience or have migrants for sexual partners. Infection rates amongst migrants in western and southern Africa have also been found to be comparatively higher than in the general population. Truck drivers, probably the most studied group of all, have been the hardest hit. One of the most cited forms of human mobility, cross-border migration, could also occur because people with AIDS-related illnesses travel to neighbouring countries seeking better medical care. Others will migrate to seek higher paying jobs that can help support their families, some of whom may be stricken by AIDS. The need to replace workers who have died from AIDS could force governments to import skilled labour. Illegal immigrants, refugees and Internally Displaced Persons (IDPs) will be extremely vulnerable to HIV/AIDS and may come in contact with local populations or be abused by them.[13]

The argument for conflict (leading to displacement) as a vector for the spread of HIV and as an explanation for higher prevalence rates in SADC as opposed to western Africa is still weak and largely lacking in empirical evidence. Information from the UN suggests that IDPs still constitute a problem in the SADC region despite the resolution of conflict. But there is a lack of data to substantiate these assertions. The causes of displacement are diverse but inter-related: displacement is discussed as a defining feature of colonialism, whose effects have not been fully addressed. Displacement was also a distinct objective of South Africa under the apartheid regime. While armed conflict is highlighted as a major cause of displacement in the post-colonial era (wars in Angola, the DRC and Mozambique stand out), there appear to be other factors that contribute significantly to mass movement of people in the SADC region. Human rights violations, political violence and urban renewal operations such as Zimbabwe's Operation Murambatsvina (drive out filth) are a case in point. Natural disasters such as droughts, cyclones, floods and volcanic eruptions also prompt sudden movements of people to escape the peril of the fallout.[14]

The parallels with West Africa are somewhat different if conflict is defined to mean armed conflict. Most of West Africa was characterised by political violence and executions soon after the toppling of civilian post-independence governments by military officers in the 1960s and 70s. The era of the military regimes spanned more than two decades. In addition, there were several countries at a time torn by full-scale armed conflicts (civil wars) covering an entire country in most instances. West African trouble spots such as Liberia, Sierra Leone, Ivory Coast and Guinea-Bissau have experienced civil war over long periods at a time punctuated by gross abuse of human rights.

In trying to quell it, the Economic Community of West African States (ECOWAS), the equivalent of the SADC in West Africa, has fought fire with fire: military tactics have been employed to stamp out wars, led by Nigeria.[15] Even with this background, no authoritative studies have established strong correlations between HIV/AIDS and conflict.[16]

Perhaps in understanding the SADC AIDS conundrum, we should critically consider the advent of peace as a facilitator of unprecedented levels of interaction between the sub-region's peoples, for better or for worse. UNDP's 2000 SADC Human Development Report underlines the fact that relative peace and stability and improved road and rail infrastructure have facilitated more effective movement of people and goods.

Eleven inter-state highways and rail systems crisscross at least 12 countries of the region, leading to 15 ports located at the Indian and Atlantic oceans. Improved infrastructure and arteries between member states and a relaxation of visa requirements in some respects have all aided the movement of the SADC region's peoples. We may summarise the incentives for movements as such:

- Improved transport (including cheaper flights between states, since the introduction of budget airlines);

- Growth of communication systems disseminates images of places of opportunity (employment, trade, tourism etc.);

- Opening up of once-closed borders like Namibia and South Africa;

- Increasing international trade and commerce (formal and informal) and increasing free trade;

- Better educational opportunities in neighbouring states.[17]

Migration, therefore, could be categorised as involuntary induced by destabilisation or voluntary which connotes movement of people for professional or economic reasons such as truck drivers, seafarers, agricultural workers, students, teachers, sex workers, traders, members of the armed forces and mine workers.

In May 2006, further attempts were made by experts to explain the difference in infection levels between southern and western Africa. A "think tank" held in Lesotho by the SADC and UNAIDS explained the higher levels of infection in southern Africa thus: "high levels of multiple and concurrent sexual partnerships by men and women with insufficient consistent, correct condom use, combined with low levels of male circumcision are the key drivers of the epidemic in the sub-region."(Halperin and Epstein: 2006). The meeting recommended as the two major strategies national circumcision campaigns and the need for a significant reduction in multiple partnerships for men and women.

Daniel Halperin and Helen Epstein (2006) elucidate that there is now conclusive evidence of an epi-

demiological and biological nature confirming the strong correlation between male circumcision and HIV which apparently explains "much of the five-fold difference in HIV rates between southern and western Africa". They caution however that in Asia and Europe, where circumcision is also uncommon, the HIV prevalence rates remain inexplicably and comparatively much, much lower. The differences in HIV infection rates based on circumcision or lack of it have not yet been studied outside of Africa.

The immediate controversial assertion would be that southern Africans or Sub-Saharan Africans are more sexually liberal than their Arabic, North African neighbours or their European or American counterparts. However, recent demographic and health surveys suggest that on average African men typically do not have more sexual partners than elsewhere. The WHO's comparative study in the 1990s revealed that men in Thailand and Rio de Janeiro in Brazil were more likely to report five or more casual sexual partners in the previous year than were men in Tanzania, Kenya, Lesotho or Zambia. The number of women who reported having five or more partners a year was even lower.

> "Men and women in Africa report roughly similar, if not fewer, numbers of lifetime partners than do heterosexuals in many western countries," (Halperin and Epstein; 2006).

Epidemiologists have however observed that Africans of both sexes usually have more than one concurrent partnership that can overlap for months or years and cite WHO studies which show that 18%, 22% and 55% of men in Tanzania, Lusaka and Lesotho respectively reported entertaining two or more regular, year-long, sexual partnerships during the previous year. Conversely, only 3% of men in Thailand and 2% in Sri Lanka reported similar profiles (ibid).

Therefore the distinctive feature, according to Halperin and Epstein, is that the pattern of concurrent partnerships which characterises (southern) Africa is markedly different from that of serial monogamy that is prevalent in the west.[18]

Figure 2.1: AIDS deaths (2002)

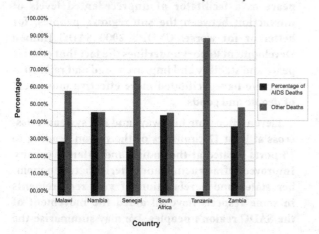

3. Senegal

Arguments that point to denial, which punctuated the early years of AIDS, as a key factor that compromised an early SADC response will also hold their own. Senegal and Uganda are credited for early mobilisation and strategic thinking on handling the advent of HIV/AIDS.

In this book's chapter on Senegal, Cheikh Ibrahima Niang provides powerful insights, using cultural and historical analysis, which speak to differences in modes and effects of colonisation between southern and Francophone West Africa, where traditional structures tended to survive and thrive in the latter as opposed to the former.

While southern Africa seems to project abuse of women and unregulated sex work, his analysis of power structures reveals a deep appreciation of women's political power in the pre-colonial societies of West Africa which still forms the bedrock of influence today. Current approaches to dealing with HIV/AIDS draw upon the local culture to develop responses and strategies which give the local communities a sense of historical and cultural continuity and expression, with women constituting a source of social mobilisation, he argues.

Unlike the SADC states, Senegal prior to the emergence of AIDS had also set up a number of political, legal and social arrangements aiming at the regulation of sex work, policies for blood transfusion safety, the management of sexually transmitted diseases, the reform of the health system, and support to women and youth movements.

With an institutional and response framework already in place, the government of Senegal was able to swiftly operationalise national multi-disciplinary approaches to deal with the epidemic, led by its Prime Minister. Niang argues that the response embraced principles of devolution, decentralisation, multi-sector planning, respect for equity and the rights of People Living With HIV/AIDS (PLWHAs), and continuous evaluation against the guiding principles of UNAIDS. The Senegalese leadership was able to mobilise actors across all spectrums, including respected religious leaders, to galvanise their communities. The success story is corroborated by other authorities who itemise the strong points as: early political engagement; a strong civil society response; and one of the earliest national initiatives for antiretroviral therapy (ART) access. Hence, funds from the Global Fund to Fight AIDS, TB and Malaria and the World Bank's Multi-country HIV/AIDS Programme for Africa (MAP) bolstered pre-existing, strong national programmatic and financial commitments.[19] The response does have its critics though. The international HIV/AIDS Alliance asserts that the scaling-up of the Senegalese strategy lacked clear vision and strategy and was found wanting in terms of its failure to target orphans and vulnerable children and other disadvantaged

populations; it questions whether respect for the rights and dignity of PLWHAs was indeed extended as claimed; and highlights the sense that access to HIV testing and ARV treatment remained limited.[20]

The role of religion as an additional neutralising instrument might also be appreciated in curbing what might be described as deviant behaviour. Certainly, it appears no coincidence that mainland Tanzania has a much higher HIV-prevalence rate (at 7% in 2004) than the predominantly Islamic island of Zanzibar (less than 1% prevalence and 4.7% incidence in 2004; UNAIDS; 2005), despite regular interaction between inhabitants of both land masses and with tourists. Senegal watchers have cited religion as an important factor, provided some flexibility is exercised in terms of how the moral code is applied. The involvement of Islamic and Christian protective norms, such as abstinence before marriage, fidelity and care of those affected early on are strong considerations in the success of the Senegalese response. Senegal, despite the prevalence of religion, was also apparently able to promote the use of condoms through church elders. Those who could not abstain were advised to use condoms. The dialogical culture in Senegal is highlighted as one of the cardinal approaches that led to effective networking amongst various interests to subvert AIDS.[21]

4. SADC in perspective: political, economic integration in the age of HIV/AIDS

It is a strange paradox in some ways that the SADC, a regional body that has shown so much promise in terms of democratisation, integration and common problem-solving, is the one saddled with a crisis that seems from time to time to defy any efforts at reversal.

With a population of 240 million people and endowed with mineral wealth ranging from oil, natural gas, copper, diamonds, cobalt, to phosphates and uranium, this region of Africa is also blessed with incredible hydroelectric potential in shared water courses.[22]

It is the relatively more stable part of the Sub-Saharan continent and is distinctive in the way it led the democratisation process through generally acceptable electoral processes in the 1990s. Guided by a common framework of principles and developmental goals, the SADC seeks to build common political and economic institutions to be able to compete in a highly globalised world market. It forms part of the vision of the Organisation of African Unity (OAU) the forerunner of the African Union (AU), to develop Regional Economic Communities (RECs) as building blocks for an integrated continent. Other RECs include ECOWAS, the Economic Community of Central African States (ECCAS) and the Arab Maghreb Union (AMU). To its credit, the SADC has managed its shared resources through a set of protocols and institutions that play critical distributive and allocative functions and avert potential conflict over resources and other contentious matters.

The events that led to the formation of the SADC began in 1970 with the idea of a military alliance of three countries – Botswana, Tanzania and Zambia – called the Frontline States (FLS). The alliance was created to fight for the liberation of territories under white minority rule; i.e. Angola, Mozambique, South West Africa (now Namibia), Rhodesia (now Zimbabwe) and South Africa with the aim of realising fundamental freedoms for all peoples. It became formally operational in 1975 with Mozambique and Angola, now independent, becoming the fourth and fifth members of the FLS respectively. In 1979, with Rhodesia on the verge of liberation, the FLS was transformed into the Southern African Development Co-ordinating Conference (SADCC) embracing the newly liberated territories. The SADCC was officially launched in 1980 in Lusaka, Zambia with the focus on economic cooperation and installing majority rule in South Africa and Namibia, the last bastions of apartheid.[23]

With the emergence of globalisation, the SADCC was reconstituted in 1992 and renamed the Southern African Development Community (SADC). Namibia and South Africa became its newest members. The SADC's founding treaty was based on deeper economic integration and democracy.[24] Its formation was in response to envisaged threats to human development in the sub-region and the need to develop strategies to avert these. Some of these were:

- The need to create mechanisms to address civil wars within member states;

- The limited size of the economies, which made countries individually unattractive to investment and integration therefore a natural choice if the region was to remain competitive in a globalised environment;

- The relatively small population size of most SADC countries meant the per capita cost of

providing infrastructure was high but could be reduced if countries cooperated in developing new infrastructure;

- Lastly, the emergence of HIV/AIDS, TB, malaria and other infectious diseases across borders called for collaboration at all levels between nations.[25]

Despite making headway in areas such as environmental management, transport, energy, peace and security, the SADC was, through its first decade of existence, unable to satisfy the general measure of human progress in the Human Development Index (HDI), which is composed of three elements of human development: longevity, education level and living standards.

The Development Policy Research Unit (DPRU) of the University of Cape Town explains that measuring HDI relies on proxy indicators. For instance, longevity is proxied by life expectancy, education by levels of enrolment and adult literacy rates and living standards by income. The DPRU indicates further that the average HDI value for the SADC region in 1998 was 0.538, which was considered to be a medium human development level (The value of the human development categories range from 0.800-1.000 (high); to 0.500 to 0.799 (medium) and 0.000-0.499 (low).

Seychelles, with a HDI value of 0.808, Mauritius with 0.782 and South Africa with 0.718 had the highest levels of human progress in the region, while Mozambique (0.350), Malawi (0.393) and Angola (0.419) had the lowest. The studies show that the value of SADC-specific HDI declined 5.3% between 1995 and 1998, indicating relatively slow progress toward improved living standards, education levels and longevity. The sharpest declines were in the DRC (-0.065), South Africa (-0.040) and Angola (-0.029).[26] The SADC attributes the negative trends in HDI mainly to HIV/AIDS (SADC; 2003).

Table 4.1: SADC human development categories (based on HDI values)

High human development category	Seychelles
Medium human development category	Mauritius, South Africa, Swaziland, Namibia, Botswana, Lesotho and Zimbabwe
Low human development category	DRC, Zambia, Tanzania, Angola, Malawi and Mozambique

Source: DPRU Policy Briefs No. 01/p13, May 2001.

The gross combined enrolment ratio at primary, secondary and tertiary levels rose between 1980 and 1995 from 38% to 51%. It, however, dipped to 51.14% in 1998. The adult literacy rate for the SADC increased from 48% in 1970 to 71% in 1995. The levels dropped to 67.32% in 1998. Adult literacy rates were highest in Angola, Mozambique and Malawi (58%, 57.7 % and 41% respectively).

Gross Domestic Product (GDP) the element in the HDI that measures living standards showed that the Seychelles (10 600), Mauritius (8 312) and South Africa (8 488), were the highest earners while Zambia (719), Malawi (523) and Tanzania (480) were the lowest.

The Regional Indicative Strategic Development Plan (RISDP), a 15-year regional integration development framework launched in 2004, now targets an annual economic growth rate of at least 7%, which is believed to be necessary to halve the proportion of people living in poverty by 2015.[27] The RISDP and Strategic Indicative Plan for the Organ on Politics, Defence and Security Cooperation (SIPO) represent more recent efforts by SADC to achieve its integration aims while collectively tackling its major challenges of infrastructural development, poverty reduction and combating disease (including AIDS), among other things.

4.1 SADC strategic framework 2000-2004

Confronted with the urgent need to integrate and compete in the global market and at the same time mitigate the impact of AIDS, SADC developed its first major response framework on HIV/AIDS for the period 2000-2004, which facilitated a number of processes including defining and promoting best practices, programme delivery, research and policy, capacity building and development of standards. However, the regional response could not adequately operationalise a multisector approach as only a limited number of its 21 sectors based in 14 countries in reality implemented any form of strategy.

The plan also lacked in-depth knowledge of the non-health impacts of HIV/AIDS. This limited scope was demonstrated by the body's inclination toward charging the responsibility for managing AIDS affairs to the SADC Health Sector Coordinating Unit (SADC-HSCU). Some other key shortcomings of the framework, as identified by a technical review of the plan in 2002, included:

- Failure to include the food security and finance sectors in the plan, despite being central to the region's development;

- Although some success was noted in the development of the SADC Code of Conduct on HIV/AIDS and employment, mechanisms for monitoring among member states were not put in place, hence discrimination against PLWHAs remained unchecked at national levels;

- The development of the strategic plan had not been supported by the necessary resources to effect implementation;

- The plan lacked the skills and capacity to mainstream HIV/AIDS. Most SADC sectors were saddled with other functions and could not cope with an additional task (SADC: 2003).

4.2 The new SADC strategic framework and plan of action, 2003-2007

In the new vision of 2003-2007, the SADC evidently broadened its understanding of the epidemic's impacts and its technical teams interacted more with new research and issues emerging from civil society and the private sector. The revised strategy was also aided in part by a restructuring exercise that collapsed the multiple sectors into technical clusters housed in one secretariat in Gaborone, Botswana.

SADC sectors dealing with a wide range of development issues, including health, environment, mining, trade, investment and tourism,[28] underwent a major restructuring exercise to concentrate its operations under the secretariat in Gaborone. Four directorates were established to lead all its functions. An HIV/AIDS unit was also established at the secretariat, within the Department of Strategic Planning, Gender and Policy Harmonisation. Each of the four directorates at SADC was assigned an HIV/AIDS specialist who would report to the unit head and who would in turn report to the chief director.

SADC national committees were recommended to lead activities at national levels, which included coordinating and mobilising the national consensus on regional responses, implementation and monitoring. The National AIDS Councils would be the secretariat to the national technical committees on AIDS-related matters. The SADC framework would also complement national and regional efforts at resource mobilisation.

Operational budgets were allocated to the Department of Strategic Planning, Gender and Policy Harmonisation, the Directorate for Social and Human Development and Special Programmes, the Directorate for Trade, Industry, Finance and Investment, the Directorate for Infrastructure and Services, the Directorate of Food, Agriculture and Natural Resources, and the Organ on Politics, Defence and Security. The new plan, devised by a group of consultants, identified five key cross-cutting areas in which to direct the efforts of its streamlined secretariat and directorates:

- **Human capital:** the SADC needed to recognise that the depletion of human capital would have consequences for social, economic and political activity;

- **Public goods:** the SADC's activities depended on the effectiveness of public administration and the supply of goods, and therefore strategies for addressing the erosion of state capacity were required;

- **Intersectoral relationships:** SADC policies needed to address interlinkages between the political, economic and social aspects of the pandemic to be effective;

- **Investment strategies:** the SADC needed to ensure that investments in different programme areas were coordinated and were supportive of each other in the response to the pandemic. The application of labour-saving technology could compensate for the losses in human capital for instance in the agriculture sector.

- **Integrating gender:** SADC policies needed to mainstream gender matters, delving deeper into the power and social relations between men and women. Women were the more prolific group in agriculture labour in the region; they not only played a bigger role in raising children and passing on life skills but were also more generally central to the economy. They, regrettably, are also the group that is disproportionately affected by the HIV/AIDS pandemic.

SADC's vision for 2003-2007 hence aimed to achieve the following:

- To reduce the incidence of new infections among the most vulnerable groups within the SADC;

- To mitigate the socio-economic impact of HIV/AIDS;

- To review, develop and harmonise policies and legislation relating to HIV prevention, care and support, and treatment within the SADC;

- To mobilise and coordinate resources for a multi-sectoral response to HIV/AIDS in the SADC region.

This time the regional body also emphasised the need for harmonisation,[29] monitoring the implementation of the SADC framework in addition to keeping tabs on member states' adherence to regional, continental and global commitments. Lastly, greater emphasis was laid on ensuring that gender was mainstreamed (SADC: 2003).

It is important to state that although the regional response came much later, member states of the SADC had operationalised their national responses targeting HIV prevention, care and support, and the mitigation of the socio-economic impact of HIV/AIDS since the mid-1980s. Their primary reference point was the WHO's Global Programme on AIDS assisted by other multilateral and bilateral donors. The early national responses were essentially health-focused and it was not until the 1990s that the multi-sector approach was adopted and mechanisms developed. Meanwhile, pressure for increased investment in health began to grow from lobby groups and activists across the globe. African governments were not spared.

4.3 AIDS resource flows

While there has been increased donor funding flows to AIDS interventions and African governments have shown a measure of political commitment, these developments are still to be translated into action through adequate resource allocation. The last two to five years have seen various countries introduce programmes to provide free ART in the public sector, financed through their own country and/or foreign sources. Despite the fact that governments have increased nominal allocations towards HIV/AIDS, empirical evidence has shown that over the years, public resources allocated to health have been decreasing owing to over-reliance on donor aid. Dependency on donor funds raises concerns about the sustainability of massive treatment programmes over decades.[30]

Even countries with enough domestic resources to shore up large-scale AIDS prevention, treatment and care interventions, such as South Africa, have experienced problems of limited absorptive capacity which affects the overall execution of its programme. Differences in provinces' readiness, capacity and political will are leading to significantly varied results in the ARV rollout, with the worst-

Figure 4.1: Development aid for HIV/AIDS: How much is going to which countries?

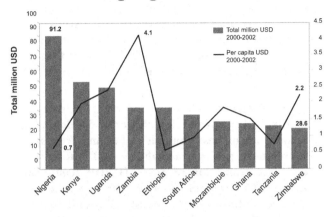

Source: OECD/UNAIDS special study: Aid Activities in Support of HIV/AIDS Control for 2000-2002

performing provinces covering only 10% of those newly in need of care (Ndhlovu & Daswa 2006:2). Specifically, readiness and capacity are often a function of visionary leadership and strong managerial skills (De Renzio, 2004:5).

Most governments have failed to adhere to the Abuja Declaration (2001) which stipulates that they allocate 15% of their national budgets to the health sector. But their ambitions to adhere to international norms do not appear diminished.

SADC member states, like other African countries, have in this regard linked their strategies to the Millennium Development Goals (MDGs). But given the myriad challenges facing the sub-region and Africa in general, and the relatively limited resources available, there is grave doubt whether some of the goals will be achieved. In the context of AIDS, we may draw some encouragement from the availability of treatment – albeit limited – and increased investments in health (and dutifully consider treatment as a moderating variable). However, we must also be mindful that socioeconomic analysis warns of the monumental task required to meet global developmental targets.

In fact recent reports indicate that the extent of HIV/AIDS is such that southern Africa is unlikely to meet the Millennium Development Goal 6: halving and reversing the spread of HIV/AIDS (malaria and other diseases) by 2015. Treatment not withstanding, indications thus far also suggest that it will be extremely ambitious to expect universal access to anti-retroviral drugs (ARVs) by 2015. And although the number of people on ART in low- and middle-income countries almost doubled in 2005 from 720 000 to 1.3 million, new infections far outstripped

this figure at 4.9 million in the same year (UN General Assembly 16th session, 2006).[31]

Tuberculosis-related deaths have soared since 1990 and the prevalence rates are still in the double digits in most countries. Despite some gains in orphan education, the AIDS factor is complicated further by the region's anticipated failure to meet the Millennium Development Goal 1: redress extreme poverty and hunger. Food insecurity and child malnutrition are likely to remain relentless adversaries for the foreseeable future. Similarly, maternal health is compromised by the relatively high mortality rate among mothers, which is being attributed mainly to HIV/AIDS.

Figure 4.2: Are African states meeting the Abuja declaration?

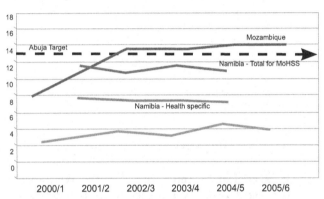

Source: Idasa, Funding the Fight, Budgeting for HIV/AIDS in developing countries, 2004 page 235.

There is more hope that Africa may meet its targets in some areas demanding gender equality such as access to education, but we are still a long way from achieving parity in employment.[32] The situation of orphans continues to deteriorate with southern Africa, again, bearing the brunt: 13 million orphans will need support as they strive to reach adulthood. Further, people with HIV/AIDS-related diseases continue to occupy more than half of all hospital beds in the high-prevalence countries of Sub-Saharan Africa, straining available services beyond capacity in most instances. Health professionals are at risk of infection due to inadequate infection control measures; they are also poorly paid and have been leaving Africa in droves for lucrative opportunities in western countries (ibid). Africans, especially southern Africans, are therefore caught in a complex reinforcing vortex of disease, poverty, food insecurity, poor infrastructure and low literacy rates, among other things, all of which lead to a massive governance challenge (UNAIDS; 2006).

This suggests that it has taken us well over 20 years to begin to realise that AIDS is a much larger epidemic than simply a health crisis affecting only one sector or a handful of countries. Years of formulating and reformulating strategies have brought us to a point where notions of governance and human security are beginning to play their part in the analysis of the pandemic's trajectory and impacts and hopefully are starting to inform our future responses.

To fully appreciate this discussion, we must first critically interrogate the related concepts of governance and democratic governance and how they are being related to HIV/AIDS in current academic discourse. We shall steer the discourse round to the role the electoral process plays in democratic governance and how it is affected by the pandemic.

5. HIV/AIDS and democratic governance

5.1 Defining governance

It is critical to emphasise that the relationship between HIV/AIDS and governance is highly complex and calls for focus in terms of how we interrogate the related issues. Extreme caution has to be exercised not to get caught up in the often confusing discourse on governance and the more normative notion of democratic governance. There is a plethora of literature that indicates that these concepts lack global consensus on their constituent elements. Hyden, Court and Mease (2004: 12) are instructive in this regard: "despite the recent popularity of governance at both practical and theoretical levels, the concept continues to mean different things to different people."

In several bodies of literature, governance as a tool is understood to facilitate a strategic developmental interaction between state and non-state actors in the management of the political, economic and social affairs of a country.[33] Much of today's understanding of the term revolves around the thought that governance is a non-hierarchical form of coordinating policy-making.

Mayntz (2003) traces the modern theory of political governance back to post-World War II when conflict-wary governments sought to steer their nations to result-defined social and economic goals.

Over the decades the use of terms such as coordination, network and decentralisation punctuated theoretical discussions on governance. The concept grew in significance in international discourse in the 1980s promoted by the World Bank and other multilateral donors. African scholars assert that the continent interrogated these concepts at about the same time.

The Khartoum Declaration of 1988, for instance, highlighted the promotion of human development, restoration of basic human rights and freedoms, overcoming political instability and intolerance and decentralisation of power (UNDP 2000). The African Charter for Popular Participation and Transformation crafted at Arusha, Tanzania in 1990 went further to emphasise accountability of leadership, press freedom and economic justice as key elements of governance.

There is some consonance in the manner in which the UNDP, the AU, the IMF and the World Bank articulate governance as a concept, each agreeing that it can be broken into different domains, all of which have policy import. These broadly encompass political, economic and social domains. The acceptance of human rights as core elements of governance by the World Bank albeit under considerable pressure from bilateral donors has moved the major international players to some common ground on the definition of the concept and its indicators in this regard (Hyden et al: 2004).

However, Hyden, Court and Mease (2004) argue that international development agencies have tended to avoid the political character of governance in their indicators because their official terms of reference for a long time barred them from working with political entities. This disconnection caused the political feature of governance "to lose its distinction in relation to the economy". More recently, there has been a convergence of opinion on political governance as the arena in which policy is formulated. UNDP elaborates: not only does political governance revolve around conditioning the quality of governance more generally, it has important constituent elements including basic political rights, freedom of expression, supremacy of the rule of law, broad participation of citizens in local governance and community forums and competitive, free and fair elections[34] (UNDP 2000), all of which facilitate the involvement of non-state actors in policy processes.

It is certain that the early attempts at analysing governance overlooked the African context: African scholars will agree that policies on the continent are usually externally defined by multilateral institutions and should not therefore see themselves as "conditioning" economic governance through politics based on their own actions only.

In fact, in later publications, the UNDP undertakes to include corporate and global governance as overriding phenomena which affect the way national governments determine their priorities. It asserts that local decisions are not always the result of national government actions but come under considerable influence from global capital. In most cases national entities, including governments, must negotiate with transnational companies and multilateral and bilateral partners to enable the allocative and distributive functions of their political, economic and social policies to take root.

Economic governance, in this sense, involves decision-making processes that affect a country's economic activities and its relationship with other economies. Economic governance also includes other key players such as trade unions, chambers of commerce, reserve banks and farming communities, the International Monetary Fund (IMF) and the World Bank (UNDP; 2000; p. 12). It is this aspect of governance that should ensure that access to the basic necessities of life, such as education, food security, welfare and health, i.e. all goals of human development, is delivered.

Finally, administrative governance is identified as the arena in which rules are implemented. There are four important observations to be made from these definitions:

- Governance can be divided into distinct domains; political, economic, administrative and corporate/global contexts all of which buttress human development;

- Governance is underpinned by a set of principles or values, which may be informed by internationally defined human rights instruments, and/or in the case of many developing states, indicators imposed by multilateral and bilateral agencies;

- Governance represents a horizontal form of policy interaction characterised by different modes of coordinating individual actions, or basic forms of social order;

- Governance is broader than government, as it embraces non-state actors in policy processes that may lead to sustainable human development.

5.1.1 "Good" or democratic governance

While there has not been much disagreement on the characteristics of governance, there was, for a long time, less consensus on what constituted "good governance" a post-cold war era concept that responded to the demands of global multilateral institutions or their beneficiaries. This post-cold war discourse was penned on political conditionalities which rewarded democratising regimes with loans and development aid and punished authoritarian and neo-patrimonial regimes with economic sanctions (UNDP: 2000). Conditionalities included the liberalisation of the political spectrum, accountability, transparency and observance of the rule of law.

Hyden et al. (2004: 2) observes that international organisations have made stronger attempts to reach consensus on what constitutes "good" governance largely based on an array of measures reflecting western historical experiences of democracy, and impliedly takes no account of Africa's own interpretations of the concepts.

To understand how this plays out in the discourse on democratisation in Africa we turn to respected intellectual Moletsi Mbeki, who emphasises that in fact Africa's much celebrated wave of democratisation in the 1990s had significant external interventions and was not primarily a result of pro-democracy actions by local organisations.[35] Mbeki's arguments reinforce undercurrents from within African academia and activism that posit that the model of democracy adopted by African countries is an imposition by multilateral agencies through the complex web of conditionalities that demand liberal market environments conducive to economic colonisation.

5.1.2 Democratic governance in Africa in the face of HIV/AIDS

Supporters of western democracy boast that the system has an unequalled record as the most accomplished form of governance in which political and socio-economic human rights are respected and conflicts resolved peacefully (NIMD: 2004). It is argued that democracies facilitate broad avenues for redress, contestation, expression and participation and hence present the best option for dealing with HIV/AIDS, taking into account the political, social and economic rights of those living with the disease.

Proponents and critics alike will however converge on one line of argument: democracies appear to be more difficult to consolidate in periods of poor economic performance, poverty and disease. Also, decision-making of an emergency nature may sometimes be stalled by uncompromising opposition standpoints in the legislature. Certainly decisions relating to an epidemic such as HIV/AIDS might also suffer, depending on the leverage the party in power has (Strand, Matlosa, Strode and Chirambo; 2005). It would also be unrealistic to assume that the rules in a democracy are applied fairly to poor people, women or minorities. Often this imbalance will arise as resources and opportunities are not always equitably allocated in areas which would be broadly empowering for the disadvantaged, leading to the unintended consequences of illiteracy, poverty and so on.

Democracies can also be unsettled by power alternations. The highly unstable situation in Malawi for example provides some invaluable lessons on the vulnerability of democracy in this regard. Since the election of the current president, Dr Bingu Wa Mutharika, in 2004 by a slender margin, his tenure has been undermined by incessant efforts by the opposition to impeach him. Although he has survived most attempts and appears to be gaining in popularity generally, long drawn out deliberations on impeachment for a long time diverted attention from key issues, such as debt cancellation and AIDS relief.

Authoritarian regimes or nominally democratic states have tended to act more swiftly and decisively against HIV/AIDS. Uganda, Thailand, Cuba and the North African states are some of those that can boast of low prevalence or a significantly reduced level of current and new infections. The trouble with authoritarianism arises when the government in power decides to ignore HIV/AIDS or any other matter of public policy concern: there may be no alternative avenues to challenge such an administration. Its weaknesses notwithstanding, therefore, we have to accept in the end that democracy in its many variants remains the dominant system of governance in the world today.

In this regard, the UNDP has added an even sharper normative edge to the concept of good governance by applying (western inspired) democratic values more critically. Good governance is now equated with democratic governance; embracing such institutions as freedom of expression and association, vibrant civil societies, gender equity and equality, rule of law, fundamental human rights, media freedom and free and fair elections.

5.2 Democratic governance principles in the context of HIV/AIDS

Drawing on the plethora of literature and Idasa's own experiences of democracy, this book embraces, with some reservations, the global interpretation of "good" or democratic governance in the context of HIV/AIDS as constructed by the UNDP. The constituent elements of democratic governance in this regard, with Idasa's embellishments, will be defined by the following principles:

UNDP 1: People's human rights and fundamental freedoms are respected, allowing them to live with dignity.

Idasa 1: Idasa's interpretation and working definition of democracy encompasses a commitment to social justice that is captured in our mission statement; democratic transition must be accompanied by a substantive improvement in the material conditions in which people live and work. In relation to public health, a balance must be struck between respecting the rights of those who are infected as well as the rights of those who are not. The individual's rights to privacy about their HIV status and treatment for AIDS are as fundamental as their right to protection from HIV. Any political intervention that imposes on any of these rights must be legitimised through public deliberation and due legal process.

UNDP 2: People have a say in decisions that affect their lives.

Idasa 2: Participation – or "active citizenship" as it is called in Idasa's mission statement – is fundamental to a modern, working democracy. The right to access to information and to participative processes at all the key moments in the policy- and law-making cycle – such as the annual budget process – are critical levers to social upliftment. Only by creating political space for poor people to have their voices heard will institutions of governance be responsive to the needs and interests of the most vulnerable members of society. Thus, policies on HIV/AIDS must be formulated and debated in a transparent process that allows PLWHAs and other stakeholders extra opportunity for participation and influence. At the very least, the opportunity for people to choose between alternative political interventions as proposed by contending parties in free and fair elections is paramount.

UNDP 3: People can hold decision-makers accountable.

Idasa 3: Those in power must be answerable for the decisions they take; the citizenry must have the capacity to be able to demand it. A variety of procedural and legal, as well as cultural and social, levers will drive a different relationship between those in power and the governed. We assert that the practice of transparent government, backed by effectively implemented "right to know" law and policy, will enable people to demand the highest standards from those in public office. Where decision-makers fail to fulfil promises or implement inefficient policies in the fight against HIV/AIDS, those ultimately responsible must agree to stand down if their (in)actions have undermined their credibility in the eyes of stakeholders or the public in general. A number of institutional arrangements can affect such accountability, of which free and fair democratic elections is the most common.

UNDP 4: Inclusive and fair rules, institutions and practices govern social interactions.

Idasa 4: The rules of the democratic game must be clear and known; if their origin is inclusive and involves the participation of all major stakeholders in society, they will attain the necessary level of legitimacy to encourage democratic tolerance and respect for the institutions of governance. Key civil and political freedoms, such as the right to freedom of expression and assembly, and the right to administrative justice to counteract abusive or arbitrary use of public power, will create the framework for a democratic society. In turn, in the arena of public health, inclusive and fair rules, institutions and practices govern social interactions between those who are and those who are not infected and/or directly affected by HIV and AIDS.

UNDP 5: Women are equal partners with men in private and public spheres of life and decision-making.

Idasa 5: Women have the fundamental right to equality, procedurally and substantively. Democracy demands that the rights of women are fully respected and protected. Due to being particularly vulnerable to the epidemic, women's experiences of being directly or indirectly affected by the epidemic must be prioritised in all decision-making.

UNDP 6: People are free from discrimination based on race, ethnicity, class, gender or any other attribute.

Idasa 6: Similarly, the right to equal treatment and protection against unlawful discrimination is fundamental to a modern democracy based on universal norms and standards. The potential stigma of HIV/AIDS raises significant dangers of discrimination. As a means to reduce the stigma attached to HIV/AIDS, the right to non-discrimination for those living with the virus should be elevated to the same level as other fundamental rights given to other categories of the population. HIV/AIDS is of no lesser concern or importance to society as a whole if it mainly affects one or more population segment that is relatively marginalised from power.

UNDP 7: The needs of future generations are reflected in current practices.

Idasa 7: The rights of children that are articulated so clearly in international law must be respected in the national sphere. The principal driver of change in this regard is to ensure that children can enjoy the right to a quality education, and that choices about the allocation of resources prioritises education and takes account of the barriers to the realisation of the right to education, such as food insecurity and inadequate public transportation. By the same token, the different decisions on prioritisation of resources and rights that go into formulating HIV/AIDS policy must also take into consideration the needs of today's AIDS orphans and the sustainability of society beyond their generation.

UNDP 8: Economic and social policies are responsive to people's needs and aspirations.

Idasa 8: The policy-making environment must be geared to permit people and civil society organisations to intervene before policy is finalised. Citizens are the best witnesses to their problems and needs; space must be created to allow their voices to be heard when designing prescriptions. On public health, government policy on HIV/AIDS must adapt in accordance with perceived incidence and estimated prevalence of HIV, and experienced illnesses and deaths from AIDS.

UNDP 9: Economic and social policies aim at eradicating poverty and expanding the choices that all people have in their lives.

Idasa 9: Endemic poverty and chronic unemployment undermine human dignity, drive human insecurity and thereby dilute and threaten the democratic dividend. The eradication of poverty must, therefore, be the number one priority of government, in partnership with all major social stakeholders. On the most vulnerable groups in society, government policy on HIV/AIDS must also address the structural problems that impact on the prevalence of HIV and reduce the receptiveness in people to treatment against AIDS. Only a person who has both information and realistic alternatives is truly empowered to change a behaviour that fuels the epidemic.[36]

Given this elaborate background, there are several ways in which the link between HIV/AIDS and democratic governance may be analysed assuming the impact of Anti-Retroviral Therapy (ART) is not optimistically factored-in:

- Growth is stunted through reduced Gross Domestic Product (GDP) as productive citizens die. Household incomes are stretched due to funeral, medical and legal costs. AIDS hence makes a significant contribution to poverty as earning power is lost by the sick and by households with deceased bread winners. The economic security of millions is threatened. Economic under-performance affects citizen confidence in the government of the day and, more critically, in the political system itself. Further, increased AIDS deaths amongst the working class could reduce tax bases and therefore the financial resources available to finance budgets.

- More generally, rising mortality rates may increase demands on public health and welfare expenditure as AIDS continues to infect millions. Health services struggle to cope with this unprecedented load while budgets are stretched beyond limits. Spending on health is highly reliant on donor funding, which raises questions about sustainability and endurance in addressing AIDS as a "long wave" crisis. The health security of nations is compromised.

- Poor economic performance may lead to democratic reversals which happen from time to time: Armed conflict or other forms of destabilisation may lead to economic and social collapse or poor productivity due to loss of skilled labour to more stable economies. Food (security) emergencies may occur and increase vulnerability to HIV as women and men trade sex for scarce commodities. Instances of sexual abuse might also increase the incidence of HIV.

- Due to limited availability of antiretroviral drugs, AIDS relief could be apportioned along ethnic or partisan lines, generating tension between working classes and various tribal groups, possibly exacerbating corruption and fomenting dissent amongst the marginalised.

- PLWHAs are targets of violence, including the psychological violence of stigma and discrimination. Gender-based violence increases female vulnerability to HIV infection. People living with AIDS withdraw from the electoral process for fear of violence or due to stigma. Similarly, there is public humiliation of people (perceived) to be living with AIDS who would seek elective office. This phenomenon exacerbates this feeling of personal insecurity.

- With the higher concentration of deaths from AIDS normally in the 15-49 age cohort, there is a strong likelihood that voting age populations will be depleted, affecting participation levels negatively. Millions of potential voters could be constrained by illness and care-giving and could therefore be rendered unable to navigate complex procedural processes that are required for citizen and voter registration. Lack of legitimacy can in turn spawn political conflict and instability as opponents seek legal and illegal means to challenge outcomes.

- AIDS could lead to political opportunism, allowing for leaders with simplistic solutions to manipulate public opinion regardless of whether they uphold democratic governance principles or not.

- The burden of orphans could similarly be overwhelming, not only tearing family systems apart but also stretching the state and civil society's resources. With millions of children in the streets, the possibilities of increased crime could rise.

- Lastly, HIV/AIDS could undermine the effectiveness of democratic institutions due to loss of skills, experienced personnel and reduced productivity. The impact of HIV/AIDS on the political society reduces the capacities of the military, political parties and government departments. Service delivery is affected, resulting in citizen protests. Skilled personnel are depleted from the ranks of electoral management bodies, political parties and parliaments, affecting institutional memory, democratic confidence and integrity. Weak governance increases chances of instability.[37]

We can assume that there will be other related arguments that will galvanise the discourse on governance and AIDS more generally. However our aims in this project are restricted to the institutional capacity and effectiveness of our democratic institutions and the participation of citizens in procedural processes in the face of HIV/AIDS. In the next section, therefore, we begin to illustrate the impact of

HIV/AIDS on the central institution of elections and discuss the democratic governance implications that will likely arise as a result of this new knowledge.

6. Overview of findings

The place of the electoral system in governance has been discussed in detail and its sensitivities and democratic relevance articulated at length. We take note that electoral systems come in many forms, can influence different outcomes and may require varying levels of expertise, organisation and financial capacity to sustain. While the criteria for designing electoral models constitute varied elements, in this section we shall focus mainly on the question of sustainability.

6.1 FPTP, MMP vs PR

Our examination of the First-Past-The-Post (FPTP), Mixed Member Proportional (MMP), Parallel and Proportional Representation (PR) electoral systems indicates clearly that the first two systems, in their current form as instituted in the SADC region, are highly vulnerable to HIV/AIDS.

SADC countries using these two systems have experienced an unusually large proportion of by-elections caused by Members of Parliament (MPs) dying of undisclosed ailments. Because records of the actual causes of deaths of elected representatives are often unavailable, there are a number of steps we have taken to explain the impact of the AIDS pandemic on electoral systems. We have done this by:

- Comparing and analysing trends in the deaths of elected leaders during the "pre-AIDS" period and the "AIDS era";

- Analysing the age cohorts of the deceased leaders (do they fall within the sexually active age group of 20-60 years?);

- And finally aggregating the causes of by-elections in countries that employ the FPTP and MMP systems (was there an increase in the number of by-elections caused by illness in the "AIDS era" compared to the "pre-AIDS era"?).

Although these steps do not conclusively attribute deaths to AIDS they do help us draw inferences on the pattern of deaths and their correlation to trends in AIDS deaths in the national population. High mortality among younger politicians (aged 40-55) provides a strong basis to link the deaths that have been attributed officially to "long" or "short illness" to the influence of the pandemic. Following this we expand the discussion by addressing the political and economic consequences of the pandemic resulting from its effect on the electoral system. These costs are best exemplified by assessing the FPTP and MMP systems which employ by-elections to fill vacancies. It is less useful to use the PR system because vacancies are filled by appointment from the party lists.

6.1.1 FPTP and MMP countries: Malawi, Tanzania, Zambia and Zimbabwe

We observe that the trends in countries which had severe epidemics in the 1990s, such as Malawi, Tanzania, Zambia and Zimbabwe, reflect a higher level of attrition amongst MPs. We also notice that death far outstrips resignations, defections, retirement or appointments as causes of parliamentary vacancies in countries that are also high-HIV prevalence zones.

We observe that the frequent deaths of MPs and other political representatives as a result of illness have only become commonplace in the last 15 years in Zambia for instance. As a result, the number of by-elections generated by the natural deaths of incumbent MPs and councillors has also increased during the same period. While only 6.44% of the 46 by-elections held between 1964 and 1984 were caused by MPs dying natural deaths, the numbers rose dramatically between 1985 and 2006: in that period at least 60% of the 146 by-elections held were due to deaths of incumbent MPs. It can of course be argued that parliament size changed during that period but that does not discount the fact that the rate of deaths still remains high.

Our research in Malawi also shows that there was a steady rise in the number of legislators who died in the 1994-1996 period – which was the height of the AIDS pandemic – compared to the 1999-2004 period. A total of 42 MPs died between 1994 and 2006. Of the 193 MPs at the end of 2005, 87 (45%) were below 50 years of age and 138 or about 72% were below 60 years of age. These figures suggest that the house is full of people who are still in the prime of their lives and will fall within the "vulnerable" category. An official statement in 2000 by the then Speaker of the National Assembly disclosed that 28 MPs in Malawi had died of HIV/AIDS-related complexes. Malawi

Figure 6.1: Causes of vacancies in national Parliaments

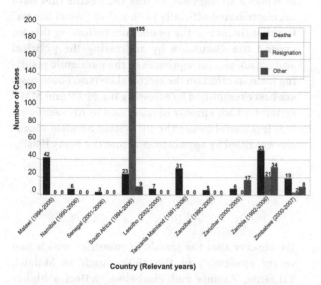

leader Morgan Tsvangirai's MDC: 62 seats to 57 seats (of 120 elective seats).

A succession of 29 by-elections had been held by 2005, with 19 having been caused by the deaths of MPs as a result of undisclosed illnesses. At least one vacancy was caused by the resignation of an MP on account of ill health, another was appointed to higher office. Additional reasons for the vacancies that led to by-elections were the dismissal of an MP. Six constituencies Buhera North; Hurungwe East; Mutoko South; Chiredzi North; Gokwe North; and Gokwe South had their results nullified by the high court following petitions by losing candidates. The sitting MPs appealed to the Supreme Court but the case was still being heard by the time of the 2005 parliamentary elections.

Figure 6.2: Age cohort and numbers of deceased MPs 1990-2003 Zambia

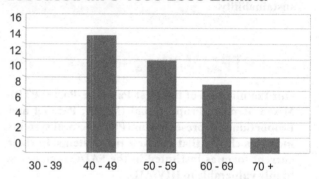

Source: Chirambo, 2003; 2006.

lost seven MPs in a single year (2005). Twenty three MPs died between 1994 and 1999 and 12 between 1999 and 2004.

In Tanzania, a total of 31 MPs died between 1991 and 2006. As in the other countries, no information is available on the actual cause of death in cases where illness is involved. Four MPs are listed as victims of car accidents and shootings, while the rest died from undisclosed "long" and "short" illnesses. Mortality at the House of Representatives in Zanzibar is relatively low at five deaths between 1990 and 2005. The disparities between Zanzibar (less than 1% prevalence and 4.7 incidence in 2004 (UNAIDS; 2005)), and Tanzania mainland (7% HIV prevalence rate) in terms of prevalence rates might be explained by the influence of religion or geographical position and size, among other things. Zanzibar is a much smaller area to barn-storm with AIDS campaigns. In addition, deviant behaviour in a place where everybody knows everybody else will very likely be frowned upon. In particular, the influence of Islam coupled with strong management of the pandemic and its link to the spread of HIV/AIDS is a matter requiring further investigation.

There is further evidence provided by Zimbabwe in terms of the instability of the FPTP system in the face of HIV/AIDS. Zimbabwe held its most competitive parliamentary election in 2000, upon the birth of the Movement for Democratic Change (MDC) which rigorously tested the liberation party the Zimbabwe African National Union Patriotic Front (ZANU-PF). The ruling ZANU-PF headed by founding president Robert Mugabe won a relatively slender victory over

6.1.2 The Parallel and PR systems: Senegal, Namibia and South Africa

Senegal generally exhibits prevalence rates among the general population that vary between 0.7% and 9% (UNAIDS, 2006),[38] which is still far below the Sub-Saharan levels. During Senegal's 2001-2006 parliamentary session, only three MPs died. This figure does not indicate a substantial increase in deaths when compared with prior legislatures, particularly those before the HIV/AIDS pandemic. It has also not been established that there has been a high mortality in elected representatives of local government.

In the same vein, Namibia does not show any significant trends that may be linked to an unusual phenomenon such as HIV/AIDS. It may be argued that this is because the Namibia epidemic may be comparatively less severe.[39] Also, data from the apartheid era was not made available to us. Records from the country's parliament indicate that between 1990 and

2006 six sitting MPs died. Four of these were from the National Assembly and two from the National Council. None died from illnesses related to HIV/AIDS according to the causes of death issued to the media. Press reports at the time of the MPs deaths gave as the causes complications from diabetes, vehicle accident, long and short illnesses and heart attack. The death rates among the 98 elected members of both houses have remained relatively low. As in South Africa, the PR system employed at national level is relatively cheaper to manage when vacancies occur as no by-elections are required.

Data from the parliament of South Africa suggests that 227 MPs departed (resigned, were appointed to higher positions or were dismissed) between 1994 and 2006. Twenty three of the vacancies arose as a result of deaths. There is no information on the causes of deaths and no evidence to suggest that the trends mimic the so-called AIDS mortality profile, where relatively younger people (aged 50 and below) die at a faster rate than relatively older people (50 and over). The relatively lower death rates have been explained as to do with the extent of medical cover extended to parliamentarians in South Africa.[40]

While this might be a factor, it should also be noted that other countries also have similar medical aid schemes. But the fact that senior parliamentarians from other SADC states have on occasion been flown to South Africa or abroad for advanced medical attention in some instances indicates a disparity in the capacity and quality of medical care.[41]

6.1.3 MMP: Lesotho and South Africa (local government)

While South Africa appears insulated from the financial costs of replacing deceased leaders, it has held by-elections at a local level to replace directly elected councillors under the MMP system employed at the local government level. The electoral system used for local government elections is as follows: (a) for local and municipal councils (Category A and Category B respectively) 50% of ward councillors are elected directly through the FPTP system and the other 50% through the PR model in order to achieve overall political proportionality; and (b) at the district level (Category C) 40% of the councillors are directly elected by eligible district residents while 60% of the councillors are indirectly elected in that they are appointed representatives of local and municipal councils (Strand, Strode, Matlosa & Chirambo: 2005). In 2001, a total of 79 by-elections were held. Of these 27 were in KwaZulu-Natal and

nine in Gauteng. A study undertaken by Michael Sachs[42] provides reasons for the by-elections held by province. The Sachs report indicates that of the 79 by-elections in 2001, 34 were caused by a councillor's resignation, 33 resulted from the death of a councillor and 12 were the result of the expulsion of a councillor either from the party or the council concerned. It has to be stated that in Africa, generally, MPs and councillors will enjoy a much higher standard of living than the general population and will also have access to better medical services. These deaths would have occurred despite all that.

To further underline the vulnerability of the MMP system we turn to the Kingdom of Lesotho where deaths amongst MPs and other factors continue to generate costly by-elections despite a change in the electoral model. Eight by-elections were held in the kingdom between 2002 and 2005, the period in which the modified MMP electoral model was instituted.[43] Seven of the MPs had been elected through the FPTP system and one through the PR system.

6.2 Average ages of MPs and vulnerability factors

Nuances in this discussion suggest that the younger MPs are the more vulnerable and will continue to be susceptible in the absence of holistic strategies to maintain a relatively AIDS-free future leadership. On the basis of the current information provided by the respective national assemblies, Zambia has the youngest parliamentarians on average at 46 years; followed by Namibia and Malawi at 51 years, Tanzania has a relatively higher average of 54, while South Africa and Senegal come in at 55 years.

In analysing the ages of the parliamentarians in relation to their vulnerability to HIV/AIDS, we need to bear in mind that the epidemic is "a long wave event". We started discussing its trajectory from the mid-1980s when most countries recorded their first cases. This was a time when HIV risk perception would have been relatively low in the general population and the leadership. This phase was followed by long periods of denial by many countries around the globe as to the extent of the epidemic amongst their people. Stigma and discrimination were rife; ignorance and myths predominant.

This would have been the phase in which most of the parliamentarians who were 40 years old in 1987 for instance will be 60 years old today. In short, it may be naïve of us to simply categorise 18-49-year-olds in the present day as being potential casualties of HIV/AIDS. It is highly likely that many of the older MPs who may have died of AIDS in the 1990s contracted the virus in the early 1980s. Therefore, a person who is in their sixties by 1999 or in the next millennium might quite easily have carried the virus leading to their eventual death.

In Zambia for instance, we see a concentration of deaths amongst the 40-49 and 50-59 age cohort between 1990 and 2003. Most of these people would have been younger and vibrant in the 1980s and therefore more vulnerable to HIV/AIDS given their presumably more sexually active lifestyles at the time. This was the period in which ARV access was almost non-existent. In the rare situations when it was available much later in the late 1990s, it was pro-hibitively expensive.

To underline this point, we turn to the experi-ence of one of the champions of HIV/AIDS in the world today. Judge Edwin Cameron of South Africa is the only high-profile figure to disclose his HIV status. Unlike the subjects of this study, he is not an elected official. He was born on 15 February, 1953.[44] He disclosed his status in 1999 when he was 46 years old during a job interview with the Judicial Service Commission. A high court judge at the Supreme Court of Appeal, Cameron was 54 in 2007 and by his own assertion, has had the benefit of treatment, job security and support of family, friends and col-leagues, factors that could explain his longevity as a PLWHA.[45] There would have been many less for-tunate citizens and political elites within the SADC region who had limited or no access to ARVs, par-ticularly in the early to mid-1990s.

6.3 Loss of representation

The immediate political cost of the death of an MP is the constituency's loss of representation. Depending on the time it takes to replace the deceased through by-elections, this might disadvantage the masses. MPs are expected to drive development at constitu-ency level, even though they may not always have the resources to do so. Any long period without representation alienates the affected districts. On the Tanzania mainland, six constituencies Kisesa, Mbeya Vijijini, Ulanga Mashariki, Kasulu Mashariki, Rahaleo and Kilombero had no MPs by the December 2005 general elections. Their MPs had died during the 2000-2005 parliamentary sitting. During the 1995-2000 parliaments, ten MPs died.

In Malawi, it took more than a year for by-elec-tions to be conducted in the six constituencies that

fell vacant after the 2004 elections. Lack of finances is understood to be the main reason. The lack of capacity of Malawi to finance elections from its own vault was revealed when local government elections scheduled for 2005 were postponed. A crunching food security crisis for the predominantly agrarian economy meant that the state was unable to raise enough funds to support its local polls, resulting in a constitutional crisis. In the case of parliamentary vacancies, the requirement by law is that a by-elec-tion be held within 90 days of a seat being declared vacant. The MEC is required to prepare special budg-ets to justify central treasury funding, which are often not approved in time. Hence, the reality is that the timeframes for holding by-elections have not been adhered to. The implication of this is that the voices of ordinary people, often expressed through vibrant elected representatives, are silenced for an unusually long time. In cases where an MP is also responsible for assisting in donor and state interven-tions in community-based projects, the benefit to the constituency may be affected by his/her absence.

A very real consideration of the prospect of too many by-elections within months or weeks of each other is poor attendance by the electorate. Voting consumes a substantial amount of an individual's time; it can be frustrating to spend long periods in queues or at a campaign rally. Poor turnouts will raise problems of legitimacy for the winners as they may be seen to represent only relatively few people.

6.4 Parliaments: changing power configurations in national parliaments of Zambia and Zimbabwe

We note that disease in general, and HIV/AIDS in particular, contributes to power shifts in countries operating the FPTP electoral model. This phenom-enon is best exemplified by Zambia and Zimbabwe where elections have become increasingly competi-tive. The effect of natural deaths, combined with vacancies generated by expulsions, resignations or floor-crossing by members, compelled Zimbabwe to hold 14 by-elections following the 2000 legislative polls. Eight of the by-elections arose because par-liamentary representatives had died prematurely of undisclosed illnesses.

In the 2000 Zimbabwean parliamentary elections ZANU-PF won 62 seats of the 120 elective seats while the opposition MDC secured 57 seats. A lone seat went to the other opposition ZANU-Ndonga party. Through victories in most by-elections, ZANU-PF increased its parliamentary strength from 62 to 67 seats by 2004. It secured five extra seats from the MDC whose portfolio shrank within the same period from 57 to 52 seats.

Figure 6.3 Seats breakdown per Parliament

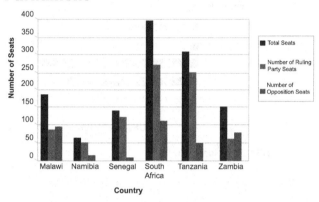

Source: Malawi, Namibia, Senegal, South Africa, Tanzania and Zambia parliaments. Compiled by Idasa.

Death has now become the biggest cause of vacancies in the Zimbabwe parliament. Between 2004 and 2007, 19 of the 29 by-elections held were due to MPs dying from undisclosed illnesses. The effect of numerous by-elections is that the opposition parties have generally lost the majority of the polls, partly perhaps due to their inability to compete with a well-resourced ruling party. In Zambia, the opposition also lost ground after entering parliament in the 2001 general elections with a combined slender majority. The by-elections that followed in succession several months later were won mainly by the ruling Movement for Multi-party Democracy (MMD). There is nothing undemocratic about this,

one might add. But it is an important observation regarding how a disease may contribute to tipping the balance of power.

For example, table 6.1 indicates that of the 29 by-elections held between 26 June 2001 and 12 April 2006, the ruling MMD gained 14 seats from the opposition out of a pool of 16 held by the opposition following the general elections of 2001.

Thus the MMD's strength increased from 46% to 54% representation in parliament between the 2001 and the 2006 presidential and parliamentary general elections. Conversely, the parliamentary representation of the two larger opposition parties that could present the stiffest challenge to the MMD in general elections, the UPND and UNIP, dropped from 49% to 43% and 8.7% to 6% respectively. These two examples clearly show how numerous by-elections, whether generated by HIV/AIDS or not, are likely to favour the ruling parties and significantly alter the balance of power. This, as asserted above, would impact on political party policy leverage determining governance priorities.

6.5 Economic costs

There is a high cost to the Treasury in holding numerous by-elections. In December 2005 the six by-elections in Malawi cost an estimated MK65 million ($US474 799.12), which translated into approximately MK10.8 million ($US78 889.70) per constituency. Each by-election held in Zambia cost US$235,849 on average.[46] In Tanzania, by-elections cost between $US300 000 and $US500 000 depending on the size of the voting district. The MMP in Lesotho is equally vulnerable: the seven by-elections held in Lesotho since the country modified the electoral model in 2002 from FPTP to an MMP system

Table 6.1: Power shifts in Zambian parliament between 2001 and 2006									
	MMD	UPND	FDD	UNIP	HP	PF	ZRP	INDPT	Totals
2001 election seats	69 (46%)	49 (32.7%)	12 (8%)	13 (8.7%)	4 (2.7%)	1 (0.7%)	1 (0.7%)	1 (0.7%)	150 (100%)
Seats lost	2	7	1	4	2	1	0	0	15
Seats retained	11	1	0	0	0	1	0	0	13
Seats gained	14	0	1	0	0	1	0	0	16
Net gain	12	-6	0	-4	-2	0	0	0	
Pre-2006 election seats	81 (54%)	43 (28.7%)	12 (8%)	9 (6%)	2 (1.3%)	1 (0.7%)	1 (0.7%)	1 (0.7%)	150 (100%)
Source: Foundation for Democratic Process									

each cost approximately R1million (US$143 601[47]). Three by-elections were the result of the deaths of MPs. Although wards are smaller and therefore less costly, the cumulative effect of holding many by-elections in terms of South Africa's MMP system at local government level could prove daunting. A ward poll can cost approximately R30 000.00 ($4000 at the rand-US dollar exchange rate at the time of writing).[48] Countries such as Malawi and Zambia have had their national elections substantially supported in financial terms by foreign donors, which may render the prospect of increased by-elections more onerous.[49]

Table 6.2: Average cost of by-elections

Country	Electoral system	Average cost of by-elections
Tanzania mainland	FPTP	US$416.000
Zanzibar	FPTP	US$45,000
Zambia	FPTP	US$235,849
Malawi	FPTP	US$78,889
Lesotho	MMP	US$143,601[50]

Source: Compiled by Idasa

The costs illustrated above only relate to the state's allocations to the EMB. These costs will cover the provision of air/road transport to deliver ballots; design and printing of ballots; setting up temporary shelters for electoral staff; allowances for election and presiding officers; lighting for the polling stations; booths; communication; advertising on television, radio and newspapers; posters; public education of a direct nature; discursive programmes for political parties, among other things.

The table above does not include costs incurred by civil society and donor agencies in relation to election monitoring and voter and civic education activities. Neither do they include expenditure by political parties on repeated campaigns. Finances will be needed by political parties to cover road/air transport; television and newspaper advertising; public meetings; salaries or stipends for support staff and cadres; t-shirts for promoting candidates; paying political party monitors, among other things. Cash-strapped political parties will obviously be outpaced by the more powerful entities. If neither the competing political parties or the civil society monitors are able to achieve sufficient coverage of all electoral events, the likelihood of post-election conflict might rise as independent voices and "judges" will be seen to be absent from the electoral process, undermining the credibility of the outcomes.

Figure 6.4: Average cost of national elections per voter

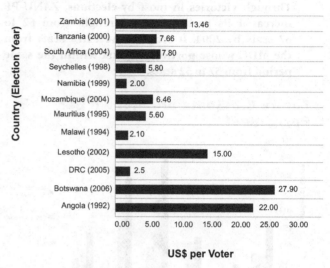

Source: EISA 2006; Idasa: 2002

6.6 Parliamentary debates on HIV/AIDS

Despite the now rather distinct manner in which elected MPs have been dying in countries severely affected by AIDS, we do not see any significant levels of debate within parliament that suggests that the institutions have even attempted to investigate mortality amongst their members let alone deploy in-house strategies to minimise the impact. Parliaments in Namibia, Malawi, Tanzania, Senegal, South Africa and Zambia have interrogated many aspects of the HIV pandemic, including high costs, drugs, rape and deliberate transmission of the HI virus, orphaning, behaviour change, preventative methods, budget allocations and culture, among other things. While evidence exists that MPs in Tanzania for instance have encouraged each other to go for VCT, there is no public disclosure or records of how many have actually volunteered for tests.

The high attrition rates from death within parliaments has not however been lost on some publics: the Medical Association of Zambia initiated a debate on mandatory HIV testing for all presidential and parliamentary candidates in 2005, as the country's 2006 general elections approached. Despite the media storm that followed, relatively lukewarm responses in terms of parliamentary discussions were observed. Human rights activists argued that such a move would violate the rights of MPs.

And while Senegalese MPs interviewed for this study profess to be actively involved in HIV/AIDS initiatives in their local communities, the parliament does not have institutionalised approaches to deal with members who are PLWHAs. The low prevalence status of Senegal might encourage a sense of low risk perception as exemplified by the MP who remarked that AIDS does not constitute a major priority: "At this moment, it must all the same be recognised that sectors like education, agriculture and the fight against poverty have priority over the other ones…"

The debate on VCT for elected representatives also emerged in Namibia. Former Swapo MP, Ben Ulenga, who was Deputy Minister of Local Government at the time, stirred a heated debate when he announced his intention in 1996 to take a test for HIV. He also alleged that half the national parliament was infected by the virus. His negative results did not inspire others to follow suit. In the seven countries being studied that have released preliminary results, there is not a single elected member or cabinet minister known to be HIV-positive. This contradicts the statistics just presented.

The South African parliament is also cagey on the matter. Perhaps what is even more surprising is that Malawi, a country whose speaker was on record as having attributed 28 of the 31 deaths amongst MPs (by the year 2000) to AIDS-related illness, does not appear to have had any significant reference to the impact of the epidemic on the national assembly and its representatives. Such blatant disregard may quite easily be interpreted as denial. This denial may be a direct result of stigma and discrimination in politics otherwise referred to herein as "political stigma".

6.6.1 Political ostracism and political rights

In all the countries studied, there appears to be an inherent fear of disclosure due to the potential loss of economic benefits that come with being a politician. Disclosure of one's HIV status has been equated with "political suicide" or becoming "a political liability" to the party. A salient feature noted in our research in Zambia is the use of HIV/AIDS as a weapon in electoral politics. Opposition candidates who are perceived to be sick are undermined and destroyed before the eyes of the electorate. Weight loss is closely associated with AIDS and has caused opposition parties to cast doubt on the health of leading candidates and incumbents alike. In our post-research stakeholder meetings with the ruling

MMD and opposition parties in July 2006 in Zambia this was further underlined by top party officials. No party was willing to adopt a candidate who was HIV-positive or was perceived to be positive, as they were seen to be liabilities (Chirambo: 2006). In Malawi, some political party candidates were reluctant to dwell on HIV/AIDS during the campaign for the 2004 presidential and parliamentary elections for fear of being associated with the illness. Senegalese MPs were equally reluctant to pursue an open policy on their HIV status. As indicated in the foregoing, Namibia and Tanzania are not any different.

We take note therefore of the silent exclusionary practices of political elites who have taken to marginalising fellow aspirants to elective office at the remotest sign of illness. Political ostracism should, in our view, be considered a real threat to people's political rights. It has led to the highly improbable record of non-disclosure amongst senior elected officials in government and parliamentary structures. To date, no elected official is on record as carrying HIV, presumably for fear of rejection by their political parties and the electorate. Particularly, pervasive denialism amongst leaders severely undermines their moral authority to address HIV/AIDS as a public policy emergency.[51] Generally, pervasive denialism permeates societies at all levels. These are matters that require the help of high-level actors to generate a new wave of sensitisation in the echelons of power and start regional and national attitude shifts amongst elites.

6.7 Impact of HIV/AIDS on electoral management, administration in Africa

The impact of HIV/AIDS on EMBs has to be understood in three ways:

- The loss of core staff, which might affect efficiency and institutional memory;

- The loss of part-time staff who were mainly drawn from the public service's teaching profession compromises continuity, undermines the quality of work and raises costs as training is then needed for new staff;

- The rapid rise in numbers of deaths renders the voters' roll unmanageable.

Studies are showing a severe impact of AIDS on the public sector and in particular the teaching profession. An estimated 200 000 of Sub-Saharan

Africa's 650 000 teachers are projected to die of AIDS. At least half of the positions in the education sector are vacant at present. It is suggested that globally it will cost up to $1billion annually to compensate for the loss and absenteeism of teachers resulting from AIDS.

The sum effect of AIDS on the teaching profession is summarised as follows:

- Infected teachers lose six months of professional working time before developing full-blown AIDS;
- Teachers experience on average 18 months of increasing disability prior to leaving the school system.

The wholesale loss of teachers has wider implications for the affected countries. Firstly, experts assert that the teaching profession constitutes the largest segment of public workers, the public sector being the largest employer in Africa. The attrition of teachers, including university professors, means the next generation of young people will be exposed to poorer quality education. Younger citizens will also find it exceedingly difficult to meet the requirements of highly competitive job markets or will experience difficulties in launching their own entrepreneurships.[52]

In Zambia, it is projected that the HIV/AIDS epidemic is likely to reduce the number of teachers from an expected 59 500 to only 50 000 by 2010, while teacher absenteeism due to HIV-related illnesses will cost 12 450 teacher/years over the next decade. Studies by the Human Sciences Research Council (HSRC) in South Africa indicate that 4 000 teachers died in 2004 while 45 000 more, about 12.7% of the workforce, were HIV-positive. Of those who died of AIDS, 80% were under the age of 45. The study was conducted at 1 700 schools. Ten thousand of the 45 000 HIV-positive teachers needed ARVs (The Star, 05/04/05). A study titled "The Impact of HIV/AIDS on the Human Resources in Malawi's Public Sector" conducted by the Malawi Institute of Management (MIM) for the government of Malawi and the UNDP illustrates a grave situation of morbidity, absenteeism and attrition due to HIV/AIDS among civil servants.

Except for Namibia, where the Electoral Management Body (EMB) advertises temporary work to the general public to assist in elections, the other SADC countries in this study usually utilise teachers for backup during the polls. As conducting elections requires experienced staff, the vulnerability of support personnel to the disease is likely to reduce the Independent Electoral Committee's ability to rely on them to bring their accumulated experience and skills to bear on future elections.

6.8 Impact of HIV/AIDS on voter registers

6.8 1 Institutionalised citizen and voter registration systems

"The impact of HIV/AIDS has forced electoral management bodies to face a number of problems regarding the voters' roll. The number of registered voters on the voters' roll is not a true reflection of what is on the ground. Our voters' rolls are bloated with dead voters."
M. Ngwembe, Commissioner Malawi Electoral Commission (Chirambo & Caesar, 2003. p. 128).[53]

The countries in this study have varying levels of development in terms of their electoral institutions. Some, like Tanzania, only established a voters' roll in 2005. Others, like Malawi, have highly controversial rolls that cannot be reconciled with the country's population size, particularly with their Voting Age Population (VAP). Zambia has changed registers at least three times in two decades and only launched a biometric system in 2006. For a long time, the Zambian citizen registration and voter registration systems have not been directly compatible; they are two different processes that are independently managed. Senegal also instituted a digitised citizen ID and voter registration mechanism in 2007. South Africa has a technologically advanced and well established citizen and voter registration systems which allows it to timeously remove dead voters from the registers. Rather than compare systems that are in effect incomparable, we choose to contrast the problems associated with not having an institutionalised citizen and voter registration system in the age of AIDS with the benefits of investing in one. In this regard, we contrast Malawi with South Africa.

6.8.1.1 Malawi

The case of Malawi is a compelling one in as far as defining how a country struggling with the installation of a credible citizen, voter and death registration system is challenged to deal with high attrition rates amongst its population. Firstly, the death registration system in Malawi is at best colonial. When citizens in rural outposts die, their deaths are relayed to the chiefs and it is through them that confirmation of death is captured by the government. This system will not respond expeditiously to the high attrition associated with AIDS. This will lead to the electoral roll, which should eliminate the names of all registered voters on receipt of a death certificate, to be highly unreliable. In the 1999 general elections, the Malawi Electoral Commission registered 5 071 822 voters. The MEC claimed to have removed 106 086 registered voters from the roll in the five years prior to the 2004 general elections. A highly disputed figure of 6 668 839 registered voters was announced for 18 May 2004 presidential and parliamentary elections, despite the removal of dead voters.[54]

The National Statistics Office (NSO) projections during the same period suggested that there were 5 594 081 people aged 18 years or older in Malawi who were eligible to vote. In short, the MEC could not adequately explain where the extra one million registered voters came from.

> "Our projections [based on the last (1998/99) national population census] are [that] the population has grown at an average rate of 3.2 per cent", observed the NSO. [sic:] "But if you calculate the average rates at which the Commission's figures are based, you will find that they are way above the normal population growth rate."

Mainly because of the system's failure to account for all its citizens and its voters, dead or alive, the results of Malawi's 2004 elections were highly controversial especially as the eventual president, Dr Bingu Wa Mutharika, won by a slender majority with an opposition-controlled parliament. The results have led to the relatively weak mandate that Mutharika has had to endure, surviving several impeachment initiatives by the opposition in the process.

6.8.1.2 South Africa

The case of South Africa is radically different. Equipped with bar-coded IDs and with electronic compatibility between citizen and voter registers, South Africa purges dead voters on a monthly basis. The dataset from the Independent Electoral Commission in South Africa contains the following:

The number of registered voters at the end of 1999, 2000, 2001, 2002 and 2003; the total number of deceased registered voters for 1999, 2000, 2001, 2002

and 2003, for each gender and each age cohort (18–19; 20–29; 30–39: 40–49; 50–59; 60–69; 70–79; 80+); the number of registered voters at the end of 1999, 2000, 2001, 2002 and 2003, for each gender, each age cohort (as above), each province and each municipality; and the total number of deceased registered voters for 1999, 2000, 2001, 2002 and 2003, for each gender, each age cohort (as above), each province and each municipality.

The data is extremely powerful as it provides absolute numbers of deceased voters at all levels of governance. Based on this dataset, it was established in our South African study that 1 488 242 of the country's registered voters died between 1999 and 2003 out of a total of 20 674 926 people who were on the voters' roll for the 2004 general elections. Deaths are concentrated in the 20-49 years and 60-79 years age groups. We argue that the sharp increases in mortality in some cases up to 200% among registered voters between the ages of 20-49, particularly among women in the 30-39 year bracket, can to a large extent, if not wholly, be explained by AIDS.

We based our argument on the strong correspondence between the profiles that our analysis generated and those that have been described by the expert demographers in the field of HIV/AIDS.

Figure 6.5: South Africa: Increase (in %) in relative numbers of deaths among registered voters between 1999-2003, per age and sex

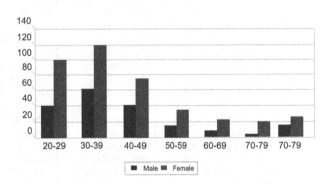

Source: IEC

6.8.1.3 Namibia and Senegal

In Namibia, while no evidence of voter attrition to the extent exhibited by South Africa exists, there are strong perceptions by political actors, particularly the opposition, that AIDS has had some influence on the electoral process but there is no empirical evidence to support this belief. The Congress of

Matrix of electoral management systems in SADC and Senegal

	Malawi	Namibia	Senegal	South Africa	Tanzania	Zambia
Citizen registration system	No citizen register Death registration not institutionalised (done by local chief)	National identity card	New digitised ID system introduced	Digitised bar coded ID system	National ID system available	ID system available
Voter registration system	Voter register available but size unknown (controversial)	Voter register available	New biometric register established in 2006	Digitised electoral register	No register until 2005 when Permanent Voters Register was introduced	New biometric register introduced in 2006
Purging of dead voters	Problematic and slow because the country does not have a civic register. However, each voter's status must be verified by a district commissioner, village headman, chief or other prominent person	It is provided that monthly updates should be made but this has shown to be ineffective and not constant, especially in rural areas	Until 2000, there was continuous registration. This process did not fully account for deceased voters or changes to personal details of electors. For the 2007 elections, the Ministry of Interior made a totally new register of electors. Each Senegalese citizen who meets the legal requirements had to register and obtain a voter's card and national identity card	The Independent Electoral Commission (IEC) of South Africa assures us that all dead voters were purged from the voters' roll before the 2004 elections	Deaths are reported to village chiefs and to home affairs ministry	The ECZ removes illegally registered persons, dead people or those who change locations. In this system, any citizen or relative can go to the ECZ to lodge a request to remove an individual from the voters' roll citing reasons, including death or ineligibility as in the case of foreigners
Delimitation of constituencies	The Malawi Electoral Commission is also responsible for the demarcation of constituency boundaries and this is contained in Section 72(2) of the Constitution and the Electoral Commission act of 1998 S. 8 (1)Article 106 on Regional Council Elections states that: (1) Each region shall be divided into constituencies the boundaries of which shall be fixed by the Delimitation Commission in accordance with the provisions of an Act of Parliament and this Constitution: provided that there shall be no fewer than six and no more than twelve constituencies in each region	Article 106 on Regional Council Elections states that (1) Each region shall be divided into constituencies the boundaries of which shall be fixed by the Delimitation Commission in accordance with the provisions of an Act of Parliament and this Constitution: provided that there shall be no fewer than six and no more than 12 constituencies in each region	According to the law, the CENA sets up departments, the embassies and the consulates reporting structures in the regions that can help them fulfil their mandate. In the past (for the elections of 2000), the ONEL (that has been replaced by the Commission Electorale Nationale Autonome), had created 10 regional bodies and 40 departmental ones on the tops of which they themselves nominated 9 000 delegates in order to represent them in each polling station	The Electoral Commission Act 51 of 1996 states in chapter 2 (5) (1)(m) that the IEC's functions include the demarcation of wards in the local sphere of government or to cause them to be demarcated	Article 75(1) (3) and (4) of the Constitution of the United Republic of Tanzania empowers the NEC to demarcate the URT into constituencies and to review the delimitation of constituencies at least once every 10 years	In terms of Article 77 [Constituencies and Elections]: (1) Zambia shall be divided into constituencies, for purposes of elections to the National Assembly so that the number of such constituencies, the boundaries of which shall be such as an Electoral Commission prescribes, shall be equal to the number of seats of elected members in the Assembly

	Malawi	Namibia	Senegal	South Africa	Tanzania	Zambia
Establishment of electoral commission	The Constitution of Malawi mandates the establishment of an Electoral Commission that is independent of any external authority (Constitution 1994, Articles 75, 76(4)). The Electoral Commission Act 1998 provides for the setting up of the Malawi Electoral Commission (MEC)	Through the promulgation of the Electoral Act (Act No. 24 of 1992) the ECN was established to direct, supervise and control national, regional and local elections in a fair and impartial manner.	In 2005, a law establishing the Autonomous National Electoral Commission (CENA) was passed. The CENA is a permanent structure with legal status including some financial autonomy. According to the law, it is responsible for the enforcement of the electoral law in order to ensure that legislation is complied with, to guarantee the transparency and the sincerity of the vote by guaranteeing the free expression of the rights of both voters and candidates	The IEC was established by statute (IEC Act, No. 150 of 1993) as an interim body with the mandate to organise and rule on the "freeness and fairness" of the 1994 elections. It was then made a permanent body through the Electoral Commission Act, No. 51 of 1996 with the mission to strengthen, promote and safeguard constitutional democracy through the delivery of free and fair elections in which every voter is able to record his or her informed choices	The National Electoral Commission (NEC) is an autonomous government institution. It was established in 1993 under Article 74(1) of the Constitution of the United Republic of Tanzania, 1977.	In terms of Article 76 [Electoral Commission]: (1) The President shall, in accordance with the provisions of this Article, establish an Electoral Commission to supervise the registration of voters and the conduct of the Presidential and Parliamentary elections and to review the boundaries of the constituencies into which Zambia is divided for the purposes of elections to the National Assembly.
Appointment of electoral commission officials	The Commission is chaired by a judge nominated by the Judicial Service Commission but appointed by the State President. There are also six other commissioners who are nominated by political parties but appointed by the State President for a four-year renewable term	The ECN is headed by five commissioners who have been appointed by the President.	The CENA is managed by a President who is assisted by a vice president and general secretary and includes twelve members. Its members are selected from independent authorities known for their moral integrity, their intellectual honesty and their impartiality	Five commissioners who have been appointed in terms of par. 6 of the Electoral Act. (Electoral Commission Act, No. 51 of 1996)	The Commission has seven members appointed by the President. The Chairman of the Commission must be either a judge of the High Court or of the Court of Appeal	The Commission consists of a Chairperson and not more than four other members appointed by the President, subject to ratification by the National Assembly (Section 4 (1) (b)), for a term not exceeding seven years
Recruitment of temporary staff of electoral commission	The Commission does not have a permanent structure. At elections, Returning Officers are appointed and in most cases District Commissioners act as Returning Officers. To conduct elections efficiently and effectively, the MEC relies on the large pool of public servants from various ministries.	In order to conduct elections, the ECN appoints Returning Officers, Counting Officers and Presiding Officers. During elections permanent staff is temporarily extended. The members of the team supporting the body of management of elections are often recruited mainly among teachers and middle public executives.	The members of the team of support to the body of management of elections are often recruited mainly among the teachers and the middle public executives	In terms of recruiting temporary staff to assist with elections the IEC has a formal arrangement with the Department of Education so that 98% of the presiding officers and deputy presiding officers are drawn from the ranks of teachers	There are 58 permanent staff members of the NEC. However, during election time the number grows to around 90; some people are taken from other government departments to do temporary work for the Commission	The ECZ usually hires a temporary workforce from the Local Authorities, the Ministry of Education and other government ministries and departments countrywide to carry out electoral functions as and when the need arises
Voting age	18	18	18	18	18	18
Source: Country reports; compiled by Idasa						

Democrats (CoD) was concerned that the voters' roll would be outdated due to the high death rates caused by HIV/AIDS. The CoD insists that the Electoral Commission of Namibia (ECN) undertake "immediate and consistent" updating of the roll, rather than "waiting to the last minute" before an election.[55] Delays in dealing with dead electors will escalate if left unattended, the CoD argues. Both the UDF and CoD are in agreement that HIV/AIDS was negatively affecting voter turnout, pointing to bedridden, hospital-bound potential voters who would be marginalised, for instance. In Senegal, the scenario is less compelling as based on the estimated prevalence rate of 1% among adults the number of PLWHAs on voter registers would be insignificant.

6.9 Impact of HIV/AIDS on political parties

6.9.1 Implications for party structures

We stated earlier that there were three levels at which HIV/AIDS may impact on political party structures:

- Organisational: The loss of cadres and members affects electioneering capacity;
- Financial: Loss of members reduces subscriptions;
- Leadership: The loss of a patron can spell the end of a party or compromise its electoral viability and financial status.

The single common feature emerging from preliminary research on political parties in several of the six countries studied is poor record-keeping amongst the entities. Membership cards are often distributed without charge; therefore using a decline in subscription as a proxy indicator for member attrition is futile. However perceptions of loss to HIV/AIDS amongst members are expressed in Namibia, Malawi, Zambia and South Africa by party and government officials alike.

> It is now an acknowledged fact that political parties, which are an essential part of any multi-party democracy, are affected by HIV/AIDS. Almost all political parties in this country have been losing leaders at various levels due to HIV/AIDS-related illness and deaths.[56]

In our 2005 study, the leading political parties in South Africa, including the African National Congress (ANC), the Democratic Alliance (DA) and the Inkatha Freedom Party (IFP), did acknowledge that HIV/AIDS does or could strain party structures, creating an increased need to replace cadres who have died, especially HIV/AIDS. Although no discernible functional defects have arisen in the party structures, a loss of seniority and experience was reported. A more direct impact acknowledged by religious-based parties such as the African Christian Democratic Party (ACDP) is the time HIV/AIDS-related deaths have committed political leaders to in terms of officiating at recurrent funerals of cadres. This might affect their organisational capacities.

Malawi provides some data on attrition in the structures of its founding party, the Malawi Congress Party (MCP). Confidential correspondence shows that the party lost at least 22 members of its district committees, at least 13 members of its regional committees and not fewer than eight members of its central executive committee between 1987 and 1993. In Senegal, an analysis of parties' programmes and structures shows a poor interest in matters relating to AIDS and health (political parties lack specific structures relating to health and HIV/AIDS issues). During the 2007 presidential campaign, only one candidate mentioned AIDS in a public declaration. This is explained by the low prevalence of HIV in the West African country.

In Namibia nearly all the party spokespeople interviewed indicated that HIV/AIDS has affected their campaign capacity with the loss of key activists, organisers or candidates. The Democratic Turnhalle Alliance's (DTA's) Secretary-General Gende[57] acknowledged that the party's administration had been "dysfunctional", because "highly skilled officials who had been trained through NGOs and the party throughout the years had passed away or were sick in bed and cannot perform." The United Democratic Front (UDF)'s Goreseb[58] underlined that "even the death of one party activist is a notable loss" and could stretch the limited resources of small political parties. Some of the strongholds of the South West African People's Organisation (Swapo), the ruling party, will have been depleted of potential supporters. Areas such as the Caprivi Strip have the highest prevalence rates at 42.6% and are also predominantly controlled by Swapo in terms of voting proclivities.

In Tanzania, political parties foresee the epidemic as having a much larger impact on them in the future and since they do not have the mechanisms to track its impact within party structures, they believe it is a problem requiring strategic planning and further research.

6.10 Impact of HIV/AIDS on political participation

6.10.1 Stigma, discrimination as impediments to citizen participation

Finally we come to the "side effects" of AIDS in our societies: stigma and discrimination. Stigmatisation is defined by UNAIDS as "a process of devaluation within a particular culture or setting where attitudes are seized upon and defined as discreditable or not worthy" (Panos/Unicef, 2004). Essentially this means a group of people are cast aside based on the assumption that they are different or apart from the normal social order. It connotes a sense of shame arising from the apparent violation of a set of values or norms by an individual or group. Discrimination is the exclusion that follows this process and can be institutional in character.

AIDS sickness has been highlighted in Tanzania, Zambia, Namibia, Malawi and South Africa as an impediment to political participation. Although the levels of stigma and discrimination differ from country to country, it was only in South Africa that PLWHAs expressed fears about their status compromising their engagement with the wider public in an election. We can explain this by appreciating the mature nature of the epidemic in other African countries, where longer periods of living with the epidemic may have led to greater awareness within their communities. Also, the higher literacy levels would explain higher levels of tolerance.

In our South Africa study, stigma and discrimination resonated as the single most dominant determinants of lack of participation in elections by PLWHAs and care-givers in rural KwaZulu-Natal. Focus group discussions with PLWHAs and caregivers, who were all registered voters for the 2004 election in urban and rural areas of KwaZulu-Natal, yielded seemingly well-founded fears that communities will further ostracise or marginalise those infected and affected if they appeared at major public events. The participants' opinions are corroborated by the findings of studies on stigma and discrimination, particularly the South African Department of Health study of 2002, that HIV/AIDS remains a taboo topic among some South African communities, especially in the rural enclaves. The sense of stigma, it seems, is strongest where people are symptomatic; participants said that most members of the communities would not stand in the same queue with someone with visible signs of disease e.g. body rashes or sores.

Although we cannot say how many people stayed away due to AIDS, the disparities between turnout and Voting Age Population present further opportunities for us to interrogate the gaps in registration and voting and the underlying causes.

Quite often, as stated earlier, assessments of voter turnouts are misleading because they are calculated against registered voters. In such instances, even when registration levels are low, the turnout may appear high. However, when turnout is calculated as a percentage of Voting Age Population, we get a much more comprehensive picture of participation. The figures below clearly show these disparities.

Based on these discussions, we concluded that in South Africa people who have visible signs of HIV/AIDS and those who have publicly declared their status are more likely to withdraw from public voting, particularly if they are located in a rural area. There is nothing to suggest that PLWHAs have lost the will to participate in political life. In fact, the majority of participants expressed a desire to participate but said they were constrained by attitudinal and structural factors. Structural factors included lack of transport, toilets, seating facilities and running water at polling stations. These results are not representative of the opinions of all PLWHAs but they are indicative of such attitudes across several countries. It needs to be reiterated that the value of qualitative studies is in the depth and wealth of information that is drawn from our units of analysis rather than the number of people involved in the discussions or interviews.

6.10.2 Public opinion

The Afrobarometer network, in its Compendium of Trends in Public Opinion in 12 African countries, provides useful insights into citizen perceptions of government performance on meeting key governance indicators including health and HIV/AIDS. The barometer conducted its round one surveys between July 1999 and March 2001; round two surveys between May 2002 and September 2003; and round three surveys from March 2005 to March 2006. The countries covered by the surveys were: Botswana, Ghana, Lesotho, Malawi, Mali, Namibia, Nigeria, South Africa, Uganda, Zambia and Zimbabwe. The surveys have since included Benin, Cape Verde, Kenya, Madagascar, Mozambique and Senegal. The minimum sample size in each country is 1 200, which its experts explain is sufficient to produce a confidence interval of plus or minus 3% points at a confidence level of 95% (Bratton & Cho: 2006).

It may perplex observers that despite the gravity of HIV/AIDS, poor people, who would normally be considered the most affected by the epidemic, regard the epidemic as less important in relation to other concerns such as food security or access to medical care for other debilitating illnesses (TB, malaria, cholera). Understandably, citizens in a country like Senegal or other low-prevalence West African countries such as Ghana are unlikely to place AIDS as their main priority in the face of immediate threats to their wellbeing (unemployment, crime, food insecurity, etc). Their counterparts in the SADC region will similarly respond to questions on less stigmatising diseases more openly. Cholera, malaria and TB decimate their victims much faster than the slow onslaught characterised by the array of opportunistic infections that define AIDS. A cholera epidemic for example will constitute a clear and present danger to society requiring swift policy responses from the government given also the international embarrassment that comes with this so-called "disease of poverty".

Indeed, it is also conceivable that not many people would wish to associate themselves with an epidemic that attracts discrimination even through mere perception of illness. It is quite possible that the major-

ity of the respondents did not wish to be seen to be ill, as a demonstration of concern about AIDS might imply. We have seen from Idasa's multi-country studies that political elites will not disclose their HIV status unless it is sero-negative. This "secrecy" is what renders public opinion surveys in matters of a deeply personal nature limited in their effectiveness.

The flip side of this discussion is that in the same survey, two-thirds of all adult respondents in 2005 on average thought their governments had performed well on AIDS. Afrobarometer reports that respondents in 2005 gave governments better grades (70%) for HIV/AIDS management than for any other social policy.[59]

The flow of optimism obviously does not reflect reality as rightly indicated by the Afrobarometer. As already discussed, the incidence of AIDS continues to rise even as its prevalence in some countries, such as Uganda, Kenya and Zimbabwe, is reportedly declining. The Afrobarometer attributes this to possible misinformation due to the relatively low infection rates in West Africa; the availability of ART; and persistence of social taboos amongst the local communities and political elites alike.

We should not perhaps underestimate the impact of the introduction of ART on local communities as this represents a major departure from the 1980s/90s scenario when AIDS was seen to represent a swift progression to a painful death, encouraging increasing abandonment of sufferers. And while politicians are notable absentees in the VCT circles, they still dominate the airwaves with pronouncements on government delivery of drugs and PLWHAs-friendly policies at both national and regional levels.

The accompanying evidence of ART on the ground, albeit limited, could be having profound effects on perceptions regarding governments' commitment (although donor funding also plays a significant part in this). As stated earlier, even as the incidence of HIV is rising, the number of people on ART in low- and middle-income countries almost doubled from 720 000 to 1.3 million in 2005, the year in which Afrobarometer concluded its round three.

7. Observations and recommendations

There are a number of worrying revelations in this study: the large number of younger voters who have died in a space of five years in South Africa; the rise

Figure 6.6: Voter turnout as a percentage of registered voters (2004-2006)

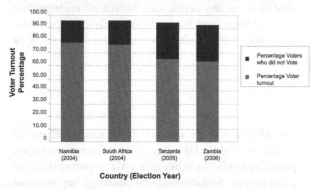

Figure 6.7: Voter turnout as percentage of voting age population (2004-2006)

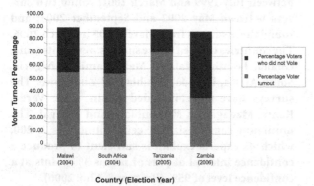

in deaths amongst MPs in Malawi, Tanzania, Zambia and Zimbabwe and more generally; the loss of representation attributed to these deaths; the effect on the capacity of parliament and potential effect on institutional memory; the impact on small or under-resourced opposition parties and the implications for democratic accountability. There should also be concerns about the deep-seated stigma and discrimination amongst the political elite in several countries under study and finally the economic costs generated by HIV/AIDS through multiple by-elections all of which provide a strong basis to argue for new interventions to redress the situation. Such interventions will need to transcend traditional health approaches and in fact challenge us to deal with our democratic deficits in tandem with AIDS activities. In that sense, the following proposals and observations may serve to help countries absorb the shocks of HIV/AIDS as well as consolidate their electoral profiles:

7.1.1 Electoral engineering and public choice

Firstly, there is a need to modify the FPTP system given its susceptibility to HIV/AIDS. This could mean either waiving the requirement for by-elections or adopting a PR system. This route is of course not as straightforward as it sounds. Adopting a PR system comes with concerns around poor accountability as MPs will not be directly elected by the people. The MMP system provides some modicum of compromise but is itself quite vulnerable to by-elections as demonstrated in Lesotho. Electoral reform is a long-term enterprise requiring wide consultation through a constitutional review process and depending on how soon political actors can reach consensus on AIDS as one of the key threats to a sustainable democracy, it may be a while before we actually see any changes. Our recommendation, given the complexities and multiple considerations for reform that need equitable attention, is that countries operating the FPTP, MMP and Parallel systems may need to modify their systems to include MP substitution. A viable option would be to simply allow political parties to replace the deceased through appointment.

We noted that electoral systems also have impacts on human development. Majoritarian systems record comparatively lower human development levels than the proportional models. This further challenges nation-states to carefully consider their choices. In the age of AIDS it is prudent to tailor new electoral models toward a goal that seeks to contribute to the upliftment of people's general welfare. In this regard, experts have to assess all imperatives in order to arrive at a home-grown model.

7.1.2 Political parties

Secondly, it is certain that there is no place for people living with HIV in political party leadership. The stigma and discrimination that is now known to exist amongst the political elite will require innovative solutions. Failure to address this situation may compromise the many efforts by AIDS service organisations aimed at building a strong leadership required to tackle the problem of AIDS. New strategies need to be adopted that encourage political parties to deliberately infuse PLWHAs into their ranks. This is particularly possible in countries using the PR and MMP systems. However, FPTP countries could also exploit the slots for nominated MPs to appoint PLWHAs. The presence of dominant parties such as the ANC in South Africa and the Botswana Democratic Party (BDP) in Botswana, which are not in immediate threat of losing an election, provides a genuine opportunity to dramatically impact on stigma and discrimination in politics and society in general by adopting a person living with HIV/AIDS as a candidate for parliament or local government.

At a more strategic level, political parties will need to develop succession plans where none exist and initiate workplace programmes with strong information, education and communication components on the political, economic and social dynamics of AIDS in addition to the personal health matters. There is now evidence in South Africa for instance of the IFP embarking on an elaborate HIV/AIDS programme aimed at providing care and support to affected members, details of which were not available at the time of writing.

7.1.3 Parliaments

It is surprising that despite what might be described as a very noticeable trend of deaths from undisclosed illnesses amongst MPs, none of the parliaments have discussed the effects of HIV/AIDS on parliamentary capacity and institutional memory. Instead debates have focused on society at large. Parliamentary bodies are best placed to commission internal investigative processes on MP attrition and solicit appropriate strategic support from experts in civil society organisations (CSOs), academia and the development sector. Workplace policies with strong all-encompassing information, education and communication strategies need to be instituted to help develop pools of AIDS competent MPs.

Training and knowledge-building is needed for parliamentarians to enable them to act on the political, social and economic challenges faced by their constituencies and employ that knowledge in their oversight functions. We take cognisance of the fact that not every parliamentarian will treat HIV/AIDS as a priority. There is therefore a need to identify champions in parliamentary bodies who would form the core of strategic parliamentary interventions.

7.1.4 Public participation in parliamentary process

Parliaments at present are generally quite removed from the people. They are Europeanised institutions whose language of instruction is often restricted to people with a western education. Parliaments are in addition located in national capitals and will be completely out of reach of ordinary rural and peri-urban folk. Even where they are accessible, entering the public gallery of parliament as a passive observer requires certain adherence to dress codes, not to mention there is limited space available. We would encourage greater interaction between parliamentarians and PLWHAs and other CSOs to help define and solve the problem. Issues such as discrimination in politics, employment and financial services require legislative interventions and are fundamental to reversing the impact of HIV/AIDS. At present, few parliaments have the budget to hold public hearings and these will normally be held by specific committees.[60] But public hearings remain important in engaging the broader public on matters of HIV/AIDS and governance and therefore funds should be set aside to facilitate them.

7.1.5 Legislative protection of PLWHAS

While parliaments have contributed to a legislative response by instituting provisions for the criminalisation of wilful transmission of HIV, there is clearly a need for further state interventions in ensuring that discriminatory practices in the employment, banking industries and for that matter in the political sphere are eliminated. Exclusionary tendencies are deeply entrenched in the practices of insurance companies, employment agencies and lending organisations and these replicate themselves in the area of electoral politics.

Underlining the fact that HIV/AIDS is a manageable ailment, and therefore requires accommodative considerations by all sectors through a well-structured legislative intervention, could help minimise institutional stigma and discrimination across many fields including politics.

7.1.6 Voter participation

The research suggests further that there are roles for the EMBs in the HIV/AIDS field. The impact of stigma and discrimination on participation, though only indicative in rural South Africa, deserves attention as it may be more extensive than this study suggests, with ramifications for the involvement of individuals infected and affected in politics. EMBs could assist by incorporating non-discriminatory messages in their voter education campaigns which encourage more people to participate in elections and ensure there is tolerance to a greater degree of people who are ill. Only the Zanzibar Electoral Commission encouraged political parties to deploy AIDS awareness messages during the 2005 election in Tanzania.[61] Setting up special voting mechanisms for the disadvantaged might also be a consideration as is the case in South Africa. Such facilities should not be exclusively tailored to PLWHAs to avoid accentuating stigma and discrimination; they should rather seek to engage all persons with disability and those challenged by ill health, among others.

7.1.7 Electoral governance

Countries in Africa that do not have institutionalised and directly compatible citizen and voter registration systems will be unable to determine the extent to which HIV/AIDS has undermined their political institutions. This will impact on their electoral planning and more generally on their long-term developmental visions. We can see from the case of Malawi that doubts about the size of the voters' roll can contribute to weak political mandates and instability. Investment in new technologies is recommended to ensure timeous deletion of dead voters to avert unnecessary post-election conflict.

7.1.8 AIDS service organisations

It is time that traditional NGOs dealing with HIV/AIDS took on board new research perspectives that could inform their actions toward the MDG targets. One of the lessons from this study is that AIDS is not a problem of one specific industry, requiring only sector-specific responses. It challenges us to continually review our strategies based on fresh knowledge. Donor support for innovative social and political research may prove important in galvanising the key policy actors who, from time to time, appear to lose sight of the relevance of HIV/AIDS as a long-term adversary.

Appendix: Impact of HIV/AIDS on democratic governance (adapted, POKU: 2007)

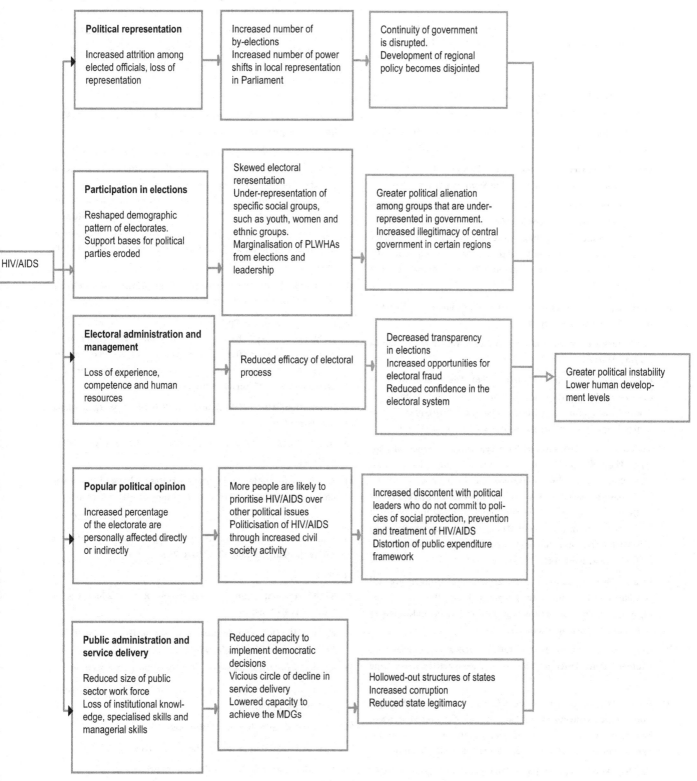

Endnotes

1   Barnett and Whiteside explain that the epidemic comes in successive waves, the first being HIV infection; followed several years later by a wave of opportunistic infections and finally a third wave of illness and death.

2   UNAIDS/WHO global reports (2002-2005); Iliffe J. (2006) The African AIDS Epidemic. A History. Oxford. James Curray Ltd.

3   Daniel Halperin & Helen Epstein (2006): The Role of Multiple Concurrent Partnerships and Lack of Male Circumcision.

4   SADC and International Cooperating Partners: Framework on Regional Support to HIV and AIDS in Southern Africa. 2006.

5   Life expectancy at birth is the average number of years a person can expect to live at current levels of mortality. These estimates are the outcome of modelling by the UN and national estimates for some countries may differ significantly, e.g. Botswana estimates its life expectancy to be currently 55 years compared to the UN figure of 36.

6   Workshop report on Human Mobility, Migration and HIV/AIDS, Idasa 2002. www.idasa.org.za

7   The factors are prevalent in all of the countries in the region to varying degrees.

8   Daniel Halperin & Helen Epstein (2006): The Role of Multiple Concurrent Partnerships and Lack of Male Circumcision. www.healthdev.org/eforums/editor/assets/accelerating-prevention/daniel_halperin's% 20key_paper_FINAL%20 VERSION.pdf

9   According to expert sources, both types have a range of subtypes. They will both be transmitted sexually, through blood and through mother to child transmission and will cause "clinically indistinguishable AIDS". Experts note however that HIV-2 is less easily transmitted and the period between initial infection and illness is longer in the case of HIV-2. HIV-2 is concentrated in West Africa and rarely found elsewhere. The pre-dominant virus is HIV-1(www. avert.org).

10 In a number of countries in the region, adult women are still considered to be "minors" for purposes of inheritance and owning property. This makes them highly dependent on male relatives (husbands, fathers and brothers).

11 Chirambo K. & Caesar M (Eds) (2003): AIDS and Governance in Southern Africa; Emerging Theories and Perspectives. Idasa: Cape Town.

12 Daniel Halperin & Helen Epstein (2006): Tthe Role of Multiple Concurrent Partnerships and Lack of Male Circumcision. www.healthdev.org/eforums/editor/assets/accelerating-prevention/daniel_halperin's% 20key_paper_FINAL%20 VERSION.pdf

13 Crush J., Frayne B., & Grant M. (2006) Linking Migration, HIV/AIDS and Urban Food Security in Southern and Eastern Africa. RENEWAL. IFPRI, SAMP. www.queensu.ca/samp. Crush et al caution against stigmatiszing migrants as bearers of disease and enacting restrictive laws in that regard: rather, there is need to direct HIV/AIDS interventions such as education, prevention, voluntary counselling and testing, and treatment and care at them as part of a holistic strategy of dealing with the pandemic.

14 IRIN: Southern Africa: Conflict, Development and Natural Disasters Fuel Internal Displacement. 14 February 2006, United Nations Office for the Coordination of Humanitarian Affairs-integrated Regional Information Networks (IRIN).http://www.reliefweb.int/rw/rwb.nsf/db900sid/KHII-6M25GM?Opendocument

15 Niedan C., (2006): West African Conflict Roots Examined. 10/3/03. http://www.pittnews.com/home/index.cfm?event

16 IRIN reports that: "experts have long assumed that the violence, wide-scale rape and refugee crises are the inevitable by-product of war that fuel HIV/AIDS epidemics, but an analysis of HIV prevalence surveys from seven Sub-Saharan African countries with similar recent histories found no evidence that higher HIV infection rates accompany conflict. The study is available at (http://www.thelancet.com/journals/lancet/article/PIIS0140673607610150/fullt

17 IRIN report at (http://www.thelancet.com/journals/lancet/article/PIIS0140673607610150/fullt

18 Halperin and Helen Epstein differentiate the two practices as such: the tendency to have one relatively long term (a few months or longer) partner after another (concurrent partnership)…or more "once off" casual and commercial sexual encounters that occur everywhere" (serial monogamy).

19 International HIV/AIDS Alliance.http://aidsalliance.org/sw44583.asp?usepf=true

20 International HIV/AIDS Alliance.http://aidsalliance.org/sw44583.asp?usepf=true

21 See also, Information and Library Services Exchange. http://www.kit.nl/exchange/html/2001_2_harnessing_senegal_s_ap.asp

22 Southern African News Features no. 39, August 2007: SARDC.

23 Chirambo K & McCullum H. Reporting Elections in Southern Africa: A Media Handbook: SARDC 2000.

24 Ibid.

25 SADC regional Human Development Report 2000; UNDP; SADC;SAPES Trust

26 Human Development Indicators in the SADC Region, DPRU Policy Brief No. 01/p13, May 2001

27 Southern African News Features no. 39, August 2007: SARDC

28 SADC Update, 04/18/01. http://www.africa.upenn.edu/Urgent_Action/apic-041801.html

29 The focus areas of harmonisation were:

•   Care and treatment including the use of ARVs

•   Nutrition, nutritional therapies and traditional herbs

•   Human resource needs in all sectors in the context of HIV/AIDS

•   Regional issues of HIV/AIDS such as migrant population/mobile labour, refugees and displaced populations

- Harmonisation of procedures, regulations and laws of transit at borders and ports

- Bulk procurement of drugs and medical supplies of HIV/AIDS

- Regional guidelines for clinical trials

- Guidelines for programme intervention in High Transmission Areas such as border sites and high traffic sites

- Sustenance of human capital in the context of HIV/AIDS in the region

- Policy guidelines on how to increase access to care and treatment of the most vulnerable social groups

- Mainstreaming

30 Forthcoming: Impact of AIDS on National Budgets in Africa: Cape Town: Idasa.

31 Scaling Up HIV Prevention, Treatment Care and Support (2006). UN.

32 Chipika J. T.(2007) Current Macroeconomic Frameworks, Challenges and Alternatives for the Attainment of the Millennium Development Goals: http://www.sarpn.org.za/document/d0002654/index.php

33 Cheema, G.S. (2000) in Good Governance: A Path to Poverty Eradication; defines governance as " a set of values, policies and institutions by which a society manages its economic, political and social processes at all levels through interaction among government, civil society and private sector," UNDP.

34 Author's italicisation.

35 Moeletsi Mbeki's address to the opening of the European Association of Centres of African Studies Conference, Leiden University in the Netherlands, 11 to 14 July 2007. Mbeki is deputy chair of the South African Institute of International Affairs. He refers also to the post-colonial era as a period of partnership between western donors and emergent African dictators in plundering mineral and intellectual wealth and the destruction of indigenous institutions that were critical to political and social mobilisation; the African nationalist party was one significant casualty.

36 ZHDR (2002) Human Development Report, Oxford: Oxford University Press. First quoted Strand P., Matlosa K., Strode A., & Chirambo K (2005) HIV/AIDS and Democratic Governance in South Africa: Illustrating the Impact on the Electoral Process. Idasa: Cape Town. With thanks to Richard Calland, manager of Idasa's Economic Governance Programme (EGP) and staff for additional input into the nine principles.

37 Statement by Peter Piot, Executive Director of UNAIDS 2001. http://www.africaaction.org/docs01/piot0110.htm

38 See Niang et al (Forthcoming); HIV/AIDS and Democratic Governance in Senegal: Illustrating the Impact on Electoral Processes. Cape Town. Idasa: "These rates, considered as relatively low in the Sub-Saharan African context, however conceal substantial disparities between the various regions of the country".

39 Barnett and Whiteside explain that the epidemic comes in successive waves, the first being HIV infection; followed several years later by a wave of opportunistic infections and finally a third wave of illness and death.

40 Mattes R. & Strand P (2007) AIDS Impact Research at DARU: HIV/AIDS and Society: Building a Community of Practice. Cape Town.

41 In 2005, the speaker of the National Assembly of Malawi was flown to South Africa for further medical treatment. Similarly, leading politicians from Zambia often access medical aid from South Africa or in Europe.

42 Sachs M. (2002) By Elections in 2001: A Statistical Review. UMRABULO. Issue number 14 in April ANC. www.anc.org.za/ancdocs/pubs/umrabulo/umrabulo14/elections.html

43 By-elections costs include, transport, printing of ballot papers, allowances or election officers, presiding officers, tents, lighting, distribution of voters' registers, transport (air and land), among others.

44 http://concourt.law.wits.ac.za/judges/jdcameron.html

45 http://www.beatit.co.za/episode9.php.

46 According to the Electoral Commission of Zambia's Deputy Director, Priscilla Isaacs, (telephone interview, 2004): and official statement to Idasa released in 2007.

47 Using the rate of 1 USD= 6.9637 rand, September 25th, 2007

48 By-elections costs include, transport, printing of ballot papers, allowances or election officers, presiding officers, tents, lighting, distribution of voters' registers, transport (air and land), among others.

49 Tsie B., (2000). Electoral Sustainability and the Cost of Development. Johannesburg: EISA

50 Using the rate of 1 USD= 6.9637 rand, September 25th, 2007

51 Chirambo K (2006): Democratisation in the Age of HIV/AIDS: Understanding the Political Implications. Cape Town: Idasa.

52 Academy International Affairs Working Paper Series: (2006) Mitigating HIV/AIDS Impacts on Teachers and Administrators in Sub-Saharan Africa. Washington: www.napawash.org

53 The actual size of the voters' roll is not known due to discrepancies in both citizen and voter registration. Malawi does not have an established citizen registration and identification system and has therefore found it difficult to determine just how many of its people are of voting age. Malawi's voters' roll is hence not regularly updated. In 1999, a total of 5 071 822 voters were registered (national population of 11 million) and of these 2 417 713 were registered in the southern region, 1 975 203 in the central region and 678 906 in the northern region. However in April 2004, the MEC announced that 6 668 839 voters had registered for the May 18, 2004 presidential and parliamentary elections.54 These figures were challenged by opposition political parties and other institutions with the National Statistical Office taking the lead. It described the figure as "bogus" because it did not conform to

the country's natural demographic trends. The result of Malawi's problematic voters' roll is a weak mandate for the new government and post-election conflict over outcomes. Malawi has been preoccupied with impeachment tensions since the last presidential polls.

54 Some records show a figure of 6.7 million registered at this time.

55 Ibid

56 Kapembwa Simbao, (former) Deputy Minister of Health, Zambia, in his opening speech at the Idasa/FODEP/INESOR policy forum on AIDS and elections, 2005.

57 Interview on 13 April 2006.

58 Interview on 20 April 2006.

59 Bratton M., & Cho W., (2006) Working Paper No.60. Where is Africa Going? Views from Below. A Compendium of Trends in Public Opinion in 12 Countries, 1999-2006. Cape Town: Idasa/CDD/MSU

60 Caesar M., & Myburg M (2006) Parliaments, Politics and AIDS; Comparative Study of Five African Countries. Cape Town: Idasa.

61 Zanzibar and Tanganyika form one state under the Union of the Republic of Tanzania.

References

Books

Bang P. H. (2003) Governance as Social and Political Communication. Manchester University Press.

Barnett T. and Whiteside A. (2002) /AIDS in the Twenty-First Century: Disease and Globalisation. New York: Palgrave Macmillan.

Braman S. (2003) Communication Researchers and Policy-making. Massachusetts Institute of Technology.

Bratton M. & Cho W. (2006) Working Paper No.60. Where is Africa Going? Views from Below. A Compendium of Trends in Public Opinion in 12 Countries, 1999-2006. Cape Town: Idasa/ CDD/ MSU

Bumler J. G. (1996) Introduction to Political Communication. Module Two: Unit 12. MA in Mass Communications. Centre for Mass Communication Research. Leicester University.

Caesar M., & Myburg M (2006) Parliaments, Politics and AIDS; Comparative Study of Five African Countries. Cape Town: Idasa.

Cheema, G. S. (2000) In Good Governance: A Path to Poverty Eradication. New York: United Nations Development Programme (UNDP).

CHGA (2004), Q & A on HIV/AIDS and Governance in Africa. Addis Ababa: Commission for HIV/AIDS Governance in Africa/Economic Commission for Africa.

Chirambo K. & McCullum H. (2000) Reporting Elections in Southern Africa: A Media Handbook: SARDC.

Chirambo K. (2003) Impact of HIV/AIDS on Electoral Processes in Southern Africa. Presentation to the UNDP/Idasa Satellite Conference, Nairobi, September. Idasa.

Chirambo K. and Caesar M. (eds) (2003) HIV/AIDS and Governance in Southern Africa: Emerging Theories and Perspectives. Cape Town: Idasa.

Chirambo, K. (2004) AIDS and Electoral Democracy: Implications for Participation, Political Stability and Accountability in Southern Africa. Johannesburg: EISA.

Chirambo K. (2005) AIDS & Electoral Democracy: Insights into Impacts on Africa's Democratic Institutions. Pretoria: Institute for Democracy in South Africa. Cape Town: Idasa.

Chirambo K. (2006) Democratisation in the Age of HIV/AIDS: Understanding the Political Implications. Cape Town: Idasa.

De Renzio P. (2004) The Challenge of Absorptive Capacity: Will Lack of Absorptive Capacity Prevent Effective Uuse of Additional Aid Resources in Pursuit of the MDGs? Report on seminar at DFID, Overseas Development Institute, London.

Fay B. (1993) Elements of Critical Social Science. In Hammersley, Social Research: Philosophy, Politics and Practice. London: SAGE.

Halloran J. (1995) Media Research as Social Science. Module One: Unit 2, in MA in Mass Communications, Centre for Mass Communications Research: Leicester University.

Hammerssley M. (1993) Social Research: Philosophy, Politics and Practice. London: SAGE.

Hansen A., Cottle S., Negrine R. & Newbold C. (1998) Mass Communication Research Methods. London: Macmillan Press Ltd.

Hunter S. (2003) Who Cares? AIDS in Africa. New York. Palgrave Macmillan.

Hyden G., Court J. & Mease K. (2004) Making Sense of Governance: Empirical Evidence from 16 Countries. London: Rienner.

Illiffe J. (2006) The African AIDS Pandemic: A History. Oxford: James A Curray Ltd. University.

Lodge T. (2004) Handbook of South African Electoral Laws and Regulations. Johannesburg: EISA.

Meehan E. J. (1988) The Thinking Game: A Guide to Effective Study. New Jersey; Chatam House.

Matlosa K., Chiroro B. & Letsholo S. (2007) Politics of Electoral System Reform and Democratisation: Contemporary Trends in Southern Africa. Johannesburg EISA, conference paper.

Ndhlovu N. & Daswa R.(2006) Review of progress on the Comprehensive Plan for HIV and AIDS for South Africa. Occasional papers. AIDS Budget Unit, Idasa, Cape Town.

Parsons W. (1995) Public Policy: An Introduction to the Theory and Practice of Policy Analysis. Cheltenham: Edward Edgar Publishing Ltd.

Poku N. (2007) PowerPoint presentation to Idasa's second Governance and AIDS Forum, Cape Town: May 22-24.

Reynolds A., Reilly B. & Ellis A. (eds) (2005) Electoral System Design: The International IDEA Handbook. Stockholm: IDEA.

Simbao K. (2005) Opening speech at the Idasa/ FODEP/INESOR policy forum on AIDS and Elections, quoted in Chirambo K. AIDS & Electoral Democracy: Insights into Impacts on Africa's Democratic Institutions. Cape Town: Idasa.

Strand P., Matlosa K., Strode A. & Chirambo K. (2005) HIV/AIDS and Democratic Governance in South Africa: Illustrating the Impact on Electoral Processes. Cape Town: Idasa.

Tredoux C. & Durrheim (eds) (2002) Numbers, Hypotheses & Conclusions: A Course in Statistics for the Social Sciences. Cape Town: UCT Press.

Tsie B. (2000). Electoral Sustainability and the Cost of Development. Johannesburg: EISA.

Youde J. (2001) All the Voters Will be Dead: HIV/ AIDS and Democratic Legitimacy and Stability in Africa. Iowa.

Official sources

IDEA. (2000) The Functioning and Funding of Political Parties in the SADC Region: An Overview; Conference on Sustainable Democratic Institutions in Southern Africa. Stockholm: IDEA.

Human Development Indicators in the SADC Region, DPRU Policy Brief No. 01/p13, May 2001

Idasa/HEARD/DARU. (2002) AIDS and Democracy Workshop for Researchers Report.

NAC. (2004) The HIV/AIDS Epidemic in Zambia: Where are we now? Where are we going? Lusaka: September.

NAC. (2004) HIV/AIDS Communication Strategy. Lusaka: May.

National Intelligence Council. (2005) Mapping Sub-Saharan Africa's Future, Conference Report.

Nelson Mandela/HSRC Study of HIV/AIDS, (2002) Cape Town: Human Sciences Research Council.

Nepad. (2003) Nepad Health Strategy. Pretoria: Nepad.

NIMD. (2004) Institutional Development Handbook. A Framework for Democratic Party-Building. Hague: Netherlands Institute for Multiparty Democracy.

Principles for Election Management, Monitoring and Observation in the SADC Region. (2003) Johannesburg: EISA.

SADC Human Development Report. (2000) Challenges, Opportunities for Regional Integration. UNDP/SAPES.

SADC (2003) HIV/AIDS Strategic Framework and Programme of Action 2003-2007: Managing the HIV/AIDS Pandemic in Southern African Development Community, July, 2003

SADC and International Cooperating Partners: Framework on Regional Support to HIV and AIDS in Southern Africa. (2006).

SADC Parliamentary Forum. (2001) Norms and Standards for Elections in the SADC Region. Windhoek: SADC-PF.

SARDC. (1999) Zambia Democracy Fact file. Harare: SARDC.

SARDC/SADC-Parliamentary Forum. (2002) The SADC MPs Companion on Gender and Development in southern Africa. Harare: SARDC.

SARDC. (2007) Southern African News Features no. 39, August.

Scaling Up HIV Prevention, Treatment Care and Support. (2006). UN.

UNAIDS/WHO global reports (2002-2005).

UNDP. (2000) Zimbabwe Human Development Report. Governance. UNDP.

Zambia National Women's Lobby Group. (2001) End of Year Report January – December; Submitted to Netherlands Embassy; p 19.

Newspaper articles

New York Times (2001) AIDS permeates Uganda Politics Too. March 12, Ian Fisher.

Star (2005) 11 Teachers a day die of AIDS, April 1; Ndivhuwo Khangale & Sapa

Interview

Priscilla Isaacs, (telephone interview, 2004)

Articles from websites

Academy International Affairs Working Paper Series. (2006) Mitigating HIV/AIDS Impacts on Teachers and Administrators in Sub-Saharan Africa. Washington: www.napawash.org

Chipika J. T (2007) Current Macroeconomic Frameworks, Challenges and Alternatives for the Attainment of the Millennium Development Goals.

http://www.sarpn.org.za/document/d0002654/index.php

International HIV/AIDS Alliance.http://aidsalliance.org/sw44583.asp?usepf=true

Crush J., Frayne B. & Grant M. (2006) Linking Migration, HIV/AIDS and Urban Food Security in Southern and Eastern Africa. RENEWAL. IFPRI, SAMP. www.queensu.ca/samp

Halperin D. & Epstein H. (2006) The role of Multiple Concurrent Partnerships and Lack of Male Circumcision.

www.healthdev.org/eforums/editor/assets/accelerating-prevention/daniel_halperin's% 20key_paper_FINAL%20 VERSION.pdf

Information and Library Services Exchange.

http://www.kit.nl/exchange/html/2001_2_harnessing_senegal_s_ap.asp

IRIN news report: Malawi: Illegal Orphanages Mushroom.

http://www.irinnews.org/report.aspx?reportid=61374

Matshalaga N. & Powell G. (2002) Mass Orphanhood in the Era of HIV/AIDS: Bold Support for Alleviation of Poverty and Education May Avert a Social Disaster.

http://www.pubmedcentral.nih.gov/articlerender.fcgi?artid=1122118

Mayntz, R. (2003), From government to governance: Political steering

in modern societies. Presented at the Summer Academy on IPP at

Wuerzburg, September 7-11 2003. http://www.ioew.de/gov.../SuA2Mayntz.pdf

http://www.ioew.de/governance/english/veranstaltungen/Summer_Academies/SuA2Mayntz.pdf

Niedan C. (2006) West African Conflict Roots Examined. (2003).

http://www.pittnews.com/home/index.cfm?event

Panos/UNICEF. (2004). Stigma, HIV/AIDS and Prevention of Mother-to Child Transmission: A Pilot Study in Zambia, Ukraine, India and Burkina Faso.

Sachs M. (2002) By Elections in 2001: A statistical Review. UMRABULO. Issue number 14 in April ANC.

www.anc.org.za/ancdocs/pubs/umrabulo/umrabulo14/elections.html

SADC Update, 04/18/01. http://www.africa.upenn.edu/Urgent_Action/apic-041801.html

Statement by Peter Piot, Executive Director of UNAIDS 2001.

http://www.africaaction.org/docs01/piot0110.htm

UNAIDS; Report on the Global AIDS epidemic (2006) UNAIDS. www.unaids.org/en/hiv_data/2006globalreport/default.asp

Willan S. (2004) Recent Changes in the South African Government's HIV/AIDS Policy and its Implementation. HEARD; University of Natal.

http://afraf.oxfordjournals.org/cgi/content/abstract/103/410/109?etoc

Malawi

Alister C. Munthali, Wiseman Chijere Chirwa and Peter Mvula

1. Introduction

The Malawi study focused on the potential impact of the HIV/AIDS epidemic on electoral governance, with special attention to the potential impact on: the voters' roll, the management of the electoral process, electoral administration and management, the country's electoral system, political parties, and the financial and human cost. It is believed that, with increased HIV/AIDS incidence, Malawi will need more resources to spend on by-elections because of the increased number of deaths occurring at leadership levels. Thus, the First-Past-The-Post (FPTP) electoral system that Malawi uses is expensive and inappropriate. Also, with the increased prevalence of HIV/AIDS and the related deaths, the voters' roll will, if not regularly updated, become ever more bloated with "ghost voters". Malawi, therefore, needs an efficient and effective electoral administration and management system for dealing with the potential risk to electoral governance. At the moment, the Malawi Electoral Commission (MEC), which is the electoral management body, heavily relies on civil servants, teachers and other public workers to serve as election officers and monitors. The commission lacks its own field staff for the administration and management of the electoral process. As will be shown later, some studies in the country have shown the negative impact of the HIV/AIDS epidemic on this group of people.[1] In the event of this group being heavily affected by HIV/AIDS, the electoral administration and management system of the country will lose top professionals from among its ranks, those in possession of much-needed skills and expertise. The skills and knowledge relating to the conduct of elections will be lost.

The HIV/AIDS epidemic has, therefore, both a financial and human cost. As some elected officials die from the complications of such illness, the cost of holding by-elections in the country will increase, resulting in the funding of elections becoming heavily dependent on external donors. About 80% of the country's development budget and 40% of the recurrent budget is donor supported,[2] with donors funding more than 60% of the election budget. The financial cost will, therefore, sap not only the country's budget, but also the donor support that the country receives. The increased attention paid to the HIV/AIDS epidemic will be accompanied by the diversion of resources from other sectoral programmes to programmes aimed at mitigating the effects of the epidemic. HIV/AIDS has already been shown to probably be the single largest donor-funded sector in the country at the moment. For example, figures of donor funding distributed to a total of 26 ministries or government institutions indicate that, between 2004 and 2005, the National AIDS Commission (NAC) received more donor funding than any other institution in the country. The Ministry of Agriculture, Irrigation and Food Security came second due to the government response to the food shortages that the country has faced over the current and preceding years (see Appendix 1).

1.1 Aims of the Malawi study

The aims of this study are:

- To facilitate an informed debate on electoral system reform by means of the exchange of best practice between Malawi and selected other African countries;

- To generate further debate about how national resources are affected by the application of current electoral models;

- To enable an informed policy dialogue on the greater participation of People Living With HIV/AIDS (PLWHAs) and other marginalised groups in political/policy processes (including elections);

- To mobilise leadership awareness and stimulate stronger political engagement at both community and constituency levels aimed at dealing with problems arising from stigma and discrimination;

- To contribute to the development of a more comprehensive external HIV/AIDS policy for the electoral management bodies concerned, especially the MEC; and

- To engender public awareness of the broader implications of the pandemic for strategic interventions.

Funding for the HIV/AIDS programmes falls within the framework of "democratisation aid" or "aid for democracy". Though much of such funding comes from the Global Fund for the Fight Against HIV/AIDS, Tuberculosis and Malaria, there is also a sizeable amount that comes from the governance support of institutions, such as the United Nations Development Programme (UNDP) and the European Union (EU). Good governance, which includes issues of electoral governance, people's participation, the interface between civil society and the state, local governance, state accountability and transparency, and access to justice and the rule of law has become a major element of "democratisation aid" both to Malawi and to many other African and other third-world nations in general. The principle of good governance, as outlined in the UNDP 1997 policy framework, *Governance for Sustainable Development* (UNDP, 1997), holds that good governance is, among other positive qualities, participatory, transparent and accountable, while also being both effective and equitable. Such governance promotes the rule of law, ensuring that the political, social and economic priorities are based on broad consensus within society and that the voices of the poorest and the most vulnerable are heard in decision-making over the allocation of resources in the development process. The UNDP's "democratisation aid" thus fits into such a framework. While all other donors have their respective frameworks for the granting of "democratisation aid", such perceptions might change according to the evolving dynamics of the donor's foreign policy aims. However, the prudent management of resources and their equitable distribution are important pillars of good governance. Democratic systems are seen to be best suited to good governance, resulting in the expression of interest in electoral governance as a vehicle for ushering in democratic systems. The support provided to initiatives that leads to the strengthening of democratic processes, an improvement in their accountability and transparency, enhanced local governance, competitive politics, the strengthening of civil society, and the refinement of the interface between the state and the citizenry all fall within the good governance framework. All such support is threatened by the HIV/AIDS pandemic.

The incapacity of Malawi to fund elections from its own resources was shown in 2005 by the postponement of the local government elections, which should have taken place in that year. Due to the prevailing food shortage, the country was unable to raise adequate funding to support the holding of local polls, resulting in a constitutional crisis. The human cost also amounted to a loss in representation, such as in cases where a Member of Parliament (MP) or a ward councillor died or fell chronically ill. Though the electoral law in the country requires that a by-election be held within ninety days of the demise of an MP, in reality three to six months have been known to pass before such by-elections could be held. The failure to keep to the allotted timeframe has often resulted from the inadequate funding of both the MEC and the electoral process itself, as, in the event of by-elections, the former is required to

prepare special budgets to justify central treasury funding, which often are not approved in time.

Therefore, the Malawi study uses the voters' roll as a focal entry point to investigations into the potential impact of HIV/AIDS on electoral governance in the country. As well as fieldwork, the study uses information taken from, among other institutions, the MEC voters' roll, National Statistical Office (NSO) demographic data, NAC HIV/AIDS prevalence figures, as well as from various studies of HIV/AIDS and electoral governance in the country.

2. Methodology

The activities and tools employed to capture comprehensively the issues under investigation included consultations with stakeholders, a literature review, an examination of existing data and primary data collection by means of a structured questionnaire, administered by post, focus group discussions (FGDs) and the observation of certain by-elections and political party campaigning that occurred between October and December 2005.

2.1 Consultations with stakeholders

After an initial project meeting in Pretoria in June 2005, the research team started immediately conducting interviews with those involved with institutions concerned with electoral processes and management in Malawi.

The institutions were visited to alert them to the need to participate in the study, as well as to identify participants for a reference group. Dates were determined for a meeting with the group, once constituted.

2.2 Literature review and use of secondary data

Visiting the potential reference group members allowed the researchers to collect and review HIV/AIDS-related literature, which significantly helped in the development of relevant data collection instruments. The data collected from the MEC complemented that gleaned from the districts.

2.3 Stakeholders' workshop

A stakeholders' workshop was held on 5 October 2005 at the Sun and Sand Holiday Resort in Mangochi, for which the main agenda was to introduce Idasa's HIV/AIDS and governance research project, especially its study into 'The impact of HIV/AIDS on the electoral process in Malawi' to be jointly conducted by the Centre for Social Research (CSR) and Idasa. The workshop provided an opportunity to discuss the adaptation of the South African methodology and draft data collection instruments to Malawian conditions.

The stakeholders fell into six categories:

- Officials drawn from the central policy-making executive committees of the seven political parties represented in the Malawi Parliament and of one major party without a parliamentary seat;
- Representatives of the AIDS advocacy groups (PLWHAs), including the NAC;
- Members of human rights bodies and civil society organisations (CSOs) involved with civic and voter education;
- MEC participants;
- Members of the parliamentary committee on health and research department; and
- Academics with experience of elections and the democratic process.

2.4 Fieldwork

In reviewing the study instruments, questionnaires were circulated, at the end of November 2005, among all the districts for the election officers to complete before collection three weeks later by the researchers, who would then verify the information provided. In one northern, two central and three southern districts, FGDs relating to the political participation of those living with HIV/AIDS and their care-givers were held.

2.5 Challenges

During the data collection phase, due to the non-delivery of some forms, replacements could be completed only after the visits made by the researchers to the district. Some forms had also been rendered temporarily inaccessible by being locked away. Mortality-related data from 1994 to 2000 was neither available at district level, nor from the MEC, making

the discerning of death-related trends problematic before 2004. MPs failed to participate in stakeholders' workshops due to their unanticipated demand for Parliament-set hefty allowances. Dealings with PLWHAs were comparatively unproblematic. A representative of PLWHAs groups was sent to both the inception and dissemination workshops. When organising FGDs with PLWHAs and their care-givers, help was sought from CBOs and support groups that customarily deal with PLWHAs.

3. HIV/AIDS in Malawi

3.1 Demography and epidemiological data

After the first case of AIDS in Malawi was diagnosed in 1985 at Kamuzu Central Hospital in Lilongwe, the number of those with HIV rapidly grew in the next decade. The HIV prevalence among pregnant women attending antenatal clinics was estimated at 2% at the end of the 1980s, with an alarming increase to 26% by 1998.[3] While urban Malawi has been seen to suffer the most from the epidemic, the rural areas has also experienced an increase in the number of cases. For example, in 1992, HIV prevalence rates in rural Malawi were estimated at 6% among antenatal women, which increased to 18% by 1998. By the end of the 1990s, antenatal HIV prevalence figures levelled off at about 25% in urban areas, with increases still being observed in semi-urban populations.[4]

According to the 2005 sentinel surveillance survey, the HIV prevalence rate among people aged 15 to 49 years was estimated at 14.0% – a decrease from 14.4% in 2003. Sentinel surveillance surveys have been used in Malawi to estimate the prevalence of HIV. The more recent population-based Demographic and Health Survey (DHS) conducted in 2004/5, which involved the sampling of blood from people aged 15 to 49 years, found a relatively lower HIV prevalence of 11.8%. The 2004 DHS figures further show that the prevalence of HIV is 30% higher among women at 13.3%, compared with that among men of 10.2%. Among adolescents aged 15 to 19 years old, prevalence is higher among female adolescents (3.7%) than among males (0.4%).

As well as gender differences in HIV prevalence, the 2004 DHS figures further show that the epidemic is urban-based, with adult prevalence in such areas reaching 17.1%, compared to 10.8% in the rural areas. Regionally, HIV prevalence is highest in the Southern region at 17.6%, compared to the Northern and Central regions, where prevalence is estimated at 8.1% and 6.5%, respectively.

Similarly, more HIV is encountered in the richest quintile and among those who have attained relatively high educational qualifications, indicating that those with more disposable income tend to be more at risk of HIV and sexually transmitted infection (STI).[5] Figure 3.1 summarises the trends in HIV prevalence for the period 1996 to 2005.

Figure 3.1: Trends in HIV prevalence

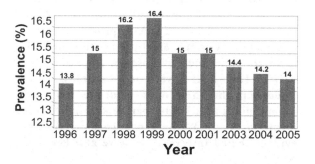

Figure 3.1 shows that, while in 1996 the HIV prevalence rate was estimated at 13.8%, the rate increased to 15% in 1997 and 16.2% in 1998, reaching its peak in 1998 at 16.4%. After 1999, HIV prevalence started declining, with the 2005 sentinel surveillance survey estimating it at 14%. The prevalence of HIV in Malawi has clearly stabilised over the last seven years.

According to the NAC, about 100 000 infections occur annually, of which at least half occur among people aged from 15 to 24,[6] with about 90 000 deaths occurring annually.[7] In 2005 the total number of people infected with HIV was estimated to stand at 930 000, including children younger than 15, with 30% of the infected living in urban areas, while 60% live in rural areas. Despite most Malawians (over 80%) living in rural areas, prevalence is low in such areas. Although HIV prevalence has recently stabilised, the epidemic remains a major threat to Malawians.

3.2 Impact of the epidemic

Using several studies conducted into the impact of HIV/AIDS at household, community and national levels, it has been estimated, at national level, that, prior to the epidemic, 22 000 deaths occurred a year, with the number skyrocketing to 80 000 deaths a year[8] due to the epidemic.

Most HIV/AIDS-related deaths affect the economically productive youth. HIV/AIDS is usually characterised by chronic illness and consequent death. Households affected by the illness spend a great deal on medical care, drugs and funerals. Businesses also incur financial loss from having to pay sick leave privileges and having to train replacement staff.[9] As shall be shown later, the loss of young people due to HIV/AIDS have also heavily affected the civil service.[10]

HIV/AIDS have also affected the average life expectancy of 54 years, with it declining to 39 years, the fifth lowest in the world, by 2000. The negative impact on Malawi's fight against tuberculosis can be seen in that, in 1985, somewhat more than 5 000 cases of tuberculosis were reported, while in 1999 the total number of reported cases of tuberculosis stood at 24 396, with this number rising to 27 000 in 2004, with 70% of tuberculosis patients being estimated by the Ministry of Health to also be HIV positive.[11]

The death of young economically active youth results in the increased vulnerability of the orphans and elderly left behind. According to the National Plan of Action for Orphans and Other Vulnerable Children, 2005–2009 just more than 1 008 000 children were recorded as orphans in 2005, half of whom had been orphaned by HIV/AIDS.

According to the DHS of 2000, 20% of Malawian households care for one or more orphans. The HIV/AIDS epidemic has resulted in an increasing number of child- and female-headed households; orphaned children being disposed of as property; elder-headed and fragmented households; and early marriages. Due to poverty and the inability to otherwise sustain themselves, many orphans have dropped out of school and become engaged in risky behaviours.[12]

3.3 Multisectoral response

3.3.1 Government's policies, strategic efforts

The national response to the HIV/AIDS epidemic has been informed by well-developed plans and frameworks. Medium-term Plans I and II guided Malawi's response to the AIDS epidemic for the period 1989 to 1999, after which the National HIV/AIDS Strategic Framework (NSF) was developed for the period 2000 to 2004. Thereafter the National HIV/AIDS Action Framework 2005–2009 was formulated, which still directs the national response.

During the first years of the AIDS epidemic, while

the late Dr Hastings Kamuzu Banda was the life president of Malawi, public debate about issues, such as sexuality, relating to HIV/AIDS was discouraged. Nevertheless, the National AIDS Committee, set up by the then government, coordinated the national response, setting up blood-screening centres in all the major cities and instituting a comprehensive HIV/AIDS awareness campaign. After the National AIDS Control Programme was set up in 1988, the first medium-term plan for the period 1989–1994 focused on blood-screening, public awareness and the setting up of an epidemiological HIV surveillance infrastructure.

The second medium-term plan, for 1995–1999, focused on the human resources shortage, the mobilisation of resources for the fight against HIV/AIDS and the setting up of care and treatment programmes for PLWHAs.

For the period 2000–2004, Malawi developed the NSF to direct the national response to the AIDS epidemic, building on the progress made during the implementation of the medium-term plans. The overall goal of the community-based multisectoral NSF was to reduce the incidence of HIV and STIs and to improve the quality of life of those infected and affected by HIV/AIDS. The strategic framework contained eight components, namely culture and HIV/AIDS; youth, social change and HIV/AIDS; socioeconomic status and HIV/AIDS; despair and hopelessness; HIV/AIDS management; HIV/AIDS and orphans, widows and widowers; the prevention of HIV transmission; and HIV/AIDS information, education and communication.[13]

Structural changes occurring at the time of implementation included the setting up, in July 2001, of the donor-recommended NAC outside the Ministry of Health to replace the National AIDS Control Programme.[14] At the same time, the NAC, the Ministry of Health and other stakeholders, with donor support, also jointly developed policies, interventions and guidelines for the delivery of HIV/AIDS services by both public and private sector, as well as CSOs involved with the prevention of mother-to-child transmission (PMTCT) of HIV, counselling and testing, Antiretroviral Therapy (ART), the treatment of opportunistic infections and community and home-based care.

Simultaneously, the wide-ranging National HIV/AIDS Policy was developed by means of consultation to provide the guidelines for such programmes and interventions.[15] Other policies, such as the National Orphans and Other Vulnerable Children Policy and the Antiretroviral Equity Policy, were also developed

during this period. The evaluation of the NSF (2003) revealed that considerable progress was made in the prevention of transmission and behavioural change; treatment, care and support; impact mitigation; mainstreaming, partnerships and capacity building; research, monitoring and evaluation; resource mobilisation and utilisation; and policy coordination and programme planning, which priority areas were carried forward into the National HIV/AIDS Action Framework (NAF) planning for the period 2005 to 2009.

After the NSF ended in October 2004, Malawi developed the NAF to guide the expanded, multisectoral national response for the period 2005–2009. The overall goal of the consultation-based NAF was to prevent the spread of HIV by providing access to treatment for PLWHAs and by mitigating the health, socioeconomic and psychosocial impact of HIV/AIDS.[16] High-level government commitment and leadership, the 'three ones' principle, multisectoral and multi-stakeholder partnerships, the greater involvement of PLWHAs, gender considerations and evidence-based interventions were also key to the NAF.

The NAF implementation strategies included the behavioural change interventions strategy; the mainstreaming of HIV/AIDS both in the public and private sectors and CSOs; the building of capacity in all stakeholder organisations; the mobilisation of resources; and the implementation of a comprehensive monitoring and evaluation system.

Nationally, Malawi has made much progress in the treatment, care and support of PLWHAs. HIV testing and counselling (HTC) services are key to influencing behaviour change, providing access to care and support programmes, such as ART and PMTCT services, delivered in both 'stand-alone' and integrated sites offering outreach services,[17] with the former largely being provided by the Malawi Counselling and Resource Organisation (MACRO) and the latter by the government and Christian Health Association in Malawi (CHAM). The national guidelines for HTC instruct that such essential services be freely offered in all publicly funded health facilities. According to the 2004 DHS, only 13% of women aged 15 to 49 years and 15.1% of men aged 15 to 54 years reported knowing the results of their HIV tests.[18] HIV testing has increased from 149 940 in 2002, to 215 269 in 2003, to 283 467 in 2004.[19]

The number of sites offering HTC services has also increased from 70 in 2002 to 146 by December 2004,[20] due to an increase in the number of those seeking HTC, the mandatory testing of mothers attending antenatal clinics, the increase in the number of HTC centres and the introduction of free antiretrovirals.[21]

3.3.2 The private sector

The Malawi Business Coalition Against HIV/AIDS (MBCA), launched in 2003, coordinates and provides a voice for private-sector response. Despite its initial urban base, which was largely limited to multinational organisations, the MBCA was restructured to accommodate both small and medium-scale companies, which comprise 75% of Malawian business. From its relatively small beginnings of only 15 members in 2003, its membership had grown to 20 in 2004 and 65 by 2006.

The many mandates of the MBCA include helping member companies to devise HIV/AIDS policies; the training of peer educators; the provision of HIV/AIDS-related training programmes to the business sector; and the mainstreaming of HIV/AIDS and antiretroviral training for the private sector, as well as helping to mobilise private-sector resources. The MBCA asks companies to contribute a minimum 2% of their budget to HIV/AIDS-related programmes, which accords with the National HIV/AIDS Policy which requires the same commitment from the government ministries. The coordinating role played by the MBCA in the private sector validates its representation of the sector in national HIV/AIDS forums.[22]

3.3.3 Civil society activities

CSOs, in the form of umbrella organisations and faith-based forums, also play a key role in coordinating non-profit civil society response to the HIV/AIDS pandemic. The Malawi AIDS Network (MANET) and the National Association of People Living with HIV/AIDS in Malawi (NAPHAM) coordinate HIV-related organisations. Civil society also participates in national HIV/AIDS programmes, playing a major role in developing the National HIV/AIDS Policy as part of the national multisectoral team constituted to draft such policy, as well as in the development of the NAF and operational guidelines for programmes such as PMTCT, HTC and ART.

Mostly international umbrella NGOs, which are the epicentres of information dissemination at community level, facilitate the trickling down of funds to the communities through CBOs and build the capacity of local assemblies and CBOs through skills

transfer. Civil society has been key to creating awareness about the HIV/AIDS epidemic and in complementing government delivery of HTC, ART and PMTCT.

HIV/AIDS is a serious public health and development problem in Malawi, as in many other Sub-Saharan African countries. HIV prevalence, which is still very high at about 14%, is lowest among children younger than 15 years of age. However, the institutionalisation and adoption of orphans is now on the increase due to the HIV/AIDS epidemic. The annual mortality rate has more than tripled, with most hospitals afflicted by HIV/AIDS-related illnesses. With most existing studies having focused on the economic and social aspects of the problem, its yet relatively unexplored impact on democratic governance will form the focus of this study.

4. HIV/AIDS and democratic governance

4.1 Historical perspective

Malawi is in southern Africa, bordering on Mozambique in the east, south and southwest, Zambia in the west and Tanzania in the north. The 1998 Population and Housing Census determined that the population was 9.9 million, of which 51% were female and 49% male. Currently, Malawi's population is estimated at 12.9 million. From 2000 to 2004 the annual population growth was estimated at 2.25%.[23] Between 1966 and 1998 the country's population more than doubled from 4.04 million to 9.9 million, while between 1987 and 1998 the population grew by 24%, with an annual growth rate estimated at 2.0%.[24] About 86% of Malawi's population live in the rural areas, with 14% living in the urban areas, showing a marked increase over the 1977 and 1987 censuses findings of 8.5% and 11.0%, in respect of the country's urban-based population.

Administratively, Malawi is divided into a northern, central and southern region, comprising 28 administrative districts. Nearly half of the country's population (47.0%) live in the south, while 41.0% and 12.0% live in the centre and north, respectively. The 1998 Population and Housing Census further showed that approximately 44% of the population were aged below 15 years of age, with 52% between 15 and 64 years and 4.0% above 65 years of age. The dependency ratio for Malawi is therefore 0.906.[25]

Malawi was a British colony from 1891 until 1961, when the country came to govern itself for the first time, with subsequent independence being declared in 1964 under Kamuzu Banda as its first president. After Malawi became a Republic in 1966, it developed into a one-party state, with Banda, in 1971, being declared its life President. Though the 1971 national Constitution entrenched an independent judiciary and Parliament, with a tripartite separation of government powers, in reality such powers were overridden by the absolute powers of the life president, who was also empowered to select the MPs.[26]

From 1964 to 1994, Banda's one-party state, over which he had absolute power, was characterised by the general abuse of human rights and the absence of fundamental freedoms. Opponents to Dr Banda's autocracy were dealt with ruthlessly by his Malawi Congress Party (MCP) followers. In March 1992, the Catholic bishops in Malawi published the first open challenge to Banda's 30-year rule in the form of a pastoral letter calling for the introduction of multiparty politics and the rule of law. Several pressure groups, notably the United Democratic Front (UDF) and the Alliance for Democracy (AFORD), were formed; leading political figures were arrested; and labour unrest and university student protests prevailed. About the same time, major donors froze non-humanitarian aid to Malawi, trying to force Banda's government to adopt a multiparty system of government and to embrace the rule of law. Together with the severe drought at the time, Malawi's economy was hard-hit, resulting in serious devaluation of the Kwacha, the national currency, and a rampant increase in inflation.

In 1993 Banda felt compelled to hold a referendum, in which about 66% of Malawians voted in favour of the introduction of multiparty politics. The UDF, led by Banda's one-time Secretary General in the MCP, Elson Bakili Muluzi, won the first multiparty general elections held in 1994.

As Muluzi neared the end of his second and last term in office, he tried unsuccessfully to alter the Constitution so that he could extend his presidency for a third term. When Muluzi opposed Bingu wa Mutharika as presidential candidate for the UDF during the 2004 elections, the latter won with a minority of parliamentary seats.

A few months later, Mutharika, an economist and former Secretary General of the Preferential Trade Area (PTA) of the Common Market for Southern and Eastern Africa (COMESA), resigned from the UDF, the party which had brought him to power. Later, Mutharika formed and became president of the Democratic Progressive Party (DPP). His departure from the UDF meant that the ruling party was relegated to opposition status, which the Malawi Constitution allows by being silent on the matter, hence creating a grey area that is open to abuse. Due to such constitutional inadequacy, Mutharika's newborn DPP assumed the position of "ruling party" by virtue of its leader remaining the state president.

4.2 Implications of HIV/AIDS for democratic governance

While Malawi is a poor country and has some of the world's worst health indicators, there have been improvements in the recent past. Such improvements have however been negatively affected by HIV/AIDS. The overall fertility rate for Malawi is currently estimated at 6.0 children a woman,[27] which is a decrease from 6.7 in 1992 and 6.3 in 2000.[28] The maternal mortality rate (MMR) in 1992 was estimated at 620 maternal deaths for 100 000 live births, which rose to 1 120 deaths for 100 000 in 2000 and then decreased to 984 deaths for 100 000 live births in 2004.[29] Such figures are considered high.

The infant mortality rate in 1960 stood at 205 deaths for 1 000, but declined to 117 in 2000. The under-five mortality rate currently stands at 188 for 1 000 live births.[30] While the infant and under-five mortality rates are on the decrease, they might start increasing again as a result of HIV/AIDS. The life expectancy rate has been on the decrease since the early 1990s, estimated at 40 years in 2000,[31] a drop from 48 in 1992.[32]

The precipitous drop in overall life expectancy in the region is mainly due to the HIV/AIDS pandemic, which is mostly claiming the lives of those most economically productive between the ages of 15 and 49 years.[33] Malawi, as is the case with most countries in Sub-Saharan Africa, is one of the countries with the highest levels of HIV infection in the world.

How, then, has the epidemic affected democratic governance? It has had potentially devastating results, in terms of the soaring numbers of orphans and its negative impact on the health, and hence the economy, of the country.

However, public opinion surveys, such as the Afrobarometer, have shown that Malawians still do not rank HIV/AIDS highly, with only those who have personally suffered loss tending to consider it a priority, while others tend to consider employment, crime and education to be of greater concern. Such perception might be due to the stigma and discrimination associated with the disease. To make HIV/AIDS a campaign issue and a priority for Malawian voters, intensive voter education is needed for evidence-based interventions linking HIV/AIDS to politics.

The media can play a key role in sensitising voters to HIV/AIDS issues, with leading newspapers, such as *The Chronicle, The Nation* and *The Daily Times*, dedicating whole pages to the coverage of such issues. Despite the increase in coverage of many public issues, including HIV/AIDS, since the 1990s, the coverage of technical subjects still remains shallow, due to the lack of institutionalised training for Malawian journalists geared towards generating high-quality democratic discourse.[34]

The failure to disclose the presence of AIDS when first diagnosed in the country, due to fears that it might lead to political instability, led to pressure having to be exerted by the World Health Organisation and Malawi's chief medical officer.[35] When Muluzi became president, with the introduction of democracy, notable changes occurred.

Under Banda's one-party system, CSOs were constrained to minimal advocacy of basic human rights issues, including. HIV/AIDS.[36] However, since the setting up of democratic governance in the early 1990s, many CSOs have become involved with promoting human rights and the active implementation of HIV/AIDS-related programmes. However, key political anchors of democratic governance, such as the Ministries of Education, Finance, Justice, Home Affairs and Parliament, continue to suffer the depredations of the epidemic in terms of staff attrition.

The HIV/AIDS epidemic has retarded economic development, resulting in greater economic inequality, despite the start of irreversible 'democratic waves' in most African countries, including Malawi, from the early 1990s onwards.[37]

5. Impact of HIV/AIDS on electoral system

Previous studies of the HIV/AIDS epidemic have focused on how it has retarded economic development, rather than on its impact on the electoral system. This study, in contrast, examines how the death of an MP affects the electoral system and parliamentary configuration, in the light of how much it costs to run by-elections.

In terms of the former single-party system, public policy mostly constituted presidential directives, with political participation being severely circumscribed. MCP candidates could only participate in the elections subject to the approval of the life president, who was empowered to nominate MPs, resulting in many candidatures being unopposed. Dulani has described elections held under the one-party system as "farcical shows".[38] The FPTP electoral system, which is the legacy of British colonial rule, is still used in Malawi. However, the introduction of multiparty democracy in 1994 has enabled Malawians to participate in, and thus influence, the democratic political process, including both presidential and parliamentary election outcomes. In 1995 Malawi also adopted a Constitution that promotes the holding of periodic elections.

5.1 Elections, electoral systems

The Parliamentary and Presidential Elections Act (PPEA) of 1993 and the Constitution of the Republic of Malawi of 1994 provide for a simple plurality electoral system (FPTP), with Section 96 (5) of the PPEA (Cap.2:01) stating that "subject to this Act, in any election the candidate who has obtained a majority of the votes at the poll shall be declared by the Commission to have been duly elected". However, Section 80(2) of the Constitution states that a president shall be elected by "a majority of the electorate through direct, universal and equal suffrage". While the PPEA emphasises the majority of the votes, the Constitution refers to the majority of the electorate, which it fails to define. Broadly speaking, an electoral system comprises the rules and regulations governing the conduct of elections, the institutional arrangements for the administration and management of elections, and the translation of votes into seats in Parliament. The difficulty in precisely defining the impact of the HIV/AIDS pandemic on such aspects of the electoral system is particularly felt in relation to the rules and regulations and the institutional arrangements made in terms of the electoral system. As the lack of data regarding how HIV/AIDS affects Malawian electoral bodies and those institutions involved with elections complicates this challenge, the following sections provide an overview of the major deficiencies in the Malawi electoral system that might fall prey to the increased incidence and prevalence of HIV/AIDS.

The 1994, 1999 and 2004 general elections have brought to the fore shortcomings with the FPTP electoral system in Malawi which significantly affect political participation. Such shortcomings include high levels of wasted votes, minority rather than majority rule, the failure to address gender inequalities and the entrenchment of regionalism.

5.1.1 The question of representation

The FPTP system suffers from lack of representation. Candidates elected under the system are answerable to and representative of all constituency members, regardless of whether they voted for them or not – accordingly, all Malawians are represented. However, in reality, as Chingaipe has argued, elected representatives are largely influenced by party leadership and consensus, "even though individual conscious and constituency interests are at marked variance with party positions".[39] In the past, some purported representatives of the masses have acted contrary to the wishes and aspirations of the people whom they represent for reasons of party discipline and politicking.

For example, in 1997 most MCP and AFORD members boycotted Parliament for a period of nine months, in line with party demands,[40] despite their representing CSOs with opposing views. While every constituency, and hence every Malawian, is represented in the legislature, overall, MPs fail to consult members of their constituencies, adhering to the party line of thinking.

5.1.2 Minority candidates and problems of governance and leadership legitimacy

The winner in the FPTP system does not have to amass the most votes, but only a simple majority, even when many voters vote for someone else. The result is the election of minority supported candidates for both the presidency and Parliament, which brings into question the legitimacy of leaders elected in terms of the FPTP system. The results of the 1994, 1999 and 2004 presidential and parliamentary elections illustrate this issue.

In both 1994 and 1999 Bakili Muluzi of the UDF won the presidency with less than 50% of the votes, which raised many questions. Section 96(5) of the PPEA states that a candidate with most of the votes at the poll will be declared duly elected. Section 80(2) of the Constitution, however, stipulates that a president shall be elected by "a majority of the electorate through direct, universal and equal suffrage," but fails to define the electorate. The majority of the electorate has been interpreted as the proportion of Malawians eligible to vote. Since Dr Muluzi did not win the support of "the majority of the electorate" in 1999, the losing candidates launched a legal battle.

In 2004 the five presidential candidates were Gwanda Chakuamba of the Republican Party (RP), representing the seven-party Mgwirizano Coalition; Justin Malewezi, an independent (IND) candidate; James Mpinganjira of the National Democratic Alliance (NDA); Bingu wa Mutharika of the UDF; and John Tembo of the MCP. Dr Hetherwick Ntaba of the New Congress for Democracy withdrew his candidature, instead joining the UDF. Figure 5.1 shows the results of the 2004 presidential elections.

Figure 5.1: Results of the 2004 presidential elections (n=3,323.801)

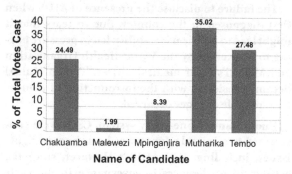

As can be seen from the results of the 2004 presidential elections presented in Figure 5.1, President Bingu wa Mutharika was elected by only 35% of the vote, followed by John Tembo at 28% and Gwanda Chakuamba at 25%. Malewezi and Mpinganjira together polled just over 10% of the votes. Overall, Mutharika got only 21% of the vote,[41] showing that the opposition lost a chance to win both the presidential and parliamentary elections. The combined votes of the other four losing candidates, namely Tembo, Chakuamba, Mpinganjira and Malewezi, amount to more than 60% of the votes, showing that Mutharika was elected by a mere minority.

The 2004 parliamentary elections resulted in a similar scenario, with constituencies such as 013 naming 11 candidates: four independents and one each from AFORD; the NDA; the National Unity Party (NUP); the Movement for Genuine Democracy (MGODE); the MCP; the RP; and the People's Transformation Party (PETRA). The results of these elections in constituency 013 in 2004 are shown in Figure 5.2.

Figure 5.2 clearly shows that the candidate who rep-

Figure 5.2: Results of parliamentary elections in Constituency 013 (total number of votes cast = 21512)

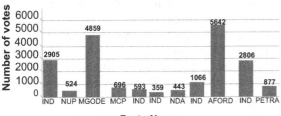

Table 4.1: Voter turnout, 1993–2004

Year	Percentage turnout			
	1993	1994	1999	2004
North	71	85	93	64
Centre	71	81	90	61
South	65	78	94	56
National	69	80	92	59

resented AFORD in the 2004 elections was declared winner, despite receiving only 26.2% of the votes cast. In 2004, out of 193 seats contested in the legislature, 103 representatives of the constituencies were elected by minorities, meaning that in 103 constituencies, most of the members of these constituencies opposed the election of "their representatives". In 1999 this occurred in only 29 constituencies.[42]

The Constitution of the Republic of Malawi does not allow for a rerun, as other countries experiencing such inconclusive results might. As Dulani has argued, one of the major problems with the current FPTP is that it has resulted in the delivery of inconclusive and unrepresentative results and so does not render democratic outcomes in terms of majority rule. Despite most votes being cast for the losers, they are essentially wasted, potentially leading to voter disenfranchisement.[43]

Figure 5.2 shows that in constituency 013 a total of 21 512 people voted, with only 5 642 people voting for AFORD electing a representative, implying that 15 870 votes were essentially lost. Demands for electoral reform in favour of more democratic outcomes urge the setting up of the principle of majority rule.

No definition yet exists of who should form the government, with the party producing the winning president tending to form the government.[44] In 2004 the MCP produced the highest number (57) of MPs, followed by the UDF at 50, 39 INDs and 15 from the RP. Even though the MCP had the most MPs, the party did not produce a winning president. Such a scenario, as Dulani,[45] Chirwa[46] and Chingaipe[47] have argued, creates problems of governance, especially for minority-led governments, hence the need for definitive rules and regulations.

Minority and inclusive results are not necessarily due to voter apathy, as general election results indicate increased popular participation in elections for the period between the referendum of 1993 and general elections of 1999. However, there was a decline in voter turnout in 2004, as shown in Table 4.1.

The political transition in Malawi has clearly not translated into prosperity for most Malawians.[48] Levels of poverty have been on the increase over the last 15 years against the backdrop of reduced life expectancy resulting from HIV/AIDS; peasant agricultural incomes have fallen; wage employment has not increased; educational standards have deteriorated; and hunger is common.

Enfranchisement is seen as only a means of advancing political leaders to self-serving positions, with the increasing incidence of HIV/AIDS still further reducing voter turnout, thus compounding an already existing problem.

Turnout figures for general and by-elections do not yet indicate voter fatigue, with such figures varying annually among constituencies, unmarked by specific patterns. The personal and political strengths of the individual candidates, the intensity of the campaign, and the number of voters in the particular constituencies all affect the turnout figures.

5.1.3 Promotion of regional and ethnic divisions

The past three Malawian elections have shown that the regional support for parties and the origin of its leadership largely determine electoral outcomes. The Northern, Central and Southern regions of Malawi are strongholds of the AFORD, the MCP and the UDF, respectively. In 1994 AFORD took all the seats in the Northern region, while the MCP and UDF won most of the seats in the Central and Southern regions, respectively. In 1999, however, parties upset the established pattern by invading others' political strongholds.

In 1999 the newly-formed AFORD–MCP alliance influenced how the parties performed regionally. Though intended to disrupt regionalism by promoting national unity, that year's electoral results still showed regional voting patterns, reflected in Figure 5.3.

While AFORD won all the Northern seats and three seats in the Central region, in 1994, it lost five

Figure 5.3: The 1994 and 1999 parliamentary elections in Malawi

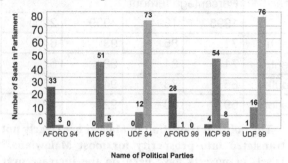

Name of Political Parties

■ North ■ Central ■ South

Source: Patel, 2000

seats in the 1999 elections to the MCP and UDF, when, due to the grand alliance, the former won some seats in the North and South. Despite some parties making unexpected inroads in certain geographical areas, regionalistic voting patterns still prevailed in the later elections.

In 2004, as well as the three parties with prior parliamentary representation, the representatives of some new parties were also voted into office: the RP (15); the NDA (8); the People's Progressive Party (6); MGODE (3); PETRA (1); and the Congress for National Unity (CONU) (1).[49]

Currently the geographical spread of constituencies comprise 33 in the North, 72 in the Centre and 87 in the South. As Dulani argues, democracy might be endangered if such a spread translates into "one-party dominance for a predominantly Southern region party in national politics".[50] The current electoral system promotes regional and ethnic fiefdoms and cleavages, as shown in the 1993 referendum and the later general elections.

5.1.4 Under-representation of women

In 1997, the Southern African Development Community (SADC) set 2005 as the year by which 30% of the government decision-making posts in member states should be occupied by women. At the time of writing, the 27 women in the 193-member legislature represent only 14% of the whole, so that Malawi falls short of the SADC-set standard. As the FPTP electoral system encourages open competition, it discourages women from participating in national politics and elections, which directly depends on the campaign-directed availability and access to resources.[51] Countries with a Proportional Representation (PR) system have more women in Parliament than those using the FPTP system.[52]

5.1.5 The rise of independent candidates

The rules for holding primary elections are not clearly defined, with parties usually imposing candidates who are loyal supporters of party leadership and the sitting MPs,[53] despite the electorate openly opposing such nominations. The number of INDs has grown significantly, due to the frustrations of would-be MPs and the desire of the electorate to exercise its freedom and to hold their parties accountable.[54]

This practice of choosing candidates has led to a lot of frustration among the aspirants who have instead chosen to run as INDs instead of using a party ticket. In the 2004 elections The 372 INDs in the 2004 elections largely came from the Southern region, the traditional UDF stronghold.

5.2 Economic, political cost

5.2.1 Political cost

Conducting largely donor-supported by-elections is costly, especially in terms of skills. The level of parliamentary debate is enhanced by the mingling of new and experienced legislators, though the death of the latter might affect not only the level and type of such debate, but also parliamentary power shifts. By-elections are inevitable following the death of a legislator, which might result in a loss of the seat for the previously represented party, especially if small and under-funded.

5.2.2 Lack of development

In Malawi, parliamentary representation amounts to supporting the constituency by means of development projects, which is lost on the death of an MP. The inevitable delays resulting from by-elections also result in loss of representation. For example, after the 2004 elections, six seats fell vacant in the national assembly, taking over a year to fill by means of by-elections.

5.2.3 Costs associated with by-elections

In December 2005 the six by-elections in Malawi cost an estimated MK65 million (US$474 800), which translated into approximately MK10.8 million (US$78 890) per constituency.[55] As Matlosa and Patel have argued, as by-elections have to be held within

90 days of the death of any MP, such replacement costs are very high, with associated delays being interpreted as unconstitutional.

5.3 Electoral system reform debate

As the current electoral model has failed to de-escalate conflict, redress regionalism or promote inclusive, consensual politics Matlosa and Nandini urge the need for review, especially due to the HIV/AIDS epidemic. Leading CSOs, such as the Malawi Electoral Support Network, a coalition of election-concerned NGOs, recommend adopting a combined electoral system.[56]

The MEC admits that the shortfalls of the FPTP system are a source of regional or tribal tensions and instability.[57] In 2006 the commission conducted a study, financially supported by the Konrad Adenauer Foundation (KAF), whose aim was "to contribute towards the consolidation of democracy in Malawi by creating enabling institutions and legal instruments for the conduct of regular, free, fair, credible, transparent and accessible elections through a broad-based public debate and national dialogue in Malawi on the current electoral system,"[58] allowing for electoral reform.

The Mixed Member Proportional (MMP) system would seem the best option for Malawi, ensuring that a certain proportion of parliamentary seats be occupied through constituency voting, while the rest are guided by the List PR system, which would promote female participation. The relative cheapness of this system stems from by-elections being necessary only in the case of vacancies previously occupied by the FPTP. Adoption of the MMP would require amendment of the Constitution in terms of the reinstatement of section 64 on recall of MPs, or of section 62(1) to reflect a Constitution based on both the FPTP and PR systems.[59]

FPTP systems are attractive due to their simplicity, the ability to produce winners and because they often produce single-party governments that are more secure than coalitions. Though broad-based political parties tend especially to benefit regionally and ethnically divided societies, Malawi does not appear to have benefited from such advantages.[60] Instead of providing a clear-cut choice for voters between two main parties,[61] the number of political parties and INDs has proliferated, with the winning candidates garnering fewer votes than the losing

candidates combined, and with the former representing the minority.

6. Impact on parliamentary configuration

Results of the parliamentary elections suggest that elections in Malawi provide real opportunities to change or replace representatives. Out of the 187 contested seats[62] in the 20 May 2004 parliamentary elections, 59 were retained by incumbents, while 128 were won by new challengers.[63] Opposition INDs triumphed over 23 MPs who filled key positions as ministers or deputy ministers.

While the incumbent governing party has tended to dominate presidential and parliamentary by-elections, with, from 1994, the UDF winning the presidency, parliamentary elections have experienced a very high turnover rate at party level, as can be seen in Table 6.1.

Table 6.1: Turnover in composition of Parliament, 1994-99		
Party	Seats by 1994 GE out of 177	Re-elected in 1999
MCP	55	19
AFORD	35	10
UDF	86	43
1999-2004		
Party	Seats by 1999 GE out of 177	Re-elected in 2004
MCP	64	31 (one not consecutively)
AFORD	29	3
UDF	93	22
Source: Research Department, Malawi National Assembly		

Note:

- Several MPs were re-elected to the 2004 Parliament, based on different political affiliations, with altered party affiliations.

- The 2004 Parliament is characterised by shifts and swings in the political allegiance of members.

In all by-elections between 1994 and 1999, the party retained those seats won during the general elections. However, from 1999 to 2004 the governing UDF, having consolidated power, won three former-ly-held MCP seats. All six by-elections of December 2005 were won by the newly formed DPP, led by the incumbent President Mutharika. One smaller party, the People's Progressive Movement (PPM), which won six seats during the general elections, lost one to the DPP during the by-election, with the remainder being ex-UDF.

Such turnover also reduced representativeness by changing the parliamentary configuration and minimising the contribution made by the smaller parties in terms of an alternative voice and plurality of ideas and representation. The legislative processes and parliamentary debate then become increasingly dominated by the leading party, enabling it to con-solidate its power, as the UDF did when it won more seats through the by-elections held between 1999 and 2004. Among the controversial bills it tried to push through were the Open Term and Third Term proposals aimed at repealing the two consecutive terms required for the presidency, which were nar-rowly defeated as they required a two-thirds major-ity that the UDF was unable to amass. The same period saw extensive Constitutional amendments, requiring only a simple minority vote in the house, including those governing local government and decentralisation and allowing for the impeachment of high court judges.[64]

Certain Constitutional amendments appear to have been motivated by partisan interests or political advantage, rather then national interests. For exam-ple, in 2001, Senate-related Sections 68 to 72 and Section 210, dealing with its composition, vacancies, functions and powers, the scrutiny of legislation, and dissolution were repealed.[65] Such sections provided for a Senate enabling participation by chiefs, women, and other interest and specialised groups in the leg-islative process. Such cost-cutting measures would allow local government and the decentralisation programme to empower the local levels, facilitating community participation in key decision-making relating to development policy.

In reality, the abolition of the Senate undermined the scrutinising of legislation and executive deci-sions undertaken by the country's special groups. Since the amendment was made, civil society has opposed it by petitioning Parliament and political parties. Between 2003 and 2006, the Church and Society Programme of the Livingstonia Synod of the Church of Central Africa Presbyterian spearheaded

the lobby for reinstating the Senate and recalling it into the Constitution, including at the constitutional conference review at the end of March 2006.[66]

In 1995, Parliament repealed Section 64 providing for the recall of MPs by way of petitions, requiring signatures by at least half the registered voters in a constituency, submitted to the Speaker.[67] Parliament unanimously voted for repealing the much abused section, which allowed anyone conflicting with an MP to follow the said route, which inadequately provided for the verification and authentication of the signatures concerned. The repeal, which made political representatives less accountable to their constituents, also reduced the power of the elector-ate over their elected representatives.

The only meaningful mechanism by means of which the electorate can hold their representative accountable is now through the ballot at the end of the tenure of office five years after the elections. CSOs have so far failed to reinstate the recall provi-sion, despite, in March 2006, their jointly with the chiefs submitting the issue to the Law Commission for consideration during the Constitutional review process.

6.1 Parliament and HIV/AIDS

6.1.1 Death rates

Figure 6.1 shows the number of Malawian MPs who died between 1994 and 2005. More legislators died from 1994 to 1999 than from 1999 to 2004, with seven legislators dying since the 2004 parliamentary elections. Some of the deaths might have been due to HIV/AIDS-related causes. No inferences could be made from the ages at which the MPs concerned

Figure 6.1: Number of deaths of MPs, 1994-2005

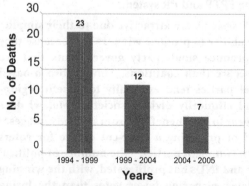

Source: Malawi Parliament

died, as such information was not in parliamentary record. However, in 2000, the then Speaker of the National Assembly, Sam Mpasu, officially disclosed that 28 Malawian MPs had died of HIV/AIDS.[68]

The current Malawi Parliament is dominated by the relatively young. Of the 193 MPs at the end of 2005, 87 (45%) were below 50 years of age, with 138 (about 72%) being younger than 60. Hence, most MPs are still in their prime and vulnerable to HIV infection, being sexually active.

6.2 Parliamentary debates on HIV/AIDS

The commitment of MPs to the fight against HIV/AIDS is shown in the type of HIV/AIDS-related parliamentary debate held.

6.2.1 Parliamentary debates 2001-2003

Parliament is required, in terms of the Constitution, to sit at least three times annually: in May/June (for six weeks), November/December and February/March. During each sitting, after the opening presidential address, ministerial debates on matters of national interest, including HIV/AIDS, are held, with questions being directed by the MPs at the ministers responsible for particular portfolios.

Minister of Health Aleke Banda emphasised HIV/AIDS-related issues during his ministerial parliamentary address in June 2001. The October 2001 presidential opening speech then announced the setting up of both the NAC outside the Ministry of Health and the state-faith community task force, intended as a permanent forum for HIV/AIDS-related dialogue. Some MPs, during the later parliamentary discussions, acknowledged their responsibility for conducting HIV/AIDS voter education, with two even requesting their fellow legislators to ask local leaders, church elders and sheikhs to preach about AIDS. While one MP urged Malawians to observe the seventh Biblical commandment: "Thou shall not commit adultery" (Ex. 20:14), another attested that forests are being depleted by the wood used for coffins for those who have died from AIDS. The 2001 parliamentary sittings also emphasised the needs of orphans and the need for a reduction in medicine prices, as antiretrovirals were proving too expensive for ordinary Malawians at MK2 500 (approximately US$18) a month. The failure of awareness campaigns to transform behaviour was also said to be of concern.

With support from the Global Fund for the Fight Against HIV/AIDS, Tuberculosis and Malaria, Malawi started implementing a free antiretroviral programme in June 2004. As of November 2006, more than 70 000 people have been placed on antiretrovirals.[69]

During the June 2002 parliamentary sitting, Yusuf Mwawa, the then Minister of Health and Population, acknowledged the devastating effects of HIV/AIDS on communities in terms of the death of those who should be most productive and the increasing number of orphans. Of hospital admissions, 60% suffered from HIV/AIDS-related illnesses. Having explained government efforts to control the HIV/AIDS epidemic, including the expansion of treatment of opportunistic infections, VCT, ART and PMTCT services and the setting up of a National Blood Transfusion Service, he called on people to change their behaviour. MPs also interrogated the Minister of Health about HIV/AIDS-related issues, such as the grant received from the Global Fund and why Malawi had not yet developed a national HIV/AIDS policy. Also, the high prices of antiretrovirals, resulting in the need for heavy subsidisation or even their free provision, required donor funding to be sought. Inquiry was made into whether the Ministry considered using traditional medicines to cure AIDS, as traditional healers claimed. The transmission of HIV through blood transfusion, mother-to-child transmission, and work-related risks affecting AIDS health workers were debated.

During the June 2003 parliamentary sitting, HIV/AIDS-related discussion centred on the provision of antiretrovirals, with one MP asking for the Minister of Health to consider antiretroviral provision to MPs who subjected themselves to free HIV testing as an example for the public. Despite the introduction of free ART, elected leaders have been reluctant to publicly disclose their status after testing, showing lack of awareness and openness among the parliamentarians themselves. Neither has there thus far been interrogation of strategic approaches to broader management of the pandemic in the workplace, nor consideration of the institutional elements which would mitigate the impact of the HIV/AIDS pandemic on the National Assembly. Malawi now has a comprehensive national HIV/AIDS policy which promotes HIV testing, including the mandatory testing of pregnant mothers, encourages notification and discourages discrimination against PLWHAs.[70]

7. Electoral administration and management

An electoral system entails "institutionalized procedures for the choosing of office-holders by some or all of the recognized members of an organization".[71] The legitimacy of the electoral process hinges on the electorates' and candidates' perception that the process has been conducted in a way that does not in advance ensure a certain outcome: in a democracy there should be certainty about the process, but uncertainty about the results.[72] To ensure legitimacy, the electoral process must be regulated by Constitutional rules and special legislation, as well as by cultural norms developed to govern the behaviour of the actors. The electoral process necessitates rules for the electoral formulae, constituency demarcation, electorate definition, candidate nomination, political party registration, and electoral campaign conduct. Elklit (1999)[73] identifies twelve steps in the electoral process:

12 steps of the electoral process

1. The legal framework of the electoral process.

2. The establishment of adequate organisational management structures, including the mandate, autonomy and capacity vested in the MEC.

3. Constituency and polling district demarcation.

4. Voter education and voter information.

5. Voter registration.

6. Nomination and registration of political parties and candidates.

7. Regulation of electoral campaigning.

8. Polling.

9. Counting and tabulating the vote.

10. Resolving of electoral disputes and complaints.

11. Election result implementation.

12. Post-election handling of election material.

The electoral process is long, starting from the finalisation of the last election, with the polling itself forming only the eighth step of the process. In this section after first considering certain steps in the process, as managed in Malawi, we look at how the HIV/AIDS epidemic has affected the management and administration of the electoral process.

7.1 Structures, staff and legal framework of the Malawi Electoral Commission

7.1.1 Legislative framework

Several legislative instruments govern electoral conduct, with both the Constitution of the Republic of Malawi in section VII, paragraphs 75–76, and the Electoral Commission Act providing for the setting up of the MEC. Section 40(3) of the Constitution further provides for the right of Malawians to participate in elections secretly, freely and fairly. The Electoral Commission Act, the Local Government Act and the PPEA also spell out the MEC structure and functions.

The PPEA mandates the MEC to prepare for and conduct elections. The Act further details the functions of the MEC, including conducting elections freely and fairly and dealing with electoral disputes and conflicts equitably and liaising with electoral stakeholders on the conduct of elections. The MEC is also responsible for managing the voters' roll, including registering voters and candidates; providing voter education, electoral personnel and voting materials; regulating electoral campaigning; and conducting and announcing the results of the electoral process.

Section 76 (2) of the Constitution empowers the MEC with the responsibility for demarcating constituency boundaries. The number of constituencies has grown from 53, at the time of declaration of independence in 1964, to the current 193, as shown in Figure 7.1.

The rapid growth in the number of constituencies

Figure 7.1: Number of constituencies in Malawi 1964-1998

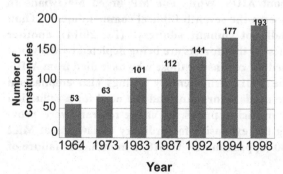

since 1992 has been unconstitutional and non-standardised,[74] leading to much debate. Opposition parties accused the ruling UDF and the MEC of aiming the demarcations at ensuring that the former won in most of the constituencies.

7.1.2 Structures, staff of Electoral Commission

The MEC, first set up in 1993, has always drawn its commissioners from the different political parties. Though first located in the Office of the Clerk of Parliament in the National Assembly, after the 1994 elections an independent secretariat, staffed full-time and charged with electoral administration and accompanying electoral processes, was set up. Apart from being chaired by a judge nominated by the Judicial Service Commission, six other commissioners, all of whom are appointed by the state president, are nominated by political parties for a four-year renewable term. The Public Appointments Committee of Parliament sets the terms and conditions for the appointment of commissioners and might recommend their removal to the president.

The MEC is serviced by a Secretariat, headed by the Chief Elections Officer, who is supported by deputies for finance, administration and electoral services. Though the MEC has three regional offices, one in each region, the commission lacks a permanent structure. During elections, returning officers are appointed, with, in most cases, district commissioners acting as returning officers, empowered to manage elections in their districts alongside the district elections supervisory teams (DESTs).[75]

The returning officer is also responsible for managing any conflicts that arise during elections at district level.[76] MEC effectiveness is hampered by the temporary nature of district structures, resulting in increased demands for more permanent, costly electoral structures.[77] All returning officers and members of the DESTs are civil servants, who are critical for voter registration and poll-related duties, such as the counting of votes.

Secretariat headquarters and the three regional offices are staffed by about 150 people. For the MEC to conduct elections efficiently and effectively, it therefore relies heavily, especially in the rural areas, on teachers from the Ministry of Education, members of the Malawi Police Force and other civil servants.

7.2 Internal impact of HIV/AIDS

7.2.1 Malawi Electoral Commission

The MEC relies on its specially trained core staff and temporarily employed public servants to manage elections, so might suffer from the loss of trained personnel who take extensive sick leave.

7.2.2 Commission's response

Due to the slow reactions of the MEC to the HIV/AIDS epidemic, the commission is only now consulting with different stakeholders regarding streamlining HIV/AIDS management. Though an HIV/AIDS-related taskforce is investigating how to respond to the HIV/AIDS epidemic both within the commission and among the electorate, the commission has not yet devised a policy governing HIV/AIDS management in the workplace.[78]

7.3 External impact of HIV/AIDS

Public servants who staff the electoral process, if heavily affected by the HIV/AIDS epidemic, will negatively affect the management of elections. Two major studies undertaken in 2001, *The Impact of HIV/AIDS on the Human Resources in the Malawi Public Sector*, conducted for the government and UNDP by the Malawi Institute of Management (MIM) and *The Impact of HIV/AIDS on Primary and Secondary Schooling in Malawi*, conducted by the Centre for Educational Research (CERT), highlight how seriously the civil service has been affected by the HIV/AIDS epidemic.

The former study indicates overwhelming morbidity, absenteeism and attrition figures due to HIV/AIDS afflicting civil servants, which might impede the management of the electoral process, through staff losses incurred, which might lead to loss of institutional memory, the depletion of skills and increased retraining costs. Such retraining could detract from the quality of delivery by increasing the likelihood of error. Mistakes could be costly, since they might bring into disrepute the integrity of both the MEC and the poll itself.

The MIM report indicates that certain social groups, particularly the poor, the youth, women, and, increasingly, children, are showing a disproportionately high level of vulnerability to the devastating impact of HIV/AIDS. Those public sector employees on whom the MEC has come to rely and whom it has trained might not be available for the next election due to ill health or death.

The next section illustrates how staff in the Ministry of Education and the Malawi Police Force are key in performing MEC activities, so as to see how the epidemic might indirectly affect the management and administration of the elections.

7.3.1 Reasons for attrition of teachers in the Ministry of Education and how this affects pre-election and polling phases

The 2002 GoM/UNDP study examined attrition among teachers in the Ministry of Education, as revealed by its records, which is the largest supplier of personnel to MEC during elections. The study found that between 1990 and 2000 the Ministry lost 5 188 qualified teachers and other support staff due to deaths, dismissals, redundancy and retirement.

Though retirement accounts for most staff attrition, as shown in Figure 7.2, death, which has soared since 1993, is also a key cause. Although the cause of death varies, such rampant increase is linked to the HIV/AIDS pandemic.

The increase in the number of deaths started approximately a decade after the first case of AIDS was diagnosed in 1985. The study under review states that the number of teachers retiring prematurely due to ill health accounted for 1.7% of the annual attrition figure. The MEC has to train teachers to replace those lost through death or illness.

Around 1994 the Government of Malawi (GoM) ordered all civil servants, including teachers, who had reached retirement age to retire, which accounts for retirement being a major cause (51.7%) of staff attrition, closely followed by deaths (45%).

Figure 7.2: General attrition by cause and year among qualified teachers and support staff (n=5188)

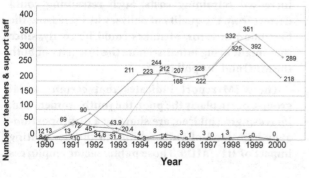

Between 1990 and 2000 the Ministry of Education lost 766 temporary teachers, most of whom had completed a secondary school education, with 650 (84.8%) dying during the same period, as can be seen in Figure 7.4.

Figure 7.5 shows the death-related attrition rate by sex and age group of the 2 196 reviewed.

Most deaths occurred in the age group 25–44 years, among those younger than 40, with HIV/AIDS being the most likely major cause.[79]

Figure 7.3: Causes of attrition among teachers and staff, Ministry of Education 1990-2000

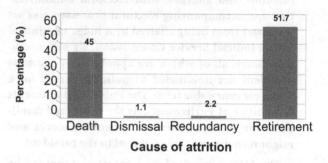

Figure 7.4: General attrition by cause and year among temporary teachers (n=766)

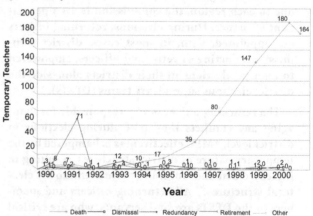

Figure 7.5: Death-related attrition in the Ministry of Education (n=2196)

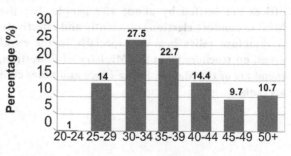

In the study by Kadzamira *et al* of the impact of HIV/AIDS on Malawian primary and secondary schools, an increase in teacher mortality was detected, with such mortality being found to be six times higher in the three urban schools sampled than in the three rural schools. The study also found that most deaths were of those younger than 40[80] with such findings agreeing with those of the MIM study.

The MIM study further analysed the number of AIDS-related cases occurring among professionals, including teachers in the Ministry of Education between 1995 and 2000, as shown in Figure 7.6. Between 1995 and 2000, of the total number of deaths (2 265) of professionals recorded in the Ministry, 9.8% were HIV/AIDS-related, with the proportion being highest in 1995, but remaining relatively constant thereafter.[81]

Figure 7.6: Estimation of number of HIV/ AIDS-related deaths in MoE 1995-2000

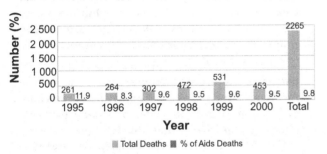

Source: Government of Malawi and UNDP

7.3.2 Malawi Police Service

The Malawi Police Service plays a crucial role in maintaining law and order and escorting and guarding election materials during elections in Malawi. The GoM/UNDP 2002 study found that death was the major cause of attrition in the service. Of the total 3 628 employees lost between 1990 and 2000, 46% were due to death, 27% to retirement, 16% to dismissal, 6% to redundancy and 5% to resignation. Figure 7.7 shows the trends in the causes of attrition among policemen between 1990 and 2000.[82]

The trend through the years (see Figure 7.7) shows that attrition through death has been on the rise. Further analysis of the data showed that 16% of deaths reported in the Malawi Police Force were AIDS-related.[83]

The MEC has had problems in updating the voters' roll as the system does not allow the timely purging of deceased voters. During the 2004 elections, both the NSO and the opposition parties challenged the

Figure 7.7: General attrition by cause in Malawi Police Service (n=3 628)

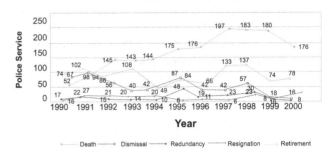

figures on release of the voters' roll as they felt that the figures had been deliberately inflated so as to allow the UDF, the then ruling party, to win the elections. The MEC was thus forced to clean up the voters' roll, with the final figures of registered voters, after more than a million voters had been purged from the roll, closely approximating the projections made by the NSO. The correct and timely compilation of the voters' roll and its subsequent maintenance requires well qualified and skilled personnel, especially as the registration of births and deaths is not centralised.

Neither the chronically ill nor their care-givers might be able to travel to polling stations to register, a problem that is compounded by the fact that personnel involved with registration do not visit homes in Malawi. The time lapse that occurs between registration and actual voting might lead to an inability to vote due to chronic illness.

8. Impact on political parties and policy proposals

In EISA Research Report no. 21, Patel notes the critical role played by political parties in the democratisation process, finding that they are "key to the institutionalisation and consolidation of democracy".[84] Political parties are usually the primary mechanism for citizens' active participation in national political institutions. Therefore, they should genuinely promote alternative policies, in terms of internal democracy and popular organisation, rather than simply empower individuals with no particular agenda.

Many political parties that participated in the first independent elections did not survive thereafter, as Malawi became a single-party MCP system until 1992, when the pressure groups AFORD and UDF formed, turning into political parties after the 1993 referendum which was aimed at determining whether Malawi should become a multiparty system. This section examines how the HIV/AIDS epidemic has affected the functioning and policy-making of the more than 30 currently operating political parties.

8.1 Difficulties determining impact on political parties

In assessing the impact of the HIV/AIDS epidemic on the institutional capacity of Malawian political parties, the present study is limited by four factors. First, most of these parties, apart from the MCP, have emerged only over the last ten to twelve years. Of the nine parties that won parliamentary seats in the 2004 elections, only three were more than ten years old: the MCP was founded in 1959 and AFORD and the UDF were both founded in 1992. The rest had been founded within three years prior to the elections. As such, most parties in Malawi are institutionally fluid and weak, with simple structures and lacking records that might otherwise constitute an institutional memory.

Second, a 1998 study showed that no Malawian party keeps membership lists, so that they do not know their own size and also fail to distinguish between members and supporters, therefore making determining how the HIV/AIDS epidemic is affecting their numbers and sizes difficult.[85] The parties lack both set requirements and registration systems for members. Though parties with local-level organisational structures are broad-based, most parties are active only during elections.

Third, a study of inter- and intra-party conflict in Malawi published in 2002 showed that, instead of political parties being broad-based coalitions with shared views,[86] they are largely mere vehicles for seizing power and gaining access to state resources. The parties, characterised by ethno-linguistic and regionalist differences, tend to be manipulated to suit their leaders' personal ambitions.

Most district party members stated that their parties kept no records of dead members or the cause of death, and had scant recall of how many had died. The lack of written policy proved their institutional incapacity. The legal framework governing party registration, regulation and conduct comprises:

• Section 40 1(a) of the Constitution, which

entrenches the right to form, join and participate in the activities of, as well as to recruit members for, a political party, while 1(b) allows campaigning for a political party or cause.

• The Political Parties (Registration and Regulation) Act (2:07), which provides the legal framework for the registration and deregistration of political parties.

• The PPEA (2:01),which outlines the conditions and methods, including nomination of candidates, in terms of which political parties can participate in parliamentary and presidential elections.

• The Communications Act No. 41 of 1998, which ensures political parties have equal access to the media during elections.

All parties registered must conform to the universal political rights enshrined in the Constitution and not be founded along racial or ethnic lines. However, almost all the major parties in Malawi are regionally based, drawing their major membership and support from the ethnic groups in those regions, usually the source of origin of their founder or current leader.

When the HIV/AIDS epidemic especially affects a particular rural/urban geographical area, it therefore tends largely to affect the party that draws much of its support from that area or from a particular ethnic group. Given that the HIV prevalence in Malawi is higher in the urban than in the rural areas, the parties with a large urban base will clearly be worse affected than those with predominantly rural bases, with the most vulnerable being the UDF, with its large urban support base in the South. Equally susceptible would be the elitist class-based parties with largely middle-class urban support, such as PPM, PETRA, and the Malawi Forum for Unity and Democracy (MAFUNDE).

Fourth, constitutionally, political parties are neither required to register nor are they subject to regulation by a parliamentary act. As political parties started to register before the Constitution came into force at the beginning of the political transition from one-party to multiparty politics in the early 1990s, their registration is governed by the 1993 Political Parties (Registration and Regulation) Act (2:07). Patel observes that "the law does not define political parties as such, although references are made to them in many sections of the Constitution".[87] The Act, which stipulates that a party may comprise no fewer than 100 members, requires any application for party registration to contain the party's constitution and manifesto, plus the names and addresses of interim executive committee members.

Parties are registered with the Registrar of Political Parties in the Registrar General's office. Malawi has seen many parties formed, led by veteran politicians who personalise and own all associated vehicles and infrastructure. Figure 8.1 shows the increase in the number of political parties in Malawi since 1994, resulting in the more than 37 political parties registered in 2006.

Figure 8.1: Number of political parties

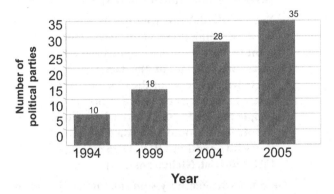

Due to the lack of a political party regulatory mechanism, these institutions fail to record their membership and policies, so it is difficult to determine how the HIV/AIDS epidemic is affecting the composition and membership of individual parties.

The fluidity of party membership compounds the problem, with no distinction drawn between party members and supporters, which are characterised by the unrecorded, unrestricted movement between parties. All political parties will be affected similarly by HIV/AIDS due to such freedom of movement.

8.2 Potential effects on leadership structures

Leadership levels are likely to be badly affected by HIV/AIDS. Currently, there are 37 registered political parties in Malawi. Between August 2004 and September 2005 some of the parties merged or disbanded, while many became dysfunctional shortly after the May 2004 elections. In terms of their structures and functions, the parties are governed by their individual constitutions that describe their hierarchies and administrative structures.

In most cases, the hierarchical structures start with branch committees at village level, rising through the following committee levels: area (ward for some);

constituency; district; region; to the national, which may have different names depending on the individual party. For example, some parties prefer to call their branches zones, while others, such as the PPM and AFORD, do not have regional committees.

Most parties have both hierarchical and administrative structures, with the latter rising from chairperson/governor at the local (branch or zone) level to the national president/chairperson. As well as all positions having either one or two deputies and vice-heads, there are secretaries general, treasurers, publicity secretaries, organising secretaries, press secretaries, legal advisers and directors for specific areas, such as women, youth and foreign affairs. Most parties also have various internal committees at the different levels, including disciplinary, fund-raising, publicity and special events committees.

As the subsequent section shows, all the parties involved with this study reported having lost some personnel at different structural levels, though, due to the absence of comprehensive records, it is difficult to determine the degree and effects of the losses incurred. For example, scattered confidential correspondence between the district officials and the national executive of the MCP show that the party lost 22 members from its district committees, at least 13 members from its regional committees, and eight members from its central executive committee between 1987 and 1993.

The records, which are not comprehensive, do not state the cause of death, so how many were AIDS-related is unknown. However, of the 22 deaths at district level, 19 occurred between 1990 and 1993, and of the 13 at regional level, 11 occurred during the same period, with all eight at national executive level also occurring during this period. Such a pattern suggests a connection with the effects of the pandemic felt at the time. The connection of the deaths to the most vulnerable age group would have been much clearer if the ages at which the deaths occurred were known.

8.3 Integrity of electoral process

Almost all Ntcheu and Mzimba district party officials interviewed for the study expressed the opinion that, though the effects of the HIV/AIDS pandemic were generally severe, they did not challenge the integrity of the 2004 general elections, due to few of the electorate not being able to vote as a result of AIDS-related ailments.

Since all eligible Malawians may vote, district officials strove to ensure the participation of PLWHAs and their care-givers in the elections. Chiefs can facilitate the registration and voting of all those who are bedridden if the MEC takes the appropriate lead.

8.4 Party capacity to campaign

District party officials from the UDF, RP and MCP interviewed for this study acknowledged that some PLWHAs who were party members could not campaign on behalf of their parties due to HIV/AIDS-related illness, resulting in the immediate despatch of replacements. Some of those who had to be replaced were seasoned campaigners, who were unable to attend campaign rallies and even vote due to their illness.

Identifying replacements was difficult and time-consuming, according to some UDF respondents. Campaigning was disrupted for those attending the funerals of relatives/friends, although not to a significant extent, it appears.

8.5 Party practice

Political parties claimed to deliberately include HIV/AIDS issues in their campaigning after they became aware that many were ignorant about HIV transmission and prevention. Party officials then started to advise the electorate to use condoms during sexual intercourse, to remain faithful to their spouses, to attend VCT, to seek medical attention if HIV positive and to avoid stigmatisation and discrimination. Parties also encouraged PLWHAs to register and vote, as they were entitled to do.

The inclusion of HIV/AIDS prevention and treatment messages in campaigning was best exemplified by the president of the UDF, Dr Bakili Muluzi, whose slogan was "Tipewe! Tipewe Edzi chifukwa ilibe mankhwala", which means "Let us avoid AIDS, because it has no cure!"

The *Mail & Guardian* of 21–27 May 2004 reported that AIDS was a key issue in Malawi's general elections, with nearly all political parties, including the MCP, promising universal access to ART, despite the country's limited resources and the fact that antiretrovirals were not freely available at the time.[88]

The emphasis on HIV/AIDS treatment by political parties not only showed awareness of the pandemic, but also indicated political opportunism, appealing to men, women, the youth and PLWHAs. However, their lobbying on the issue did not appear to attract votes, probably due to pervasive denial (De Waal, 2006). Instead, development seemed to attract the most attention during the 2004 polls:

> … They want to hear about schools, hospitals and bridge construction. They want to hear about food distribution. They did not vote because we talked about AIDS. People love immoral behaviour and they do not want to be reprimanded in public. [UDF official, Mzimba District]

> But people did not vote for us because we were telling them about AIDS. People want to hear about development in most cases. We talk about the fact that our party will take care of the sick and other related issues. But these did not make people to vote for us. Those who wanted to vote for us would have voted for us any way with or without HIV/AIDS messages. [MCP official, Ntcheu District].

Despite such negativity, some officials emphasised the need to include HIV/AIDS in campaigns to maintain the health of their supporters.

8.6 Implications for policy, programme development

Few programmatic, or even ideological, differences exist among Malawian political parties,[89] so that they are not mobilised around matters of national importance, such as HIV/AIDS. In a study done in 2004 on HIV/AIDS and leadership, it was found that while some parties, such as the UDF and PPM, devoted sections of their manifestos to HIV/AIDS, it was still a peripheral issue,[90] not clearly formulated in terms of written party policy, programmes and strategic plans.[91] [92] Without regular conventions and conferences, consultation processes are ill-defined, with most crucial political decision-making lacking a democratic vote. Both the KAF and the Netherlands Institute for Multiparty Democracy (IMD) have to develop capacity aimed at formulating related party programmes and policies.

Malawi political parties lack ideological commitment:

> Rather than promoting political norms, beliefs and values, political parties in Malawi are structured as 'issue pushers' that appear incoherent, unsystematic

Table 8.1: Focus areas in party manifestos		
Party	Manifesto Title	Key Coverage and Emphasis
MCP	*Reconciliation, Reconstruction and Development*	• Economic and social development • Agricultural development • Private sector development • Infrastructural development • Fiscal development • Democracy and good governance: separation of powers • Gender equality, women empowerment • Social policies: education, health and social welfare
Mgwirizano Coalition	*Governance for Sustainable Development*	• Good governance and democracy: separation of powers, respect for human rights, rule of law • Anticorruption fight • Economic development • Agricultural subsidies • Sound international relations • Social and economic equity in development • Gender equity: protection of widows, women and orphans • HIV/AIDS policies • Private sector development • Fiscal discipline, effective revenue generation and management • Vocational and skills education • Improved health, especially primary health care
NDA	*Towards Prosperous Malawi*	• Gender equity: protection of widows, women and orphans • Fight against corruption • Economic development • Agricultural subsidies • Sound international relations • Social and economic equity in development • Good governance and democracy: separation of powers, respect of human rights, rule of law • Fiscal discipline, efficient revenue collection • Spiritual and ethical issues • Family welfare
UDF	*Forging Ahead with Social and Economic Transformation – Unity, Democracy and Development*	• Poverty alleviation • Sound economic management • Robust international and local trade • Infrastructural development • Good governance, democracy and human rights • Youth development • Gender equity • Private sector development • Fight against unemployment • Free education, increased literacy and vocational education

and not committed to ideologies. That is, besides the availability of ideological resources in the country such as the existence of more than 80 per cent of the peasantry in the countryside, a sizeable workforce, students, the mass of farmers and the emerging political elite, parties fail to articulate particular interests of these social strata….Instead of cultivating class-based interests, world views, political norms, values and beliefs, these parties merely optimise regionalism and ethnicity.[93]

Nevertheless, political parties in Malawi refer to the contents of their campaign manifestos, though differing very little from one another, as expressions of policy and as the points of "difference" between them.[94] A brief overview of some of the key party manifestos for the 2004 elections provides evidence of such similarities.

Most Malawian parties clearly lack specified HIV/AIDS policies or programmes. However, pandemic-related issues are touched on in the general statements on social policies, especially those relating to women, gender, children and orphans. The reference to widows and orphans is a tacit admission of the effects of the HIV/AIDS epidemic on Malawian society. Similarly, the focus on the improvement of health care and health facilities acknowledges the pressure created by the pandemic and related illnesses on the country's health care system.

The contents of party manifestos are not translated into, or extracted from, written policy documents. As Patel has observed, "even after a decade of democratic transition, Malawi's political parties are based on personalities rather than ideologies, and it is difficult to distinguish one party from another on the basis of what they stand for."[95] The result is that "in spite of the political party system gaining ground in the country, the choice for the voter is severely limited….Parties do not offer much choice to the electorate in terms of policies and ideologies…"[96]

No clear evidence exists of party policy platforms being used to guide action once the parties are elected to the government, as party messages are relatively weak in terms of substantive national matters, instead centring more on personalities. As the African Union Election Observer Mission said, in relation to the 2004 elections,

The nature of the campaign was of great concern. The campaigns did not focus on issues as such but on personalities and character assassination. The use of language was often intimidating, provocative and insulting. The practice of handouts was a disturbing feature. The Observer Team will be happy to see a culture emerging in Malawi of clean and dignified campaigns that address issues and help the voters make informed decisions as they exercise their right to choose leaders.[97]

Non-delivery on campaign promises is identified as an issue of concern by academics and CSOs,[98] although the Malawi public generally has been rather apathetic about such issues. To date, no evidence exists of an organised public outcry, protest, open demands or any demonstration of concern over such non-delivery on campaign promises. If anything, these are confined to individualised expression of concern.

9. Political opinion, civic participation

Using Afrobarometer survey data from Rounds one (1999), two (2003) and three (2005) surveys, this section explores how Malawians prioritise HIV/AIDS in relation to other major problems that they face and for which they demand government intervention.

Figure 9.1 shows what respondents felt to be the most important problems that the government needed to address in 1999: economic (39%); food security and supply (15%); personal security (12%); and health (10%).[99] No problems were acknowledged by 3% of the respondents.[100]

It is apparent from Figure 9.1 that in 1999 the most important problems that Malawians felt should be addressed by the government were economic and financial in nature at 39% and this was followed by food security and food supply-related problems at 15%, personal security problems at 12% and then health-related problems at 10%. The rest of the problems, as can be seen in Figure 9.1, were mentioned in fewer than 10% of the cases. It is also important to note that 3% of the respondents either said that there were no problems or that they did not know any problems.[101]

Clearly, generally health, including HIV/AIDS, was not perceived as a major problem requiring government intervention. Despite the fact that HIV

Figure 9.1: Most important problem

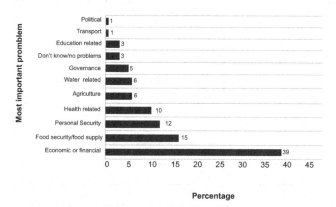

Source: Afrobarometer Surveys

prevalence was at its peak at the time, most respondents assigned priority to economic and survival-related food security issues.

Table 9.1 shows that respondents felt that food shortages/famine and farming-related problems, unemployment and poverty were the most important problems that needed to be addressed by the government in the 2003 and 2005 rounds of the Afrobarometer surveys. Such prioritisation is understandable in the light of Malawi experiencing a severe famine prior to 2005.

The number of respondents who regarded health as the most important problem in 1999 (10%) decreased to 4.3% in 2003, and then 3.1% in 2005. In a country where 52% of the respondents live below the poverty line,[102] the prioritisation of poverty is not surprising.

Table 9.1 also shows that in 2003 only 0.5% of the respondents considered AIDS as the most important problem that the government needed to address, with the percentage dropping still further to 0.3% in 2005, despite nearly all Malawians aged 15–49 years old having heard about HIV/AIDS[103] and the increase in the number of orphans due to the epidemic.[104]

In a qualitative study conducted among adolescents aged 12–19 years old, they stated that they found poverty to be the most critical problem that they faced, as it resulted in a general lack of basic necessities, such as food, clothing and school-related materials. When asked how they compared their most important problem with that of HIV/AIDS, most stated that they found HIV/AIDS to be of a more pressing nature than other issues that they had cited earlier because it is incurable, while solutions can be found for other problems; it has resulted in many children being orphaned; many of the

critically ill cannot work; and PLWHAs suffer stigma and discrimination. Some out-of-school adolescents, petty traders and street children said that AIDS was not as critical as other problems they faced in their lives because they needed to satisfy their hunger and other basic needs more immediately.[105]

The respondents in the Afrobarometer surveys were asked how long they spent caring for orphans, whether their poor physical health reduced their number of working hours and whether the degree of stress that they experienced left them feeling exhausted.

Figure 9.2 shows how much time respondents claimed to spend caring for orphans. It shows that 53% of the respondents did not care for orphans, while more than 40% spent more than five hours caring for them, 8.4% spent three to five hours, 6.6% spent one to two hours and 5.2% less than one hour. While children can be orphaned by other causes, several are orphaned due to the HIV/AIDS epidemic.

Table 9.2 shows the proportion of respondents who reported that their physical health reduced the number of work hours they put in either inside or outside their home between 2003 and 2005. While, in 2003, 43.3% of the respondents said that their physical health never reduced the amount of work that they normally did, the number that responded in this way increased to 53.6% in 2005, while the percentage of those who found this often occurring decreased from 18.7% to 12.8% over the same period.

As can be seen in Table 9.2, little change was found in the proportion of respondents who said that during the reference period their physical health always reduced the amount that they normally did inside or outside their homes. Although inconclusive, the findings seem to indicate some improvement in the physical health of Malawians. Such improvement might be due to the introduction of free antiretrovirals in 2004, as accessing antiretrovirals until then had been prohibitively expensive for many who

Figure 9.2: Time spent caring for orphans

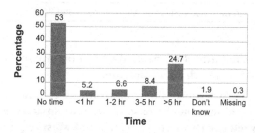

Source: Afrobarometer 2003

Table 9.1: Most important problem (n=1 200)

Most important problem	2003 (%)	2005 (%)
Nothing/No problems	0.8	.3
Management of economy	9.2	3.2
Wages, incomes and salaries	1.3	1.0
Unemployment	10.3	2.6
Poverty/destitution	12.2	3.8
Rates and taxes	0.8	2.0
Loans/credit	2.0	3.3
Farming/agriculture	11.5	12.4
Food shortage/famine	28.4	48.9
Drought	0.3	.5
Land	0.2	.2
Transportation	0.4	.5
Communications	0.6	.1
Infrastructure/roads	2.4	2.4
Education	3.8	3.8
Housing	-	.3
Electricity	0.8	.2
Water supply	3.1	6.1
Orphans/street children/homeless	1.3	.4
Services (other)	0.1	.3
Health	4.2	3.1
AIDS	0.5	.3
Sickness/disease	-	.1
Crime and security	4.0	.9
Corruption	0.8	.8
Political violence	0.2	.1
Political instability/ethnic tensions	0.4	.2
Discrimination/inequality	-	.2
Gender issues/women's rights	0.1	.2
Democracy/political rights	0.2	.2
Other	-	.4
Don't know	0.8	1.5
Total	100.0	100.0

Source: Afrobarometer Surveys: Malawi, 2003 and 2005

could not afford to spend MK2 500 (approximately US$18) a month on medication.

Table 9.3 shows the proportion of respondents who said that they were so worried or anxious that they felt tired, worn out or exhausted. Most respondents reported feeling neither worried nor anxious or only feeling so occasionally. In 2003, 15.3% reported often feeling worried or anxious, with 18.9% reported being so in 2005. While the majority were either not worried or only occasionally worried in the said period, more than a quarter of the respondents were either often or constantly worried or anxious.

Table 9.2: Amount of work normally done inside or outside the home reduced by ill health (n=1 200)

Number of times	2003		2005	
	Frequency	Percentage	Frequency	Percentage
Missing	2	.2	0.0	0.0
Never	519	43.3	643	53.6
Just once or twice	416	34.7	368	30.7
Many times	224	18.7	153	12.8
Always	37	3.1	35	2.9
Don't know	2	.2	1	.1
Total	1 200	100.0	1 200	100.0
Source: Afrobarometer Surveys				

Table 9.3: Amount of time, worry or anxiety resulted in tiredness or exhaustion

Number of times	2003		2005	
	Frequency	Percentage	Frequency	Percentage
Never	670	55.8	639	53.3
Just once or twice	282	23.5	258	21.5
Many times	183	15.3	227	18.9
Always	49	4.1	75	6.3
Don't know	16	1.3	1	.1
Total	1 200	100.0	1 200	100.0
Source: Afrobarometer Surveys				

Figure 9.3: Number of close friends and relatives who have died from AIDS

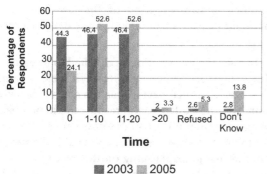

Source: Afrobarometer Survey

Table 9.4 shows the proportion of respondents and the time that the respondents spent taking care of their own illness. Even though many respondents did not rate HIV/AIDS among the most important problems encountered in Malawi, the majority (686 of the 1 200 or 57.2%) said that they spent more than five hours taking care of their own illnesses.

Table 9.5 shows the amount of time that respondents spent caring for sick household members, with 43.4% of the respondents reporting spending more than five hours taking care of sick household members. Figure 9.3 and Tables 9.2 to 9.5 generally show that, despite HIV/AIDS receiving a very low rating, there is very high morbidity among Malawians, which might indicate the impact of HIV/AIDS. When respondents in the Afrobarometer surveys of 2003 and 2005 were asked whether they had had friends and relatives who had died of HIV/AIDS in 2003, 34.9% stated that they had had, with the corresponding proportion in 2005 being 58.6%. Figure 9.3 shows the clear increase in the number of close friends and relatives who were reported to have died of AIDS. The proportion of respondents who reported no friends or relatives dying of AIDS decreased from 44.3% in 2003 to 24.2% in 2005, with an increased proportion of respondents reporting that they had lost between one and 10, 11 and 20 and more than 20 friends and relatives. These statistics might either show that Malawians are generally becoming more open about HIV/AIDS or that there is an increase in the number of deaths due to HIV/AIDS.

Most Malawians seem to prioritise immediate requirements, putting everyday survival needs first.

Table 9.4: Amount of time spent taking care of own illness

Amount of time spent	2003	
	Frequency	Percentage
No answer	2	.2
Spend no time	95	7.9
Less than 1 hour	102	8.5
1-2 hours	113	9.4
3-5 hours	131	10.9
More than 5 hours	686	57.2
Don't know	71	5.9
Total	1 200	100.0

Table 9.5: Amount of time spent caring for sick household members

Time spent	2003	
	Frequency	Percentage
No answer	5	.4
Spend no time	120	10.0
Less than 1 hour	129	10.8
1-2 hours	190	15.8
3-5 hours	184	15.3
More than 5 hours	521	43.4
Don't know	51	4.3
Total	1 200	100.0

10. HIV/AIDS impact on voter turnout

According to Section 77 of the Malawian Constitution, all Malawians who are qualified to register as voters are eligible to vote in any general election, by-election, presidential election, local government election or referendum. Such qualifications include citizenship or continued residence in the country for a period of seven years or more; being 18 years of age or older; and having residence, birthplace, employment or operating a business in the constituency where one intends to vote.

The registration process during elections has generally been marred by irregularities and logistical problems, such as shortage of registration forms and usable recording equipment and a lack of transport for delivering the required materials to registration centres.

The lack of institutionalised citizen registra-

tion systems enables under-aged people to vote in Malawi, in contravention of the law. Also, as no national death register exists, some deceased might be registered voters.

In 2004 the registration period had to be extended due to logistical problems, after civil society claimed that the scheduled period was too short. The extension was not adequately resourced; hence, some qualified potential voters did not register.[106] Similar problems were also experienced in 1999,[107] suggesting not just poor planning on the part of the MEC, but also a failure to learn from past mistakes.[108] The shortcomings undermined both public confidence in the electoral body and the integrity of the elections.

For its part, the commission argued that most of the logistical problems arose from poor funding and delays in, as well as the inadequacies of, technical and financial donor support. As well as being a tacit admission of poor planning, such an argument also shows the extent to which Malawian democratic elections have not yet been institutionalised as funding should already have formed a major component of the standard budget. Given that the Malawian Constitution requires that elections be conducted every five years, such financial shortcomings should not arise.

The HIV/AIDS epidemic would potentially affect the above development in a number of ways. First, the planning for the elections and the production and distribution of electoral materials require that the size of the voting population be known. The MEC's failure to produce and distribute adequate amounts of registration and voting material was partly a result of the fact that the size of the voting population was not precisely known. Second, the conduct, administration and management of the registration and voting processes require qualified and skilled electoral staff.

Given that the MEC does not have its own field staff for such exercises, it relies on the staff from the public services. As has been shown elsewhere in the report, such groups have been badly affected by the HIV/AIDS epidemic, with the resultant impact on the electoral system and electoral governance.

Third, the findings from the management and administration of the 2004 elections show that the MEC did not provide preferential treatment to those infected by HIV/AIDS. As most polling stations were at public schools and centres, sanitation facilities, such as toilets, though limited, were available.

10.1 Voters' roll and HIV/AIDS

The component of the electoral system most susceptible to the impact of the HIV/AIDS epidemic is the voters' roll, and its mismanagement. The Malawian voters' roll is not regularly updated, though it should be by fresh registration at the start of the electoral process. The effects of the HIV/AIDS pandemic on the country's demographic database compounds these tensions. With deaths not being reported in time and the roll not being subsequently purged of the dead voters, there is a real risk that the roll is bloated with the names of dead people.

The database on which the voters' roll is based is therefore not entirely credible as its exact size remains unknown. The absence of a civic register means that there is no system of reporting births and deaths, so that the country's demographic database tends to be out of date. The voters' roll thus inherently creates political tensions, especially when elections are announced.

In 1999, a total of 5 071 822 voters were registered: 2 417 713 in the South; 1 975 203 in the Centre; and 678 906 in the North. However, in April 2004, the MEC announced that 6 668 839 voters had registered for the 18 May 2004 presidential and parliamentary elections.[109] While opposition political parties and other national institutions challenged this figure, the most severe criticism came from the NSO, who described the figure as "bogus" because it did not conform to the country's natural demographic trends.

A mathematician and statistician at the Polytechnic, one of the constituent colleges of the University of Malawi, who was also Director of Publicity for the opposition NDA, described the figure as "absurd and a pointer to [election] rigging".[110]

The projection from the NSO at that time was that there were 5 594 081 people aged 18 years or older in Malawi who were eligible to vote: 2 635 507 from the South; 2 260 480 from the Centre; and 698 094 from the North. Figure 10.1 shows the number of voters registered in 1999 and the number of voters registered as of April 2004, as announced by the MEC and the NSO projections in this regard.

Figure 10.1 indicates discrepancies between the projected NSO figures and the figures released by the MEC in April 2004. The NSO argued at the time that:

> Our projections [based on the last (1998/99) national population census] are [that] the population has grown at an average rate of 3.2 per cent. But if you calculate the average rates at which the Commission's figures are based, you will find that they are way above the normal population growth rate.

The MEC registered some 5 071 822 voters for the 1999 general elections. The figure for the 2004 elections suggested an increase of one million, despite 106 086 registered voters being reported dead during the previous five years whose names were meant to have been removed from the voters' register. To some analysts, including the NSO, such figures did not make sense, especially when broken down into regional distributions. Malawi has three administrative regions, as shown in Figure 10.1.

Figure 10.1 also shows that the 678 906 voters registered in the North in 1999 had increased to 924 879 in 2004, according to the MEC, representing a 36% increase. In the Centre, while 1 975 203 voters registered in 1999, 2 703 621 registered in 2004, amount-

Figure 10.1: Registered voters according to different sources

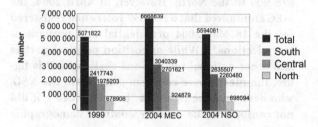

ing to another 36% increase. In the South, 3 040 339 voters registered in 2004, compared to 2 417 713 in 1999, amounting to an increase of 25%.

According to the NSO, the average population growth for Malawi is 3.2%; hence, the number of registered voters, as released by the MEC, was perceived by many as excessive. According to the *Weekend Nation* (17–18 April 2004), "either [the adult] population is unknown or 6.5 million voters are from Mars….Even if the Commission assumes a 100% registration rate – which is not possible even where people get punished for not registering – the 6.5 million figure cannot be accurate. There simply are not that many adults of 18 years and above in our country."

The management of the voters' roll in 2004 was further criticised by donors who provided technical and financial support for the elections, with the MEC using two parallel voters' rolls: one computerised and one manual, though donors had recommended only the former. The MEC argued that they lacked adequate capacity to efficiently manage such a roll, as the manual roll would be easier to use in remote rural areas.

The MEC was accused of being used by the UDF to manipulate the voters' roll so as to enhance that party's chances of winning the elections.[111] The UDF was accused of trying to get some of its supporters to register more than once, so that they could cast multiple votes in the elections[112] and also of purchasing voting certificates. No evidence of deliberate skewing of figures in favour of the southern region to advantage the governing party was found.

A weekly paper reported that "two days after the voter registration exercise closed, irregularities [had] emerged with the ruling party being accused by civil society and opposition parties of offering jobs and money, distributing starter packs, in exchange for voter registration numbers."[113] The opposition parties and CSOs argued that the voters who lost their registration certificates in this way, such as those who did not register, were disfranchised.

However, voting regulations in Malawi allow for

a person who has lost his/her voter certificate to vote, as long has his/her name can be traced on the register on the polling day. One also has to possess authenticated identification or be positively identified by the polling staff and monitors.

The MEC, due to its apparent inefficiency, lost its credibility as a trustworthy election management body. Due to the disputes arising from the registers, the MEC then started, with the help of a South African company, to clean up the voters' roll. The exercise reduced the number of registered voters from the April 2004 MEC figure of 6.7 million to 5.8 million. Figure 10.2 shows the then regional distribution.

The number of registered voters in the North and Centre, the areas regarded as the opposition strongholds, increased so much as to pose, when combined, a potential threat to the governing party, particularly in the presidential elections. At the time, the opposition parties were contemplating fielding a single presidential candidate.

The opposition parties got a court injunction postponing the voting date by two days to allow sufficient time for the stakeholders to inspect the voters' roll, as required by the PPEA. The delay, Dulani argues, arose from the failure of the MEC to operate within the prescribed rules and regulations.[114] The irregularities in the registration process and the mismanagement of the voters' roll might have affected the voters' response to, and subsequent participation in, the presidential and parliamentary elections.

Figure 10.2: Number of registered voters in 1999 and 2004

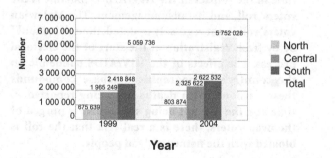

10.1.1 Voter turnout: Trends in 1993-2004

In Malawi, the 1993 referendum on whether the country should change to a multiparty state or remain a single-party state was followed by presidential elections conducted in 1994, 1999 and 2004.

Figure 10.3 shows the voter turnout during the elections.

It shows that the voter turnout for the 2004 presidential elections was much lower at 59% than the preceding 69% in 1993, 80% in 1994 and 94% in 1999. The turnout was higher in the North and Centre, at 64% and 61% respectively, than in the South at 56%, which had a negative impact on the performance of the UDF, which had previously been the dominant party in the latter area.[115]

Public disenchantment with the electoral processes is one of the major reasons contributing to low voter turnout. During the 1993 referendum and the 1994 general elections that followed, Malawians were showered with many promises which remain unfulfilled. Most Malawians choose not to participate in the electoral processes, as shown by the 2004 election results, because they do not materially benefit from the elections.[116]

10.2 Voter turnout

The economically productive 15–49 year olds, who are most active in the elections, are those who tend to be chronically ill with HIV/AIDS-related illnesses. FGDs held with PLWHAs revealed that those who fall into this group are finding it increasingly difficult to register, campaign and vote. Others might also fail to register or vote due to their having to nurse their chronically ill relatives. A special vote is needed for such cases.

10.3 Trends in HIV prevalence in Malawi

At national level, the estimated prevalence of HIV among the 15–49 year olds increased between 1985 and 1999, after which it started declining. According to the national HIV surveillance system, in 2005 the HIV prevalence was estimated at 14%. As can be seen in Figure 10.4, the rate of HIV infection has stabilised over the last seven years.

Figure 10.5 shows the prevalence of HIV among the defined population groups according to the 2004/5 DHS, with HIV prevalence at national level being estimated at 12% among the 15 to 49 year olds, with it peaking between 30 and 44 years. The prevalence of HIV among adolescents aged 15 to 19 is low,

Figure 10.3: Voter turnout as a percentage

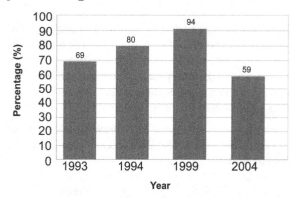

Figure 10.4: Prevalence of HIV among 15-49 year olds, 1996-2004

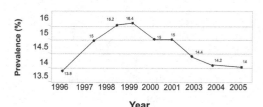

Sources: UNAIDS Secretariat, nd; Tsoka et al, 2002; National HIV Surveillance System

so they need to be targeted with strongly worded behavioural change interventions.

According to the NAC, annually about 80 000 people in Malawi die from AIDS and nearly 110 000 infections occur among young people.[117] By the end of 2003, 900 000 people were living with HIV, of whom 460 000 were women.[118] More than half of the Malawian hospital beds are occupied by HIV/AIDS patients.[119] In the absence of AIDS, the number of deaths among people aged 15 to 49 years would have remained constant from 1985 until today, at about 22 000 a year. However, due to the presence of AIDS, adult mortality figures have more than tripled. Life expectancy is similarly now reduced to 40 years, whereas otherwise it would have been 56 years.[120]

Figure 10.5: HIV prevalence among persons aged 15-49

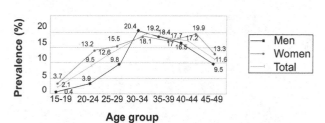

10.3.1 Malawi Electoral Commission mortality-related data

Data capturing and record keeping are problematic, as the 1999 voters' roll does not show the number of registered voters who died after the 1994 presidential and parliamentary elections. However, the 2004 voters' roll enumerates the number of deaths occurring in each district from 1999 to 2004.

Figures 10.6, 10.7 and 10.8 show the percentage of registered voters who died in each region during that period.

Figure 10.6: Percentage of voter deaths in Northern region, 1999-2004

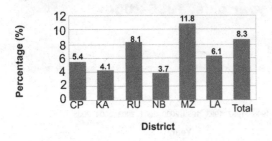

Figure 10.7: Percentage of voter deaths in Central region, 1999-2004

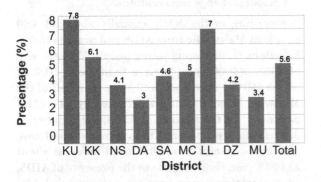

Figure 10.8: Percentage of voter deaths in Southern region, 1999-2004

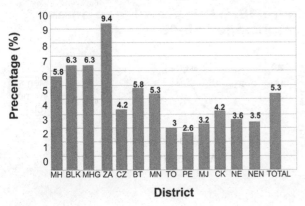

According to the MEC, a total of 803 874 voters were registered in the North in 2004, meaning that, by 2004, 7.3% (25 305) of the voters registered in the North had died. Mzimba District registered the highest percentage of deaths over this period at 11.8%, followed by Rumphi (8.1%); Likoma (6.1%); Chitipa (5.4%); Karonga (4.1%); and Nkhata Bay (3.7%).

As can be seen in Figure 10.7, the highest percentage of deaths among registered voters in the Centre during the same period occurred in Kasungu at 7.8%, followed by Lilongwe (7%); Nkhota Kota (6.1%); Mchinji (5%); Salima (4.6%); Dedza (4.2%); and Ntchisi (4.1%). Dowa and Ntcheu Districts reported fewer than 45 reported deaths. The Centre had a total of 2 325 622 voters registered, of whom 44 076 (5.6%) died over the period 1999–2004.

In the Southern region, a total of 2 622 532 voters were registered, of whom 48 153 (5.3%) registered voters had died.

As can be seen in Figure 10.8, Zomba recorded the highest proportion of deaths in the Southern region at 9.4%, followed by Balaka and Machinga, both at 6.3%. The North can be seen to have recorded the highest percentage (8.3%) of deaths out of the three regions, followed by the Centre (5.6%) and the South (5.3%). At the national level, Mzimba district in the North recorded the highest percentage of registered voters who died, followed by Zomba in the South and Kasungu in the Centre. One question that needs to be addressed is whether the HIV prevalence rates at district level are reflected in the MEC-recorded deaths of voters.

10.3.2 Voter death rate at district level

In districts where HIV prevalence is very high, more deaths are likely than in districts less affected by HIV. Figure 10.9 shows the relationship between HIV prevalence at district level and the death rates among voters, as reported by the MEC.

Figure 10.9: HIV prevalence and death rate at district level

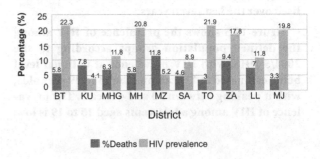

Figure 10.9 shows that Blantyre has the highest HIV prevalence rate in Malawi, followed by Thyolo, Mangochi, Mulanje and Zomba. Accordingly, Blantyre would have been expected to have the highest percentage of reported deaths in Malawi, followed by Thyolo and Mangochi. However, Mzimba, with an HIV prevalence rate of only 5.2%, which is much lower than that of Blantyre, Mangochi and Thyolo, recorded the highest percentage of reported deaths.

Though HIV prevalence is high in Blantyre, the area is urban and therefore better equipped with health care facilities to which many have access. The voter mortality percentage represents only those aged 18 years and above, while the HIV prevalence rate covers only the age group 15–49 years. As the MEC data does not show the proportion of registered voters who died and their ages, prevalence data cannot be directly compared to the percentage of deaths of voters. As a result, drawing any valid conclusions about the relationships explored in this section is difficult.

The names of voters who have died due to HIV/AIDS and other causes are not being timeously removed from the voters' roll. Hence, a system that will effectively purge deceased voters from the roll is urgently called for.

11. Focus groups: Role of stigma and discrimination

11.1 Introduction

Stigma can be defined as the act of identifying, labelling or attributing undesirable qualities to those who are perceived to be so shamefully different and deviant from the social ideal that the person or group is discredited and diminished. Discrimination refers to any distinction, exclusion or preference based on any ground. Acts of stigmatisation and discrimination might come in the form of sanctions, blame, harassment and violence targeted at others, such as those infected, or associated with, HIV/AIDS.[121]

Stigma and discrimination, which can be felt at individual, household and community level, are the two key factors that need to be addressed to effectively implement HIV prevention, care and treatment and support programmes. According to USAID, the fear of stigma and discrimination can prevent people from being tested and seeking treatment, care and support when needed; promote denial of being infected; discourage use of protection during sexual intercourse; and hinder PLWHAs from accessing basic social services, such as education, housing and employment.

Learning one's status by means of VCT is known to contribute to behavioural change, though about only 15% of Malawians aged 15 to 49 have taken such a course.[122] VCT enables the HIV-positive to access treatment, care and support programmes, such as ART, PMTCT and community home-based care services.

As of December 2005, more than 400 000 Malawians had been tested, as compared to the 149 540 tests performed in 2002. Before 2004, reluctance to undergo such testing was largely due to the inaccessibility of the costly antiretrovirals. The commencement of the free ART programme funded by the Global Fund now enables PLWHAs to live longer.

With the prevailing stigma and discrimination against those with HIV/AIDS,[123] one wonders what it is that motivates people to undergo such testing.

Those who have suffered from chronic diseases, which have resisted therapeutic interventions for some time, might decide to be tested. The desire to have children or to marry and a general awareness of vulnerability to HIV infection might lead to potential sufferers undergoing testing.

Most people who have decided to undergo testing visit VCT centres far from their place of residence due to the fear of stigma, and keep any positive results secret. HIV/AIDS-associated discrimination leads to the non-disclosure of results. The formation of PLWHA support groups, largely supported by low-profile individuals, has contributed significantly to the heightened disclosure of sero status. High-profile figures tend to avoid such groups because of the fear of stigma as reported in the Panos Southern Africa UNGASS report for Malawi. The same study also claimed that non-disclosure of status might be due to the fear of loss of employment or the possibility of being passed over for promotion.[124]

The decrease in stigma and discrimination, according to DHS 2000 data, was attributed by over 90% of the respondents to caring for AIDS-affected relatives at home. However, about half such respondents indicated that they believe that an HIV-positive co-worker should be dismissed from employment, thus suggesting some form of stigma and discrimination.

The 2004 DHS data showed improvement on these figures, with about 94% of the female and 97% of the male respondents expressing a willingness to care for HIV/AIDS-affected relatives at home.

The results of the DHS data also show that 82% of the male respondents would buy vegetables from an HIV-infected shopkeeper, 72.3% suggest an HIV-positive teacher should be allowed to teach, though 43.8% said the status of an HIV-positive family member should be kept secret. The corresponding figures for females were 66.6%, 66.6% and 64.8% respectively,[125] suggesting that, overall, women tend to be more negative towards PLWHAs. Stigma and discrimination is still deep-rooted, manifesting in many different forms with varied effects on PLWHAs and their societal interactions.

The impact of HIV/AIDS on PLWHAs and care-givers' capacity to participate in elections might mean that people lose interest in political life. PLWHAs might want to influence policy or participate in life-changing policy-making. Being ill might automatically dampen one's desire to choose a representative policy-maker. Societies might be accommodative of those PLWHAs who try to participate in public affairs. Certain mechanisms might facilitate such participation. Such were the issues discussed in the focus groups meetings held for this study.

11.2 Designing the discussions

The FGDs conducted in rural areas of Zomba, Mzimba and Ntcheu were participated in by 30 PLWHAs and care-givers, mainly the former, who comprised both eligible and registered voters. The CBOs and PLWHA support groups helped in identifying the relevant PLWHAs and care-givers. The FGDs aimed to determine whether attitudinal and structural factors prevented PLWHAs and their care-givers from participating in elections.

11.3 Structural challenges for PLWHAs and care-givers

During the FGDs, some PLWHAs expressed reluctance to take a stand on HIV/AIDS-related issues due to the stigma and discrimination that they suffer. At local community level, PLWHAs are perceived as "already dead".

In Zomba, some PLWHAs said they were too ill and weak to walk to the polling stations, which sometimes were located far from their homes. Other participants cited the long queues as discouraging their participation in the 2004 elections:

People with HIV/AIDS have got weak bodies. As a result, they cannot stand on long queues for a long time. Because of this some PLWHAs opted not to vote due to lack of a special provision to allow sick people including those who are HIV positive to be the first to vote. [FGD with PLWHAs and care-givers, TA Malemia, Zomba]

The time spent on taking care of the sick and orphans restricts participation in the elections. Funeral attendance also occupies much time that might otherwise be spent on politics, with funerals requiring up to two weeks of full-time attendance by close relatives.

Participants generally seemed to distrust politicians, regarding them as opportunists, long promising AIDS relief that failed to materialise, causing some PLWHAs in the FGDs to stay away from the polls despite registering. One Ntcheu participant equated voting with enriching the MP concerned, as, once elected, the MP would relocate to the city, neglecting his or her constituency.

While the lack of ablution facilities might have prevented some PLWHAs from voting, not all FGDs experienced such a problem.

11.3.1 Effects of HIV/AIDS-related stigma

In all the FGDs, the extent of one's illness appeared to worry the participants, causing them to withdraw from the elections, though the community's reaction to their physical condition appeared more of a problem. Some participants, feeling that their advanced stages of illness would draw curious stares and insults, stayed away from the polls to avoid embarrassment. In the Mzimba FGD, some participants said that in the 1999 general elections many PLWHAs who looked thin were questioned by other community members about why they were bothering to vote, knowing full well, as they did, that they were dying. At the Ntheu FGD, one participant commented, "Some just feel shy to go for voting because of the way they look. They think that people will just be staring at them because of their sickly looks."

Voting was generally felt to be necessary to ensure that candidates who were well equipped for dealing decisively with the pandemic were elected into office for the benefit of PLHWAs and their children.

A participant in the Zomba FGD, when seen

voting, was asked "Are you also going to vote? How long are you going to live? Do you want to die here while voting?" Another was told "You should really be attending political meetings, so that the MP can know you and the party can purchase a coffin for you when you die."

Some participants felt so hopeless and desperate that they saw no need to register. However, some PLWHAs did not feel intimidated by others' reaction to their conditions, saying "Even though some speak ill words to infected people...this does not discourage us to go for voting because we know that it is our right to do so..."

Reference was also made in the Ntcheu FGD to the children of PLWHAs being provided for by their voting for promising leaders. "We have children which we also would like to prepare their good future by electing good leaders."

In another Ntcheu FGD, participants reported encountering no problems, as many voting centres adjoined their villages, reducing congestion.

> This time around in 2004, there were a lot of voting centres set up and these areas were near to our villages...this reduced the burden of walking long distances and also congestion at the polling centres...because of this there were no problems we encountered so far. [FGD with PLWHAs and care-givers, Ntcheu]

Overall, other factors that encouraged voting were the need to elect leaders who would:

- Alleviate poverty;
- Undertake the financially burdensome care of orphans; and
- Strive to develop the road infrastructure, subsidise farming and build schools and markets.

While voting is seen as a means of ensuring the security of the next generation, optimism prevails as to its facilitating access to vital resources and infrastructure for improving the general living standards of communities.

The introduction of ART enables PLWHAs to emphasise enhancement of the quality of life rather than the inevitability of death:

> We wanted someone who could think about us...our welfare as people... We are able to access ARVs freely as compared to the past. Had it been not for these drugs, then you couldn't have found any head that you are seeing now. [PLWHAs participant in FGD, Ntcheu].

11.3.2 Participation of PLWHAs in politics

The exploitation of the contentious nature of the HIV/AIDS issue by politicians in their campaigning also raised concerns, with reference being made to certain political agents trying to discredit their opponents by dismissing them as PLWHAs.

Some participants suggested that such disparagement would be likely to discourage PLWHAs from participating in politics:

> In the absence of insults from the rest of the community members and sometimes from fellow PLWHAs, PLWHAs would more likely participate in politics. However, with the presence of insults, PLWHAs would participate less in politics. [FGD with PLWHAs and care-givers, Zomba]

While some felt the provision of readily accessible treatment had somewhat reduced stigma and discrimination, most participants felt non-disclosure was the better strategy. In relation to this, one of Ntcheu FGD participants stated that he had lost his position as a village committee member when he openly declared his HIV-positive status. "When people learned about my HIV status, they removed me from my position as a chairman...there is heavy stigmatisation which discourages us from participating in various village development activities..."

Another explained that she was delisted as a recipient of borrowed groundnut seed when her HIV-positive status became known.

Though the parliamentary committee on health and sub-committee on HIV/AIDS frequently report to the house on the national status of the epidemic, the house has not yet proposed mandatory testing. So far, no MP has disclosed his/her HIV status to serve as a role model to the nation. Fear of rejection by the electorate, ridicule by opponents and loss of political office could be the leading causes of this.

Strategic planning is needed to counter stigma and discrimination beyond the mere provision of VCT.

12. Conclusion and recommendations

This chapter has explored the impact of HIV/AIDS on electoral governance with special attention to the impact on Malawi's electoral system, electoral management and administration, the voters' roll and political parties, as well as its financial and human cost.

As has been seen, the death of a legislator automatically calls for a costly by-election, for purposes of replacing the deceased. Apart from having to depend on donor funding of elections, the long time that it takes to fill a parliamentary vacancy denies the electorate a voice and representation in the legislature for its duration.

The FPTP system, inherited from the British, has been marked by shortfalls. More resources will have to be spent on by-elections as a result of the increasing number of HIV/AIDS-related deaths of leaders. Electoral reform is urgently needed, given that the electoral system is unsustainable.

Further, the poorly staffed MEC largely depends on public servants and extra-commission staff for the administration and management of electoral processes. Death has been shown in this report to be the main factor responsible for the attrition of both teachers and police, posing a serious challenge to the MEC and the administration of elections. The MEC urgently requires an HIV/AIDS policy, due to the extensive amount of travelling and mobility undertaken during elections.

The number of deaths a year is increasing due to HIV/AIDS. While the 1980s toll was about 22 000 a year, it has now increased to 80 000. The lack of an efficient system for removing the deceased from the register has resulted in the voters' roll being bloated with names of the deceased. Malawi needs an efficient and effective electoral administration and management system for dealing with the potential threat of HIV/AIDS to electoral governance.

The electoral participation of PLWHAs should be facilitated. The creation of a special voting mechanism should be promoted by the relevant political institutions to ensure that the ill are not marginalised. Continuing civic and voter education should incorporate HIV/AIDS-related issues.

District party officials and community members have acknowledged the impact that HIV/AIDS has had on political campaigns and participation in voting. Political parties, since they rely on the electorate, should formulate their approach to management of the pandemic in terms of policy-making, party structures and membership.

Appendix 1: Some key donor-funded sectors in Malawi, 2005

Rank	Ministry/Institution	Total funding (Million US$)	% share of total donor funding
1	National Aids Commission	149.0	18.3%
2	Agriculture, Irrigation and Food Security	115.9	14.2%
3	Education, Science and Technology	107.1	13.2%
4	Health and Population	98.6	12.1%
5	Transport and Public Works	79.4	9.7%
6	Local Government and District Administration	51.8	6.4%
7	Water Development	35.6	4.4%
8	Natural Resources and Environmental Affairs	30.2	3.7%
9	Office of the President and Cabinet	29.3	3.6%
10	Finance	28.1	3.5%
11	Office of the First Vice-President	24.9	3.1%
12	Labour	14.4	1.8%
13	Economic Planning and Development	13.1	1.6%
14	Commerce and Industry	12.5	1.5%
15	Gender and Community Services	7.0	0.9%
16	National Statistical Office	4.1	0.5%
17	Youth, Sports and Culture	3.0	0.4%
18	Malawi Revenue Authority	2.4	0.3%
19	Justice	2.3	0.3%
20	Tourism, Parks and Wildlife	1.8	0.2%
Total		810.4	99.5%

Endnotes

1   For example see Government of Malawi and UNDP, 2002. *The Impact of HIV/AIDS on Human Resources in the Malawi Public Sector*, Lilongwe: Government of Malawi and UNDP.

2   See AfriMAP, 2006. *Political Participation in Malawi: A Country Study*, Johannesburg, AfriMAP.

3   Kalipeni, E., 2000. "Health and Disease in Southern Africa: A Comparative and Vulnerability Perspective", *Social Science and Medicine*, 50 (7/8).

4   Joint United Nations Programme on HIV/AIDS, 2002. *Epidemiological Fact Sheets on HIV/AIDS and Sexually Transmitted Infectious: Malawi*. www.unaids.org.

5   National Statistical Office, 2005. *Demographic and Health Survey*. Zomba: National Statistical Office.

6   National AIDS Commission, 2005. *National HIV/AIDS Action Framework, 2005-2009*. Lilongwe: National AIDS Commission.

7   National AIDS Commission, 2007. *Universal Access Indicators and Targets for Malawi*. Lilongwe: National AIDS Commission.

8   National AIDS Commission, 2005. *Malawi HIV/AIDS National Action Plan, 2005-2009*, Lilongwe: National AIDS Commission.

9   Bollinger, L., Stover, J. and Palamuleni, M.E., 2000. *The Economic Impact of AIDS in Malawi*, Washington: The Policy Project.

10 For example see Government of Malawi and UNDP, 2002. *The Impact of HIV/AIDS on Human Resources in the Malawi Public Sector*, Lilongwe: Government of Malawi and UNDP.

11 Panos Southern Africa, 2006. *Keeping the Promise? A Study of Progress Made in Implementing the UNGASS Declaration of Commitment on HIV/AIDS in Malawi*, Lusaka: Panos Southern Africa.

12 Government of Malawi, 2005. *National Plan of Action for Orphans and Other Vulnerable Children, 2005-2009*, Lilongwe: Government of Malawi.

13 National AIDS Commission, 2000. *National HIV/AIDS Strategic Framework, 2000-2004*, Lilongwe: National AIDS Commission.

14 See Putzel, J. and Munthali, A., 2004. *HIV/AIDS and Leadership in Malawi*, Final report submitted to DFID Malawi.

15 National AIDS Commission, 2003. *The National HIV/AIDS Policy*, Lilongwe: National AIDS Commission.

16 National AIDS Commission, 2005. *The National HIV/AIDS Action Framework, 2005-2009*, Lilongwe: National AIDS Commission.

17 Ministry of Health, 2004. *HIV/AIDS Counseling and Testing: Guidelines for Malawi*, Lilongwe: Ministry of Health.

18 National Statistical Office, 2005. *Demographic and Health Survey*, Zomba: National Statistical Office.

19 Malawi National TB Control Programme, 2005. *Malawi National TB Control Programme: Annual Report July 2004-June 2005*, Lilongwe: Malawi National TB Control Programme.

20 Malawi National TB Control Programme, 2005. *Malawi National TB Control Programme: Annual Report July 2004-June 2005*, Lilongwe: Malawi National TB Control Programme.

21 Munthali, A., Kadzandira, J. and Mvula, P., 2003. *Formative Study on the Prevention of Mother to Child Transmission of HIV*, Lilongwe: National AIDS Commission and UNICEF.

22 http://www.weforum.org/pdf/GHI/Malawi.pdf (accessed 27 March 2007).

23 United Nations Population Database.

24 See endnote 1 above.

25 National Statistical Office and International Food Policy Research Institute, 2002. *Malawi: An Atlas of Social Statistics*, Zomba: National Statistical Office and Washington D.C.: IFPRI.

26 See Tsoka, M.G., 2002. *Public Opinion and the Consolidation of Democracy in Malawi*, Afrobarometer Paper No. 16. Cape Town: Idasa.

27 National Statistical Office, 2005. *Demographic and Health Survey: Preliminary Report*, Zomba: National Statistical Office.

28 National Statistical Office, 1992. *Demographic and Health Survey*, Zomba: National Statistical Office; National Statistical Office, 2001. *Demographic and Health Survey*, Zomba: National Statistical Office.

29 National Statistical Office, 2005. *Demographic and Health Survey: Preliminary Report*, Zomba: National Statistical Office.

30 UNICEF, 2002. *The State of the World's Children, 2002*, New York: UNICEF.

31 UNICEF, 2002. *The State of the World's Children, 2002*, New York: UNICEF.

32 United Nations and Government of Malawi, 1993. *Situation Analysis of Poverty in Malawi*. Lilongwe: UN and GoM.

33 World Health Organization, 2002. *WHO Issues New Healthy Life Expectancy Rankings: Japan Number One in New 'Healthy Life' System*, Press Release, Washington and Geneva: WHO.

34 Panos Southern Africa, 2006. *Keeping the Promise? A Study of Progress Made in Implementing the UNGASS Declaration of Commitment on HIV/AIDS in Malawi*, Lusaka: Panos Southern Africa.

35 Putzel, J. and Munthali, A., 2004. *HIV/AIDS and Leadership in Malawi*, Lilongwe: DFID.

36 De Waal, A., 2005. *HIV/AIDS and Democratic Governance*, Paper presented at the AIDS, Security and Democracy: Expert Seminar and Policy Conference, Clingendael Institute, The Hague, 2-4 May 2004.

37 De Waal, A., 2005. *HIV/AIDS and Democratic Governance*, Paper presented at the AIDS, Security and Democracy: Expert Seminar and Policy Conference, Clingendael Institute, The Hague, 2-4 May 2004.

38 Dulani, B., 2005. "The Elections under Scrutiny: Process, Results, Lessons", In: M. Ott, B. Immink, B. Mhango and C. Peters-Berries,

(eds). *The Power of the Vote: Malawi's 2004 Parliamentary and Presidential Elections*, Balaka: Montfort Press.

39   Chingaipe, H.G., 2005. *The Electoral System, Mass Representation and the Sustenance of Political Liberalization: The Case of Malawi*, Paper presented at the Electoral Systems and Reform in Representation Conference, Sun and Sand Holiday Resort, Mangochi, Malawi, 29 June-2 July 2005, organised by the Netherlands Institute for Multiparty Democracy.

40   Chingaipe, H.G., 2005. *The Electoral System, Mass Representation and the Sustenance of Political Liberalization: The Case of Malawi*, Paper presented at the Electoral Systems and Reform in Representation Conference, Sun and Sand Holiday Resort, Mangochi, Malawi, 29 June-2 July 2005, organised by the Netherlands Institute for Multiparty Democracy.

41   See Dulani, B., 2004. The Elections under Scrutiny: Process, Results, Lessons, In: M. Ott, B. Immink, B. Mhango and C. Peters-Berries, (eds). *The Power of the Vote: Malawi's 2004 Parliamentary and Presidential Elections*, Balaka: Montfort Press.

42   Chingaipe, H.G., 2005. *The Electoral System, Mass Representation and the Sustenance of Political Liberalization: The Case of Malawi*, Paper presented at the Electoral Systems and Reform in Representation Conference, Sun and Sand Holiday Resort, Mangochi, Malawi, 29 June-2 July 2005, organised by the Netherlands Institute for Multiparty Democracy.

43   Dulani, B., 2004. The Elections under Scrutiny: Process, Results, Lessons. In: Ott, M., B. Immink, B. Mhango and C. Peters-Berries, (eds) *The Power of the Vote: Malawi's 2004 Parliamentary and Presidential Elections*, Balaka: Montfort Press.

44   Dulani, B., 2004. The Elections under Scrutiny: Process, Results, Lessons. In: Ott, M., B. Immink, B. Mhango and C. Peters-Berries, (eds) *The Power of the Vote: Malawi's 2004 Parliamentary and Presidential Elections*, Balaka: Montfort Press.

45   See Dulani, B., 2004. The Elections under Scrutiny: Process, Results, Lessons. In: Ott, M., B. Immink, B. Mhango and C. Peters-Berries, (eds) *The Power of the Vote: Malawi's 2004 Parliamentary and Presidential Elections*, Balaka: Montfort Press.

46   Chirwa, W.C. (undated). *Electoral Systems and Governance: Are Reversals Possible?* [Unpublished paper].

47   Chingaipe, H.G., 2005. *The Electoral System, Mass Representation and the Sustenance of Political Liberalization: The Case of Malawi*, Paper presented at the Electoral Systems and Reform in Representation Conference, Sun and Sand Holiday Resort, Mangochi, Malawi, 29 June-2 July 2005, organised by the Netherlands Institute for Multiparty Democracy.

48   See Kamchedzera, G., 1997, "Parliamentary Strike and Public Trust", *Lamp*, No. 9, September, Balaka: Montfort Media; Chirwa, W.C., 2005. "Malawi's 2004 Elections: A Challenge for Democracy", *Journal of African Elections*, 4 (1), June.

49   The numbers in parentheses represent the number of seats in parliament won by the parties.

50   Dulani, B., 2004. The Elections under Scrutiny: Process, Results,

Lessons, In: Ott, M., B. Immink, B. Mhango and C. Peters-Berries, (eds) *The Power of the Vote: Malawi's 2004 Parliamentary and Presidential Elections*, Balaka: Montfort Press.

51   Chingaipe, H.G., 2005. *The Electoral System, Mass Representation and the Sustenance of Political Liberalization: The Case of Malawi*, Paper presented at the Electoral Systems and Reform in Representation Conference, Sun and Sand Holiday Resort, Mangochi, Malawi, 29 June-2 July 2005, organised by the Netherlands Institute for Multiparty Democracy.

52   ECF and EISA, 2003. *Principles for Election Management, Monitoring and Observation in the SADC Region*, Johannesburg: ECF and EISA.

53   Khembo, N.S., 2004. The Anatomy of Electoral Democracy in Malawi: Neo-authoritarianism in a Multiparty State, In: J. Minnie, (ed.) *Outside the Ballot Box: Preconditions for Elections in Southern Africa, 2004/5*, Windhoek: Media Institute for Southern Africa.

54   Khembo, N.S., 2004. The Anatomy of Electoral Democracy in Malawi: Neo-authoritarianism in a Multiparty State, In: J. Minnie, (ed.) *Outside the Ballot Box: Preconditions for Elections in Southern Africa, 2004/5*, Windhoek: Media Institute for Southern Africa.

55   *The Nation* Editorial, 2005. "By-elections Litmus Test for Politics after the 2004 General Polls", 10 December.

56   Chirwa, W.C., 2006. *Malawi Political Participation: A Review by AFRIMAP and Open Society Initiative for Southern Africa*, Johannesburg..

57   Msosa, A.S.E., 2006, Foreword, In: K. Mtlosa and N. Patel, *Towards Electoral System Reform in Malawi*, Occasional Paper No. 10, Lilongwe: Konrad Adenauer Stiftung and Blantyre: Malawi Electoral Commission.

58   Matlosa, K. and Patel, N., 2006. *Towards Electoral System Reform in Malawi*, Occasional Paper No. 10, Lilongwe: Konrad Adenauer Stiftung and Blantyre: Malawi Electoral Commission.

59   Matlosa, K. and Patel, N., 2006. *Towards Electoral System Reform in Malawi*, Occasional Paper No. 10, Lilongwe: Konrad Adenauer Stiftung and Blantyre: Malawi Electoral Commission.

60   For the merits and demerits of the system and its applicability to the Malawi case see Bakken, M., 2005, "Electoral Systems Design and Effects on Representation and Regionalization in Malawi", PhD thesis, University of Bergen, Norway.

61   IDEA, 2005. *Electoral System Design: The New International IDEA Handbook*.

62   Six seats were not contested, one because a candidate from one party had died just prior to the election, and the others due to various election-related administrative problems, ranging from misprinted ballot papers to legal contestations.

63   Figures compiled by the National Initiative for Civic Education (NICE) Project Management Unit (PMU) are available in M. Ott, B. Immink, B. Mhango, and C. Peters-Berries (eds), 2004. *The*

Power of the Vote: Malawi's 2004 Parliamentary and Presidential Elections, Balaka: Montfort Press.

64 For details on these, see Chirwa, W.C., 2006. *Malawi Political Participation: A Review.* Johannesburg: AFRIMAP and Open Society Initiative for Southern Africa.

65 Act No. 4 of 2001.

66 Moses Mkandawire, Civil Society Presentation to the Constitutional Review Conference, March 2006.

67 Act No. 6 of 1995.

68 Mwafulirwa, S., 2007. "AIDS Fight: Abstinence is Normal", *Daily Times*, 11 January 2007.

69 National AIDS Commission, 2007. *Universal Access Indicators and Targets for Malawi*, Lilongwe: National AIDS Commission.

70 National AIDS Commission, 2003. *The National HIV/AIDS Policy*, Lilongwe: National AIDS Commission.

71 Rokkan, S., 1970. *Citizens, Elections, Parties: Approaches to the Comparative Study of the Processes of Development*, New York: McKay.

72 Przeworski, A., 1991. *Democracy and the Market*, Cambridge University Press.

73 Elklit, J., 1999. "The Danish March 1998 Parliamentary Election," *Electoral Studies*, 18.

74 Patel, N., 2000. The 1999 Elections: Challenges and Reforms, In: M. Ott, K. Phiri and N. Patel, (eds) *Malawi's Second Democratic Elections: Process, Problems and Prospects*, Blantyre: CLAIM.

75 The district elections supervisory team comprises district education managers, the district information officer, police in charge, the district investigations officer, the director of administration and the director of development and planning.

76 English, K., 2005. The management of the 2004 electoral process. In: M. Ott, B. Immink, B. Mhango and C. Peters-Berries, (eds) *The Power of the Vote: Malawi's 2004 Parliamentary and Presidential Elections*, Balaka: Montfort Press.

77 English, K., 2005. The Management of the 2004 Electoral Process, In: M. Ott, B. Immink, B. Mhango and C. Peters-Berries, (eds) *The Power of the Vote: Malawi's 2004 Parliamentary and Presidential Elections*, Balaka: Montfort Press.

78 Personal communication with an official from the Malawi Electoral Commission, 28 March 2007.

79 Government of Malawi and UNDP, 2002. *The Impact of HIV/AIDS on Human Resources in the Malawi Public Sector*, Lilongwe: Government of Malawi and UNDP.

80 Kadzamira, E.C., Maluwa-Banda, D., Kamlongera, A. and Swainson, N., 2001. *The Impact of HIV/AIDS on Primary and Secondary Schooling in Malawi: Developing a Comprehensive Strategic Response*, Zomba: Centre for Educational Research and Training.

81 Government of Malawi and UNDP, 2002. *The Impact of HIV/AIDS on Human Resources in the Malawi Public Sector*, Lilongwe:

Government of Malawi and UNDP.

82 Government of Malawi and UNDP, 2002. *The Impact of HIV/AIDS on Human Resources in the Malawi Public Sector*, Lilongwe: Government of Malawi and UNDP.

83 Government of Malawi and UNDP, 2002. *The Impact of HIV/AIDS on Human Resources in the Malawi Public Sector*, Lilongwe: Government of Malawi and UNDP.

84 Patel, N., 2005. *Political Parties: Development and Change in Malawi*. EISA Research Report No. 21, Johannesburg: EISA.

85 Kadzamira, Z.D., Mawaya, A. and Patel, N.A., 1998. *Profile and Views of Political Parties in Malawi: A Final Report*, Zomba: KAF.

86 Maliyamkono, T.L. and Kanyongolo, F.E. (eds), 2003. *When Political Parties Clash: Cases Studies from Malawi and Tanzania*, Dar er Salaam: TEMA Books.

87 N.A. Patel, 2005, *Political Parties: Development and Change in Malawi*, EISA Research Report No. 21. Johannesburg: EISA. For more general problems of political parties in Malawi see Kadzamira, Z.D., Mawaya, A. and Patel, N.A., 1998. *Profile and Views of Political Parties in Malawi: A Final Report*, Zomba: KAF; Meinhardt, H. and Patel, N., 2003. *Malawi's Process of Democratic Transition: An Analysis of Political Developments Between 1990 and 2003*, Lilongwe: KAF; Khembo, N., 2004. "Political Parties in Malawi: From Factions to Splits, Coalitions and Alliances", In: M. Ott, B. Immink, B. Mhango, and C. Peters-Berries (eds), 2004. *The Power of the Vote: Malawi's 2004 Parliamentary and Presidential Elections*, Balaka: Montfort Press.

88 *Mail & Guardian*, 2004, "AIDS High on Malawi Poll Agenda", 21-27 May.

89 Patel, N.A., 2005. *Political Parties: Development and Change in Malawi*. EISA Research Report No. 21, Johannesburg: EISA.

90 Putzel, J. and Munthali, A., 2004. *HIV/AIDS and Leadership in Malawi*, Lilongwe: DFID.

91 Kadzamira, Z.D., Mawaya, A. and Patel, N., 1998, *Profile and Views of Political Parties in Malawi: A Final Report*, Zomba: KAF; Maliyamkono, T.L. and Kanyongolo, F.E. (eds), 2003, *When Political Parties Clash: Cases Studies from Malawi and Tanzania*, Dar er Salaam: TEMA Books; Meinhardt, H. and Patel, N., 2003, *Malawi's Process of Democratic Transition: An Analysis of Political Developments Between 1990 and 2003*, Lilongwe: KAF; Khembo, N., 2004. "Political Parties in Malawi: From Factions to Splits, Coalitions and Alliances", In: M. Ott, B. Immink, B. Mhango, and C. Peters-Berries, (eds) 2004, *The Power of the Vote: Malawi's 2004 Parliamentary and Presidential Elections*, Zomba: Kachere Books; Patel, N., 2005, *Political Parties: Development and Change in Malawi*. EISA Research Report No.21. Johannesburg: EISA.

92 Interviews, W.C. Chirwa, Wallace Chiume, former Secretary General and former Acting President, AFORD, 9 September 2005; Chirwa vs Kate Kainja, former Secretary General, MCP, 10 September, 11 September, 2005; Chirwa vs Paul Maulidi, former Secretary General, UDF, 13 September, 2005.

93 Khembo, N., 2004, "Political Parties in Malawi: From Factions to Splits, Coalitions and Alliances", In: M. Ott, B. Immink, B. Mhango, and C. Peters-Berries (eds), 2004, *The Power of the Vote: Malawi's 2004 Parliamentary and Presidential Elections*, Balaka: Montfort Press.

94 Examples: Malawi Congress Party (MCP), *Reconciliation, Reconstruction, and Development*, Lilongwe: MCP; Mgwirizano Coalition, *Governance for Sustainable Development*, Blantyre: Mgwirizano Coalition; National Democratic Alliance (NDA), *Towards Prosperous Malawi*, Blantyre: NDA; United Democratic Front (UDF), *Forging Ahead with Social and Economic Transformation – Unity, Democracy and Development*, Blantyre: UDF.

95 Patel, N., 2005, *Political Parties: Development and Change in Malawi*. EISA Research Report No. 21, Johannesburg: EISA, p. 58.

96 Meinhardt, H. and Patel, N., 2003, *Malawi's Process of Democratic Transition: An Analysis of Political Developments Between 1990 and 2003*, Lilongwe: KAF, p. 32.

97 "African Union", 2004, Statement of the African Union Observer Team on the Presidential and Parliamentary Elections in the Republic of Malawi held on 20 May 2004.

98 See, for example, Kamchedzera, G., 2004, "Parliamentary Strike and Public Trust", In: *The Lamp*, (9), July-September, Balaka: Montfort Media; Lwanda, J., 2004, "*Makwacha*: The Violence of Money in Malawi Politics", *The Lamp*, (46); Lwanda, J., 2004, "Changes in Malawi's Political Landscape between 1999 and 2004: *Nkhope ya Agalatia*", In: M. Ott, B. Immink, B. Mhango, and C. Peters-Berries, (eds), 2004, *The Power of the Vote: Malawi's 2004 Parliamentary and Presidential Elections*, Zomba: Kachere Books; Dzimbiri, L., 1999, "Socio-political Engineering and Chameleon Politics in Malawi: The Period of Transition", *African Currents*, (16); Dzimbiri, L., 1998, "Democratic Politics and Chameleon-like Leaders", In: K.M.G. Phiri and K. Ross (eds), *Democratisation in Malawi: A Stocktaking*, Blantyre: CLAIM.

99 Tsoka, M.G., 2002. *Public Opinion and the Consolidation of Democracy in Malawi*, Afrobarometer Paper No. 16, Cape Town: IDASA.

100 Tsoka, M.G., 2002. *Public Opinion and the Consolidation of Democracy in Malawi*, Afrobarometer Paper No. 16, Cape Town: IDASA.

101 Tsoka, M.G., 2002. *Public Opinion and the Consolidation of Democracy in Malawi*, Afrobarometer Paper No. 16, Cape Town: IDASA.

102 National Statistical Office, 2005. *Integrated Household Survey, 2004-2005*, Zomba: National Statistical Office.

103 National Statistical Office and ORC Macro, 2005. *Malawi Demographic and Health Survey, 2004*, Zomba: National Statistical Office and Calverton, USA: ORC Macro.

104 Government of Malawi, 2005. *National Plan of Action for Orphans and other Vulnerable Children, 2005-2009*. Lilongwe: Government of Malawi.

105 Munthali, A., Moore, A., Konyani, S. and Zakeyo, B., 2006. *Qualitative Evidence of Adolescents' Sexual and Reproductive Health Experiences in Selected Districts of Malawi*. Occasional Report No. 23, New York: The Guttmacher Institute.

106 *The Nation*, 9 January 2004, "Voters fail to register in Mzimba Centres"; also *The Daily Times*, 20 January 2004, "Voter registration extended".

107 Patel, N., 2000. The 1999 Elections: Challenges and Reforms, In: M. Ott, K. Phiri and N. Patel, (eds) *Malawi's Second Democratic Elections: Process, Problems and Prospects*, CLAIM: Blantyre.

108 Dulani, B., (2004). The Elections under Scrutiny: Process, Results, Lessons, In: M.Ott, B. Immink, B. Mhango and C. Peters-Berries. *The Power of the Vote: Malawi's 2004 Parliamentary and Presidential Elections*, Balaka: Montfort Press.

109 Some records show a figure of 6.7 million registered at this time.

110 W.C. Chirwa, 2004, "Malawi's 'Bogus' Voter Statistics", in *Election Talk: A Fortnightly Policy Brief from the Electoral Institute of Southern Africa*, (11), May.

111 See *The Weekend Nation*, 17-18 April, 2004, and *The Nation*, 9 January 2004, "Three Fined for Registering Twice"; *The Daily Times*, 20 January 2004, "Voter Registration Extended"; *Tamvani*, 31 January–1 February 2004, "*Bungwe la EC Likukondera* UDF-CHRR".

112 See Dulani, B., 2004. The Elections under Scrutiny: Process, Results, Lessons, In: M. Ott, B. Immink, B. Mhango and C. Peters-Berries, *The Power of the Vote: Malawi's 2004 Parliamentary and Presidential Elections*, Balaka: Montfort Press.

113 The agricultural inputs comprising fertilisers and seeds are given to smallholder peasant farmers as start-up packages. See *The Weekend Nation*, January 31-1 February 2004, "The UDF Plot: CCJP, Parties Accuse UDF of Buying Certificates".

114 See Dulani, B., 2004. The Elections under Scrutiny: Process, Results, Lessons. In: M. Ott, B. Immink, B. Mhango and C. Peters-Berries, *The Power of the Vote: Malawi's 2004 Parliamentary and Presidential Elections*, Balaka: Montfort Press.

115 See Dulani, B., 2004. The Elections under Scrutiny: Process, Results, Lessons, In: M. Ott, B. Immink, B. Mhango and C. Peters-Berries, *The Power of the Vote: Malawi's 2004 Parliamentary and Presidential Elections*, Balaka: Montfort Press.

116 Kamchedzera, G., 1997. "Parliamentary Strike and Public Trust", *The Lamp*, (9), July-September.

117 Ministry of Health and National AIDS Commission, 2004. *Report of a Country-wide Survey of HIV/AIDS Services in Malawi*, Lilongwe: National Tuberculosis Control Programme, HIV/AIDS Unit and National AIDS Commission.

118 UNAIDS, 2004. *Country Fact Sheets: Malawi*.

119 National AIDS Commission, 2003. *National HIV/AIDS Policy*, Lilongwe: National AIDS Commission.

120 National AIDS Commission, 2005. *Malawi HIV/AIDS National Action Plan, 2005-2009*, Lilongwe: National AIDS Commission.

121 MANET+, 2003. *Voices of Equality and Dignity: Qualitative Research on Stigma and Discrimination Issues As They Affect PLWHAs in Malawi*, Lilongwe: MANET.

122 National Statistical Office, 2005. *Demographic and Health Survey, 2004*, Zomba: National Statistical Office.

123 Panos Southern Africa, 2006. *Keeping the Promise? A Study of Progress Made in Implementing the UNGASS Declaration of Commitment on HIV/AIDS in Malawi*, Lusaka: Panos Southern Africa.

124 Panos Southern Africa, 2006. *Keeping the Promise? A Study of Progress Made in Implementing the UNGASS Declaration of Commitment on HIV/AIDS in Malawi*, Lusaka: Panos Southern Africa.

125 The National AIDS Commission, Monitoring and Evaluation Section.

References

"African Union", 2004, Statement of the African Union Observer Team on the Presidential and Parliamentary Elections in the Republic of Malawi held on 20 May 2004.

AfriMAP, 2006. *Political Participation in Malawi: A Country Study*, Johannesburg, AfriMAP.

Bakken, M., 2005, "Electoral Systems Design and Effects on Representation and Regionalization in Malawi", PhD thesis, University of Bergen, Norway.

Bollinger, L., Stover, J. and Palamuleni, M.E., 2000. *The Economic Impact of AIDS in Malawi*, Washington: The Policy Project.

Chingaipe, H.G., 2005. *The Electoral System, Mass Representation and the Sustenance of Political Liberalization: The Case of Malawi*, Paper presented at the Electoral Systems and Reform in Representation Conference, Sun and Sand Holiday Resort, Mangochi, Malawi, 29 June-2 July 2005, organised by the Netherlands Institute for Multiparty Democracy.

Chirwa, W.C. [undated]. *Electoral Systems and Governance: Are Reversals Possible?* [Unpublished paper].

Chirwa, W,C., 2004, "Malawi's 'Bogus' Voter Statistics", in *Election Talk: A Fortnightly Policy Brief from the Electoral Institute of Southern Africa*, (11), May.

Chirwa, W.C., 2005. "Malawi's 2004 Elections: A Challenge for Democracy", *Journal of African Elections*, 4 (1), June.

Chirwa, W.C., 2006. *Malawi Political Participation: A Review by AFRIMAP and Open Society Initiative for Southern Africa*, Johannesburg.

De Waal, A., 2005. *HIV/AIDS and Democratic Governance*, Paper presented at the AIDS, Security and Democracy: Expert Seminar and Policy Conference, Clingendael Institute, The Hague, 2-4 May 2004.

Dulani, B., 2005. "The Elections under Scrutiny: Process, Results, Lessons", In: M. Ott, B. Immink, B. Mhango and C. Peters-Berries, (eds). *The Power of the Vote: Malawi's 2004 Parliamentary and Presidential Elections*, Balaka: Montfort Press.

Dzimbiri, L., 1998, "Democratic Politics and Chameleon-like Leaders", In: K.M.G. Phiri and K. Ross (eds), *Democratisation in Malawi: A Stocktaking*, Blantyre: CLAIM.

Dzimbiri, L., 1999, "Socio-political Engineering and Chameleon Politics in Malawi: The Period of Transition", *African Currents*, (16).

ECF and EISA, 2003. *Principles for Election Management, Monitoring and Observation in the SADC Region*, Johannesburg: ECF and EISA.

Elklit, J., 1999. "The Danish March 1998 Parliamentary Election," *Electoral Studies*, 18.

English, K., 2005. The Management of the 2004 Electoral Process, In: M. Ott, B. Immink, B. Mhango and C. Peters-Berries, (eds) *The Power of the Vote: Malawi's 2004 Parliamentary and Presidential Elections*, Balaka: Montfort Press.

Government of Malawi, 2005. *National Plan of Action for Orphans and Other Vulnerable Children, 2005-2009*, Lilongwe: Government of Malawi.

Government of Malawi and UNDP, 2002. *The Impact of HIV/AIDS on Human Resources in the Malawi Public Sector*, Lilongwe: Government of Malawi and UNDP.

IDEA, 2005. *Electoral System Design: The New International IDEA Handbook*.

Joint United Nations Programme on HIV/AIDS, 2002. *Epidemiological Fact Sheets on HIV/AIDS and Sexually Transmitted Infectious: Malawi*. www.unaids.org.

Kadzamira, E.C., Maluwa-Banda, D., Kamlongera, A. and Swainson, N., 2001. *The Impact of HIV/AIDS on Primary and Secondary Schooling in Malawi: Developing a Comprehensive Strategic Response*, Zomba: Centre for Educational Research and Training.

Kadzamira, Z.D., Mawaya, A. and Patel, N.A., 1998.

Profile and Views of Political Parties in Malawi: A Final Report, Zomba: KAF.

Kalipeni, E., 2000. "Health and Disease in Southern Africa: A Comparative and Vulnerability Perspective", *Social Science and Medicine*, 50 (7/8).

Kamchedzera, G., 1997, "Parliamentary Strike and Public Trust", *The Lamp*, No. 9, September, Balaka: Montfort Press.

Khembo, N.S., 2004. The Anatomy of Electoral Democracy in Malawi: Neo-authoritarianism in a Multiparty State, In: J. Minnie, (ed.) *Outside the Ballot Box: Preconditions for Elections in Southern Africa, 2004/5*, Windhoek: Media Institute for Southern Africa.

Khembo, N.S., 2004. "Political Parties in Malawi: From Factions to Splits, Coalitions and Alliances", In: M. Ott, B. Immink, B. Mhango, and C. Peters-Berries (eds), 2004. *The Power of the Vote: Malawi's 2004 Parliamentary and Presidential Elections*, Zomba: Kachere Books.

Lwanda, J., 2004, "Changes in Malawi's Political Landscape between 1999 and 2004: *Nkhope ya Agalatia*", In: M. Ott, B. Immink, B. Mhango, and C. Peters-Berries, (eds), 2004, *The Power of the Vote: Malawi's 2004 Parliamentary and Presidential Elections*, Zomba: Kachere Books.

Lwanda, J., 2004, "*Makwacha*: The Violence of Money in Malawi Politics", *The Lamp*, (46).

Malawi Congress Party (MCP), *Reconciliation, Reconstruction, and Development*, Lilongwe: MCP.

Malawi National TB Control Programme, 2005. *Malawi National TB Control Programme: Annual Report July 2004-June 2005*, Lilongwe: Malawi National TB Control Programme.

Maliyamkono, T.L. and Kanyongolo, F.E. (eds), 2003. *When Political Parties Clash: Cases Studies from Malawi and Tanzania*, Dar er Salaam: TEMA Books.

MANET+, 2003. *Voices of Equality and Dignity: Qualitative Research on Stigma and Discrimination Issues As They Affect PLWHAs in Malawi*, Lilongwe: MANET.

Meinhardt, H. and Patel, N., 2003. *Malawi's Process of Democratic Transition: An Analysis of Political Developments Between 1990 and 2003*, Lilongwe: KAF.

Mgwirizano Coalition, *Governance for Sustainable Development*, Blantyre: Mgwirizano Coalition.

Ministry of Health, 2004. *HIV/AIDS Counseling and Testing: Guidelines for Malawi*, Lilongwe: Ministry of Health.

Ministry of Health and National AIDS Commission, 2004. *Report of a Country-wide Survey of HIV/AIDS Services in Malawi*, Lilongwe: National Tuberculosis Control Programme, HIV/AIDS Unit and National AIDS Commission.

Mkandawire, M. Civil Society Presentation to the Constitutional Review Conference, March 2006.

Msosa, A.S.E., 2006, Foreword, In: K. Mtlosa and N. Patel, *Towards Electoral System Reform in Malawi*, Occasional Paper No. 10, Lilongwe: Konrad Adenauer Stiftung and Blantyre: Malawi Electoral Commission.

Mtlosa, K. and Patel, N., 2006. *Towards Electoral System Reform in Malawi*, Occasional Paper No. 10, Lilongwe: Konrad Adenauer Stiftung and Blantyre: Malawi Electoral Commission.

Munthali, A., Kadzandira, J. and Mvula, P., 2003. *Formative Study on the Prevention of Mother to Child Transmission of HIV*, Lilongwe: National AIDS Commission and UNICEF.

Munthali, A., Moore, A., Konyani, S. and Zakeyo, B., 2006. *Qualitative Evidence of Adolescents' Sexual and Reproductive Health Experiences in Selected Districts of Malawi*. Occasional Report No. 23, New York: The Guttmacher Institute.

National AIDS Commission, 2000. *National HIV/AIDS Strategic Framework, 2000-2004*, Lilongwe: National AIDS Commission.

National AIDS Commission, 2003. *The National HIV/AIDS Policy*, Lilongwe: National AIDS Commission.

National AIDS Commission, 2005. *Malawi HIV/AIDS National Action Plan, 2005-2009*, Lilongwe: National AIDS Commission.

National AIDS Commission, 2007. *Universal Access Indicators and Targets for Malawi*. Lilongwe: National AIDS Commission.

National Democratic Alliance, *Towards Prosperous Malawi*, Blantyre: NDA.

National Statistical Office, 1992. *Demographic and Health Survey*, Zomba: National Statistical Office.

National Statistical Office, 2001. *Demographic and Health Survey*, Zomba: National Statistical Office.

National Statistical Office, 2005. *Demographic and Health Survey, 2004*, Zomba: National Statistical Office.

National Statistical Office, 2005. *Integrated Household Survey, 2004-2005*, Zomba: National Statistical Office.

National Statistical Office and International Food Policy Research Institute, 2002. *Malawi: An Atlas of Social Statistics*, Zomba: National Statistical Office and Washington D.C.: IFPRI.

National Statistical Office and ORC Macro, 2005. *Malawi Demographic and Health Survey, 2004*, Zomba: National Statistical Office and Calverton, USA: ORC Macro.

Ott, M., Immink, B., Mhango, B. and C. Peters-Berries, C. (eds), 2004. *The Power of the Vote: Malawi's 2004 Parliamentary and Presidential Elections*, Balaka: Montfort Press.

Panos Southern Africa, 2006. *Keeping the Promise? A Study of Progress Made in Implementing the UNGASS Declaration of Commitment on HIV/AIDS in Malawi*, Lusaka: Zambia.

Patel, N., 2000. The 1999 Elections: Challenges and Reforms, In: M. Ott, K. Phiri and N. Patel, (eds) *Malawi's Second Democratic Elections: Process, Problems and Prospects*, Blantyre: CLAIM.

Patel, N.A,, 2005. *Political Parties: Development and Change in Malawi*. EISA Research Report No. 21, Johannesburg: EISA.

Przeworski, A., 1991. *Democracy and the Market*, Cambridge University Press.

Putzel, J. and Munthali, A., 2004. *HIV/AIDS and Leadership in Malawi*, Lilongwe: DFID.

Rokkan, S., 1970. *Citizens, Elections, Parties: Approaches to the Comparative Study of the Processes of Development*, New York: McKay.

Tsoka, M.G., 2002. *Public Opinion and the Consolidation of Democracy in Malawi*, Afrobarometer Paper No. 16. Cape Town: Idasa.

UNAIDS, 2004. *Country Fact Sheets: Malawi*.

UNICEF, 2002. *The State of the World's Children, 2002*, New York: UNICEF.

United Democratic Front (UDF), *Forging Ahead with Social and Economic Transformation – Unity, Democracy and Development*, Blantyre: UDF.

United Nations and Government of Malawi, 1993. *Situation Analysis of Poverty in Malawi*. Lilongwe: UN and GoM.

World Health Organization, 2002. *WHO Issues New Healthy Life Expectancy Rankings: Japan Number One in New 'Healthy Life' System*, Press Release, Washington and Geneva: WHO.

Abbreviations

AFORD	Alliance for Democracy
ART	Antiretroviral Therapy
CHAM	Christian Health Association in Malawi
CBO	community-based organisation
CERT	Centre for Educational Research and Training
COMESA	Common Market for Southern and Eastern Africa
CONU	Congress for National Unity
CSO	civil society organisation
CSR	Centre for Social Research
DEST	district elections supervisory team
DHS	demographic and health survey
DPP	Democratic Progressive Party
EU	European Union
FGD	focus group discussion
FPTP	First Past The Post
GoM	Government of Malawi
HTC	HIV testing and counselling
IMD	Institute for Multiparty Democracy
IND	Independent (candidate/member of Parliament)
KAF	Konrad Adenauer Foundation
MACRO	Malawi Counselling and Resource Organisation
MAFUNDE	Malawi Forum for Unity and Democracy
MANET	Malawi AIDS Network
MBCA	Malawi Business Coalition Against HIV/AIDS
MCP	Malawi Congress Party
MEC	Malawi Electoral Commission
MGODE	Movement for Genuine Democracy
MIM	Malawi Institute of Management
MK	Malawi Kwacha (Malawi Currency)
MMP	Mixed Member Proportional (system)
MMR	maternal mortality rate
MP	Member of Parliament
NAC	National AIDS Commission
NAF	National HIV/AIDS Action Framework
NAPHAM	National Association of People Living with HIV/AIDS in Malawi
NDA	National Democratic Alliance
NGO	non-governmental organisation
NSF	National Strategic Framework
NSO	National Statistical Office
NUP	National Unity Party

PETRA	People's Transformation Party
PLWHAs	people living with HIV/AIDS
PMTCT	prevention of mother-to-child transmission
PPEA	Parliamentary and Presidential Elections Act
PPM	People's Progressive Movement
PR	Proportional Representation
PTA	preferential trade area
RP	Republican Party
SADC	Southern Africa Development Community
STI	sexually transmitted infection
UDF	United Democratic Front
UNDP	United Nations Development Programme
VCT	voluntary counselling and testing

Namibia

Graham Hopwood, Justine Hunter, Doris Kellner

1. Introduction

In 1990, Namibia gained independence, experiencing a successful transition from authoritarian to democratic rule. The young democracy is among the countries worst hit by the HIV/AIDS pandemic. The United Nations (UN) recognises that the pandemic challenges both social and economic development in Namibia. The pandemic constitutes the key obstacle to Namibia achieving its Millennium Development Goals (RoN, 2004a), which, as such, might undermine the realisation of *Vision 2030*, the Namibian long-term development framework (UN, n.d.).

The most relevant demographic statistics and epidemiological data are used to analyse how the pandemic affects the electoral processes in Namibia. A causality analysis leads into exploring the effects of the pandemic. The chapter ends with a comprehensive discussion of the multisectoral response to HIV/AIDS in Namibia.

2. Methodology

The research carried out in Namibia involved five different key methodological approaches to collecting information:

1. The *comprehensive overview of available literature* included an analysis of the legal and constitutional framework; the status of the voters' roll with regard to deceased voters; key documents on HIV/AIDS in Namibia; records of parliamentary debates and on deceased Members of Parliament (MPs) and regional councillors; party manifestos; research papers; newspaper articles; information on the administration and management capacities of the Electoral Commission of Namibia (ECN); and election results and voter turnouts.

2. Largely structured *in-depth interviews* with key informants have been conducted with the ECN; the Ministry of Health and Social Services (MoHSS); political party representatives; public servants; and civil society activists.

3. *Focus group discussions* (FGDs) with people living with HIV/AIDS (PLWHA) have been used to enrich the qualitative analysis of citizens' perceptions and their ability to participate in elections and civil society.

4. To determine the impact that HIV/AIDS has on civic participation and to correlate public perception with government actions, a detailed analysis of *public opinion survey data* from the Afrobarometer has been carried out.

5. A *post-research stakeholder meeting* was held to help with reviewing the preliminary findings and to ensure that the information presented is relevant, appropriate and accurate, allowing it to be used for policy design to mitigate the effects of HIV/AIDS on the electoral process.

Owing to the stigma and secrecy that surrounds HIV/AIDS and the absence of precise illness-related information, determining whether a person has died of an AIDS-related illness is difficult. Ascertaining how many by-elections have resulted from AIDS is just as difficult. Proxy-indicators, like age at death, might indicate whether deaths might be AIDS-related. The study does not imply that any civil servant, parliamentarian or councillor died from AIDS. Questions that are proxy-indicators are used in the Afrobarometer survey data.

3. HIV/AIDS in Namibia

3.1 Demographic and epidemiological data

According to the *2001 Population and Housing Census* (Central Bureau of Statistics, 2003), Namibia had a total population of 1 830 330 people in 2001, with the 2005 estimate for the total population being 2 030 000 people. With one of the lowest population density ratios in the world at 2.1 people a square kilometre, most Namibians live in the five north–central regions. HIV/AIDS has profoundly affected Namibian demography, reducing the population growth rate (3.1% a year) in the decade before independence to 2.6% a year. Because of the pandemic, Namibia's life expectancy declined from 61 to 49 between 1991 and 2001 (RoN/UN System in Namibia, 2004: 6). Since the mid-1990s AIDS has been the leading cause of death. The high percentage of mortality due to AIDS seems to be underestimated, since by far most deaths blamed on tuberculosis (TB) and other infectious and parasitic diseases were most probably caused or complicated by HIV (El Obeid, Mendelsohn, Lejars, Forster and Brulé, 2001: 35–36).

Women face a greater risk of HIV infection due to their biological vulnerability and their generally lower societal status (Phororo, 2002: 5). Namibia also has more than 120 000 orphans, which is likely to increase to more than 250 000 (AIDSBRIEF, 2004b: 8; UNICEF, 2005: 4).

Vision 2030 aims to transform the country from a lower-middle income country to a more highly developed nation by 2030 by means of a series of seven five-year development plans. The solid progress made towards meeting several Millennium Development Goals and Targets, such as achieving universal primary education and promoting gender equality, is undermined by the deteriorating HIV/AIDS situation (RoN/UN Systems in Namibia, 2004: 3).

The MoHSS (RoN/MoHSS, 2005: 1) identifies those most at risk: the mobile populations; young women and girls along transport routes; sexually active youth; uniformed service members; and commercial sex workers, noting that all who have unprotected sex with a partner of unknown HIV status are at risk. Risk factors include high unemployment; poverty; cultural norms; alcohol abuse; gender discrimination; and stigma. According to its 2001 impact projections, the MoHSS estimates that the rapid growth in HIV prevalence which occurred in the last few years of the previous century will soon be reflected in increased morbidity and mortality, with 38% of boys and 48% of girls who are assumed to be HIV negative on their 15th birthday dying before their 40th (MoHSS, 2001: 40). The long incubation period of the pandemic means that its full-scale impact will manifest itself only within the next decade or so.[1]

Figure 3.1: HIV prevalence among pregnant women, biennial surveys, 1992-2004, Namibia

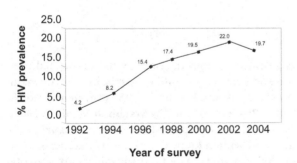

Source: MoHSS, 2005: 10.

The National HIV Sentinel Survey, which is conducted among pregnant women, has so far given the most reliable information on the pandemic in Namibia, due to its early detection of changes or trends and its ability to discern meaningful differences in disease rates and trends between sentinel sites.[2] Namibia has followed internationally accepted guidelines developed by the World Health Organisation (WHO). The weakness of the system lies in its incapacity to produce national prevalence rates, as it is biased against gender and age factors coupled with the geographical accessibility of sites.

The first AIDS cases in Namibia were reported in 1986. Since 1992, the MoHSS has biennially conducted a sero surveillance survey of all women visiting a participating antenatal clinic (ANC) for the first time during the current pregnancy during the sampling periods. Namibia was found to have experienced a steep rise from its 1992 level of 4.2%,[3] followed by a levelling of the pandemic, which does not clearly indicate whether the country's pandemic has stabilised. In 2004, the prevalence of HIV was estimated at 19.7%, compared with 22.0% in 2002 (see Figure 3.1). Accordingly, the 2004 sero-sentinel survey represents the first clear decrease in HIV prevalence since the start of ANC surveillance by the MoHSS in 1992. Apart from monitoring trends in HIV prevalence over the past 12 years, the MoHSS seeks to improve overall representativeness by including additional sites, bringing the total number of participating sites to 24 in 2004 (RoN and MoHSS, 2005).

Figure 3.2: HIV prevalence among ANC attendees by age group, 2004

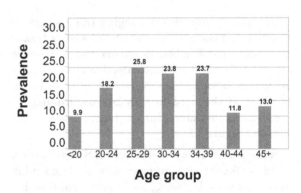

Source: MoHSS, 2005: 9.

Both site-specific longitudinal data and HIV trends by age group, including the sexually active age groups (15–34 years), show a slight decline of the HIV prevalence rate in Namibia. Positive behavioural patterns learned while young are increasingly being upheld, thereby favourably affecting the prevalence rates among the older age groups (Nanaso, 2005b: 7).

According to the *Namibia Demographic and Health Survey 2000*, awareness of AIDS is almost universal in Namibia, with 98% of women and over 99% of men saying they had heard of it (MoHSS, 2003). Nevertheless, according to the MoHSS (Ron and MoHSS, 2005: 17), trends in HIV prevalence must be examined carefully, as they might not be influenced only by policies and prevention efforts, but also by the survival time of PLWHAs[4] and risk behaviour change.[5]

Though the rate of infection might be slowing, Namibia is experiencing increasing numbers of PLWHAs, who, by falling severely ill or dying, result in an increase in the number of orphans and vulnerable children (OVC) (Nanaso, 2005a: 9; RoN and UN System in Namibia, 2004: 20).

Figure 3.3: HIV prevalence among ANC attendees by site, 2004

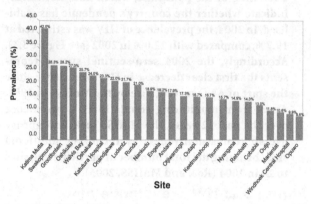

Source: Nanaso, 2005b: 6.

Site-specific prevalence, ranging from a high of 42.4% in Katima Mulilo in the Northeast (a transit area bordering Zambia, Botswana and Zimbabwe, countries that all have high infection rates) to 8.5% in Opuwo in the isolated Northwest, provides clear evidence of the need to translate the findings of the sero-sentinel survey into regionally comparative data (see Figure 3.3).

While a decreasing or levelling trend was observed in 16 of the 21 sites compared in 2002, an additional five sites, including Swakopmund and Walvis Bay (Keulder and LeBeau, 2006), have increased in prevalence. Particular prevention interventions are necessary in those areas where the pandemic is still expanding or only slowly stabilising (Nanaso, 2005b: 7; RoN and MoHSS, 2005: 17).

To approximate the number of PLWHAs in a region, the prevalence data is used with the regional census data, adjusted for population growth since the census in 2001 and for the proportion of the population that is sexually active. The number of those likely to have developed AIDS has been estimated on the basis that 15% of PLWHAs are likely to have developed the terminal condition (Nanaso, 2005b: 9).

Though costly population-based surveys can more

accurately assess the levels of HIV prevalence in a country than can ANC surveillance systems, as they use a representative sample of both men and women in reproductive ages, no such population-based survey has yet been undertaken. The lack of such a survey has been described as "the single largest obstacle to progressive and coordinated research in Namibia" (Van Zyl, 2003: 17).

Apart from the sentinel survey, the MoHSS publishes yearly epidemiological reports which include AIDS-related hospitalisation and deaths (like MoHSS, 2000).[6] The *Namibia Demographic and Health Survey* conducted by the MoHSS in 1992 and 2000 offers a representative sample of people and households across Namibia. Though the behavioural surveillance survey provides valuable health-related data relating to HIV/AIDS awareness, the level of stigma associated with the pandemic and the frequency of testing, it implies nothing about the HIV status of the respondents (MoHSS, 2003).

Similar survey instruments to the Afrobarometer do not directly question the interviewees' HIV/AIDS status or the status of those in their care (Strand and Chirambo, 2005: 122). Moreover, the voluntary counselling and testing (VCT) service centres managed by the Council of Churches in Namibia (CCN) and Catholic AIDS Action (CAA) cannot serve as surveillance centres, due to their unsystematic approach. The *Human Development Report, 2000/2001* argues that under-reporting of HIV/AIDS deaths is generally widespread and that the total number of infections can, therefore, only be estimated (UNDP and UN Country Team, 2000: 11).

3.2 Causality analysis

High rates of unprotected sex with an infected person and mother–to–child transmission are the main causes of Namibia's high HIV prevalence (RoN, 2004a: 25–26; RoN and UN System in Namibia, 2004: 20–23). Many Namibians have multiple sexual partners and seldom know their own HIV status or that of their partners. The high prevalence of sexually transmitted infections (STIs) increases the risk of transmission, as does the sexual exploitation of women, including intergenerational sex.

Widespread alcohol abuse decreases self-control, increasing risky sexual behaviour. Many lack accurate HIV/AIDS-related information, so that stigma and discrimination are common. The low status of women, unemployment and connected high mobility have added to the spread of HIV/AIDS.

3.3 Effects of the epidemic

AIDS-weakened capacities of families, communities and institutions are likely to lead to decreased household income and agricultural productivity, worsening poverty. Households face stigma and discrimination, expensive health care and funerals, and having to care for orphans (Phororo, 2002: 9). Though first felt at household level, the effect of the pandemic is then experienced by the community and, ultimately, the economy. Reduced productivity, increased health care expenditures, reduced savings and human capital investments in term of skill loss will occur (UNDP and UN Country Team, 2000: 12).

Increased mortality rates will result in a decreased population rate and changed age structures (UNDP and UN Country Team, 2000: 12), with AIDS-related morbidity and mortality eroding the capacity of governance institutions to function effectively (RoN and UN System in Namibia, 2004: 54–55). Key areas of democratic governance that have been influenced by AIDS include: the electoral system; electoral administration and management; political parties; voter participation; and the accuracy of voters' rolls.

3.4 Multisectoral[7] response to HIV/AIDS in Namibia

3.4.1 Government policies, strategic efforts

The National AIDS Control Programme (NACP), based within the MoHSS, coordinates and manages HIV/AIDS patient care and preventive activities (Nanaso, 2005b: 9). Post independence, the government introduced both a short-term plan and the first medium-term plan (MTPI) of action aimed at raising awareness, articulating political commitment and implementing management structures (Nanaso, 2005b: 9). Through the launch of its second medium-term plan (MTPII) at the turn of the century, the government sought to create a broad national response by including all stakeholders in a nationwide multisectoral exercise (UNDP and UN Country Team, 2000: 13).

MTPII set up the National AIDS Coordination Programme (Nacop) to replace NACP. Nacop aimed to strengthen preventive efforts; ensuring that HIV-positive Namibians have access to services which are responsive to their needs; teaching prevention, home-based care and self-protection; setting up national and regional programme management

Figure 3.4: The MTPII structure

NATIONAL AIDS CO-ORDINATION PROGRAMME
(NACOP)

National AIDS Committee (NAC)
Cabinet Ministers/Governors General Secretaries of CNN and NANAWO

National Multi-sectoral AIDS Co-ordination Committee (NAMACOC)
Technical operations committee responsible for implementation

National AIDS Executive Committee (NAEC)
NAEC is part of MOHSS and is responsible for advising and supervising the implementation of NAC and NAMACOC decisions

Source: Ceasar-Katsenga and Chirambo, 2005: 12.

structures; and ensuring continuous support by both national and international communities in addressing the socioeconomic effect of the pandemic (RoN, 1999).[8] The highest policy-level body is the National AIDS Committee (Nac), which is tasked with setting major policy and strategic directions. The National Multisectoral AIDS Coordination Committee (Namacoc) is the technical operations committee, responsible for intersectoral coordination and central implementation. Under the leadership of Namacoc, the Take Control Namibia HIV/AIDS Campaign uses television, billboards, radio and print media to create awareness.

The National AIDS Executive Committee (NAEC) advises and supervises the implementation of Nac and Namacoc decisions, monitoring all HIV/AIDS-related activities throughout the country (Caesar-Katsenga and Chirambo, 2005: 9–10). The second national development plan (NDP II) complemented the strategies laid out in MTPII, bringing the targets in line with the indicators developed for the Namibian application to the Global Fund to Fight HIV/AIDS, TB and Malaria (GFATM)[9] (Nanaso, 2005b: 10).

To campaign for support among the private sector in the fight against HIV/AIDS, a *Menu of Partnership Options* was compiled in 2002. Addressing HIV/AIDS as a crosscutting issue, the overarching development framework *Vision 2030* highlights the need for leadership at all levels, a multisectoral approach, the promotion of policies to combat stigma and discrimination, the inclusion of HIV/AIDS in all development plans, and greater understanding of the effect of the pandemic on different sectors.

In 2003, the review of MTPII concluded that, though much progress has been made, the capacity to plan, coordinate, and monitor the national and local responses, in particular the multisectoral response, needed strengthening (Nanaso, 2005b: 11). HIV/

AIDS is not yet systematically mainstreamed in the relatively underdeveloped multisectoral response.

The review guided the formulation of the current third medium-term plan (MTPIII). MTPIII aims to broaden the response to HIV/AIDS, as well as focusing on areas previously neglected (RoN, 2004b). The five-year plan set for 2004 to 2009 has ambitious goals, ranging from providing treatment for HIV/AIDS patients and pregnant women to drastically reduce the number of HIV infections (AIDSBRIEF, 2004a: 8–10). With a mid-term review planned for 2007, the Nac and Nacop will be responsible for monitoring and evaluation (M&E) of the process at all levels.[10]

The Namibian HIV Charter of Rights (Lac, n.d.); an HIV/AIDS Policy for the Education Sector;[11] a National Code of HIV/AIDS in Employment, which was compiled in cooperation with the AIDS Law Unit at the Legal Assistance Centre (Lac) and the National Policy on OVC, are in place. Policies and guidelines have been developed for a wide range of health interventions, such as prevention of mother–to–child transmission (PMTCT), post-exposure prophylaxis, access to antiretroviral therapy and VCT. The percentage of HIV-infected pregnant women receiving treatment for reducing the risk of mother–to–child transmission increased from 7% in 2003 to 25% in 2005.

By late 2005, 35% of PLWHAs in an advanced stage of the illness were receiving antiretroviral combination therapy, while 71% were receiving antiretrovirals.12 Cabinet recently approved plans for the production of generic HIV/AIDS drugs within Namibia to boost affordable public treatment, as articulated by the Treatment Action Forum at the AIDS Law Unit/Lac (Caesar-Katsenga and Chirambo, 2005: 6–7).

Through Nacop, the government distributed 11.2 million condoms in 2000 and 2001 by way of family planning services, health services, government sectors, non-governmental organisations (NGOs) and private companies (UNAIDS, n.d.). Free female condoms have also been made widely available throughout the country. The Ministry of Women's Affairs and Child Welfare (MWACW) has set up a trust fund for OVC, who do not receive any other kind of help (AIDSBRIEF, 2004b: 9; RoN and UN System in Namibia 2004: 12; UNICEF, 2005: 10). However, the Orphans Law needs to be restructured to facilitate access to funding (NDI and Sadc PF, 2004: 18). Throughout the country, regional AIDS coordinating committees (Racocs) have been tasked with the synchronisation and monitoring of HIV/AIDS-related activities (Caesar-Katsenga and Chirambo, 2005: 14).

Local and regional governments coordinate well with NGOs where councils show commitment to addressing the problem of HIV/AIDS. However, regional councils require more resources to fulfil their mandate (Caesar-Katsenga and Chirambo, 2005: 18, 21, 30–31; NDI and Sadc PF, 2004: 34). Joint programmes, including multipurpose centres, OVC interventions and youth skills training, have been coordinated by local authorities and their umbrella bodies (Caesar-Katsenga and Chirambo, 2005: 21–22, 30).

The response to HIV/AIDS requires more leadership and commitment at all levels and among all stakeholders (RoN and UN System in Namibia, 2004: 22), as well as the multisectoral coordination of HIV/AIDS prevention, care and support. An environment must be created in which PLWHAs are more open to declare their status (RoN and UN System in Namibia, 2004: 22). The issue of HIV/AIDS tends to be regarded as less important than economic challenges, such as poverty and unemployment.

Key decision-makers seem to lack knowledge of the illness, which can be seen in the way in which MPs debate and deal with issues such as the confidentiality of PLWHA (AIDSBRIEF, 2004a: 10). Public awareness needs to be raised to overcome stigma (Caesar-Katsenga and Chirambo, 2005: 16; NDI and Sadc PF, 2004: 22–23). Parliament lacks a standing committee on health (NDI and Sadc PF, 2004: 22–23),so that, despite the public sector being the largest single employer in Namibia, the affect of HIV/AIDS on government institutions remains under-researched (Van Zyl, 2003: 14).

Though the government has not developed multisectoral workplace policies for the public sector, the office of the Prime Minister is in the process of developing a Charter of Rights on HIV/AIDS for the public service sector, in cooperation with the AIDS Law Unit/Lac. Only some individual ministries have developed workplace HIV/AIDS-related programmes for both their target group and their own staff (Caesar-Katsenga and Chirambo 2005: 20). In 2003, the government launched national guidelines and training programmes for antiretroviral therapy and introduced access to antiretroviral therapy in the public sector. The government covers the cost of antiretroviral medicines for members of the Public Service Employees Medical Aid Scheme and their dependants, so that many HIV-positive public servants are taking life-prolonging drugs. However, membership in the medical aid scheme is not compulsory.[13] Public servants with medical aid and people with private medical aid are able to access treatment, thereby dividing the Namibian society into those who can afford to live with AIDS and those who cannot (Caesar-Katsenga and Chirambo, 2005: 16).

To harmonise and systematically mainstream the approaches, the HIV/AIDS Unit at the Office in the Prime Minister called a *Workshop on Workplace Programmes for the Public Service Sector* at the end of April 2006.[14]

3.4.2 Civil society activities

The umbrella organisation Namibia Network of AIDS Service Organisations (Nanaso) records that 240 organisations employ 840 full-time staff, 300 part-time staff and nearly 15 000 volunteers (Nanaso, 2005b: 12). However, about 35% of the organisations involved in fighting the pandemic are very small and have no full-time staff at all. Many agencies work only in one or two regions (Nanaso, 2005b: 17). Of the organisations actively seeking to create an enabling environment, 69% are engaged in prevention and 58% are focused on mitigating the effect of AIDS. While 42% focus on providing access to treatment, care and support, 17% are involved in integrated and coordinated programme management (Nanaso, 2005b: 18).

The umbrella body CCN and its member churches have set up HIV/AIDS committees and VCT centres throughout Namibia, as well as trained pastors in counselling (UNAIDS, n.d.). The Church Alliance for Orphans (Cafo) is an interfaith organisation, representing a wide network of faith-based organisations and congregations, all active in the care of OVC (AIDSBRIEF, 2004b: 10).

Namibia's largest civil society AIDS service organisation CAA records 84 full-time staff and 1 600 volunteers. The AIDS Law Unit/Lac has helped to set up a human rights approach to the pandemic and to develop workplace policies (Caesar-Katsenga and Chirambo, 2005: 19). The Namibia Planned Parenthood Organisation (Nappa) advocates for the rights and access of young people to information, education and counselling services on sexual and reproductive health (UNAIDS, n.d.). The National Social Marketing Programme (Nasoma) uses commercial marketing techniques to promote condoms; while the Social Marketing Association (SMA) provides information and education on HIV/AIDS through radio shows and health awareness events at village level (UNAIDS, n.d.). Based in northern Namibia, Hope

Namibia reaches people with general information, education and condoms. The Johanniter Hilfswerk organisation conducts courses in home-based care, manages several clinics and schools and offers support to OVC (AIDSBRIEF, 2004b: 5). Furthermore, the Namibian network of PLWHA Lironga Eparu ("Learn to Survive"), launched in 2001, mobilises communities. Apart from civil society activists, traditional leaders are involved in HIV/AIDS activities, where they strongly influence societal attitudes and behaviour (Caesar-Katsenga and Chirambo, 2005: 19; NDI and Sadc PF, 2004: 28).[15] In civil society, the print media also forms a "powerful agenda-setting agent" (Keulder, 2006: 10).

The Tenor Institute for Media Analysis concludes, "looking at the media coverage on HIV/AIDS … one might be forgiven for thinking that there is no pandemic at all" (Keulder, 2006: 10). The only media attention paid to the pandemic is in the form of media campaigns, such as the Take Control Campaign.

3.4.3 The private sector as latecomer

Though the private sector organises HIV/AIDS-directed funds and develops relevant workplace programmes, the former has still to gain momentum (RoN and UN System in Namibia, 2004: 24). The umbrella body Namibian Chamber of Commerce and Industry (NCCI) has set up an HIV/AIDS desk to spearhead several initiatives. The Namibian Business Coalition on AIDS (Nabcoa) undertakes the coordination and facilitation of business activity to best address the pandemic, as well as devising a strategy for small and medium-sized enterprises (Phororo, 2003: 11).[16]

The Hanns Seidel Foundation concludes that "the private sector still continues to believe that HIV/AIDS is not their responsibility" (Phororo, 2003: 10). Concern has been expressed about the inactivity of the business community in this regard (AIDSBRIEF, 2004a: 12).

Smaller companies lack the resources to set up HIV/AIDS programmes (Phororo, 2003: 12–14), while some of the larger companies, such as the Ohlthaver & List (O&L) Group, are implementing HIV/AIDS workplace programmes. Only a few of the Namibian parastatals with written policies or guidelines run specific campaigns for their employees and participate in HIV/AIDS campaigns. Tertiary education institutions, such as the University of Namibia (Unam), the Polytechnic of Namibia and the Namibian College of Open Learning (Namcol), reach out to young, sexually active adults on HIV/AIDS issues (AIDSBRIEF, 2004b: 12–13).

With a growing number of development partners[17] joining the fight against HIV/AIDS, coordination will become one of the key priorities for the government. The duplication of efforts and loss of resources at the expense of the beneficiaries must be avoided.

4. Impact on electoral systems

Since the UN-supervised election of 1989, which paved the way for Namibia's independence, Namibia has held regular presidential, National Assembly (NA), regional and local elections. Despite occasional administrative problems and reports of intimidation, the elections have largely been regarded as free and fair by international observers.

4.1 Elections, electoral systems

Four types of elections and three different electoral systems are used in Namibia (see Table 4.1).

Table 4.1: Electoral systems and frequency of Namibian elections

Type	Frequency (last election)	System
Presidential election	Every five years (November 2004)	Majority (50%+1)
National Assembly election	Every five years (November 2004)	PR (list)
Local authority election	Every five years (May 2004)	PR (list)
Regional council election	Every six years (November 2004)	FPTP

The electoral system is inherited from Namibia's pre-independence history. UN Security Council Resolution 435 of 1978 was instrumental in attaining Namibia's independence as it set out a plan for UN-supervised elections for the Constituent Assembly (CA) that heralded independence.

The *Constitutional Principles* brokered by the Western Contact Group (consisting of Canada,

France, West Germany, the UK and the US) in 1982 set out the post-independence dispensation, including regular multiparty elections and respect for human rights. Though neither Resolution 435 nor the *Constitutional Principles* specified the system for the CA election, the UN secretary-general's office confirmed in 1985, after talks between South Africa and the Contact Group, that the proportional representation (PR) system would be used. Resolution 435 was eventually implemented in 1989 and Namibia's first genuinely democratic elections were judged free and fair by the UN (Hopwood, 2006: 33).

Due to the success of the UN-supervised 1989 elections, the CA opted to continue using the PR system, and the South West Africa People's Organisation (Swapo) abandoned its preference for a single-member constituency system and a unicameral Parliament in exchange for concessions on other issues, including an executive presidency. With the adoption of the Constitution on 9 February 1990, article 49 enshrined the party list and PR system for the NA elections. As the Constitution did not prescribe an electoral system for local authority elections, the proposed ward system was abandoned in 2002 in favour of a party list system.

In the presidential elections, a single-member majority (SMM) of 50%, plus one vote, is used[KC4]. According to article 28 of the Constitution, if there is no clear majority, then further ballots will be held, until a candidate gains over 50% of the vote. The Constitution further states that elections for regional councillors should follow a single-member plurality system (SMP) (article 106), or the first-past-the-post system (FPTP), meaning that the candidate with the most votes in a constituency wins the seat[KC5]. The National Council (NC) comprises two members elected by each regional council (article 69).

Voters (meeting the criteria of citizenship, voting age and a minimum period of one-year residence in their constituency for the local elections) are eligible to vote on voting day only upon presenting their voter's card and must vote within their constituency for both regional and local elections.

4.1.1 Proportional representation system

Set up according to article 44 of the Constitution, the NA is the highest law-making body of Namibia. The 72 seats of the NA are filled in accordance with the PR system, with the president being empowered to appoint an additional six individuals, who lack voting rights, based on their expertise in an advisory capacity. Parties are required to submit their party list, containing a minimum 24 and maximum 72 names of candidates, to the ECN on a predetermined date before the election. As there is no legislative provision for selection of such candidates for both the NA and local authority elections, the selection process has sometimes been controversial (Hopwood, 2006: 37).

4.1.2 First-past-the-post system

Regional council elections are administered on the FPTP system. As with the local authorities, such councils are decentralised institutions formed to bring democracy closer to the people they serve and to whom they are directly accountable within their jurisdiction. Each region in Namibia has its own council, consisting of between six and twelve councillors, with one councillor being elected for each constituency, which is responsible for its development and administration. During the first sitting of the regional council, a governor is elected directly by the members, as are two councillors to represent the region in the NC. Table 4.2 shows the parties which have held parliamentary seats since independence.

Table 4.2: Parties with parliamentary seats since independence

Abbreviation	Full name	Period
ACN*	Action Christian National	1990–95
NNF	Namibia National Front	1990–95
DCN	Democratic Convention of Namibia	1995–2000
DTA	Democratic Turnhalle Alliance	1990–2010
Mag*	Monitor Action Group	1995–2010
FCN	Federal Convention of Namibia	1990–95
NPF	National Patriotic Front	1990–95
UDF	United Democratic Front	1990–2010
Swapo	South West Africa People's Organisation	1990–2010
COD	Congress of Democrats	2000–10
RP	Republican Party	2005–10
Nudo	National Unity Democratic Organisation	2005–10

*The ACN was renamed Monitor Action Group (Mag) in 1995.
Source: Guide to Parliament, 2005.

4.1.3 The accessibility of suffrage

Held concurrently with presidential elections over two days, the first day of the elections has been declared a public holiday to facilitate voting. With women representing 52% of the electorate, the issue of gender balance in Parliament has received increasing attention over the years, gaining in momentum with the 50/50 Campaign in 2004. Implemented by the Namibian Women's Manifesto Network, the campaign lobbied for gender balance in Parliament, specifically through the implementation of the "zebra list" system (the alternation of male and female candidates on party lists) and the implementation of the National Gender Policy. The campaign also addressed other related issues, including the representation of people living with disabilities, and the securing of a living wage for domestic workers and adequate pensions. In the campaign, the electorate was encouraged to vote for parties that would work towards gender equality and the empowerment of women in the regions[18] by:

- Developing the gender policies of regional councils in consultation with the community to ensure that development and service delivery strategies are gender-sensitive and supportive of gender equality;
- The setting up of regional gender desks or committees to administer the implementation of gender policy; and
- Gender budgeting in regional councils to ensure the equitable distribution of resources.

The campaign further challenged political parties to elucidate on their position regarding:

- Programmes to eliminate poverty;
- The promotion of the economic independence of women;
- The accessibility of affordable housing, land and water;
- The provision of affordable and safe childcare facilities;
- The combating of violence against women and children;
- The provision of support for prevention programmes;
- The provision of treatment and care for PLWHAs;
- The promotion of reproductive and sexual health and the rights of girls and women;
- The promotion of accessible education and lifelong learning; and

- The promotion of the sharing of domestic responsibilities between men and women.

The 50/50 Campaign has thus spearheaded a holistic approach to the relationship between development and inclusive politics, focusing particularly on issues affecting women.

4.2 Economic, political costs

The total budget provision of N$60.5 million for the 2004 presidential, NA and regional council elections was allocated as follows: N$30 million to the ECN; N$20 million to the Namibian Police Force; N$8 million to the Namibian Defence Force; and N$2.5 million to the Namibian Broadcasting Corporation. While the PR list system is not as expensive as the FPTP system, under which by-elections must be held whenever members die or resign, both systems

are contentious in their response to HIV/AIDS. The costs associated with the effect of HIV/AIDS on electoral systems are either tangible quantitative (financial) costs or intangible qualitative costs.

4.2.1 Costs associated with by-elections

The effect of HIV/AIDS on the electoral system is difficult to gauge, primarily due to the policy of non-disclosure, in which no MPs have apparently died of HIV/AIDS-related illness. The ECN has also not kept official records of Namibian by-elections.

No statistical comparison is possible of the mortality rate of MPs pre- and post-Independence. Table 4.5 shows that the post-1999 records of regional council by-elections indicate that 32 by-elections have been held. Specified illness (illnesses generally unrelated to HIV/AIDS) is distinguished from

Table 4.3: Gender representation in the National Council

Party	1992–98		1998–2004		2004–10	
	Female	Male	Female	Male	Female	Male
Swapo	1	17	2	22	6	18
DTA	0	8	0	1	1	0
UDF	0	0	0	1	0	1
Total	1	25	2	24	7	19

Source: Guide to Parliament, 2005.

Table 4.4: Gender representation in the Constituent/National Assembly

Party	1989–90		1990–95		1995–2000		2000–05		2005–2010	
	Female	Male	Female	Male	Female	Male	Female	Male	Female	Male
CAN/Mag	0	3	0	3	0	1	0	1	0	1
CoD	0	0	0	0	0	0	3	4	2	3
DCN	0	0	0	0	0	1	0	0	0	0
DTA	1	20	1	20	2	13	2	5	0	4
FCN	0	1	0	1	0	0	0	0	0	0
NNF	0	1	0	1	0	0	0	0	0	0
NPF	0	1	0	1	0	0	0	0	0	0
Nudo	0	0	0	0	0	0	0	0	0	3
RP	0	0	0	0	0	0	0	0	0	1
Swapo	4	37	4	43	12	47	16	45	18	43
UDF	0	4	0	4	0	2	1	1	1	2
Total	5	67	5	73	14	64	22	56	21	57

Source: Guide to Parliament, 2005

Table 4.5: Regional council by-elections held since 1999								
Year	Total number of by-elections	Venue	Death: Specified/ unspecified illness	Resignation: Incapacity/ Other ventures	Other	Unknown	Political party of previous councilllor	Political party of successor
1993	5	Kabe, K'hoop Rural, Arandis, Aroab, Olukonda	Unspecified	1		1 1 1	Unknown Unknown Unknown Unknown Unknown	Swapo DTA Unknown Unknown Unknown
1994	1	Ompundja				1	Unknown	Unknown
1995	2	Gobabis, Okongo					Unknown Unknown	Swapo Unknown
1996	1	Katima Mulilo			Councillor expelled		DTA	Swapo
1997	1	Ompundja				1	Unknown	Unknown
1998	2	Kapako, Rundu Urban	Unspecified			1	Unknown	Swapo
1999	2	Wanaheda, Walvis Bay Urban			Political posting Political posting		Swapo Swapo	Swapo Unknown
2000	2	Gobabis, Rundu Urban	Unspecified		Nullified		DTA Swapo	Swapo Swapo
2001	5	Rehoboth, Kapako, Oshikango, Karibib, Rundu Urban	Unspecified Unspecified Unspecified	Incapacity	All removed		Swapo Swapo Swapo Unknown	Swapo Swapo Swapo Unknown
2002	0							
2003	4	Windhoek West, Kapako, Oshikango, Reho Urban West	Unspecified Unspecified Specified		Other		DTA Swapo Swapo DTA	Swapo Swapo Swapo DTA
2004	7	Otjinene, Tsumkwe, Omatako, Aminius, Okakarara, Grootfontein, Tsumeb	Other Other Other Other Other Other	Political posting			DTA DTA DTA DTA DTA Swapo Swapo	* Swapo Swapo Nudo Nudo Swapo Swapo

* Note: The Otjinene by-election voting process was suspended midway, as ballot papers ran out. Due to the regional council elections scheduled for four months later, an extra by-election was not held.
Source: Electoral Commission of Namibia, *The Namibian, 19 July, 2004*.

unspecified illness (where reference is made to only a "long" or "short illness", which might serve as euphemisms for AIDS).

The results indicate one specified case of illness and eight unspecified cases of illness. Furthermore, there was one resignation due to incapacity ("illness"), one case in the pursuit of other business and seven cases involving political ventures.

The high incidence in 2004 of resignation to embark upon other ventures is due to the splintering of the National Unity Democratic Organisation (Nudo) from the Democratic Turnhalle Alliance (DTA) to form an independent political party. Political posting, where the incumbent was promoted to an ambassadorial position, accounted for three by-elections. The causes of the other by-elections are unknown. Of the total of 32 by-elections, eight (25%) might thus be blamed on AIDS. Since 1989, one NC member died from a heart attack, while another died, as reported in the media, due to a "short illness".

Table 4.6 depicts the deaths of CA/NA MPs since 1989, with the one case of specified illness being distinguished from one unspecified. Of the total five deaths, one might thus be AIDS-related. The death rate is relatively low, with deaths unrelated to HIV/AIDS, such as vehicle accidents, accounting for three of the five deaths.

Table 4.6: Deaths of Constituent/National Assembly MPs

	Total	Vehicle accident	Illness: Specified	Illness: Unspecified
1989–90	1	1		
1990–95	0			
1995–2000	2	1	1	
2000–05	2	1		1

MPs, due to their high incomes, have access to life-prolonging medication, about which they know considerably more now than before 2003, when treatment first became more readily available.

4.2.2 Political costs

Political costs incurred can, at this point, largely not be quantified, as such costs include:

• The loss of institutional knowledge and capacity

at political party level;

• A decrease in the potential future leadership base of political parties;

• The loss of members of the electorate;

• A potential shift of power from opposition to ruling parties or vice versa, because of losing by-elections (in this study, such shifts are largely attributable to factors other than HIV/AIDS, including shifts in the political environment); and

• The potential political cost of a stagnation of constituency issues and "loss of representation" in a constituency during the first declaration of a vacancy and the filling of that seat by way of a by-election within three months, in terms of the Regional Councils Act No. 22 of 1992.

4.2.3 Economic costs

While comparatively easy to quantify, the costs of individual elections in Namibia are, however, sometimes difficult to ascertain due to more than one election being held simultaneously to cut costs.

Table 4.7: Budget: Presidential and National Assembly elections, 2004

Description	Expenditure US$
Remuneration: Coordinators; area managers; returning offices; polling/counting officials	3 503 142
Electronic voters' register operators, including materials and supplies	393 692
Transport of personnel and materials	1 270 642
Other services: Printing of ballot papers, advertisements, maps and manuals; venue rental; equipment and installation of equipment	1 488 786
Voter education	571 831
Total US$	7 228 093
* Forex rate of 6.5	

Savings for presidential by-election are possible on only pro rata voter education and ballot paper printing. Regional council by-elections cost an average U$77 000, at a forex rate of 6.5.

Table 4.8: Budget: Local authority elections, 2004	
Description	Expenditure US$
Remuneration: coordinators; area managers; returning offices; polling/counting officials	843 881
Materials and supplies	67 253
Ballot papers	22 559
Voter education	77 841
Total US$	1 011 534

4.3 Electoral system reform debate

Electoral system reform might result in the adoption of the mixed member proportional (MMP) electoral system, due to difficulties with the PR system, which have been debated since the mid-1990s (Hopwood, 2006). Though benefiting the smaller parties, the latter system is criticised for its lack of accountability, because of a party list system in which:

- The selection and sorting of names on party lists is highly centralised;

- MP representation of regions in the NA is undefined;

- NA MPs are more likely to be accountable to their party than to the electorate;

- MPs are likely to tow the party line to ensure their political careers; and

- The prevalence of MPs in the Executive limits the availability of MPs for service on committees.

As any electoral system reform would entail substantial constitutional amendment, it would therefore need to be addressed sensitively and considerately. Any such reform should be contextualised within Africa and incorporate the experiences of other countries on the continent.

Legislative reform stems from a Cabinet decision in 2002 which called for the complete redrafting of electoral legislation in Namibia. Proposals forwarded to the National Planning Commission were approved in March 2006. In 1999, the tendered ballot was extended to absentee voters in foreign countries and continuous registration gave rise to the Electoral Amendment Act of 1994. The Act further stipulated that all future ballot papers used in the list system were to contain photographs of nominated candidates or of party leaders.

Though HIV/AIDS has not emerged as an electoral reform issue, further considerations include a postal voting system and the Namibian equivalent of South Africa's special vote facility.

5. Electoral administration and management

5.1 Structures, staff, legal framework of Electoral Commission of Namibia

In Namibia, the responsibility for the administration of elections is divided between two bodies: While the ECN directs and supervises the electoral process, the Directorate of Elections administers registration, polling and related activities on behalf of the Commission and works under its authority. In elaborating the implications HIV/AIDS might have on electoral management, this chapter will investigate the potential impact on the core functions of the ECN.

5.1.1 Structures and staff

The ECN is headed by five commissioners appointed by the president. As part of the voter registration process, the commission appoints a supervisor of registration and registration officers in each constituency and each local authority area. Furthermore, the ECN might employ additional staff to help the supervisors and registration officers. To conduct elections, the ECN appoints returning officers,[19] counting officers and presiding officers,[20] mostly through public advertisement (EISA, 1999: 35).

The head of the Directorate of Elections is appointed on the commissioners interviewing five candidates, of whom they recommend at least two candidates to the president. In 2003 President Sam Nujoma confirmed Philemon Kanime, the Chief Executive Officer of the ECN, as Director of Elections. The director is responsible for the administrative and clerical work of the commission. Between elections, the directorate employs core administrative staff, including a deputy director and chief control officer, chief clerks, secretaries and typists. During elections, temporary staff, including "unemployed literate people" reflecting "the social composition of the population", are employed (EISA, 1999: 15). Accordingly, the directorate commits itself to affirmative action and gender awareness (Tötemeyer, 1996: 19). During elections, the directorate is subdivided into sections that appoint their own support team. The vast distances in Namibia necessitate the use of regional coordinators. Besides, political parties may appoint their representatives as election agents to observe and monitor polling stations and as counting agents (EISA, 1999: 36).

5.1.2 Legislative framework

Through the promulgation of the Electoral Act (Act No. 24 of 1992) the ECN was set up to direct, supervise and control national, regional and local elections in a fair and impartial manner.[21] According to the Act, the ECN's duties include: the supervision and control of the registration of voters; the supervision of the preparation, publication and updating of a national voters' register and a local authority voters' register; the supervision and control of the registration of political parties; and the supervision, direction and control of the conduct of elections.

Though not specifically included as part of its mandate in the Electoral Act (Hopwood, 2006: 36), the commission also oversees voter education in cooperation with NGOs, such as Lac and the Namibia Institute for Democracy (Nid). Until 2000, the commission was located within the office of the prime minister, after which it was set up in its own right and given its own budget. Electoral commissioners became more transparently selected. On candidates' application in response to the posts advertised in two daily newspapers, a selection committee recommends eight short-listed applicants to the president, who chooses five (Hopwood, 2006: 36).

The setting up of the Directorate of Elections as the administrative arm of the ECN has been determined by a government notice of 19 November 1992 (Tötemeyer, 1996: 16).

5.2 Internal impact of HIV/AIDS

5.2.1 Internal impact on ECN

Idasa's *HIV/AIDS and Democratic Governance in South Africa* reviews literature on the impact of HIV/AIDS on the internal functioning of workplaces

(Strand and Chirambo, 2005: 85–88), indicating what the impact on electoral commissions will be like.

The taking of additional sick leave by HIV-positive employees is likely to affect both productivity and costs. Accordingly, the increased levels of morbidity might pose a threat to the effective administration of elections. High rates of mortality or early retirement have also been identified as potential threats to the effectiveness and competence of electoral commissions.

With the loss of skilled, experienced employees, staff will need to be trained at extra cost. Increased absenteeism due to AIDS-related illnesses, the attendance of funerals and having to take care of sick family members might also hinder the internal functioning of commissions. The effective administration of elections is also likely to be seriously affected by lower staff morale, making for a negative impact on the employment equity profile. On the basis of the literature review carried out by Idasa, this section will investigate to what extent the ECN has already been negatively affected by the pandemic, and, if so, whether the Namibian electoral body has developed a strategic plan for effectively countering such effects.

Getting AIDS-related mortality information tends to be difficult, as PLWHAs have, according to the National Code on HIV/AIDS in Employment, the legal right to confidentiality regarding their HIV status in the workplace, with disclosure of such status possible only with the employee's written consent (MoL, 1998). As most of their personnel are employed only temporarily during voter registration and elections, the ECN staffs only 25 permanent employees, of whom most (15) are women, who suffer most from the pandemic. As 21 of its permanent staff are between the ages of 25 and 49, the ECN is likely to be vulnerable to the effects of HIV/AIDS among young and middle-age adults.[22] With some permanent staff being part-time students, only 20% are highly skilled.[23]

During the past five years, two permanent staff died due to illness while employed by the ECN, with no indication of either having died from an AIDS-related illness. Therefore, AIDS seems to have had little effect, as yet, on the permanent staff. Neither has increased absenteeism, due to illness, caring for sick family members and attending funerals, been observed.[24] Nonetheless, anecdotal evidence in the regard was provided by the former Director of Elections, Joram Rukambe. Though unaware of any AIDS-related mortality during his tenure at the ECN from 1998 to 2003, he recalls that absenteeism

Table 5.1: Supplementary registration and polling staff, 2004 local authorities elections

	Government officials	Unemployed citizens	Female staff (%)	Male staff (%)
Supplementary registration staff	161	1 084	57.5	41.9
Polling staff	319	1 215	59.6	40.4
Source: ECN, 2004: v.				

Table 5.2: Supplementary registration staff, 2004 presidential and National Assembly elections

	Total	Government officials	Unemployed citizens	Female staff	Male staff
Regional coordinators	13	12	1	4	9
Area managers	26	21	5	5	21
Constituency supervisors	10826	81	77	37	71
Supplementary registration officers	2 906	453	2 453	1 724	1 181
Source: ECN, 2005: 46.					

increased due to frequent attendance of funerals.[25]

As the temporary staff noticeably outnumbers the permanent staff, the composition of the short-term workforce employed by the ECN during the 2004 local authority elections and the 2004 presidential and NA elections is now reviewed. The ECN report on the local authority elections states that, for the supplementary registration process before the elections, 1 245 officials (57.5% females and 41.9% males) were appointed, of whom 161 were government officials and 1 084 were unemployed at the time of appointment. The polling staff for the local authority elections comprised 40.4% males and 59.6% females, of whom 319 were government officials and 1 215 were unemployed at the time of appointment (see Table 5.1).

Before the 2004 presidential and NA elections, 13 regional coordinators were recruited for supplementary registration purposes, with most being females and/or unemployed at time of appointment (see Table 5.2).

The election and polling officials recruited included 13 regional coordinators, 26 area managers, 108 returning officers, 1 368 presiding officers and 6 066 polling officials, who were largely recruited in response to vacancies advertised in local newspapers. In 2004, about 7 000 (44% male and 56% female) were appointed from more than 30 000 applicants, with the minimum requirement being a grade 12 secondary school qualification or grade 10 with experience (see Table 5.3) (ECN, 2005: 47).

Table 5.3: Presiding and polling officials, 2004 presidential and National Assembly elections

	Female staff (%)	Male staff (%)
Presiding and polling officials	56	44
Source: ECN, 2005:47.		

As most temporary staff come from the highest HIV prevalence age cohorts,[27],[28] the pandemic is likely to reduce their numbers. With public jobs being advertised before every election, previously employed candidates still have to reapply for temporary positions, despite the ECN preferring to appoint those with experience of electoral procedures. Proving increased levels or mortality or morbidity among temporary staff is very difficult.[29] However, as the ECN encourages returning officers, one for each constituency, to reapply for their positions in writing, increased levels of morbidity and mortality among the returning officers might be more apparent. Some returning officers were unable to reapply due to their employers not giving their consent.[30] As most temporary staff have no experience of elections, the cost of training has to be factored in, regardless of the probable increased loss of skilled, experienced staff due to HIV/AIDS. The ECN learned from the 2004 presidential and NA elections to limit the appointment of the unemployed youth, in favour of "experienced and active retired officials who have done management and administration before" (ECN, 2005: 63).

5.2.2 ECN's response to internal impact

HIV-positive employees are protected by the National Code on HIV/AIDS in Employment (MoL, 1998). Though the ECN has no formal workplace policy on HIV/AIDS, apart from that which applies to the public service in general, awareness has been created on an *ad hoc* basis. Rukambe,[31] Director of Elections from 1998 to 2004, increased HIV/AIDS awareness during staff meetings and has also spoken privately with employees in this regard.

5.3 External impact of HIV/AIDS

Idasa's literature review (Strand and Chirambo, 2005: 85–88) shows that the administration of elections might not be negatively affected only by increased levels of morbidity, mortality and absenteeism, but also by an increased demand for service delivery.

5.3.1 Pre-election phase

Idasa argues that the sharp increase in mortality due to the pandemic will pose considerable problems for the accurate and timely compilation and maintenance of the voters' register (Strand and Chirambo, 2005: 91–93). If the ECN does not manage this process as well as it should, inaccuracies on the register could facilitate electoral fraud. Protecting the integrity of the voters' register against unrecorded deaths and other problems is possible only with regular reregistration (Keulder and Wiese, 2003: 5).

General voter registration, which should take place at least once every ten years, occurred in 1992 and 2003. A supplementary registration of voters was also instituted a month before the 2004 National Elections (ECN, 2005: 7). Before the elections, and after supplementary registration, the ECN continued to update the register. According to the ECN, more than 200 temporary employees were recruited to update the voters' roll, during which exercise the names of 4 833 deceased were removed from the register to tally with the names available from the Ministry of Home Affairs and Immigration deceased persons' register (ECN, 2005: 14).

Continuous registration, in which post offices were used as fixed registration points, was abandoned in 2001,[32] due to serious errors having occurred on the voters' roll (Hopwood 2006: 37).[33] However, electoral law reformers are considering reviving continuous registration on a regional level.[34]

The high final figure of 878 869 on the voters' register for the 1999 elections aroused suspicion, as it meant that over 90% of the eligible population registered. Yet, the registration figure for the 2004 presidential and NA elections, based mainly on the 2003 general registration, was 978 036 – again, a very high proportion of the voting age population (ECN, 2005: 60).

The high figures are surprising, as Namibians are not obliged to register as voters. Though Namibian citizens are required to have two cards, one proving their status as a registered voter and another proving that they are Namibian citizens, voters can use any one of a variety of identity documents to register or, if such documents are not available, they can use sworn statements verifying the voter's identity. More than 30% of those registering for the 1999 NA elections, especially among young and rural voters, used sworn statements (Keulder, Van Zyl and Wiese, 2003: 5). Such heavy reliance on sworn statements might facilitate fraud (Hopwood, 2006: 37).

Both the 2003 reregistration and the 2004 voting processes introduced a number of technical innovations. To get more information about registered voters, a registration form, using additional data entry fields and photographs, was introduced (Keulder and Wiese, 2004: 10–11).

Legislative reforms were proposed to restrict the use of sworn statements to those potential voters with valid birth certificates (Keulder and Wiese, 2004: 15). To speed up both the registration and the voting process, the ECN provided the polling stations with a computerised voters' register in place of manual paper-based voters' registers (ECN, 2005: 13).[35]

Since 2000, Namibia's electoral administration has been provided with two registers: one for local authority elections and the other for regional, NA and presidential elections. The Electoral Act (Act No. 24 of 1992) prescribes that the Ministry of Home Affairs and Immigration must supply the ECN with monthly death returns, enabling it to update its registers accordingly. However, staff shortages have led to delays in processing death returns, making it difficult to keep the registers up to date.

In a 2006 stakeholder meeting convened by Nid and Idasa, ECN representatives indicated that the deletion of the names of dead voters took so long because about 25 people had to deal with a large volume of death certificates from Home Affairs. Even if the death rate among registered voters was high, the data could not be computed on time.

A voter is also required to tell the ECN of any change of residence. The supervisor of registration appointed for each local authority area or constituency must submit a voters' list to the director of the ECN on the 15th of each month. Updated lists are then made available for inspection at the ECN or any other place specified in the Government Gazette during the first seven days of each month (Keulder et al., 2003: 7), during which time the names of those not found eligible to vote can be removed from the list. By law, the ECN is required to make the register public ahead of elections. According to the ECN, before the 2004 National Elections took place, the national voters' register was finalised and certified and copies made available for inspection by the public at specific places in every constituency.

The call for public inspection has been made to ascertain that the names of all qualifying individuals have been included and to allow for final objections to be made against the inclusion of those names that should not be on the voters' list (ECN, 2005: 7–11). The cumbersome task of going through the long printed lists raises concern about the effectiveness of this process (Keulder and Wiese, 2004: 1).

The ECN is also required by law to allow political parties enough time to inspect the final voters' roll. However, before the 2004 presidential and NA elections, the ECN granted political parties too little time to inspect the final voters' roll, which had been provided in hard copy of the computerised voters' register.[36]

Published by the Institute for Public Policy Research (IPPR), a research report on the 1999 voters' roll and a research paper on the 2003 Windhoek West by-election voters' registration roll has helped to identify problems recurring within the datasets (Keulder et al., 2003; Keulder and Wiese, 2004). According to the findings, both voters' registration rolls contain double entries and dubious cases, stemming mainly from the data-recording process at the different registration points (Keulder and Wiese, 2004: 7). The 1999 voters' registration roll was replaced by the ECN's reregistration of all eligible voters in 2003.

The substantial number of inaccuracies caused by technical shortcomings identified in the 1999 voters' roll might indicate how accurately the 2003 voters' register was compiled and has been maintained. Analysis of the 1999 voters' registration roll highlighted the most common mistakes in the database (Keulder et al., 2003: 12–14): duplicate or multiple entries; inadequate biographical information;

incomplete entries; inaccurate data entry; and ghost voters.

The problem of ghost voters, which has been identified as one of the most serious shortcomings of the voters' roll (Keulder et al., 2003: 14), is likely to have increased with the rise in the number of HIV/AIDS-related deaths. However, Keulder and others acknowledge that the extent of the problem is unknown. To solve the problem, the ECN depends on the help of the Ministry of Home Affairs and Immigration.

According to Keulder et al. (2003: 16–18), the accuracy of the voters' roll could be improved by extending the network to include alternative sources of information about deaths. Ideally, legislation that makes it compulsory to tell the ECN of all deaths should be drafted (Keulder et al., 2003: 17). The problem of a large percentage of individuals declaring themselves eligible to vote by means of sworn statements remains, given the slow rate at which the Ministry of Home Affairs and Immigration issues identity documents.

The Ministry of Home Affairs and Immigration failed to supply the ECN continuously with monthly death returns from 1998 to 2003.[37] The Ministry also provides the ECN with individual documents and files instead of a database, thereby overloading the ECN's limited permanent staff with work.

The ECN gave computers to the Ministry of Home Affairs and Immigration so that the latter could process information on the dead more quickly. Even if the Ministry of Home Affairs and Immigration were to supply the ECN with regular updates, the lists might be incomplete, since deaths are not always reported in the rural areas (Keulder et al., 2003: 14; UNDP and UN Country Team, 2000: 21). Children and young adults under the age of 18, as well as those not registered, who died of AIDS-related illnesses are also excluded from the ECN's death statistics.

The ECN has finalised the statistics, drawn from the Death Register of the Ministry of Home Affairs and Immigration (see Table 5.4), of all the registered deceased whose names have been removed from the voters' register for the period July 2003 to August 2005. As the aim of such statistics is only to identify registered voters who have died, to enable the removal of their names from the register, the statistics do not indicate the cause of death. The death statistics, which are translated into regionally comparative data, indicate the gender of the deceased, but not the age ranges involved. As it could not be established whether deaths were disproportionately high

Table 5.4: Death statistics: Total number of names of the deceased removed from the voters' register, July 2003 to August 2005

Region	Population by region (2001)	HIV prevalence by region (%)	Female deceased registered voters	Male deceased registered voters	Total: Deceased registered voters in each region	Death rate registered voters in each region (%)
Caprivi	79 826	42.6	545	561	1 106	1.39
Erongo	107 663	27	275	393	668	0.62
Hardap	68 249	14.9	408	494	902	1.32
Karas	69 329	18.7	255	364	619	0.89
Kavango	202 694	18.2	629	662	1 291	0.64
Khomas	250 262	16.7	626	911	1 537	0.61
Kunene	68 735	9.5	104	118	222	0.32
Ohangwena	228 384	18.2	1 335	1 429	2 764	1.21
Omaheke	68 039	13.8	229	220	449	0.66
Omusati	228 842	20.8	1 225	1 360	2 585	1.13
Oshana	161 916	24.9	919	955	1 874	1.16
Oshikoto	161 007	19.7	837	900	1 737	1.08
Otjozondjupa	135 384	22.8	297	340	637	0.47
Total	1 830 330		7 684	8 707	16 391	

Source: Electoral Commission of Namibia. Death Statistics; Hopwood, 2006: 3; Nanaso, 2005b: 8.

among young adults, no strong indication is given of whether AIDS was primarily responsible.

The total number of registered deaths among eligible voters is, inevitably, higher in densely populated regions, such as Kavango, Khomas, Ohangwena, Omusati, Oshikoto and Otjozondjupa, requiring a comparison of the regional death rate of registered voters. According to the death statistics, the Caprivi region has the highest death rate. At 42.6%, the Caprivi region also has the highest HIV prevalence rate. According to the United Nations Development Programme (UNDP and UN Country Team 2000: 23–28), Caprivi also has the lowest life expectancy (32.6 years), the lowest Human Development Index (HDI), and the highest Human Poverty Index (HPI). In 2001, according to the *2001 Population and Housing Census* (Central Bureau of Statistics, 2003), more than 50% of all deceased Caprivians died between the ages of 15 and 49, which is the age group with the highest HIV prevalence. According to the ECN's death statistics, the Hardap region has the second highest death rate among registered voters, though the HIV prevalence rate is much lower than that of Caprivi.

5.3.2 Polling phase

The Electoral Act (No. 24 of 1992) and the subsequent Amendment Act govern issues relating to the organisation of polling stations, such as the distribution of voters, the availability of suitable locations, access to polling stations, and distances to be travelled to such locations. The Act also provides for both permanent and mobile polling stations, of which the latter are especially important in sparsely populated rural areas (Tötemeyer, 1996: 49). The average polling station is expected to serve about 1 000 voters and should be within two hours walking distance (EISA, 1999: 43).[38] Being situated in schools or community halls, the permanent voting stations are equipped with toilets and seating.[39]

The tendered vote system, due to much internal migration and inadequate rural road and railway networks, provides for those who cannot vote at a polling station in the voting district in which they are registered.[40] In the system, which is used in the NA and presidential elections, people can cast their votes anywhere in the country or at diplomatic posts abroad. As tendered votes are counted in the constituency where they were cast, confusion arose in 2004 when tendered and ordinary ballots were combined and declared votes of the constituency where they were cast (Hopwood, 2006: 37).[41]

The current electoral law reform debate is considering whether the tendered vote system might be replaced by a postal voting system,[42] meaning that those who cannot go to the polls will not miss out on their right to vote. Though such a system could make democratic participation in voting as inclusive as possible, it needs to be carefully scrutinised, as it might facilitate electoral fraud. To ensure that the postal voting system will not be abused by those who do not qualify for it, the applicants for such a vote should clearly explain why they are asking to vote in this way.

A postal voting system requires formal identification of the voters, so that relying on sworn statements challenges the Ministry of Home Affairs and Immigration's ability to deliver formal identification to the voting age population. "Special vote" facilities, as already implemented in South Africa, would enable people to ask to register and vote at home in the presence of a visiting electoral officer.

5.3.3 ECN's response to external impact

The Electoral Act (Act No. 24 of 1992) provides for the ECN to make arrangements for disabled voters, who may either get help from the presiding officer or an adult family relative or friend (Tötemeyer, 1996: 49). In such a situation, the voter's decision might not be entirely secret.[43] Presiding officers may encourage disabled, pregnant or sick voters to skip the queue, or to queue separately.[44] In June 2004, the ECN set up a steering committee to plan and implement a project on the treatment of people with disabilities during elections.

From 2003 to 2005, an Election Support Consortium, consisting of the ECN, Lac and Nid, has been responsible for a voter education programme, in which each implementation partner participated according to its core competence. The initiative, apart from encouraging everyone eligible to vote to access this right, also included civic education material for people with disabilities. Strategies targeting HIV/AIDS-affected or -infected voters have not yet been implemented.

As the Act does not provide for bedridden patients who are unable to register or to visit the polls on election day, home-based care AIDS patients find it very difficult to register for elections[45] and to cast their votes (Strand, 2005: 4). Mobile polling stations have visited hospitals, prisons and old-age homes, allowing hospitalised AIDS patients to vote, but excluding patients in home-based care.[46] More flexible registration and voting times, improved access for those with special needs at polling stations, or home visits by electoral officials might help. However, such solutions are expensive.

6. Impact on parliamentary configuration

Namibia's bicameral parliamentary system was set up based on the country's Constitution in 1990. The lower house – the NA – has the power both to make and repeal laws. It comprises 72 members elected every five years, using a PR system based on closed party lists. The president also appoints six extra non-voting members for their special expertise, status, skill or experience. The upper house – the NC – has the power to review all legislation and reports passed on to it by the NA, as well as to initiate legislation on matters of regional concern.

The NC comprises 26 members who, unlike NA MPs, represent territorial constituencies. NC members are regional councillors nominated by their regional councils. Each of Namibia's 13 regions selects two representatives for the NC. Regional council elections have been held every five or six years since 1992. Since Namibia became independent on March 21 1990, Swapo has dominated both houses of Parliament (see Tables 6.1 and 6.2).

The CA, elected in November 1989 after UN-supervised elections, was transformed into the first NA (1990–1995) on independence. Swapo gained a majority of seats, but not the two-thirds majority which would have enabled the party to write the Constitution on its own. However, after subsequent elections in 1994, 1999 and 2004 Swapo gained more than two-thirds of the NA's 72 seats. Swapo has been even more dominant in the NC, set up in 1993, after Namibia's first regional elections at the end of 1992. The ruling party's share of seats increased from 19 to 24 (out of 26) in 2004.

The closed party list system used in the NA elections has been criticised for producing candidates who feel accountable to their parties ahead of the electorate. The fact that NA MPs are not rooted in constituencies influences the manner in which they

Table 6.1: Share of seats in the National Assembly since 1990

Year	Swapo	DTA	UDF	ACN/ Mag	FCN	NNF	NPF/ DCN	CoD	Nudo	RP
1990	41	21	4	3	1	1	1	–	–	–
1995	53	15	2	1	0	–	1	–	–	–
2000	55	7	2	1	0	–	0	7	–	–
2005	55	4	3	1	–	–	–	5	3	1

Table 6.2: Share of seats in the National Council since 1993

Year	Swapo	DTA	UDF
1993	19	7	0
1999	22	3	1
2004	24	1	1

Table 6.3: National Assembly and National Council MPs by age in 2000 and 2005

Age group	National Assembly, 2000	National Assembly, 2005	National Council, 2000	National Council, 2005
20-29	0	3	0	0
30-39	8	5	9	5
40-49	27	23	11	17
50-59	27	25	5	4
60-69	9	15	1	0
Over 70	1	1	0	0
Average age	51	51	44	45

contribute to debates and their accessibility to the public and civil society organisations.

Since 2000, more than 40 out of 55 Swapo MPs in the NA have formed part of the executive, either as ministers or deputy ministers, which has negatively affected the quality of debates, the functioning of the committee system (which depends on a small number of opposition MPs and Swapo backbenchers), and public perceptions of the effectiveness of MPs who are not on the executive. Though national councillors are the only MPs who directly represent the local constituents, their powers in the chamber of review are limited. They are often viewed as the "poor cousins" of the NA, and so their political influence is seen as secondary to that of the lower house.

6.1 Parliament and HIV/AIDS

The potential role of Parliament as an institution and parliamentarians as individuals in raising awareness about HIV/AIDS and creating leadership role models has largely been overlooked in official policy. Parliament as an institution has also been slow to wake up to the challenges posed by the pandemic. The government has acknowledged the need to involve all public institutions in efforts to reduce the level of HIV infections. In the preface to MTPIII, Health Minister Dr Amathila wrote: "Effective management and control of the HIV/AIDS pandemic call for a multi-sectoral approach" (RoN, 2004b:ii). However, in MTPI and MTPII the role of Parliament was not prominent. Only when MTPIII, outlining plans for the 2004–2009 period, was issued in 2004 were the obligations and commitments of the Legislative Sector included. In MTPIII, MPs are urged to do everything within their sphere of influence to:

- Influence public opinion and lead their constituents towards attitudes supportive of an effective national response to the pandemic, by increasing public knowledge and understanding of relevant issues;

- Ensure that legislation that they vote into being protects human rights and advances effective HIV/AIDS prevention, treatment, support and care programmes;

- Ensure political commitment and better governance essential for a rights-based response to HIV/AIDS;

- Mobilise the involvement of the government, private sector and civil society in discharging their societal responsibilities by responding appropriately to the pandemic; and

- Ensure that adequate and consistent financial resources are allocated to support and enhance effective HIV/AIDS national programmes that are consistent with human rights principles (RoN, 2004b).

MTPIII then outlines a series of commitments, including:

- legislative committees "providing an ongoing forum for parliamentarians to deepen their understanding of the pandemic";

- MPs "ensuring that HIV/AIDS is kept on the political agenda";

- parliamentarians "combining intellect, tolerance, compassion and resolve to address the most important issues that cause suffering among communities and PLWHAs"; and

- parliamentarians "demonstrating strong personal commitments" on the issue of HIV/AIDS (RoN, 2004b).

6.1.1 Death rates

Between 1990 and 2006 four sitting MPs from the NA and two from the NC died, though none died from HIV/AIDS-related illnesses, according to the causes of death announcements issued to the media. Press reports at the time of the MPs' deaths gave the causes shown in Tables 6.4 and 6.5.

Table 6.4: Cause of death, Members of Parliament, National Assembly

Year	Cause of death	Sex	Age	Political party
1997	Complications from diabetes	Male	55	Swapo
1999	Vehicle accident	Male	71	Swapo
2002	Vehicle accident	Female	65	Swapo
2005	Long illness	Female	44	Swapo

Table 6.5: Cause of death, Members of Parliament, National Council

Year	Cause of death	Sex	Age	Political party
2000	Short illness	Male	43	Swapo
2001	Heart attack	Male	47	Swapo

The death rates among the 98 elected members of both houses have remained low. Death certificates rarely give AIDS as a cause of death, instead listing the secondary infection, such as TB or pneumonia, partly because of the stigma and partly because some life insurance schemes are likely to pay out less if AIDS is cited as the cause of death.

The average age of MPs across both houses was 49 in 2000 and 50 in 2005. In the first NA (1990–1995), no deaths of sitting MPs occurred, while in both the second and the third NAs two members (2.7%) died. While no members died during the first term of the first NC (1993–1998), two (7.7%) died during the second NC (1999–2004). All sitting MPs who have died were members of Swapo, with only one being a cabinet minister.

The party list system used in the NA does not require a by-election when an MP dies. Instead, the party of the MP simply selects the next person from the party list used at the last election to take up the vacant seat. As a result, the cost of replacing an MP in the NA is minimal. However, the two deaths in the NC necessitated the holding of by-elections in the regional council constituencies represented by the late politicians. Since 1990, only one MP appears to have resigned his parliamentary seat citing ill health as a reason. The Swapo MP, who resigned in mid-2004, gave complications arising from diabetes as the reason for his withdrawal as one of the six non-voting MPs in the NA. HIV/AIDS seems to have caused minimal disruption to the working of Parliament in terms of the illness or deaths of MPs.

Though the issue of attendance, particularly in the NA, has been raised since the latter part of President Nujoma's final term in office, HIV/AIDS or more general ill health has not been used to explain the failure to achieve quorums. Instead, claims that MPs were attending to their private business and making too many foreign trips were suggested as the cause in press reports. However, this cannot be taken as an indicator of the actual HIV prevalence rate among MPs. MPs receive such high incomes that they were able to access medical treatment long before antiretroviral drugs became widely available in Namibia in 2003. The fact that no death has publicly been linked to HIV/AIDS might also indicate the degree of stigma associated with the virus and the generally impersonal way in which MPs talk about the epidemic.

6.2 Parliamentary debates

Since the late 1990s several significant, if not always well-informed, debates have taken place in the NA on the issues of testing, notification, discrimination and the availability of antiretroviral drugs.

6.2.1 Testing for HIV/AIDS

The debate over whether MPs should go public about the results of their HIV tests has been heavily influenced, if not undermined, by the consequences of a political controversy that occurred in 1996. Swapo MP Ben Ulenga, who was at the time Deputy Minister of Local Government, said, during a debate on the MoHSS's budget, that he had undergone testing for HIV/AIDS and would shortly announce the result in the NA.

During the ensuing heckling and questioning, Ulenga suggested that 50% of MPs in the NA could be PLWHAs. Ulenga also spoke about members of his own family being HIV positive. Due to the furore after Ulenga's comments, he did not return to the house to announce his test result, but left Swapo in 1999 to start an opposition party, the Congress of Democrats (CoD), which won seven seats in the 2000 to 2005 NA.

In November 2000, Home Affairs Minister Jerry Ekandjo, recalling Ulenga's announcement of four years earlier, called on the latter to reveal his status. On the next day, Ulenga distributed a letter to all MPs, to which he had attached a copy of his negative HIV test result, urging other MPs to declare their HIV status. Though several Swapo MPs were dismissive of Ulenga's challenge to publicly declare their test results, the remaining CoD MPs in the NA stated their intention to disclose their test results. However, this did not happen and the party later decided not to make a partisan point out of public testing, for fear of making other parties even more reticent on the issue.[47]

Emma Tuahepa, the National Coordinator of Lironga Eparu, the national association for PLWHAs, has called on public figures to be more open about their HIV status:

> It is unfortunate the HIV/AIDS has a face of poverty … We have our ministers, top officials and business people who are also HIV [positive]. Because they have good medical schemes their lives are prolonged. I call on them to come out in public to help fight the disease.[48]

Despite such a call, no public figures had acknowledged their HIV-positive status by April 2006. Staff and members of the NC, which, as an institution, has shown more commitment on the HIV/AIDS issue than did the NA, decided collectively to go for HIV testing on December 1 2005, World AIDS Day, to show the importance of being aware of one's HIV status.[49] However, logistical problems meant that the testing did not take place on December 1. By April 2006, another date for the tests had not yet been arranged, while talks with the NA were being held to see if the whole of Parliament could be involved in the exercise.[50]

In the light of previous reticence and hostility over the issue, and due to, apart from Ulenga, no MP having acknowledged being tested, the plan seemed unlikely to succeed in the short term. However, in March 2005, Richard Kamwi was appointed Minister of Health, since when he has more enthusiastically propounded VCT than have previous holders of the post. In May 2006, he told an HIV/AIDS awareness campaign launch, held at the Namibian Polytechnic, that he was prepared to undergo VCT, saying:

> Voluntary counselling and testing generates optimism, as large numbers of persons test HIV-negative. It reduces stigma and discrimination and enhances the development of care and support services. Counselling and testing also reduces transmission and enables access to preventive prophylaxis and to antiretroviral treatment.[51]

However, whether Kamwi would undergo public testing was unclear.

6.2.2 Notification of disease

In 1999, Health Minister Dr Amathila declared a directive on HIV/AIDS. Trying to end the "secrecy" surrounding the disease, Amathila said Southern African Development Community (SADC) health ministers had decided that HIV/AIDS should be regarded as a "public health concern" and that the disease would be "notifiable", meaning that medical practitioners could disregard the usual strictures about confidentiality concerning a patient's status. Though Dr Amathila included the policy in a ministerial statement to the NA, no debate occurred on the issue.

The notification policy, however, was alluded to in Swapo's 1999 election manifesto (Swapo, 1999). Though MPs did not question the notification policy, civil society groups immediately advised against the move, consulted among themselves and sought audiences with Dr Amathila. At no point, however, did they try to lobby MPs. The AIDS Law Unit/Lac drew up an alternative policy on the issue of notification, which was accepted by Cabinet in 2002. Though there were many positive aspects to the way in which the notification controversy was handled, apart from the Minister's statement, Parliament was completely bypassed.

6.2.3 Discrimination against people living with HIV/AIDS

In 1997, Deputy Labour Minister John Shaetonhodi tabled in the NA a National Code on HIV/AIDS and Employment, which stated that there should be no pre-employment testing and that PLWHAs should be protected from discrimination in the workplace.

The code was approved by Parliament, despite some objections from MPs, particularly Minister of Defence Malima, who said that pre-employment testing was crucial for potential recruits to the Namibian Defence Force. In 2000, the labour court ruled in favour of a prospective recruit, Haindongo Nanditume, who had been rejected by the army because he was HIV-positive. The labour court ruled that the army could still carry out pre-employment HIV tests, but the decision as to whether an HIV-positive recruit could join the army should be based on CD4 counts and a viral load test, rather than allowing for a blanket rejection.

In 2001, the NA amended the Labour, Defence and Security Acts that would enable the security forces to continue pre-employment testing for HIV as part of their medical tests for potential recruits. The CoD was the only party to vote against the amendments, on the grounds that they were discriminatory. The NC's Standing Committee on Foreign Affairs, Defence and Security later held public hearings on the amendments, at which it recommended that the Ministry of Defence revisit the criteria for army recruitment and introduce a panel of experts to advise on medical issues regarding who should be considered fit to serve in the army. However, the

committee's recommendations appear not to have been taken up by the Ministry of Defence.

The handling of pre-employment testing and the security services issue indicates the strength of the executive in the face of a weak opposition in Parliament. Concerns expressed by the CoD and parts of civil society could not stop the executive proceeding with plans to exempt the security forces from the National Code's provisions. Ultimately, only the court system was able to limit government policy.

6.2.4 Antiretroviral treatment

The provision of antiretroviral treatment provides a rare example of the government changing policy direction, after pressure from a political party, civil society and Swapo. The government had undertaken to provide antiretrovirals in specific cases, such in PMTCT, from the late 1990s. However, a general roll-out of antiretroviral drugs had then been ruled out as too expensive.

The climate on antiretroviral drug provision changed in 2002, when the Swapo-dominated Congress urged that treatment be extended to all PLWHAs. In early 2003, CoD MP in the NA, Rosa Namises, tabled a motion calling on the government to provide antiretroviral treatment at major hospitals. The motion coincided with several civil society candlelit vigils on the issue, organised by the Treatment Action Forum at Lac. While criticising CoD for using HIV/AIDS as a political issue, Dr Amathila told the NA that antiretroviral treatment would be made available to all who needed it. Though the process was still slow, at least the rollout would be general, rather than targeting specific groups.

6.3 Institutional response

Parliament as an institution has become increasingly required to do much more to raise awareness about HIV/AIDS, encouraging and supporting MPs to make a serious contribution on the issue, and providing internal resources and support for affected and infected staff. However, parliamentary response over the past 16 years has been tardy.

Three parliamentary clerks are assigned to the NA's HIV/AIDS desk, with HIV/AIDS-related issues taking up 10% of their time.[52] In the NC, which has made more progress on the issue than the NA, efforts have been spearheaded by one personally committed official, senior parliamentary clerk Samuel Kaxuxuena, who also spends about 10% of his working time dealing with HIV/AIDS-related matters.[53] As a former pastor, he also offers unofficial counselling sessions to NC staff affected and infected by the disease. However, his position as clerk is not enough to ensure that policy change takes place without the support of more senior personnel.

The NA lacks a standing committee dedicated to dealing with the issue of HIV/AIDS. Instead, the issue is only one of the many responsibilities of the Standing Committee on Human Resources, Social and Community Development, which also has to deal with education, health, housing, rural development, gender equality and child welfare. The standing committee has to set up an HIV/AIDS subcommittee. Internally, the NA has a staff committee (set up in 2003) that deals with HIV/AIDS, disseminating information about testing, health matters and condom usage among staff members.

NA staff declared that they were aware of one HIV/AIDS-related death of a colleague in the past three years. Detecting the influence of HIV/AIDS on the turnover of staff was difficult to do, as many NA employees left for other public service jobs after relatively short periods spent working for Parliament.[54] A workplace policy on HIV/AIDS is only in the planning stages. The NA has organised several training workshops for MPs, principally for members of the standing committee, and is sending MPs to the different regions to raise HIV/AIDS awareness. The programme started with the planned visit of six MPs to the Northeast of the country in May 2006. Members of the standing committee, including MPs from Swapo, the DTA, CoD, the United Democratic Front (UDF), the Monitor Action Group (Mag), and Nudo are expected to provide leadership on HIV/AIDS and to "represent the National Assembly in the fight" against the disease.[55]

The NC deals with HIV/AIDS through its Standing Committee on Habitat, which is setting up a subcommittee dedicated to dealing with HIV/AIDS. According to Kaxuxuena,[56] a longer-term plan exists to form a joint parliamentary committee on HIV/AIDS, which would include members of both houses.

Mag chairperson Kosie Pretorius has pointed to the weaknesses of the present parliamentary system:

> The first mistake made after independence was to appoint a Cabinet that is more than half of the National Assembly mem-

bers. Actually the backbenchers must be in a position to influence government, but we cannot do that. For an ordinary member, it is impossible to make a difference. You have to rubberstamp against your will because you cannot even do research.[57]

Swapo Chief Whip Ben Amathila said the main problem for backbenchers was that they lacked "assistants and researchers" to help them to make informed contributions. As a result, "everyone has to do his own little research" (*Insight Namibia*, 2004: 18-19). Some contributions by MPs have been ill-informed, while many have been defensive on the issue, failing to acknowledge that the disease has personally affected them (as it has everyone in Namibia). Only CoD leader Ulenga has formally declared his HIV status and, unfortunately, this was not done in an open and voluntary manner, but after political baiting from Home Affairs Minister Ekandjo.

7. Impact on political parties, policy proposals

With an estimated one in five of Namibian adults HIV-positive, almost 200 000 registered voters could be infected. If voters living with HIV/AIDS were to vote in one bloc, they would, consequently, significantly influence national election outcomes.

However, in the 1999 and 2004 NA elections, several of the parties avoided taking a confrontational stance on the issue. The parties' 2004 manifestos mostly offer similar policies on HIV/AIDS, phrased in language similar to that of the government. In theory, an opposition "AIDS party" would be most likely to focus on the thorny issue of the availability of antiretroviral drugs. However, since the issue was first "party politicised" by a CoD motion brought in the NA in 2003, opposition parties have not dedicated themselves to raising the issue, despite clear evidence that the antiretroviral rollout was delayed.

CoD has been the most outspoken on access to treatment and testing, though its stance has stirred minimal debate. AIDS activists operating in civil society have largely avoided using opposition parties to raise their concerns. Tending to bypass Parliament and the opposition parties, they have directly lobbied the executive instead, a route they see as more likely to produce effective and quicker responses. Though civil society groups working on HIV/AIDS rarely clash openly with the government, in 2003 one such incident made headlines. HIV-positive demonstrators (part of the national campaign group Lironga Eparu) publicly urged the then Deputy Minister of Health Kamwi to speed up the process of making antiretrovirals available at a candlelit vigil in Windhoek.

Later, Lironga Eparu National Coordinator Tuahepa said the demonstration "was really effective" in ensuring that the antiretroviral rollout was implemented with more urgency:

> Perhaps it was not the proper way to go about things according to the Minister, but for us people living with HIV/AIDS it worked really effectively. Immediately, people were treated.[58]

This section examines how the pandemic has affected the seven political parties that won seats in the 2004 NA elections, in their views of the electoral process, their capacity to campaign, their internal party practices, and the development of their policies. The findings are based on manifestos and policy statements produced since 2004 and interviews carried out with representatives of the CoD, the DTA, Mag and the UDF. Requests for interviews with senior officials from the remaining parties represented in the legislature were unsuccessful. Several parties have clearly spent little time and resources on devising HIV/AIDS-related policies or on how they might be able to reduce the negative affect of the pandemic on their ability to function as a political party, despite several politicians providing anecdotal evidence of how HIV/AIDS had eroded their ability to perform effectively.

7.1 Political parties on HIV/AIDS and elections

The history of the liberation struggle, personalities and tribal identity appear to have been primary factors in determining the way in which voters cast their ballots (Hopwood, 2006). In the words of DTA Secretary-General Alois Gende:

> You can write a very good manifesto, but people don't read manifestos – they ask who is the leader, where does he come from, is he respectable, is he a strong leader, is he from my region? (cited in Hopwood, 2005)

7.1.1 Integrity of the electoral process

After the 2004 NA election, several opposition parties complained that the polling had been unfair. Concerns about possible irregularities affecting the count prompted the CoD and the Republican Party (RP) to launch a court case seeking a recount of NA votes, which they won in March 2005. The high court found that, while there had been no conspiracy to subvert the election outcome, ECN officials had committed many errors, which could have undermined the integrity of the election. However, opposition parties also claimed that the recount, which produced a similar result to the first count, was riddled with errors.

A legal challenge of the result, emanating from the RP, was still pending at the time of writing. Despite complaints from several opposition parties about the competence levels and training of election officials, none of the parties interviewed for this chapter had considered that HIV/AIDS might have influenced the way in which the election was organised. The possible high turnover of ECN staff and the failure to build on staff experience gained in previous elections due to illness and/or death had not been considered by most party representatives as a possible reason for the ECN's reduced effectiveness. The DTA, Mag and UDF representatives felt that HIV/AIDS had not obviously affected the administration of the 2004 election.[59] However, the CoD's Secretary-General Reinhard Gertze said that the organisation of the 2004 ballot had been affected, because:

> HIV/AIDS has its impact on everything and elections are no exception … Looking at that given the percentage of people infected, certainly HIV/AIDS has a huge impact in that we are losing people who could play their role effectively not only as voters but in the administration – they could help in the ECN.[60]

Gertze was also concerned that the voters' roll would quickly become out of date due to the high death rates caused by HIV/AIDS. He wanted the ECN to undertake "immediate and consistent" updating of the roll, rather than "waiting to the last minute" before an election.[61] The problem of clearing ghost voters (those who had died since the last election) off the roll would become a major problem if it was left for five years. Both the UDF and CoD felt that HIV/AIDS was negatively affecting voter turnout, because many voters were bedridden at home or in hospital, preventing them from visiting polling stations.

Both the CoD's Gertze[62] and the UDF's Michael

Goreseb[63] have said that the depression caused by being in an advanced stage of such a serious illness would deter some HIV-positive people from voting. Goreseb has said that some voters were "so disillusioned that they no longer care about life". Swapo has the most to lose from high mortality rates, as it is the dominant party in regions such as Caprivi, which have the highest prevalence rate.

However, smaller parties whose support is concentrated in certain geographical areas, such as the UDF in the Northwest or Nudo in the East, could find their limited support bases eroded through high mortality rates in the future. Such an erosion might be particularly evident in regional council elections, in which relatively small swings in voting patterns can determine the winning candidate under the FPTP system. As a result, for example, the few constituencies held by the DTA and UDF in the Northeast could be lost to Swapo. Smaller parties are also often dependent on charismatic leaders and their support bases are vulnerable to erosion if such a leader is no longer able to be the party's dominant figure. In Namibia's case, several smaller parties are headed by tribal chiefs, including the UDF and Nudo.

7.1.2 Party capacity to campaign

With the possible exception of Swapo and Mag, the internal organisation of most parties is poor. Mag neither actively recruits members, nor does it hold formal campaign meetings before elections. Instead, Mag views itself as a pressure group, for which people will vote if they share the party's principles. Though Swapo has released no official membership figures, the party has invested in developing its membership and recording payment of membership fees.

Delegates to important congresses and meetings may be barred if they are not fully paid up Swapo members. The 1997 and 2002 Swapo congresses both passed resolutions urging the party to set up a functioning membership database. In contrast, however, most opposition parties have no meaningful membership records and only have *ad hoc* scattered structures, apart from their head office. In 2005, the CoD's Gertze conceded that the official opposition had fewer than 50 paid-up members (Hopwood, 2005). The DTA, after 29 years, still has no membership records.

The parties blame their absence of membership systems on a lack of financial and other resources. They also find the task of recruiting members highly time- and energy-consuming, when compared with the small income that they believe a paid-up mem-

bership could produce. The RP, for example, complains that many of its prospective members lack the income to pay even a minimal annual membership fee. As a result, the party distributed 10 000 free party membership cards before the 2004 elections (Hopwood, 2005).

While the political will to develop administrative capacity among opposition parties appears to be lacking, Swapo clearly receives most state funding for political parties. In the 2005/06 budget year, Swapo was due to receive N$11.7 million in state funds, while the other six parties in Parliament were expecting to receive only N$3.5 in total (Hopwood, 2006). As most parties hold scant membership data, assessing to what extent HIV/AIDS might have affected their campaigning capacity is difficult for them.

However, nearly all the party spokespeople interviewed acknowledged that HIV/AIDS has robbed them of key activists and degraded their campaign abilities, with several referring to specific party organisers or candidates who had died. DTA Secretary-General Gende[64] said the party's administration had been "dysfunctional", since "highly skilled officials who had been trained through NGOs and the party throughout the years had passed away or were sick in bed and cannot perform."

The UDF's Goreseb[65] indicated that "even the death of one party activist is a notable loss", which causes stress within the organisation, especially as small parties are financially strapped. Gertze of the CoD said that a candidate for the 2004 regional council elections had died, though it was not clear whether the death was HIV/AIDS-related. He also stated that the prevalence of HIV/AIDS made it difficult to organise meetings:

> I will call for an executive meeting and a lot of time I get people saying my brother or sister has died and I cannot attend. I suspect in many instances it is HIV/AIDS. In the leadership you can feel that the impact is there.[66]

Only the Mag MP in the NA, Jurie Viljoen, said his party's campaigning had been unaffected by HIV/AIDS. Mag, the party which emerged from the ashes of the National Party (NP) in Namibia in the early 1990s, has repeatedly stated that "the best way of fighting HIV/AIDS is moral values" (Mag, 2004b).

Since most parties have yet to develop the institutional capacity to recruit and maintain paid-up memberships, the only accurate measure of their support bases is the most recent election results. Swapo has maintained its share of over 75% of the vote at the last two NA elections, while the other parties are of negligible importance. Even the official opposition CoD only attracted 7% of the vote in 2004.

Only the ruling Swapo has a significant youth league, which accepts members up to the age of 35. Despite this being the hardest hit of age groups in terms of HIV prevalence, little evidence exists of a high death rate among Swapo Youth League leaders. Several are paid for completing their party duties or have other paid roles, providing them with the necessary resources to access antiretroviral treatment even before the 2003 rollout started.

7.1.3 Party practice

Parties have not institutionalised their response to HIV/AIDS by creating support structures or educational programmes for their members who are infected and affected. Most party representatives spoke of "informal", "*ad hoc*" or even "random" attempts to address the issue of HIV/AIDS within their organisation. None of the parties interviewed have openly HIV-positive people working in the party structures. The UDF representative said the party's management level had led by example by undergoing VCT,[67] even though this had not been done publicly. The DTA also said that its party leaders had been tested, though the results were not declared. Though the CoD stated in 2000 that the party's MPs would publicly set an example by undergoing testing, they did not do so.

The response to Ulenga's declaration that he would disclose his HIV status in 1996 and 2000 indicated the "political stigma" attached to any politician known to be HIV-positive. Because of such potential stigma, politicians are less likely to undergo public HIV testing and to lead the public campaign for VCT. Gertze said that the party had realised that making testing a party political issue could be counterproductive, as other parties would see such a move as a political challenge and could become defensive on the issue. He urged that public testing should be undergone as parliamentarians rather than as party political leaders: "One should not be very political about this thing. If we exclusively do this [go for testing] we would be challenging Swapo and other political leaders."[68]

Viljoen said that his party had not developed internal written policies on HIV/AIDS, due to its members' belief in high moral standards, implying that such policies were unnecessary for Mag.[69] None of the parties have workplace HIV/AIDS programmes for their staff, and while several said they would like to have such a policy, they pointed to the perennial lack of resources as the reason for their not making progress on the issue.

7.2 Policy proposals

In 1994, only Swapo made reference to HIV/AIDS in its manifesto for the NA elections. Five years later, three parties addressed the issue in their manifestos. The most controversial aspect of Swapo's 1999 manifesto was the proposal that HIV/AIDS be made a "notifiable" disease (Swapo, 1999). However, plans to identify PLWHAs were later dropped, after consultation with civil society. The CoD, in its manifesto, said that HIV/AIDS should be declared a national emergency and that coordination of the government's programmes should be transferred to the office of the president (CoD, 1999).

The UDF was the only party to call for subsidised drugs to be made available to PLWHAs (UDF, 1999). In the five years after Swapo's re-election in 1999, it countered opposition criticism by hastening antiretroviral rollout from 2003 onwards. In 2004 most parties included sections on HIV/AIDS in their manifestos. Swapo's 2004 manifesto stretched to 75 pages, which was much longer and more detailed than the other parties, which mostly produced mere pamphlets on the issue (Swapo, 2004). Nudo's manifesto came in second longest, at 23 pages (Nudo, 2004). Swapo policies are largely drawn from NDP II, Vision 2030 documents, and the party's resolutions at its 2002 congress. In contrast, most of the opposition parties' proposals are limited to a few paragraphs. In heading the government, Swapo is able to set out more detailed policies and, in some areas, state specific targets.

Swapo aimed to have at least one hospital in each region providing a comprehensive HIV/AIDS service by the end of 2004 and said at the time that all 35 public-sector hospitals would provide such services by the end of the 2006/07 financial year. Concerning the rollout of antiretroviral drugs, Swapo pledged that 18 000 PLWHAs would receive treatment by the end of 2007 and 25 000 by the end of 2009. Swapo also wants civil society, including PLWHAs, to take part in the planning and implementation of HIV/AIDS (Swapo, 2004).

The CoD said that it wanted all senior public officials to undergo VCT and to make their results public. The party repeated its calls for HIV/AIDS to be made a national emergency and for the campaign against the disease to be relocated to the president's office (CoD, 2004). The DTA stated that treatment for PLWHAs should be a national priority, and proposed that special care centres be set up to look after the infected (DTA, 2004). Nudo said that it would approach the HIV/AIDS pandemic on the basis of medical science rather than ideology. Though emphasising that it would promote cultural and family values, it said that it also wanted more effective sex education programmes (Nudo, 2004). The RP (2004) also adopted a moralistic approach, denouncing the government for confusing Namibian citizens about sexual behaviour, and urging the adoption of programmes based on Christian values.

Mag, a Christian rightwing party, did not refer to HIV/AIDS in its election material. However, the judgmental approach of the party was clearly portrayed in the budget debate speech of its MP in the NA, Viljoen, when he said: "A person with AIDS doesn't care and will infect as many people as possible." He also said that the government's provision of antiretroviral drugs should be regarded as "a sin tax" (Mag, 2006).

Those parties (Swapo, CoD, DTA) that take a human rights-centred approach, in which treatment features prominently, and those (RP, Mag) that focus on the perceived rights and wrongs of sexual behaviour and what are seen as family values are clearly split as regards their manifestos and policy statements. The UDF and Nudo, which gain much of their support from traditional communities, feature elements of both approaches in their manifestos. Most of the opposition parties feel that they are unable to devise detailed or innovative HIV/AIDS policies, due to their lack of resources, especially any research capacity.

Several parties have said that they are still in the process of developing and revising their positions before entrenching them in policy statements. Such procrastination might be a tacit acknowledgement that their previous statements and manifestos were limited in scope and thin on detail. DTA's Gende said that his party was still busy "redefining the policy to cope with the situation".[70] Only the UDF was able to provide a short policy statement and a manifesto (UDF, 2005), while Mag provided its sole MP's speech on the 2006/7 budget, which referred to the HIV/AIDS issue (Mag, 2006).

In a 2005 policy statement, the UDF stated that MPs "must be champions in the fight against HIV/AIDS by using their status to raise awareness and commitment" (UDF, 2005). Both the DTA and the UDF have said that all party leaders should deal with HIV/AIDS when addressing community meetings. However, politicians seem generally to have failed

to provide the required leadership in this regard in both their communities and the nation. The main progress made within the last six years concerns the move away from simply regarding HIV/AIDS as a contagious disease to viewing the pandemic in the context of human rights.

As a result, the issue of making HIV/AIDS a notifiable disease, raised by Minister of Health Dr Amathila in the late 1990s, has receded in importance. From a situation where only the UDF was mooting the possibility of providing antiretroviral drugs in 1999, a concerted rollout started in 2003. Though no attempt has yet been made to make a joint party statement on HIV/AIDS, there is scope for crossparty agreement and action on the issue.

8. Political opinion, civic participation

How Namibians prioritise HIV/AIDS-related issues and are affected in their participation in civil society activities is explored in this section. The Afrobarometer reports the results of national sample surveys on the attitudes of citizens in selected African countries towards democracy, markets and other aspects of development. In Namibia, the first round of the Afrobarometer survey was conducted in 1999 (round 1), while the next two rounds were conducted during 2002 (round 1.5) and 2003 (round 2), with the most recent round (round 3) being conducted in 2005.[71]

8.1 Political opinion

Table 8.1 shows the percentages of Namibians who thought AIDS was one of the serious policy issues that should receive attention from the government rather than other development-related issues such as poverty, unemployment and education.

Table 8.1: Percentage of Namibians who consider HIV/AIDS most important problem			
	2003 (%)	2002 (%)	1999 (%)
AIDS most important problem	28	35	14[72]
Source: Keulder and Wiese, 2003: 14; Strand and Chirambo, 2005: 119.			

The number of Namibians who regard the pandemic as one of the most important problems[73] first increased significantly between 1999 and 2002 by 21%, but then declined slightly by 7%. Overall, the pandemic was regarded as a more serious problem by larger sections of the population in 2002 and 2003 than at the end of the 1990s. Public consciousness regarding the HIV/AIDS issue has risen significantly over time in Namibia, though it declined slightly between 2002 and 2003. Unemployment remains by far the most dominant problem, with 72% regarding it as an important policy issue in 2003 (Keulder and Wiese, 2003: 13–14).

With the approval of more than two-thirds of Namibians, combating HIV/AIDS is among those policy areas where the government is perceived to be doing either fairly or very well. However, such approval of the government's performance is believed to have decreased from 2002 to 2003 by 12%, though it increased by 6% between 2003 and 2005 (see Table 8.2). Table 8.3 shows the similarity between rural respondents and their urban counterparts, as well as between how male and female Namibians view government performance.

Nevertheless, Namibians are split on whether they would support allocating extra resources to combating the pandemic, even if it meant diverting resources from other key developmental issues. In 2005, when asked to choose between two contrasting statements, 41% agreed or agreed very strongly on (A) "The government should devote many more resources to combating AIDS, even if this means that less money is spent on things like education", while 54% agreed or very strongly agreed on the alternative, (B): "There are many other problems facing this country besides AIDS; even if people are dying in larger numbers, the government needs to keep its focus on solving other problems". Thus, clearly there is less support for prioritising anti-AIDS spending (Idasa, 2006). Again, Table 8.4 shows no real distinction between urban and rural respondents, and no significant difference between male and female Namibians.

The Afrobarometer data further suggest that, between 1999 and 2005, many more Namibians proportionally have experienced personal loss in having lost a friend or a relative to AIDS-related illness, with a drastic increase of 31% between 1999 and 2003, and a significant decline by 11% between 2003 and 2005 (see Table 8.5).

Table 8.2: Positive ratings of government performance in combating HIV/AIDS, 2002-05

Ratings	2005 (%)	2003 (%)	2002 (%)
"Fairly well" and "very well"	72	66	78
Source: Idasa, 2006; Keulder and Wiese, 2003: 15.			

Table 8.5: Percentage of people who have lost a friend/relative to AIDS[74]

	2005 (%)	2003 (%)	2002 (%)	1999 (%)
Personal loss from AIDS	60	71	57	40
Source: Idasa, 2004: 2; Idasa, 2006.				

Table 8.3: Positive ratings of government performance in combating HIV/AIDS, 2005

Ratings	Urban (%)	Rural (%)	Male (%)	Female (%)	Total (%)
"Fairly well" and "very well"	71	71	72	72	72
Source: Idasa, 2006.					

Table 8.4: Statement closest to respondent's view, 2005

Statement closest to respondent's view	Urban (%)	Rural (%)	Male (%)	Female (%)	Total (%)
"Agree very strongly with A" and "Agree with A"	41	40	41	40	41
"Agree very strongly with B" and "Agree with B"	52	54	53	54	54
Source: Idasa, 2006.					

Table 8.6 shows the results of when, in 2005, respondents were asked, "How many close friends or relatives do you know who have died of AIDS?". Overall, Namibians recognise that the increasing numbers of death that they see are the result of AIDS-related illness, and they are becoming willing to talk about it more openly.[75]

Table 8.6: Number of friends/relatives known to have died of AIDS, 2005

Number of friends or relatives	Percentage
1-5	44
6-10	10
11-20	1
More than 20	0
Refused to answer	0
Do not know[76]	3
Not applicable	41

Source: Idasa, 2006.

Rather than asking respondents about their own HIV status, approximate levels of public health have been estimated by asking Namibians about their physical and mental well-being, with two sets of questions being used as proxy-indicators. Table 8.7 shows the results of when the respondents were asked, as a measure of their physical health, "In the last month, how much of the time has your physical health reduced the amount of work you normally do inside or outside your home?". As the levels of stress and depression associated with people knowing or suspecting that they are ill from HIV/AIDS-related causes tend to be high, respondents were asked "In the last month, how much of the time have you been so worried or anxious that you have felt tired, worn out or exhausted?" as a measure of their mental health. Table 8.8 shows the results in this regard.

Table 8.7: Amount of time normally worked inside/outside the home reduced due to physical ill health

Amount of time	2003 (%)	2005 (%)
Never	69	45
Just once or twice	17	29
Many times	11	22
Always	3	4
Do not know	0	1

Source: Bratton et al., 2004: 27; Idasa, 2006.

Table 8.8: Amount of time worry or anxiety resulting in feeling tired, worn out or exhausted

Amount of time	2003 (%)	2005 (%)
Never	67	38
Just once or twice	17	27
Many times	12	28
Always	4	7
Do not know	0	1

Source: Bratton et al., 2004: 27; Idasa, 2006.

According to the 2003 results, Namibians appear by far to be the healthiest people of the many nations included in the Afrobarometer survey (Bratton, Logan, Cho and Bauer, 2004: 27). The relatively low levels of severe illness compared with those of other countries might be due to HIV/AIDS only relatively recently reaching pandemic proportions in Namibia, with the number of respondents feeling often or always physically ill rising significantly by 12% between 2003 and 2005. During the same period, the number of people who felt often or always tired, worn out and exhausted increased drastically by 19%.

In 2005, respondents in rural areas reported feeling significantly more often physically ill, tired, worn out and exhausted than their urban counterparts (see Table 8.9).

8.2 Civic participation

Whether the endemic remobilised civic activism or whether people are demobilised by HIV/AIDS because they have to spend time looking after sick household members[77] or orphaned children is a concern for debate.[78] People were asked whether they provided home-based care for sick family or household members as well as orphans, and, if they did, how many hours a day they spent doing so. In 2003, only 1% of Namibian respondents said that they spent more than five hours a day caring for the sick (Idasa, 2004: 3). Despite Namibia having more than 120 000 orphans (AIDSBRIEF, 2004b: 8; UNICEF, 2005: 4), the same pattern could be observed with respect to their care (Idasa, 2004: 4). Orphans are regarded as biological children within the extended family support system. Namibians have only recently entered the phase where increasing numbers of people need care due to AIDS-related illnesses. The

Table 8.9: Amount of time health reduced

Amount of time	Amount of time normally worked inside/ outside the home reduced due to physical ill health		Amount of time worry or anxiety resulting in feeling tired, worn out or exhausted	
	Urban (%)	Rural (%)	Urban (%)	Rural (%)
Never	55	38	44	34
Just once or twice	25	31	27	27
Many times	16	25	22	31
Always	3	4	6	7
Do not know	1	1	1	1
Source: Idasa, 2006.				

Namibian health care system is better than average (Strand and Chirambo, 2005: 123). The communities contain inadequate caring networks, so that other networks, like private or church orphanages, relieve families of some of the burden (Idasa, 2004: 4). In conclusion, the burden of home-based care for sick family members or orphaned children seems to have been relatively insignificant in Namibia up till now, resulting in little or no impact on people's ability or willingness to participate in civil society.[79] Therefore, people might be "more concerned with getting a chance to earn an income, feed their families, protect themselves from crime and insecurity, and obtain basic health care, than with being saved from a largely invisible killer" (Whiteside, Mattes, Willan and Manning, 2002: v).

9. Impact on levels of voter turnout

The electoral statistics for the 2004 NA elections showed a significant increase in voter participation. As no major policy issues dominated the campaign, it appears that voters have been energised by the succession of the presidential candidate taking place in the ruling party, Swapo. President Nujoma, having completed three terms in office, had to make way for the presidential candidate Hifikepunye Pohamba (Hopwood, 2006: 41). Both Nudo and the RP broke away from the DTA in 2003 and registered with the Directorate of Elections as separate parties, thus perhaps increasing voter participation.

9.1 HIV prevalence and voter turnout

The 2004 presidential and NA elections produced a turnout of nearly 85% – the highest since the watershed 1989 founding elections. At the end of the last supplementary registration of voters, the total number of registered voters was 978 036. As the 2005 estimate for the total population was 2 030 000 people,[80] serious doubts have been raised about the close to one million who registered as eligible voters. The total number of votes cast in the 2004 NA elections was 829 269, representing an 84.8% voter turnout. According to the ECN (2005: 54), such a turnout was "a milestone in voter motivation", in comparison with the turnout for the two preceding NA elections. Table 9.1 shows the numbers of registered voters, the total number of votes cast and the percentage of voter turnout at national level for NA elections in 2004, 1999 and 1994.

Table 9.1: National Assembly elections, 2004, 1999 and 1994

Year	2004	1999	1994
Registered voters	978 036	878 869	654 189
Total votes cast	829 269	540 790	497 508
Voter turnout	84.8%	61.5%	76.05%
Source: ECN, 2005: 60.			

Table 9.2 shows voter turnout in the 2004 NA elections and regional council elections in each region.

Table 9.2: Voter turnout in 2004 National Assembly elections, 2004 regional council elections in regions

Region	Voter turnout: NA elections (%)	Voter turnout: regional council (%)
Omusati	88.12	74.2
Khomas	87.91	37.92
Ohangwena	88.03	72.32
Oshana	88.42	61.06
Kavango	79.85	56.13
Caprivi	79.7	56.64
Oshikoto	89.44	68.32
Otjozondjupa	79.59	47.24
Erongo	87.92	44.09
Karas	84.15	38.57
Hardap	72.18	50.83
Omaheke	78.16	61.81
Kunene	76.44	59.99

Source: ECN, 2005: 58–59; Hopwood, 2006: 336–340.

To consider HIV prevalence by region, the translation of the sero-sentinel survey into regionally comparative data gives the spread shown in Table 9.3.

Table 9.3: Likely HIV prevalence in each region, 2004

Region	Prevalence (%)
Omusati	20.8
Khomas	16.7
Ohangwena	18.2
Oshana	24.9
Kavango	18.2
Caprivi	42.6
Oshikoto	19.7
Otjozondjupa	22.8
Erongo	27.0
Karas	18.7
Hardap	14.9
Omaheke	13.8
Kunene	9.5

Source: Nanaso, 2005b: 8.

To examine whether the voter turnout in 2004 was lower in regions with a higher HIV prevalence than in regions with a lower HIV prevalence, the voter turnout for the 2004 NA elections is compared with the prevalence rates found among pregnant women in selected regions. Table 9.4 shows the percentages of registered voters among the adult population (18<) in each region.

The HIV prevalence rate in the Caprivi region is significantly higher than that of any of the remaining regions around the country. In the 2004 NA elections, the Caprivi had an HIV prevalence ratio of 42.6% for a total voter turnout of 79.7%. The Erongo region, with an HIV prevalence ratio of 27%, had a total voter turnout of 87.92%. The Oshana region, with an HIV prevalence ratio of 24.9%, had a voter turnout of 88.42%. The Kunene region, with a prevalence rate of 9.5%, had a total voter turnout of 76.44%. The Omaheke region, with a prevalence rate of 13.8%, had a voter turnout of 78.16%. Finally, the Hardap region, with a prevalence rate of 14.9%, had a total voter turnout of 72.18%. In conclusion, the three regions recording the highest prevalence rates had an average voter turnout of 85.3%, while the three regions recording the lowest prevalence rates had an average voter turnout of 75.6%. The average turnout in the regions recording high prevalence rates was clearly significantly higher than in those with low prevalence rates. A possible explanation for the high voter turnout in regions with high prevalence rates is that PLWHAs participated in the 2004 NA elections if their state of health allowed them to. However, this argument needs to be qualified by emphasising that, for instance, the percentage of registered voters among the adult population in the Caprivi region was significantly lower than that of other selected regions.

With a countrywide voter turnout of 53.65%, participation in the 2004 regional council elections was significantly lower than in the NA elections that took place later in the same year.[81] The three regions recording the highest prevalence rates had an average voter turnout of 53.9% while the three regions recording low prevalence rates had an average turnout of 57.5%. Accordingly, the average voter turnouts in regions with high prevalence rates was slightly lower than in those with low prevalence rates, possibly resulting from people attaching greater importance to NA elections and therefore being more willing to exert the effort to participate.

Table 9.4: HIV prevalence/voter turnout in each selected region

Region	HIV prevalence (%)	Registered voters/adult population: National Assembly elections, 2004 (%)*	Voter turnout: National Assembly elections, 2004 (%)	Registered voters/adult population: regional council elections, 2004* (%)	Voter turnout: regional council elections, 2004 (%)
Caprivi	42.6	75.6	79.7	75.6	56.64
Erongo	27.0	97.3	87.92	97.3	44.09
Oshana	24.9	81.6	88.42	81.6	61.06
Kunene	9.5	92.4	76.44	92.4	59.99
Omaheke	13.8	89.3	78.16	89.4	61.81
Hardap	14.9	98.3	72.18	98.1	50.83

Source: Central Bureau of Statistics, 2003; ECN, 2005: 58–59; Hopwood, 2006: 336–340; Nanaso, 2005b: 8.
*Registered voters in each region provided by the ECN for 2004. Regional population projections (Central Bureau of Statistics, 2006). Number of eligible voters (18<) in each region is based on proxy-indicators, as the Population and Housing Census distributes age groups as follows: 0–4; 5–9; 10–14; 15–19; 20–24; 25–29; 30–34; 35–39; 40–44; 45–49; 50–54; 55–59; 60–64; 65<.

10. Focus groups: Role of stigma, discrimination

The design of the FGDs was structured in three phases, namely: the preparatory phase; the FGD phase; and the evaluation phase. In preparation for the FGDs, the preparatory phase sought the input of various stakeholder organisations to ensure a process that would attain optimal results. Organisations sourced included those active in the field of HIV/AIDS, namely the Namibian Red Cross Society, Lironga Eparu and PharmAccess. Respondent selection criteria were set up to include the status of registered voter; as well as his/her HIV status; gender; age; level of education; employment status (income); and ethnicity. To ascertain whether there are marked qualitative differences between rural and urban respondents, FGDs were held both in Windhoek (Khomas region) and Ondangwa (Oshana region). On short notice, the northern FGDs had to be cancelled due to logistical problems, with their being held in Otjiwarongo (Otjozondjupa region) instead.

Due to the effects of non-disclosure in Namibia and the stigma associated with disclosure, respondents were sourced from among members of Lironga Eparu, a local NGO providing various support functions for PLWHAs. While the members of Lironga Eparu might inherently be more informed about, and less inhibited by, their HIV status and the effects of stigmatisation than PLWHAs who are not affiliated to a support group, such arguments are negated by the overriding consideration of status. FGDs were conducted in English and/or Afrikaans and/or the vernacular.

A translator was present at all seven FGDs to ensure that participants were able to participate in their language of choice, thus ensuring optimal qualitative results. Translators were selected according to their credibility within the relevant community, thus ensuring that participants would be comfortable and as unrestricted as possible in their participation, due to the presence of a respected community member sanctioning the FGD. To maximise group dynamics for optimal participation, FGDs were restricted to between eight and ten participants and differentiated on grounds of gender and age. A total of 64 participants, all registered voters and all PLWHAs, participated in the FGDs. Of the participants, the ratio of male to female was 1:2. FGDs were structured to solicit responses on the following themes:

• Baseline understanding of democracy and democratic systems;

• Perception of elections;

• Reasons for and (non-)participation in the 2004 elections;

• Perception of change agents; and

• Perception of election management bodies.

While pre-employment screening is not permissible in Namibia, and while HIV is not transmitted in most workplace settings, employers have been known to terminate the employment of, or to refuse employment to, PLWHAs. Fear of stigmatisation and discrimination by colleagues might also make employees reluctant to reveal their infection status. Discrimination might become more subtle and less explicit, with, for example, rather than having their employment terminated outright when their HIV-positive status becomes known, employees might now find themselves laid off for other reasons, or they might be harassed and pressured to the point where they would rather resign.[82] "AIDS denialism" entrenches the stigma and prejudice surrounding the virus, compounding people's fear of AIDS, resulting in a continued battle with the government (Haywood, 2004: 99).

10.1 The Namibian situation

According to the 2000 *Namibia Demographic and Health Survey* (MoHSS, 2003):

- The level of education and an urban setting encourage HIV/AIDS-related awareness and knowledge;
- 98% of women and over 99% of men have heard of AIDS;
- 54% of women and 53% of men know someone who has AIDS or who has died of AIDS;
- 83% of women and 87% of men are aware that a healthy-looking person can be a PWLHA;
- 26% of women and 32% of men believe that PLWHAs should be allowed to keep their status private;
- 91% of women and 92% of men would be willing to care for a relative with AIDS (due more to social obligation than to altruism);
- 67% of women and 55% of men believe that an HIV-positive teacher should keep on working;
- 45% of women and 46% of men would buy food from a vendor with HIV/AIDS;
- 81% of women and 80% of men believe that children aged between 12 and 14 should be taught how to use condoms;
- 95% of women and 97% of men think it acceptable to discuss HIV/AIDS on the radio and in the print media;
- 94% of women and 96% of men think it acceptable to discuss HIV/AIDS on television;
- 24% of women and 25% of men have undergone VCT, while younger respondents and the more educated are more likely to opt for testing;
- 67% of women and 66% of men would like to undergo testing;

- 73% of women and 67% of men know of a place where they can go to be tested;
- 43% of women and 67% of men report the use of a condom with a non-cohabiting partner; and
- 28% of women and 45% of men report the use of a condom with all partners.

According to the same survey (MoHSS, 2003), men's attitudes to condoms and contraception were found to be:

- 35% believe a condom reduces a man's pleasure;
- 25% believe a condom is inconvenient to use;
- 3% believe a condom can be reused;
- 96% believe a condom protects against disease;
- 24% believe a woman has no right to tell her sexual partner to use a condom;
- 24% believe that a woman is responsible for contraception and that it is not the concern of a man;
- 38% believe that a sterilised woman might become promiscuous;
- 52% believe that male sterilisation equals castration; and
- 47% believe that, as the woman is the one who falls pregnant, she should be the one to be sterilised.

10.2 Findings

Though the sample size is indicative rather than conclusive, it does provide a sound basis for future quantitative research into the suffrage of PLWHAs.

In designing the FGDs and selecting the participants (for an enumeration of which, see Table 10.1), more women than men use the services provided by Lironga Eparu, so that women, in their role of child-bearer, are more likely to be tested (according to sero-surveys conducted among pregnant women who attend ANCs and in hospital during childbirth). They are, therefore, more likely to seek counselling and support than are men. Male engagement in extramarital relations and possession of multiple partners tends to be culturally acceptable, as is a woman's subjection to her partner.

What is the level of knowledge of democratic processes, particularly elections?

The impact of HIV/AIDS on the electoral process can only be gauged as meaningful within the context of

Table 10.1: Details of participants included in the sample

	Participants		PLWHAs	Age group	Employment	
	Male	Female			Employed	Unemployed
FGD 1	0	9	9	30–45	1	8
FGD 2	0	9	9	18–29	2	7
FGD 3	9	1	10	30–45	2	8
FGD 4	7	1	8	18–29	1	7
FGD 5	0	9	9	20–45	5	4
FGD 6	4	5	9	30–45	2	7
FGD 7	2	8	10	18–29	1	9
Total	22	42	64		14	50

democracy and democratic processes and individual understanding of these concepts. Participants' perceptions of democracy included associations with peace; unity; independence; liberty; equal rights for all; majority rule; and a government for, of and by the people. Respondents furthermore stated a belief in the holding of elections as conducive to stabilising and peaceful change which facilitate the translation of rights into action.

Only four focus groups could identify all four types of elections held in Namibia, with the others having particular difficulty with identifying the regional council elections. Regional councils, therefore, do not seem key to decentralisation, accounting for the relatively low voter turnout in such elections. The choice of FPTP is questionable, especially due to the expense of by-elections. All participants thought that registering as a voter is essential, as doing so empowers all citizens to exercise their rights and responsibilities, to support their party of choice and to achieve a better life.

Which attitudinal and/or structural factors impede the participation of PLWHAs?

Only three female and one male respondent did not vote during the 2004 elections, as one was abroad, one bedridden and two were registered in another constituency. The latter indicates a lack of voter education and knowledge among the electorate regarding their eligibility to vote in elections outside their registered constituency. In terms of structural factors and participation, the following perceptions were recorded:

- *Queuing*: Most participants noted the very long queues, especially in the rural areas, resulting in their queueing for between four and six hours, with a maximum time of 11 hours recorded by one respondent. Three respondents, in an effort to avoid excessively long queues, tried two or more polling stations before casting their vote.

- *Distance to the polling station*: While peri-urban and rural respondents said that travelling distances were far, the urban-based respondents found the distance reasonable, given the large number of stations in towns and cities.

- *Ablution facilities*: Only 24 participants were aware of the ablution facilities available at the polling station where they cast their votes. However, most were reluctant to make use of the facilities, in case they lost their place in the queue. Peri-urban and rural participants were seldom aware of ablution facilities or the availability of potable water at the stations.

- Shade and seating are largely unavailable at polling stations. Urban residents were aware of Namibian Red Cross Society volunteers providing help and first aid to voters in need, while others noted the help given by sympathetic election officials, especially to pregnant women, women with babies and the infirm (though such help was not the norm).

- *Child care*: While no participants were unable to exercise their right to vote due to having to care for children or the ill, polling stations were regarded as inappropriate for children, due to the lack of basic services. Women with babies, however, indicated that they had had to take their babies with them when they went to vote, while leaving toddlers and older children with neighbours or relatives.

- *Political party campaigning on HIV/AIDS*: Only one participant was aware of an HIV/AIDS campaign message before the 2004 elections, stating that the CoD had promised to provide for improved service delivery and living standards for PLWHAs.

• *Government response to the HIV/AIDS pandemic:* Peri-urban and rural participants compared the prioritisation of urban HIV/AIDS initiatives with the scant attention paid to such initiatives in the rural areas.

PLWHAs tend to regard their HIV status as secondary to that of their being citizens with the fundamental human right to choose their own representatives.

What is the effect of status on political involvement?

The effect was regarded in terms of two aspects:

• *Attendance at rallies:* Only seven participants did not attend rallies to hear the latest on plans and proposed developments and to lobby for specific issues.

• *Political party membership:* Only three male participants said that they did not belong to a political party, noting their disillusionment with unfulfilled election promises.

All participants stated that they believed in their right to vote, irrespective of HIV status and degree of faith in political structures.

To what extent does the electoral structure reach the electorate on the issue of HIV/AIDS?

Peri-urban and rural participants were unaware of any voter education conducted by the ECN. PLWHAs were regarded as being excluded from both ECN administration, as well as from observation, as they were not encouraged to participate and lacked access to the correct channels. Only five participants thought that the ECN was handling the issue of HIV/AIDS satisfactorily. The participants were generally unaware of any ECN-directed HIV/AIDS specific intervention. The ECN was criticised for the long queues at polling stations; the poor communication between voters and election officials, who tended to be ill-trained; the lack of access to first aid facilities; and the excessively long voter process, especially where the ill, disabled, pregnant and mothers with small children were concerned.

What motivates PLWHAs to participate?

More discrimination seemed to occur among peri-urban and rural populations, leading to the migration of many participants to the cities. All participants had suffered stigma and discrimination, whether in personal relationships, employment, social benefits or health care provision.

Participants blamed stigmatisation and discrimination on a lack of education and information All participants disparaged traditional leaders as agents of social change, due to their apparent perpetuation of HIV/AIDS-related myths and misinformation, resulting in financial loss and delays in treatment, counselling and the need for lifestyle change. Respondents regarded them as helping only OVCs.

In contrast, community leaders, religious leaders and politicians rank highly as social change agents, as they are perceived to provide support, counselling and a voice for PLWHAs. While no participants were aware of any politician declaring their HIV-positive status, they had noted their support for VCT. Overall, their involvement of PLWHAs in elections was regarded as encouraging.

Participants were unaware of any PLWHAs or HIV/AIDS advocates among athletes and television and film stars, though they expressed a belief in the vital role played by sport in maintaining a healthy lifestyle, so that they regarded athletes as potential role models, as were television and film stars, who could help with civic education, dispelling HIV/AIDS-related myths and discrimination.

What structural changes would accommodate PLWHAs in the electoral process?

The participants argued against campaign messages targeting PLWHAs, as such messages might be interpreted as discriminatory. However, all stated that they felt that structural change would encourage the participation of PLWHAs in the electoral process. All participants, bar one,[83] supported a Namibian equivalent of South Africa's special vote facility. Participants urged an increase in the number of polling stations, suggesting that use be made of staffed support organisations, which would facilitate the participation of PLWHAs. Officials should be well-trained communicators. Scanners should be used to check names against the voters' roll. PLWHAs should be encouraged to use existing structures and networks, such as support groups, for voter education.

What is the effect of the conceptualisation of HIV/AIDS on voting behaviour?

HIV/AIDS was regarded as an issue of national concern by all respondents, due to the non-discriminatory nature of HIV and its far-reaching effects. Politicians are thought of as vital in ensuring the provision of antiretrovirals.

What is the importance of politics and political participation?

The participants reported participating in:

- **Community/local authority forums, to learn of development issues and to lobby for concerns;**
- **Volunteer services, including counselling, soup kitchens, providing treatment support in hospitals and positive speaking;[84]**
- **Political rallies and meetings, to show their support for their party and learn about tabled developments and issues; and**
- **Civic activities, such as the promotion of HIV/AIDS awareness via the electronic media and support groups.**

All participants are members of a support group, their motivation to join being attributed to:

- **Their desire to learn to live positively;**
- **Find acceptance among others like them;**
- **Receive and disseminate HIV/AIDS-related information;**
- **Help fight stigma and discrimination; and**
- **Be proactive.**

All but five participants expressed a belief that political participation can enhance one's quality of life, by being able to choose one's own leaders, so that one can feel represented and accounted for. Political actors were, however, encouraged to leave apartheid politics behind and to focus on securing a better future for all.

11. Conclusion and recommendations

Electoral system

HIV/AIDS-related concerns need increasingly to be factored into analyses of the viability of electoral systems and included in associated reform.

Electoral management and administration

As the ECN lacks formal workplace policies, it should develop policies and strategies to educate its staff about HIV/AIDS. Such awareness-raising activities should aim to reduce stigma and discrimination against PLWHAs. Accordingly, campaign informa-tion and material should be designed to inform and motivate PLWHAs. Inclusive messages should reduce HIV/AIDS stigma and discrimination among communities. Enough polling stations and transport facilities should be strategically situated to minimise the distance that people have to travel. Permanent and mobile polling stations should be equipped with functional ablution facilities and resting places, with the guarantee that those who make use of such facilities will not lose their place in the queue. Voter registration should be computerised and regularly checked against the population register and monthly death returns of the Ministry of Home Affairs and Immigration. Special votes should, if financially viable, accommodate bedridden PLWHAs at home.

Mobile polling stations for hospitalised patients should be continued and incorporated in the envisaged redrafting of electoral legislation. The envisaged postal voting system could make voting more inclusive, though it must be carefully implemented. The voter registration system is a serious challenge to both the ECN and the Ministry of Home Affairs and Immigration, as up to 30% of voters are still allowed to register and vote on the basis of sworn statements as to their identity.

Parliamentary configuration and political parties

Parliament should expedite plans to set up a Joint Committee on HIV/AIDS for members of both the NA and NC. Staff and members of both houses of Parliament should also become more active in public education campaigns within their own parties and through partisan platforms. Parliamentarians should undergo public VCT, as, if found positive they could show that HIV does not hinder their performance, thereby promoting greater acceptance of PLWHAs.

Political parties should consider institutionalising a strong internal response to HIV/AIDS and pledge part of their official state funding to creating an HIV/AIDS desk within their party headquarters. As well as coordinating the party's internal institutional response to HIV/AIDS (in creating workplace policies and strategies), it could also develop the party's policies on the issue. Parties should adopt bipartisan approaches to the issue, in the light of the significant amount of ground shared between several of the parties on the HIV/AIDS issue.

Electoral participation has not been as badly affected as some other countries have by the HIV/AIDS pandemic. Namibia is still among the countries with the highest voter turnouts worldwide.

Endnotes

1 The MoHSS (2001: 15) concedes the limitations of its impact projections, since the discovery of a cure for AIDS, or the development of cost-effective drugs, could "radically transform the situation".

2 The sample data on women attending ANCs has several disadvantages: First, the subjects are all women and, therefore, the data is only directly representative of infection rates among women. Second, the data is not representative of all women, as the results only include those of childbearing age who have become pregnant. Third, they are not representative of all pregnant women, as they only include those that attend state or public clinics. As Namibia has a relatively well-developed private health care system, middle-class women are under-represented. Fourth, younger women who are more sexually active are likely to be over-represented, while HIV-positive women are likely to be under-represented, as the HIV infection reduces fertility. Fifth, the sampled ANCs are not necessarily randomly selected and are, therefore, not necessarily representative (Whiteside *et al.*, 2002: 3–4).

3 *Prevalence* refers to the absolute number of people infected, while the *prevalence rate* is the proportion of the population that exhibits the disease at a particular time. Incidence is the number of new infections over a given period of time (Whiteside *et al.*, 2002).

4 The prevalence will increase at the same rate if the survival time increases due to the availability of antiretroviral medications and better living conditions, while the prevalence will decline if the survival time decreases, due to an increased death rate among those who are HIV infected.

5 Resulting from social or psychological trends unrelated to prevention efforts.

6 The Joint United Nations Programme on HIV/AIDS (UNAIDS) also summarises data collected by the MoHSS in yearly publications.

7 *Multisectoral* refers to the different sectoral activities of the government and civil society, such as education and health (Caesar-Katsenga and Kondwani, 2005: 9).

8 Critics argue that Nacop's coordination of responses has been ineffective, due to understaffing of the programme (NDI and Sadc PF, 2004: 37).

9 The government's first proposal to the GFATM was rejected, due to civil society not being involved; with NGOs collaboration on the application, it was approved (NDI and Sadc PF, 2004: 48).

10 The M&E component is especially important, as government recording of budgets and expenditure on MTPII was inadequate (AIDSBRIEF, 2004a: 8–10).

11 The HIV and AIDS Management Unit at the MoE has developed a workplace policy for HIV-positive teachers (MoE: 46) and introduced a new life skill programme for schools ("Window of Hope"), aimed at teaching primary school children how to protect themselves from HIV (AIDSBRIEF, 2004a: 3).

12 *The Namibian*, 2 June 2006.

13 Interview with Ella Shihepo, Special Programmes (TB, Malaria, HIV/AIDS), MoHSS, Windhoek, on 25 April 2006.

14 Interview with Kapenda Marenga, Policy Analyst: Public Service Commission, HIV/AIDS Unit: Office of the Prime Minister, Windhoek, on 21 April 2006.

15 For instance, in July 2004 the Evangelical Lutheran Church in Namibia AIDS Action, the Western Diocese and King Taapopi of Uukwaluudhi hosted an HIV/AIDS conference for traditional leaders and their communities in Tsandi in the Omusati region (AIDSBRIEF, 2004b: 3).

16 Moreover, the AIDS Care Trust of Namibia has led HIV/AIDS workplace intervention programmes with a number of private businesses and parastatals.

17 According to the *Common Country Assessment 2004 Namibia*, the international community also plays a key role in researching and providing technical know-how and global perspectives, as well as being vigilant and dynamic in coordinating efforts directed at prevention and treatment (RoN and UN System in Namibia, 2004: 23). For instance, the UN Theme Group on HIV/AIDS in Namibia has facilitated the setting up of a "Partnership Forum" to share information and support the national response.

18 *Sister Namibia*, 16(4): 9.

19 The main function of returning officers is to administer the candidate nomination procedures in the case of Regional Council and Local Authority elections (EISA, 1999: 36). Tötemeyer (1996: 54) regards returning officers "as the kingpins in the electoral process and as the most highly-ranked election official in the field".

20 Presiding officers are appointed for each polling district and ward (EISA, 1999: 36).

21 In 1989, the first National Assembly was elected under the legislative terms of the Constituent Assembly. National elections in 1994 were conducted using the 1992 Electoral Act (Act No. 24 of 1992). Since then, the Act has been amended several times by: the Electoral Amendment Act (Act No. 23 of 1994), the Electoral Amendment Act (Act No. 30 of 1998), and the Electoral Amendment Act (Act No.11 of 1999).

22 Interviews with Bock, Senior Personal Officer, ECN, Windhoek; Ushi Nauvala, Control Officer, ECN, Windhoek; and Gustaf Tomanga, Information Officer, ECN, Windhoek, on 24 April 2006.

23 Ibid.

24 Ibid.

25 Email interview with Joram K. Rukambe. International IDEA, Africa Programme, Former Director of Elections (1998–2003), on 12 April 2006.

26 Total obtained from ECN (2005: 46).

27 Teachers in the "high-risk group" with respect to HIV/AIDS are usually not temporary staff. Exceptionally, they are employed if elections take place during school holidays or on public holidays (Source: Interview with Gerhard K.H. Tötemeyer, former director of elections, 1992–1998, Windhoek, on 11 April 2006).

28 Interviews with Bock, Nauvala and Tomanga on 24 April 2006 and with Tötemeyer on 11 April 2006.

29 Interviews with Bock, Nauvala and Tomanga on 24 April 2006.

30 *Ibid.*

31 Interview with Rukambe on 12 June 2006.

32 The Electoral Amendment Act (Act No. 23 of 1994) provides for the continuous registration of voters, aiming to accommodate those previously unregistered or who have turned eighteen since the last national registration process (Tötemeyer, 1996: 23–24).

33 "Errors on a voters' list are possible: they include double registration, incorrect spelling of names, and voters registered in the wrong constituency." (Tötemeyer, 1996: 29).

34 Interview with Tötemeyer on 11 April 2006.

35 The average amount of time for finding a voter's particulars was reduced from an average of 12 minutes to a mere 30 seconds due to the computerisation (ECN, 2005: 14).

36 The paper-based voters' register provided too little information, as some pages were unreadable, with an incomplete dataset. After the elections, the request for a computerised voters' register has been rejected several times (Source: Telephonic interview with Carola Engelbrecht, civil society activist, former secretary-general of the RP, on 13 April 2006).

37 Interview with Rukambe on 12 April 2006.

38 Additional source: Interview with Tötemeyer on 11 April 2006.

39 *Ibid.*

40 *Ibid.*

41 The tendered vote system is not applicable to local authority elections.

42 Interview with Tötemeyer on 11 April 2006.

43 Due to the publicity surrounding polling stations, the personal help provided to sick voters might also increase stigmatisation.

44 Interview with Tötemeyer on 11 October 2006.

45 The Electoral Act (Act No. 24 of 1992) prescribes that voters must be present in person.

46 Interview with Tötemeyer on 11 April 2006.

47 Interview with Reinhard Gertze, secretary-general of the CoD, Windhoek, on 27 March 2006.

48 *The Namibian*, 27 February 2002.

49 Interview with Samuel Kaxuxuena, Senior Parliamentary Clerk in the NC, on 21 April 2006.

50 *Ibid.*

51 *New Era*, 18 May 2006.

52 Interview with Chippa Tjirera, principal parliamentary clerk in the NA, Windhoek, on 20 April 2006.

53 Interview with Kaxuxuena on 21 April 2001.

54 Interview with Tjirera on 20 April 2006.

55 *Ibid.*

56 Interview with Kaxuxuena on 21 April 2001.

57 *Insight*, November 2004.

58 *Ibid.*

59 Interviews with Alois Gende, secretary-general of the DTA, Windhoek, on 13 April 2006; Michael Goreseb, Spokesperson on Health for the UDF, Windhoek, on 29 April 2006; and an email interview with Jurie Viljoen, Mag Member of Parliament, on 7 April 2006.

60 Interview with Gertze on 27 March 2006.

61 *Ibid.*

62 *Ibid.*

63 *Ibid.*

64 *Ibid.*

65 *Ibid.*

66 Interview with Gertze on 27 March 2006.

67 Interview with Goreseb on 20 April 2006.

68 Interview with Gertze on 27 March 2006.

69 Interview with Viljoen on 7 April 2006.

70 Interview on 13 April 2006.

71 The sample was nationally representative, multistage and strati-fied, including 1 200 Namibians. All 13 regions were included and interviews were held according to each region's contribution to the country's rural and urban population (Keulder, 2002: 4).

72 HIV/AIDS was identified as the most important problem by more urban than rural respondents (Keulder, 2002: 30).

73 The respondents were encouraged to state up to three issues (Idasa, 2004: 4).

74 The question is regarded as "an admittedly imperfect proxy for actual contact with the AIDS epidemic". Whiteside *et al.* (2002: 10) name several restrictions, such as refusal to admit knowledge, misinterpretation of the reasons for death, or a multiple reporting of the same death.

75 "One factor that probably facilitated more candid responses was that we did not ask for specific names, but merely whether or not they knew of some friend or relative who had died of AIDS." (Whiteside *et al.*, 2002: 12).

76 The answer "Do not know" could mean that responses are unsure if they know anyone who died, know victims but do not know how many, do not know what caused the death, or do not wish to reveal the truth (Bratton *et al.*, 2004: 26–27).

77 This question also captured home-based care for patients who are not PLWHAs (Strand and Chirambo, 2005: 122).

78 Uncertainty exists as to whether the children were orphaned due to AIDS-related diseases (Idasa, 2004: 3).

79 Within the scope of the 1999 Afrobarometer survey, civic participation has been measured by means of a set of questions determining the frequency with which respondents attend the meetings held by public institutions. The frequency of attendance varies substantially. While meetings of groups concerned with local matters, such as schools and housing, are most frequently attended, attendance of meetings of local commercial organisations, self-help associations, and trade unions, is quite low. Overall, a low rate of participation has been stated (Keulder, 2002: 43).

80 The percentage of people under 15 years was 39% (Hopwood, 2006: 3).

81 The low voter turnout at regional council elections might be due to several reasons. First, it could mean that national elections are regarded as more important. Second, Regional Council elections are constituency-based, so that no tendered votes are included. Third, people might prefer to support political parties, rather than to vote for individual candidates.

82 www.aidslaw.co, accessed 6 February 2006.

83 The one exception noted that she would be too embarrassed to make use of the special vote.

84 By means of a formal organisation of PLWHAs, who make themselves available to share their experiences in public forums.

References

AIDSBRIEF, 2004a. Quarters 1 and 2, Windhoek: Institute for Public Policy Research (IPPR), Namibia Business Coalition on AIDS (Nabcoa).

AIDSBRIEF, 2004b. Quarters 3 and 4. Windhoek: Institute for Public Policy Research (IPPR), Namibia Business Coalition on AIDS (Nabcoa).

Boer, M., 2005. "Taking a Stand: Comparing Namibia's Political Party Platforms" in Hunter, J. (ed.), *Spot the Difference: Namibia's Political Parties Compared*, Windhoek: Nid.

Bollinger, L. and Stover, J., 1999. *The Economic Impact of AIDS in Namibia*. Washington: Futures Group International, Research Triangle Institute, Centre for Development and Population Activities.

Bratton, M. and Cho, W., 2006. *Where is Africa Going? Views From Below: A Compendium of Trends in Public Opinion in 12 African Countries, 1999–2006*, Pretoria: Idasa.

Bratton, M., Logan, C., Cho, W. and Bauer, P., 2004. *Afrobarometer Round 2: Compendium of Comparative Results from a 15-Country Survey*, Pretoria: Idasa.

Caesar-Katsenga, M. and Chirambo, K., (eds) 2005. *Understanding the Institutional Dynamics of Namibia's Response to the HIV/AIDS Pandemic*, Pretoria: Idasa.

Central Bureau of Statistics, 2003. *2001 Population and Housing Census National Report: Basic Analysis with Highlights*, Windhoek: National Planning Commission.

Central Bureau of Statistics, 2006. *Population Projections, 2001–2031: National and Regional Figures*, Windhoek: National Planning Commission.

CoD, 1999. *Political Declaration and Principles of the Congress of Democrats*, Windhoek: CoD.

CoD, 2004. *CoD's Programme for a Better Namibia*, Windhoek: CoD.

Directorate of Elections and Namibia Institute for Democracy, 1997. *Glossary of Electoral Terms and Related Concepts*, Windhoek: Directorate of Elections and Nid.

DTA of Namibia, 2004. *Election Manifesto of the DTA of Namibia*, Windhoek: DTA of Namibia.

ECN, 2004. *Local Authority Elections 14 May 2004 – Report*, Windhoek: ECN.

ECN, 2005. *Presidential and National Assembly Elections Report, 2004*, Windhoek: ECN.

ECN. [n.d.] *Death Statistics. Total number of deceased persons removed from the Voters' Register on the basis of the Ministry of Home Affairs and Immigration since beginning of July 2003 until end of August 2005.*

Electoral Act (Act No. 24 of 1992).

Electoral Amendment Act (Act No. 23 of 1994).

Electoral Amendment Act (Act No. 30 of 1998).

Electoral Amendment Act (Act No. 11 of 1999).

Electoral Institute of Southern Africa for the Directorate of Elections of the Republic of Namibia (EISA). 1999. *A Handbook on Namibian Electoral Laws and Regulations, 1999*, Johannesburg: EISA.

El Obeid, S., Mendelsohn, J., Lejars, M., Forster, N. and Brulé, G. 2001. *Health in Namibia: Progress and Challenges*, Windhoek: MoHSS, French Embassy in Namibia.

Haywood, M., 2004. "The Price of Denial", in Haywood, M. (ed.), *From Disaster to Development? HIV and AIDS in Southern Africa*, Johannesburg: INTERFUND.

Hopwood, G., 2005. "Trapped in the Past: The State of the Opposition", in Hunter, J. (ed.) *Spot the Difference: Namibia's Political Parties Compared*, Windhoek: Nid.

Hopwood, G., 2006. *Guide to Namibian Politics*, Windhoek: Nid.

Hunter, J., 2005. "Political Parties on the Record: Party Representatives Challenged" in Hunter, J. (ed.) *Spot the Difference: Namibia's Political Parties Compared*, Windhoek: Nid.

Hunter, J., 2005. *Spot the Difference: Namibia's Political Parties Compared*, Windhoek: Nid.

Idasa, 2004. *Public Opinion and HIV/AIDS: Facing Up to the Future?* Afrobarometer Briefing Paper No. 12, April.

Idasa, 2006. *Afrobarometer Data Namibia Round 3*, February.

Insight Namibia, 2004. *Bench Warfare*, November.

Keulder, C., 2002. *Public Opinion and the Consolidation of Democracy in Namibia*, Windhoek: IPPR.

Keulder, C., 2006. "HIV: A Forgotten Issue", *Insight Namibia*, March.

Keulder, C. and LeBeau, D., 2006. *Ships, Trucks and Clubs: The Dynamics of HIV Risk Behaviour in Walvis Bay*, Windhoek: IPPR.

Keulder, C. and Wiese, T., 2003. *Democracy without Democrats? Results from the 2003 Afrobarometer Survey in Namibia*, Windhoek: IPPR.

Keulder, C. and Wiese, T., 2004. *The 2003 Windhoek West Voter's Registration Roll*, Windhoek: IPPR.

Keulder, C., Van Zyl, D. and Wiese, T., 2003. *Report on the 1999 Voters' Registration Roll: Analysis and Recommendations*, Windhoek: Institute for Public Policy Research (IPPR).

Lac, [n.d.]. *Namibian HIV/AIDS Charter on Rights*, Windhoek: Lac.

Mag, 2004a. *Ons Saak, Ons Man*, Windhoek: MAG.

Mag, 2004b. *Programme of Principles and Constitution*, Windhoek: Mag.

Mag, 2006. *Comment on the Budget, 2006/7*, Jurie Viljoen Monitor Action Group, 30 March.

Mattes, R., 2003. *Healthy Democracies? The Potential Impact of AIDS on Democracy in Southern Africa*, ISS Occasional Paper No. 71, Pretoria: ISS, April.

Ministry of Regional and Local Government and Housing and Namibia Institute for Democracy, 2002. *The Constitution of Namibia*, Windhoek: Ministry of Regional and Local Government and Housing (MRLGH) and Nid.

MoHSS, 2000. *Epidemiological Report on HIV/AIDS for the Year 2000*, Windhoek: MoHSS.

MoHSS, 2001. *First Report of the Working Group on HIV/AIDS Impact Projections for Namibia (Year 2000 Projection Base)*. Windhoek: MoHSS.

MoHSS, 2003. *Namibia Demographic and Health Survey*, Windhoek: MoHSS.

MoL, 1998. *Guidelines for Implementation of National Code on HIV/AIDS in Employment*, Windhoek: MoL.

Namibian Women's Manifesto Network, 2004. *5% to 50% – Women and Men in Regional Government – Get the Balance Right*, Windhoek: Sister Namibia, October.

Nanaso, 2005a. *Annual Report, January–December 2004*, Windhoek: Nanaso.

Nanaso, 2005b. *Monitoring and Evaluation of the Civil Society Contribution to Tackling HIV/AIDS in Namibia*, Windhoek: Nanaso.

National Council, 2004. *Workplace HIV and AIDS Policy*, Windhoek: National Council.

National Democratic Institute for International Affairs (NDI) and The Southern African Development Community Parliamentary Forum (Sadc PF), 2004. *Survey of Legislative Efforts to Combat HIV/AIDS in the Southern Africa Development Community (Sadc) Region*, [n.p.]: NDI, Sadc PF.

Nid/Parliament of Namibia, 2005. *Guide to Parliament*, Windhoek: Nid, Parliament of Namibia.

Nudo, 2004. *Nudo of Namibia: Our Mission*, Windhoek: Nudo.

Otaala, B., [n.d.]. *Impact of HIV/AIDS on the University of Namibia and the University's Response*, Windhoek: Unam.

Phororo, H., 2000. *Why the Private Sector Should Be Concerned About HIV/AIDS*, Windhoek: Hanns Seidel Foundation.

Phororo, H., 2002. *HIV/AIDS: Who Suffers in Namibia?*, Windhoek: Namibian Economic Policy Research Unit (Nepru).

Phororo, H., 2003. *HIV/AIDS and the Private Sector in Namibia: Getting the Small Business on Board*, Windhoek: Hanns Seidel Foundation.

RoN, 1999. *The National Strategic Plan on HIV/AIDS: Second Medium Term Plan (MTPII)*, Windhoek: RoN.

RoN, 2004a. *Namibia 2004: Millennium Development Goals*, Windhoek: Office of the President, National Planning Commission.

RoN, 2004b. *The National Strategic Plan on HIV/AIDS: Third Medium Term Plan (MTPIII), 2004–2009*, Windhoek: RoN.

RoN. *Debates of the National Assembly, Third Parliament, 2000–2005.*

RoN and MoHSS, 2005. *Report on the 2004 National Sentinel Survey*, Windhoek: RoN, MoHSS.

RoN and UN System in Namibia, 2004. *Common Country Assessment, 2004, Namibia*, Windhoek: RoN and United Nations System in Namibia.

RP, 2004. *Vote RP: Henk Mudge, President*, Windhoek: RP.

Sacks, A. 2005. *The Other Side of HIV/AIDS: The Impact of the Epidemic on Voting Participation and Electoral Trends in Six Sub-Saharan African Countries*. Department of Sociology, University of Washington, Proposal for PAA 2006.

Strand, P., 2005. *AIDS and Elections in Southern Africa: Is the Epidemic Undermining its Democratic Remedy?* ISS Occasional Paper No. 110, Pretoria: ISS, July.

Strand, P. and Chirambo, K., (eds.) 2005. *HIV/AIDS and Democratic Governance in South Africa: Illustrating the Impact on Electoral Processes*, Pretoria: Idasa.

Swapo, 1999. *Election Manifesto, 1999*, Windhoek: Swapo.

Swapo, 2004. *Swapo Party Election Manifesto, 2004*, Windhoek: Swapo.

Tötemeyer, G.K.H., 1996. 'The Legal Framework and Organisational Requirements', in Tötemeyer, G.K.H., Wehmhörner, A. and Weiland, H. (eds) *Elections in Namibia*, Windhoek: FES.

Tötemeyer, G.K.H., Wehmhörner, A. and Weiland, H., 1996. *Elections in Namibia*, Windhoek: Friedrich-Ebert-Stiftung (FES).

UDF, 1999. *Manifesto*, Windhoek: UDF of Namibia.

UDF, 2004. *Society Back to the People – People Back to the Society*, Windhoek: UDF of Namibia.

UDF, 2005. *UDF's Policies Relating to HIV/AIDS*, Windhoek: UDF of Namibia.

UN, [n.d.]. *Declaration of Commitment to Accelerating and Scaling Up the Fight Against HIV/AIDS in Namibia*, Windhoek: UN.

UNAIDS, [n.d.]. *Join the Fight Against AIDS in Namibia*, Windhoek: UNAIDS.

UNAIDS, 2002. *Namibia: Epidemiological Fact Sheets on HIV/AIDS and Sexually Transmitted Infections – 2002 Update*, Windhoek: UNAIDS.

UNDP and UN Country Team, 2000. *Namibia: Human Development Report 2000/2001*, Windhoek: UNDP Namibia.

UNICEF, 2005. *Childhood under Threat in Namibia: A Supplement to the State of the World's Children Report, 2005*, Windhoek: UNICEF.

Van Zyl, D., 2003. *An Overview of HIV-related Research in Namibia since Independence*, Windhoek: IPPR.

Whiteside, A., Mattes, R., Willan, S. and Manning, R., 2002. *Examining HIV/AIDS in Southern Africa through the Eyes of Ordinary Southern Africans*, Afrobarometer Paper No. 21, Pretoria: Idasa.

Abbreviations

ACN	Action Christian National
ANC	antenatal clinic
CA	Constituent Assembly
CAA	Catholic AIDS Action
Cafo	Church Alliance for Orphans
CCN	Council of Churches in Namibia
CoD	Congress of Democrats
DCN	Democratic Convention of Namibia
DTA	Democratic Turnhalle Alliance
ECN	Electoral Commission of Namibia
FCN	Federal Convention of Namibia
FGD	focus group discussions
FPTP	first-past-the-post
GFATM	Global Fund to Fight HIV/AIDS, Tuberculosis and Malaria
HDI	Human Development Index
HPI	Human Poverty Index
IDASA	Institute for Democracy in South Africa
IPPR	Institute for Public Policy Research
Lac	Legal Assistance Centre
Mag	Monitor Action Group
M&E	monitoring and evaluation
MoE	Ministry of Education
MoHSS	Ministry of Health and Social Services
MMP	mixed member proportional
MP	Member of Parliament
MTPI	first medium-term plan
MTPII	second medium-term plan
MTPIII	third medium-term plan
MWACW	Ministry of Women's Affairs and Child Welfare
NA	National Assembly
Nabcoa	Namibian Business Coalition on AIDS
NAC	National AIDS Committee
Nacop	National AIDS Coordination Programme
NACP	National AIDS Control Programme
NAEC	National AIDS Executive Committee
Namacoc	National Multisectoral AIDS Coordination Committee
Namcol	Namibian College of Open Learning
Nanaso	Namibia Network of AIDS Service Organisations
Nappa	Namibia Planned Parenthood Organisation
Nasoma	National Social Marketing Programme
NC	National Council
NCCI	Namibian Chamber of Commerce and Industry
NDP II	second national development plan
Nepru	Namibian Economic Policy Research Unit
NGO	non-governmental organisation
Nid	Namibia Institute for Democracy
NNF	Namibia National Front
NP	National Party
NPF	National Patriotic Front
Nudo	National Unity Democratic Organisation
O&L	Ohlthaver and List
OVC	orphans and vulnerable children
PLWHA	people living with HIV/AIDS
PMTCT	prevention of mother–to–child transmission
PR	proportional representation
Racoc	Regional AIDS Coordinating Committees
RP	Republican Party
Sadc	Southern African Development Community
SMA	Social Marketing Association
SMM	single-member majority
SMP	single-member plurality
STI	sexually transmitted infection
Swapo	South West Africa People's Organisation
TB	tuberculosis
UDF	United Democratic Front
UN	United Nations
Unam	University of Namibia
UNDP	United Nations Development Programme
VCT	voluntary counselling and testing
WHO	World Health Organisation

South Africa

Per Strand, Khabele Matlosa, Ann Strode, Kondwani Chirambo

updated by Josina Machel and Christele Diwouta

1. HIV/AIDS and democratic governance

1.1 Introduction

Though South Africa held its third national elections in April 2004, with a level of confidence found usually in established democracies, the effectiveness of its democracy and its electoral processes risk being undermined by the HIV/AIDS epidemic. Civil society organisations and elected political representatives need to counter this threat by generating the necessary political will and commitment through the democratic process, which will be possible only once it is shown how the epidemic can hamper the mobilisation of resources.

1.2 HIV/AIDS and the electoral process

The Joint United Nations Programme on AIDS (UNAIDS), the arm of the UN that coordinates global efforts at fighting the epidemic, estimates that 5.3 million, or between 4.5 and 6.2 million South Africans of all ages were infected with HIV by the end of 2003 (UNAIDS, 2004). The South African government's HIV/AIDS and STI Strategic Plan for South Africa, 2007-2011 shows that approximately 5.4 million people were living with HIV or AIDS in the country in 2006 (the draft report was released in March 2007). Regardless of the sources consulted, South Africa reflects one of the highest absolute number of infected residents worldwide.

With the presence of the epidemic starting to be felt in the early 1990s, South Africa has only recently started to experience its devastating effects in a sharp increase in AIDS-related morbidity and mortality. Only a quick and extensive treatment, care and support strategy can effectively halt this tragic development. The nature, extent and variations of the epidemic in South Africa are presented and discussed in section two.

1.3 Methodological concerns

The literature review covers both national and international titles from academic, activist and official discourses on governance and the epidemic. The key documents explored include the legal and constitutional frameworks governing the electoral process and central epidemiological reports.[1] Parliamentary documentation and election manifestos of political parties were consulted, as well as Independent Electoral Commission (IEC) policy declarations. HIV/AIDS spokespeople of some of the political parties were asked to participate in semi-structured interviews to probe their policies and practices. A few centrally placed senior IEC officials were also interviewed.

Six focus group discussions (FGDs), held in three rural and three urban centres in KwaZulu-Natal, provided direct contact with 68 people either infected with HIV or otherwise directly affected by AIDS. The computer-based analysis of FGDs allows for a high degree of systematic rigour, capable of generating fairly representative results if participants are chosen correctly. Material from the focus groups interviews was used mainly to explore some of the results that were indicated by the statistical analysis. Given what was learned from analysing electoral and epidemiological data by statistical means, those concerned were asked whether they could explain how the epidemic affected their political participation.

A stakeholder dialogue held in early April 2004, attended by electoral officials, political party representatives, experts from the UNDP and UNAIDS, international and local research agencies, donor agencies, media and key government ministry representatives, subjected the research process to critical scrutiny.

The depth, strength and relevance of the analyses in the second and third parts of the report depended on the amount and quality of empirical data available. The reason for the death of an MP or local councillor or for a vacancy of a parliamentary seat due to illness is unavailable without individual consent.

When using the Afrobarometer surveys to analyse the effects of the epidemic on people's opinions and on their engagement in civil society, certain questions serve as proxies for HIV/AIDS, since direct questions about HIV status would have resulted in unreliable answers. Some of the questions therefore captured other illnesses and conditions than those caused by AIDS.

The statistical analyses of voter participation based on electoral data received from the IEC are only on the level of the nine provinces. As well as describing how frequencies vary, the statistical analysis of quantitative data explores the existence of "patterns" in the data by means of correlation analyses. Statistical correlation analysis should be performed on a large enough sample to ensure relative reliability and ease of interpretation. Whereas the analyses in sections 8 and 9 are only applied to nine cases, in section 7 the analysis is based on a sample that is representative of the whole population. The correlation analysis allowed for the deduction that the epidemic is related to the level of non-participation on a provincial level.

2. HIV/AIDS in South Africa

2.1 Introduction

To contextualise the analysis of how the HIV/AIDS epidemic affected the 2004 elections, the most relevant epidemiological data requires discussing how they were arrived at and why they differ. Demographic and developmental statistics are included, as they are vital for understanding the contextual complexity that a governance perspective implies for the epidemic.

2.2 Democracy and HIV/AIDS

The root of the word "democracy", the Greek word *demos*, refers to a group of people who take collectively binding decisions, while, as the words "epidemic" and "pandemic" (that is, an epidemic that has spread across countries), refers to a group of people who, in the case of HIV, are infected with the deadly virus. An infectious disease might be defined as an epidemic once infection rates increase rapidly in a population, as was seen in the rising HIV prevalence in South Africa throughout the 1990s, which soared from below 1% in 1990 to just under 25% in 1998 (Whiteside and Sunter, 2000).

Figure 2.1 shows the three "waves" of the epidemic. In the first stages of the epidemic, the virus spreads insidiously, subject to prejudice-based non-disclosure. Only after between four to eight years, depending on a person's general health, do the direct effects of the virus appear in those first infected. At that stage (T1), the number of those who display opportunistic diseases due to a low CD4 count (B) tends to be dwarfed by an "invincible", but much higher number, of people living with HIV/AIDS (A). At this relatively early stage of the epidemic, the impact of the disease is localised.

Figure 2.1: The impact of HIV/AIDS in epidemic curves

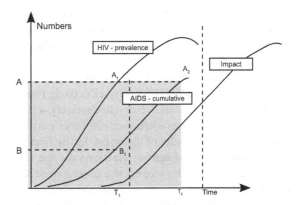

Source: A Whiteside (2001) www.uneca.org

However, if little is done to prevent further infection and to treat those who are ill, the costs of the epidemic are bound to increase dramatically. In future (T2), the epidemic might start to decline, but, even then, the detrimental effects of the epidemic on the wider society will still increase in personal grief and the undermining of households, social capital, labour resources and human skills (Whiteside and Barnett, 2002).

At this early stage, the average citizen knows little of what is happening and how effective prevention measures can affect individual behaviour, not seeing a need for state intervention and not necessarily accepting the prescribed remedies. Therefore, at this early stage, a governing party will not be able to secure power by means of a costly and demanding preventative policy – until the next election, the political incentives rather favour downplaying the crisis. Once the explicit effects of the epidemic are felt in AIDS-related sickness and death, demands for prevention and treatment may rise. The problem will then be much harder and more costly to address than it would have been earlier in the epidemic when politicians learned of the impending crisis, but lacked the political incentive to act.

The later in the process that the government finally responds, the bigger the task is of combating the epidemic. Even once successful interventions have started to reduce the scale of the epidemic, the government will still face more long-term and structural effects of the epidemic, reducing its possibilities of addressing other poverty-related issues. If a vaccine against AIDS-related diseases stopped all further infections of the virus, society would still battle with the effects of the epidemic for another 40 years (Shisana, 2002).

The sooner in the epidemiological cycle a government chooses to act, the better. However, an early response will only be possible if the government commits itself to carrying the political costs for doing so, facing the risk of losing power for pushing an unpopular policy. Such political risk might be reduced or eliminated altogether if the major parties agree to depoliticise the issue by forming a broad policy accord on HIV/AIDS policy, effectively removing it from the electoral arena. Alternatively, a party might rely on its overwhelming electoral majority and the steadfast loyalty of its voters. In the first scenario, parties do not contest elections on the HIV/AIDS issue, and, in the second, the government wins elections despite its adoption of an initially unpopular policy on HIV/AIDS, for which it will later reap the reward. (Consider figure 2.2 in this context.)

Figure 2.2: HIV prevalence rate in Thailand, Uganda and South Africa, 1990-2000

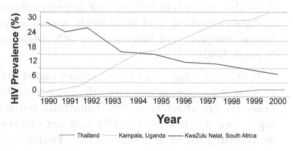

Source: UNAIDS.

The graph in Figure 2.2 shows the development of HIV prevalence rates in three countries that adopted different political responses to the epidemic. The Thai government, which was undemocratic for parts of the relevant period, reacted strongly to early signs of the epidemic, and has since managed to keep prevalence rates low. The Ugandan government, which still has to introduce competitive elections and many liberal democratic institutions, reacted strongly to realising that national prevalence rates were very high, and has since managed to reduce them considerably.

The two South African governments during the 1990s – the non-democratic apartheid government and the democratic ANC government after the 1994 elections – responded relatively late to early signs of the epidemic, so that its policies have not yet shrunk prevalence rates. Culture, political transition and the type of government all affect prevalence of the disease. The two successful scenarios are marked by strong political leadership in combating the epidemic (Van der Vliet, 2004). South African politi-

cal leaders failed to formulate and launch a strong political response to the epidemic in time to prevent the virus from causing an epidemic. However, despite the weakness of its initial response, the South African government has shown increased leadership in dealing with the epidemic and responding to the demands of its people. The HIV/AIDS and Sexually Transmitted Infection (STI) Strategic Plan for South Africa (the NSP 2007–2011), a broad plan designed to guide the country's multisectoral response to the epidemic appears to benchmark the government shift in approach from one centred on public health to a more interlinked strategy, including the broader society. The government has consulted with, and encouraged the participation of, both the public and private sectors, as well as community-based organisations (CBOs), in its plan. The goals set within the prioritised areas of prevention, treatment, care and support; human and legal rights; and monitoring, research and surveillance are achievable and measurable. The focus of the plan was also extended to the gender dynamic, the protection and promotion of human rights, and PLWHAs' access to housing employment and financial services.

2.3 Testing South Africans for HIV prevalence

The three authoritative sources of information on the national estimate of HIV infection in South Africa are the antenatal clinic data generated by the Department of Health (DoH, 2003), the survey data collected by the Human Sciences Research Council (HSRC) (Shisana, 2002) and the estimates generated by the ASSA2000 model, which partially reflect the antenatal clinic data (Dorrington, 2002: Dorrington, 2004).

The most commonly cited estimate on HIV prevalence is generated through blood tests taken from a sample of women who visit antenatal clinics provided by the public health care system, the antenatal clinic tests. The South African DoH uses this method, having conducted 14 annual tests since 1990. The HIV test is very reliable, with the response rate being close to 100%, meaning that all of the sampled women and clinics provide the information necessary for generating an estimate. Confidence intervals around the estimates are 2% or less for women who are below 35 years and slightly more than 2%, at the highest 3.5%, for women over 35 years. However, as HIV-positive women are less fertile, they are underrepresented among clinic attendees (Evian, 2003).

The clinic attendees are also not a representative sample of all South African women. The 80% of pregnant women who visit such clinics are relatively poor Africans and Coloureds, as most Indian and White women visit private clinics.

While the estimate is said to represent women 15 to 49 years old, less than 3% of the sampled women tend to be over 40 years old, which reduces the reliability of the estimate for that age cohort. The assumptions that are applied to compensate for the lack of representivity are problematic and contestable:

> The Department of Health developed a model for estimating the number of HIV-infected people in the general South African population based on the results of the survey. Certain assumptions are made and the results arrived at are only crude estimates due to the constraints of the survey. The estimates are only as good as the validity of the assumptions and the generalisability of the survey results, which are used in the extrapolation process. (DoH, 2003: 4)

The four critical assumptions made by the South African DoH are:

- The prevalence rate of HIV infection in all pregnant women in South Africa is the same as the prevalence rate among women attending public antenatal clinics;

- The prevalence rate of HIV infection in all women aged 15 to 49 years is the same as the prevalence rate among pregnant women;

- The estimate of infected males equals 85% of infected females;

- The mother–to–child transmission (MTCT) rate is 30% (DoH, 2003).

The antenatal clinic estimates are therefore only used in this study to reflect the status of women who attend the clinics.

In household surveys, a nationally representative sample of households is visited, with the inhabitants being asked to answer a set of questions, as well as to undergo an HIV test. The development of an HIV test based on a person's saliva allows for a safe, fast and less intrusive means of testing than drawing blood. The method was first used in South Africa in 2001/2002 in a research project undertaken by the HSRC and the Nelson Mandela Foundation. As the sample is representative of the whole population, it generates estimates for different population segments. However, the response rate tends to be low and biased against those without a permanent address, so underrepresents destitute South Africans, among whom HIV prevalence tends to be relatively high.

The most theoretically complex and methodologically demanding ASSA2000 model was developed by researchers at the Centre for Actuarial Research (CARE) at the University of Cape Town, which takes into account many other demographic, developmental and health-related factors than just the DoH's post-1998 antenatal clinic survey results. The data is processed, based on a set of epidemiological and demographic assumptions, all of which generate projections, which are, however, only as reliable as the data provided and to the extent that the assumptions made are reasonable. The process by which the projections are generated also lacks transparency.

Reviewing and relying on different estimates and projections of HIV prevalence requires awareness of their respective uncertainties, biases and assumptions, while not allowing them to undermine the fact that the epidemic is rife and ravaging society (Bourne, 2003). The strongest possible response is required to prevent further infections and to reduce HIV to a manageable infection through effective treatment.

2.3.1 Variance of epidemic in population

The most recent UNAIDS epidemiological update estimates that a total of 5.5 million South Africans are infected by the HI virus, a figure surpassing those of all other countries (UNAIDS, 2006).[2] According to the HSRC household report for 2005, the prevalence rate of HIV infection among those aged 2 years or older was 10.8%.

Table 2.1: Estimated national prevalence by age, race and gender, HSRC household survey 2005

Population	older than 2	15–24	15–49
African	13.3	12.3	19.9
White	0.6	0.3	0.5
Coloured	1.9	1.7	3.2
Indian	1.6	0.8	1
Male	8.2	4.4	11.7
Female	13.3	16.9	20.2
Total	10.8	10.3	16.2

Table 2.2: Prevalence among ANC attendees in 2003, 2004, 2005, by age

Age group in years	HIV prevalence (CI 95%) 2003	HIV prevalence (CI 95%) 2004	HIV prevalence (CI 95%) 2005
<20	15.8 (14.3–17.2)	16.1 (14.7–17.5)	15.9 (14.6–17.2)
20–24	30.3 (28.8–31.8)	30.8 (29.3–32.3)	30.6 (29.0–32.2)
25–29	35.4 (33.6–7.2)	38.5 (36.8–40.3)	39.5 (37.7–1.3)
30–34	30.9 (28.9–32.9)	34.4 (32.2–36.6)	36.4 (34.3–38.5)
35–39	23.4 (20.9–25.9)	24.5 (21.9–27.2)	28.0 (25.2–30.8)
40+	15.8 (12.3–19.3)	17.5 (14.0–21.0)	19.8 (16.1–23.6)

Source: DoH, 2003:8. Confidence intervals in brackets

The virus is most prevalent among the African (black) population, which, in some instances, is as much as almost six times the infection rate of the second worst affected group. The African population has experienced a steady increase throughout the development of the epidemic, while the other three groups have experienced a slight decrease or stabilisation of the prevalence rate. However, the confidence intervals overlap between some of the groups, confusing the prevalence levels between the groups. The prevalence rate is the highest in the age cohort 15 to 49 years of age, which is the most sexually active. The age span is used internationally to define the group whose prevalence rates is most commonly cited. Women are much worse affected than men, particularly in the younger age cohorts, as many biological and sociopolitical conditions make them more vulnerable to infection. Women, therefore, account for 55% of South African PLWHAs, with African women being the worst affected.

The HSRC survey estimates HIV prevalence for females to be 20.2%, which is almost double that for males, 11.7%.

Table 2.3: Population and three estimates of HIV prevalence, by provinces

Province	South African population mid-2004, %		Prevalence, 2002 in % by ASSA2000*	Prevalence, 2003 in % by DoH**	Prevalence, 2002 in % by HSRC***	Prevalence, 2005 in % by HSRC****
Western Cape	4 570 696	9.8	6.7	13.1 (8.5–17.7)	13.2 (8.0–20.0)	3.2
Eastern Cape	7 088 547	15.2	20.5	27.1 (24.6–29.7)	10.2 (7.0–14.0)	15.5
Northern Cape	899 349	1.9	12.9	16.7 (11.9–21.5)	9.6 (6.5–14.5)	9
Free State	2 950 661	6.3	26.5	30.1 (26.9–33.3)	19.4 (14.0–27.5)	19.2
KwaZulu-Natal	9 665 875	20.7	31.4	37.5 (35.2–39.8)	15.7 (12.0–21.5)	21.9
North West	3 807 469	8.2	24.8	29.9 (26.8–33.1)	14.4 (10.0–19.5)	18
Gauteng	8 847 740	19	23.8	29.6 (27.8–31.5)	20.3 (16.0–25.3)	15.8
Mpumalanga	3 244 306	7	28.1	32.6 (28.5–36.6)	21 (15.0–28.0)	23.1
Limpopo	5 511 962	11.9	20.9	17.5 (14.9–20.0)	11.5 (7.5–17.0)	11
National	46 586 607	100.1	23.4	27.9 (26.8–28.9)	11.4 (10.1–12.7)	10.8

Sources: Statistics SA, 2004: 31–32; Dorrington, 2002: 5; Shisana, 2002: 50; DoH, 2003:7. Confidence intervals in brackets.
* Prevalence among ages 18–64 years; ** Prevalence among ANC attendees, 15–49 years; *** Prevalence among ages 15–49 years, ****Prevalence among 15–49 years.

While the HSRC percentages are the best available estimates of the extent of the epidemic, they fail to reflect the level of awareness of own HIV status. According to the survey, as many as 76% of HIV-positive South Africans are not aware of being infected (Shisana, 2002).

Increasing awareness of own status might not only prolong the lives of the infected, alerting them of their need for medication, but also protect others from being infected by them. An informed constituency might constructively advocate for the elimination of stigmatisation and the development of a strong, effective political response.

2.3.2 Location of highest rates of infection

The three sources of epidemiological data differ in the estimates they present for levels of HIV prevalence in the nine provinces (see table 2.3). Though the ASSA2000 and DoH estimates are the most similar, as they build on the same antenatal clinic data, the estimates generated in the household survey deviate in some instances, such as where in the case of KwaZulu-Natal, the DoH estimate is more than twice as high as that of the HSRC.

Simplifying the data allows the ranking of the provinces according to their HIV prevalence levels.

Table 2.4: Ranking of provinces by estimated HIV prevalence

Province	ASSA 2000	DoH	HSRC	Outside margin of error
Western Cape	9	9	6	No
Eastern Cape	7	6	8	Yes
Northern Cape	8	8	9	No
Free State	3	3	3	No
KwaZulu-Natal	1	1	4	Yes
North West	4	4	5	Yes
Gauteng	5	5	2	Yes
Mpumalanga	2	2	Yes	
Limpopo	6	7	7	No

Sources: See table 2.3 above. 1 indicates the highest estimate and 9 indicates the lowest estimate.

Two provinces are similarly ranked by both the DoH and the HSRC; the same four provinces are ranked among the four with the lowest estimates;

with the differences falling within the margin of error in four cases.

2.3.3 AIDS-related sickness and deaths

A democratic government at the very least needs to be responsive and react to the frustration and devastation in society caused by increasing numbers of people falling ill and dying from AIDS-related diseases.

While Statistics SA keeps records of mortality, the latest data released at the time of this study is that of 2000, though there is no way of distinguishing whether AIDS was the cause of death (Statistics SA, 2001). Statistics SA further notes that its data tends to underrepresent the total number of deaths since some, especially in the poorer and more marginalised communities where AIDS is more prevalent, are not reported to the authorities (see table 2.5).

The term "AIDS sick" implies that a person has entered stage four of the disease, with a CD4 count of less than 200, being bedridden by AIDS-related illnesses for long stretches. Such a stage is that in which morbidity, absenteeism and mortality begin adversely to affect national economies. In the public sector in Africa, teachers are the group that provides a relatively clear picture of the catastrophic effect of the pandemic.

A 2005 HSRC study found that 12.7% of South African teachers are HIV-positive, rates which correlate with the national statistics when compared in race, gender, socioeconomic background and geographic location, with teacher absenteeism reaching astronomical rates. The provinces varied widely in AIDS-related absenteeism rates, with teachers in KwaZulu-Natal and Mpumalanga having the highest prevalence, due largely to how long the epidemic had been affecting the provincial population, and the general state of health of that population; the "older" the epidemic is, the higher the number of AIDS sick is likely to be, and the healthier the provincial population, the lower the number of AIDS sick is likely to be. The same general logic helps to explain the differences between how many people have died from AIDS-related illnesses in relation to the population in the province. Data on poverty – as a proxy for "provincial health" – seem to corroborate this interpretation. Both the Human Development Index (HDI) and the Human Poverty Index (HPI) (poverty indicators that will be introduced in the next section) correlate accordingly with the variations in AIDS-related sickness and death in the different provinces.[3]

Table 2.5: Recorded deaths by province, 1997–2000

Province	1997	%	1998	%	1999	%	2000	%
Western Cape	29 384	11.4	31 585	10.7	32 787	10.2	34 390	9.7
Eastern Cape*	30 248	11.7	36 947	12.5	43 615	13.6	49 832	14.0
Northern Cape	7 792	3.0	8 364	2.8	8 749	2.7	9 414	2.6
Free State	23 055	8.9	26 493	9.0	28 842	9.0	31 423	8.8
KwaZulu-Natal*	57 533	22.3	67 313	22.8	75 206	23.4	84 851	23.8
North West*	18 286	7.1	21 330	7.2	25 036	7.8	28 940	8.1
Gauteng	55 564	21.6	61 040	20.6	62 506	19.4	67 587	19.0
Mpumalanga	17 738	6.9	20 344	6.9	22 577	7.0	25 002	7.0
Northern Province	18 227	7.1	22 415	7.6	22 192	6.9	24 775	7.0
Total	257 827	100	295 831	100	321 510	100	356 214	100

Source: Statistics SA, 2001: 3. * Provinces with a clear trend of an increasing share of deaths nationally.
The ASSA2000 model provides more relevant data, projecting the numbers of AIDS sick and deaths by province (see table 2.6).

Table 2.6: Projected AIDS sick and AIDS deaths, by province

Province	AIDS sick in 2004, % of total population*	Projected total AIDS deaths 1990–2004, % total population*
Western Cape	0.38	0.64
Eastern Cape	1.10	1.90
Northern Cape	0.73	1.17
Free State	2.74	3.38
KwaZulu-Natal	2.31	4.56
North West	1.62	2.90
Gauteng	1.78	3.13
Mpumalanga	2.05	4.17
Limpopo	1.10	1.98
National	1.57	2.90

Source: Dorrington, 2002: 10–28. *Total population refers to the projected total provincial population in the ASSA2000 model.

2.3.4 Poverty and the epidemic

Whether the epidemic can explain variations in voter registration and turnout in the 2004 elections will be explored after a discussion of poverty levels. Poverty has been identified in the social science literature on the epidemic as one of a few crucial structural variables with a direct impact on various facets of the epidemic (Fredland, 1998; Whiteside, 2002). The HDI is a measure of people's wellbeing obtained by combining life expectancy, educational attainment and gross domestic product (GDP) indices. Values can vary between 0 and 1, where values between 1 and .8 are interpreted as high levels of human development, while values between .799 and .5 indicate medium level and values below .499 indicate low levels. The UNDP has produced several annual reports in which it ranks countries according to their respective HDI scores. Those southern African countries severely affected by the pandemic have all fallen in the ranking between 1996 and 2003 (see table 2.7), possibly due to the detrimental effect that the epidemic has had on life expectancy, which, in some instances, dropped 20 years between 1996 and 2003. If preventative efforts fail and treatment does not effectively halt the lethal effect of the virus, Botswana is projected to see its life expectancy reduced from 70 to 29 years by the year 2010, effectively wiping out decades of development that has elevated the country to one of the strongest economies and most consolidated democracies on the continent. This discussion and the projections in the literature that are presented in table 2.7 do not reflect reality, but are counterfactual statements of what life expectancy would be if, on the one hand, there was no AIDS in the population, and, on the other hand, what life expectancy could be if no efforts are made to stop the ravages of AIDS. However, though AIDS causes death, governments and societies have responded to the challenge, making the non-intervention scenarios impossible. The scenarios are, arguably, nevertheless still relevant as stark reminders of the threat posed by the pandemic.

The UNDP provides a more comprehensive and detailed account of current levels of poverty in South Africa in its *South Africa Human Development Report 2003*, subtitled *The Challenge of Sustainable Development in South Africa: Unlocking People's*

Table 2.7: AIDS-related statistics and projections from selected countries in southern Africa

	UNDP, 1996[A]		UNDP, 2003[A]		LE, 2000[B]		LE, 2010[B]		Adult preva-lence[C]
	LE	HDI	LE	HDI	AIDS	No AIDS	AIDS	No AIDS	
Botswana	65.0	71	44.7	125	39.3	70.5	29	70.3	37.3
Malawi	45.5	157	38.5	162	37.6	53.3	35.8	57.3	14.2
Namibia	59.1	116	47.4	124	–	–	–	–	22.3
South Africa	63.2	100	50.9	111	51.1	65.7	35.5	68.3	21.5
Swaziland	57.8	110	38.2	133	–	–	–	–	38.8
Zambia	48.6	136	33.4	163	37.2	58.9	38.9	62.8	16.5
Zimbabwe	53.4	124	35.4	145	37.8	69.9	32.2	72.8	24.6

Source: [A] Whiteside and Barnett, 2002, citing UNDP and the US Bureau of the Census, [B] UNDP, 2003. [C] Estimates for end of 2003, UNAIDS, 2004.

Creativity. The UNDP captures the dilemma that poverty presents to South Africa: Despite a decade of successfully sustaining and consolidating its democratic regime, the country has yet to find ways of "unlocking" the full creative potential of those of its citizens who are still trapped in poverty. Unless this unused pool of human resources is channelled and creatively developed, the social foundations for democracy will increasingly be undermined by growing poverty (see table 2.8).

Though income poverty has decreased somewhat overall, relatively large increases of poverty has occurred in the White and Indian population groups and in Gauteng. However, the national decrease of 2.6% is less than the population growth, showing that more people were living in poverty in 2002 than in 1995. The "poverty gap" presents a mixed picture. Some of those living under the poverty line have become a little less poor, whereas others are dropping further below that line. The strongest improvement was seen in Mpumalanga (by .9%), while the worst drop (1.7%) occurred in Gauteng and among Indians (2.2%). The last three indicators reflected in the table are more complex in their construction, with more obvious political implications, as they reveal the stark inequalities in South African society, showing more directly the extent to which people struggle with poverty and underdevelopment. The level of inequality of all but two (North West and Limpopo) UNDP categories has increased, so that South Africa is becoming increasingly unequal. The levels of human development are decreasing in all the provinces,[4] while levels of human poverty are increasing in all categories. The comments do not challenge any particular claims by the South African government of having improved the living conditions for South Africans (South African Government, 2003). To the extent that poverty fuels the HIV/AIDS epidemic, the macro indicators of poverty suggest that the structural context to the epidemic is increasingly undermining any other government interventions aimed at dealing constructively with the epidemic.

Correlation analyses of the different variables statistically support the argument that provinces with higher levels of poverty also have higher levels of HIV prevalence and AIDS sickness. No correlation exists between the more direct income poverty indicators or the Gini-coefficient and HIV prevalence, as such instruments are too blunt to reflect such a correlation. Only those indicators based on large-scale representations of poverty reveal a pattern. However, the HIV estimates from the HSRC responded to these indicators, though considerable correlation occurred with the other two estimates. The correlation (Pearson's r) between the DoH estimates and the HDI is .364, with a high .827 with the HPI. The correlations between the ASSA2000 estimates and such poverty indicators are very high (.55 and .91 respectively).[5]

The correlation between HIV prevalence and levels of human development and human poverty among the nine provinces in South Africa has clearly shown the relevance of including poverty as a contextual variable in any social science discussion of the epidemic (Whiteside, 2002).

Table 2.8: Poverty indicators for South Africa, by gender, race and province		Poverty %A		Poverty gap %B		GiniC		HDID		HPIE	
		1995	2002	1995	2002	1995	2001	1995	2003	1995	2001
National		51.1	48.5	17.8	18.0	.595	.635	.740	.660	16.0	22.0
Gender	Female	53.4	50.9	18.4	18.2	.560	600	–	–	15.5	21.5
	Male	48.9	45.9	17.1	17.8	.580	.625	–	–	17.5	22.5
Race	African	62.0	56.3	22.1	21.5	.540	.575	–	–	19.0	25.5
	White	1.5	6.9	1.5	2.4	.465	475	–	–	3.5	4.5
	Coloured	38.5	36.1	10.7	11.6	.490	.555	–	–	9.5	12.0
	Indian	8.3	14.7	2.2	4.4	.440	.520	–	–	5.0	5.5
Pro-vinces	Western Cape	28.6	28.8	7.5	8.5	.540	.590	.790	.760	9.5	12.0
	Eastern Cape	71.2	68.3	26.9	27.9	.610	.655	.670	.620	23.0	24.0
	Northern Cape	55.4	54.4	19.0	19.6	.600	.630	.720	.690	16.5	17.0
	Free State	63.6	59.9	20.9	20.3	.625	.645	.745	.670	14.5	22.5
	KwaZulu-Natal	53.2	50.5	18.1	18.9	.565	.610	.710	.625	16.5	27.0
	North West	59.4	56.5	22.4	21.9	.595	.585	.675	.605	23.0	25.0
	Gauteng	18.4	20.0	6.2	7.9	.530	.615	.810	.740	10.5	19.0
	Mpumalanga	59.7	54.8	20.9	20.0	.560	.610	.725	.650	19.5	26.0
	Limpopo	62.7	60.7	23.7	23.5	.640	.600	.640	.595	20.5	22.0

A) Income poverty: percent of adults who live on less than R354 a month. B) Income poverty gap: the mean shortfall of R354, in percent of that sum. C) Gini-coefficient: measures the extent of income inequality where 0 is perfect equality and 1 is perfect inequality. D) Human Development Index: a composite index of indices of life expectancy, educational attainment and gross domestic product, where 0 is low development and 1 is high development. E) Human Poverty Index: a combined index of three indicators of poverty: the probability at birth of not surviving to age 40, adult literacy rate, and the percentages of people not using improved water sources and children under five who are underweight where higher numbers indicate higher levels of poverty. Source: UNDP, 2003: 41–46

2.4 Conclusion

Irrespective of reliance on antenatal clinic data or survey data or on data generated by a statistical model, the epidemic is very serious. Two of the epidemic's three "waves" are now seriously affecting South African society: HIV prevalence is still extremely high among large parts of the population, and those who contracted the virus several years ago are dying in increasing numbers. According to Alan Whiteside's theory of the epidemiological waves, the effects of the third wave on the economy and society should now start to be seen. South Africa's political response to the epidemic has been long awaited and has already been claimed as the chief failure of the current political regime. However, despite its delay, a common approach from the public, private and CSO sector has produced a plan and programme that pro-

vides clear guidelines and achievable targets aimed at significantly reducing the prevalence rates over a period of five years. The government leadership role has motivated different sectors to engage in the governance of AIDS. Such a contribution can provide the benchmark on which future research can rely. This probe now turns to how the impact of the third wave of the epidemic can affect electoral processes more generally, and whether the effect of HIV/AIDS could be discerned in the April 2004 elections.

3. Impact on the electoral system

Much HIV/AIDS-related policy and academic discourse has focused on the implications and impact of the epidemic on socioeconomic development. All the UNAIDS global reports on the epidemic unequivocally point to HIV/AIDS being a developmental catastrophe. The analysis now introduces an alternative set of complexities and impacts, directly linked to how the epidemic undermines democratic governance more generally and how the epidemic affects the legitimacy and sustainability of electoral systems in southern Africa in general and South Africa in particular. By highlighting the significance of elections and electoral systems for a working democracy, the impact of HIV/AIDS on governance is likely to be seen to vary between countries, depending on the electoral system in place.

3.1 South Africa's electoral system

Since 1994, South Africa has used the list PR system. According to Nohlen, a pure PR electoral system is one "which, without natural or artificial hurdles, (the size of constituencies or thresholds) aim[s] at attaining the highest possible degree of proportionality" (cited in De Ville, 1996:19).

Faure and Venter (2003: 2) find:

> South Africa used the British First-Past-The-Post (FPTP) system of electing representatives for Parliament for more than eighty years. It remained essentially unchanged since its implementation of unification in 1910 until its replacement by an electoral system with the 1993 Interim Constitution and the subsequent election of April 1994. Towards the end of the 1980s, it became clear that South Africa was irrevocably moving towards some major form of political transition and a new electoral arrangement. The five years that preceded the adoption of the Interim Constitution in 1993 witnessed intensification in the debate on electoral options for the new South Africa.

South Africa's adoption of the PR model in 1994 was influenced by:

- The political compromise, which was part of the 1990s political settlement;
- Reconciliation, peace and harmony imperatives;
- A commitment to nation-building and national unity by political protagonists who participated in the multiparty talks; and

- A desire to ensure broad political representation in Parliament in a multiracial society after the centralised authoritarian system operating under the apartheid regime (see De Ville and Steytler, 1996).

However, the PR model applies in South Africa only so far as elections for the National Assembly are concerned, whereas, for purposes of local government elections, the hybrid system that combines the constituency-based FPTP electoral model with PR is applied. At national level, effort is exerted towards broadening representation in the national and provincial legislatures and nurturing and deepening reconciliation and political stability, while accessibility and accountability is emphasised at local government levels, despite the FPTP system tending to be exclusionary.

During the British colonial administration and apartheid regime, South Africa used the FPTP electoral system to split the country into electoral zones, called constituencies for purposes of election, with each constituency electing one individual to represent the electorate in that particular zone into the legislature; candidates contested elections as individuals, irrespective of whether they were independent or party-endorsed. This system was changed in 1994 in line with the political changes that ushered in a democratic dispensation marked by majority rule and the demise of apartheid. The 1996 Constitution prescribes that the electoral system must result in general in PR. Thus "the system chosen to fulfil this mandate for national Parliament was a highly proportional party list system, in which each party draws up closed and rank-ordered national and provincial lists of candidates for Parliament. Elections are held every five years" (Butler, 2004:105). Since 1994, therefore, South Africa has used list PR, in which the entire country is considered one large electoral zone or constituency, with various voting districts. Parties contesting elections prepare the following lists of candidates for the 400-member National Assembly:

- A National Assembly, or national–to–national, list, comprising 200 candidates;
- A National Assembly, or province–to–national, list, comprising 200 candidates; and
- Nine provincial, or province–to–province, lists, comprising candidates equivalent to the number of seats available in each provincial legislature (Cherry, 2004; Southall, 2004).

Having been duly constituted by means of an election, the national Parliament "elects the president who is the head of the executive branch of government, and who is responsible for governing in conjunction with the Cabinet, which he appoints" (Butler, 2004:105). Thus, unlike in the FPTP system of the apartheid era, in the present PR electoral model, political parties prepare their party lists of candidates, who, in turn, contest elections not as individuals chosen to the legislature to represent constituencies, but as party representatives who represent parties in the legislature. The allocation of seats itself is a fairly technical process, which uses the Droop quota of the threshold that is used in highest average list PR systems, with the quota being "ascertained by the following formula: total vote divided by the number of seats plus one, then one is added to the product" (Reynolds and Reilly, 1997: 140). In the seat allocation formula, the South Africa PR system provides for a fairly low threshold for party access to Parliament in the Southern African Development Community (SADC) region compared with Mozambique (5%). Such a threshold determines the inclusion and exclusion of parties in the legislature on the basis of the number of votes cast for each party contesting the elections, with each party having to pass the test of implicit threshold before gaining access to Parliament.

The South African Constitution prescribes an implicit quota, which is determined primarily by voter turnout and the calculation of seats won by each party. According to Paul Graham,[6] "the lower the voter turnout, the lower the quota, thereby allowing more parties access to Parliament; the higher the voter turnout, the higher the quota and the fewer the parties gaining parliamentary seats." Using the Droop method, "the quota of votes per seat (…) does, however, provide for an implicit threshold. The size of the implicit threshold is also dependent upon the way in which remaining seats are allocated, the number of votes cast and the number of spoilt papers" (De Ville, 1996:24). De Ville, Faure and Venter (2003: 5) aptly observe:

> for both the National Assembly and the regional/provincial legislatures the respective thresholds of various regions/ provinces differ, unless they have the same numbers of seats in comparative cases. About 1/400th of votes cast for the national party lists of the National Assembly (i.e. about 0.25%) constitutes the threshold, but the number of seats already allocated regionally is subtracted from the seats won in this way, effectively making this threshold about 0.50%. The threshold for the National Assembly as a whole is 0.24938%

The outcomes of the 1994, 1999 and 2004 elections were derived using this calculation (for the results, see tables 3.1, 3.2 and 3.3).

Table 3.1: 1994 election outcome

Political party	Proportion of seats won
ANC	62.65 252
NP	20.39 82
IFP	10.54 43
FF	2.17 9
DP	1.73 7
PAC	1.25 5
ACDP	0.45 2

Note: 7 out of 19 parties won seats in the election.

Both the political opening caused by the transition and the low threshold of the electoral model triggered the phenomenal mushrooming of political parties shown in table 3.1. The main political parties in the first democratic election were the ANC (with 63% of the votes); the National Party (with 20% of the votes); the Inkatha Freedom Party (IFP) (with 11% of the votes); the Freedom Front (with 2% of the votes); the Democratic Party (with 2% of the votes); and the Pan-African Congress (with 1% of the votes). Despite the multiplicity of parties and broad parliamentary representation, the ANC has remained a hegemonic force in South African politics, as seen in the outcome of the 1999 election (see table 3.2).

As in the 1994 election, the ANC scored a land-

Table 3.2: 1999 election outcome

Political party	Proportion of seats won
ANC	66.35 266
DP	9.56 38
IFP	8.58 34
NNP	6.87 28
UDM	3.42 14
ACDP	1.43 6
FF	0.8 3
UCDP	0.78 3
PAC	0.71 3
FA	0.54 2
MF	0.3 1
AEB	0.25 1
Azapo	0.17 1

Note: 3 more seats were contested.

slide victory in the 1999 election, snatching 66% of the total valid votes, while the main opposition – the Democratic Party – was only able to win 10%. The ANC electoral hegemony is firmly entrenched in South Africa, with the 2004 election result reinforcing the dominant party system, marked by an overwhelmingly strong ruling party on one hand and enfeebled and fragmented opposition parties on the other. As parties began to gear themselves up for the 2004 election, the ANC's primary strategy was to maintain its political hegemony, while the opposition parties aimed principally to put up a spirited fight not so much to win state power as such, but rather to narrow the margin of the ANC's already presumed victory well in advance of the electoral contest itself. The general elections held in post-apartheid South Africa in 1994, 1999 and 2004 are due to be followed by a fourth in 2009, while local government elections were held in 1995, 1999 and 2005.

and a corresponding 69.75% of seats. A direct correlation of votes and seats won by parties is rare under the FPTP system. While often criticised for lack of accountability of MPs, given their strong link to the party, rather than directly to the electorate, the PR system is reputed for its inherent values that seem to advance democratic governance, including:

- the broad representation of key political forces in the legislature;
- an inclusive political system;
- reconciliation in post-conflict societies; and
- facilitation of gender balance in the governance realm, as reflected in table 3.4.

Table 3.3: The results of the 2004 National Assembly election

Party	Total votes	%	Total seats	%
ANC	10 878 251	69.68	279	69.75
DA	1 931 201	12.37	50	12.5
IFP	1 088 664	6.97	28	7
UDM	355 717	2.28	9	2.25
ID	269 765	1.73	7	1.75
NNP	257 824	1.65	7	1.75
ACDP	250 272	1.6	6	1.5
FF+	139 465	0.89	4	1
UCDP	117 792	0.75	3	0.75
PAC	113 512	0.73	3	0.75
MF	55 267	0.35	2	0.5
Azapo	41 776	0.27	2	0.5
Note: An additional eight parties did not win seats. Source: The Independent Electoral Commission				

Table 3.4: Gender balance in the National Assembly, 1994–2004

Year	Size of Parliament	Number of women	Percentage of women (%)
1994	400	111	27.7
1999	400	120	29.8
2004	400	131	32.8
Source: Morna, 2004.[7]			

Table 3.4 shows that women's participation in the South African Parliament has grown since 1994. In a 400-seat Parliament, women occupied 111 seats, constituting 27.7% of the total, in 1994, which rose in the country's second democratic election of 1999 to 120, translating into 29.8% of the total parliamentary seats. The 1997 SADC Declaration on Gender and Development, which was signed by member states in Blantyre, Malawi, showed the commitment of SADC states to achieving equal gender representation in key organs of governance. After the 2004 election, South Africa exceeded its 2005 target of 30% women representation in Parliament. The current women representation in Parliament is 131, which translates into 32.8%, about 3% above the SADC benchmark for 2005, and about 17% shy of equal (50%) gender representation in the legislature. The electoral system has overwhelmingly influenced the positive trend in South Africa's evolving democracy. However, added to this has been the commitment of political parties to a political culture that embraces gender equality in governance. Though PR might not suffice to ensure gender equality in the legislature, commitment to gender equality by the political elite in charge of party affairs and institutionalisation of quotas for women representation in the legislature should combine to do so.

Tables 3.1, 3.2 and 3.3 show that the PR allots parliamentary seats to parties almost in direct proportion to their electoral strength, indicating the fairness and inclusivity of the system. The correlation between the party's percentage of votes won and the percentage of seats acquired is close, suggesting that the number of seats won by each party equates its electoral strength. For instance, while the ruling ANC won 62.65% of votes and 63% of seats in 1994, in 1999, it won 66.35% of votes and 66.5% of parliamentary seats and in 2004, it won 69.68% of votes

3.1.1 Political parties

Electoral contest and system have significantly influenced the existing party system. Lodge (2004: 189) asserts that "robust democracies benefit from strong parties. Strong parties attract durable support". A party system denotes procedures, rules and an institutional framework for party political contest for state power within a given political system. However, the party system is not confined to interparty and intraparty relations and how parties contest political power as such, but also extends to the articulation of party interests with the interests and demands of popular organisations in society. The *Encyclopedia of Democracy* characterises party systems as including:

- The number of parties;
- The size of parties;
- The party political configuration in the National Assembly;
- Party manifestos and programmes;
- Party relationships (alliances) with interest/pressure groups;
- Interparty relations; and
- Intraparty relations.

World-over, party systems comprise:

- the one-party system, which provides for a governance system in which the only *de jure* or *de facto* existing party has sole control of state power;
- a two-party system, or duopoly, wherein two main parties dominate and drive the political system, alternating in controlling state power through electoral contest;
- a multiparty system, in which more than two parties exist and are politically active in directing governance and, in so doing, alternate among themselves control over state power; and
- the dominant party system, in which, despite the multiparty situation, only one party is so dominant that it directs the political system and is firmly in control of state power over a fairly long period of time, allowing opposition parties little, if any, intrusion on its political hegemony (Karume, 2004; Lodge, 2004).

The political hegemony of the ruling ANC suggests that the governance of South Africa comprises a dominant party system, of which the key features are:

- The continuous electoral victories by huge margins of a dominant party over a protracted period of time, with attendant reduction in the importance of oppositional contest;
- The political hegemony of the ruling party over state institutions, including control of the largest share of the legislature and local government authorities; and
- The sole determination and direction of development policy trajectories by the ruling party, with little challenge or credible policy alternatives offered by opposition parties for a long time.

3.2 Links between HIV/AIDS and an electoral system

The electoral system in place in South Africa has ensured that, even under conditions set by the dominant party system, the National Assembly still remains broadly representative of the key political parties that, to various degrees, influence the nature of the political system. Such a feature distinguishes the dominant party system markedly from the one-party system that has prevailed in some other countries. Given that political parties play such a key role in any vibrant democracy, investigating the likely impact of the HIV/AIDS epidemic on their capacity to drive the democracy project is worthwhile, as well as is interrogating their policy approaches to the epidemic.

3.2.1 The FPTP compared to the PR

In previous sections, there have been detailed descriptions of how HIV/AIDS affects the FPTP system. Before we delve into South Africa's PR and MMP models in this regard, let us examine the trends in its neighbour, Zimbabwe, another FPTP country. Since its 2000 parliamentary elections, Zimbabwe has held 29 by-elections for the replacement of MPs. Nineteen of the by-elections were caused by deaths of MPs due to illnesses (see figure 3.1).

Figure 3.1: Reasons for by-elections in Zimbabwe, 2000-07

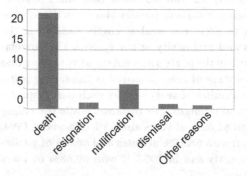

Source: ZESN; 2007.

The frequency of such by-elections suggests that they overburden the national budget. Zimbabwe, as with other FPTP countries, will urgently need to reform its electoral model in favour of the PR or MMP system, which Lesotho adopted in 2002. Mauritius adopted an MMP system after its 2005 general elections, with its National Assembly having 70 members, 62 of whom are elected by universal adult suffrage in a secret ballot. Mauritius Island is divided into 20 constituencies, each of which returns three members, while Rodrigues returns two. The other eight seats are allocated by the Electoral Supervisory Commission, according to a complex formula of "best losers", aimed at ensuring "a fair and adequate representation of each community" (EISA, 2006).

3.2.2 Cost of by-elections in Lesotho

Lesotho reformed its electoral model from an FPTP to an MMP system (Elklit, 2002; Fox and Southall, 2003; Matlosa, 2004), though its adoption of the latter has not eliminated the costs involved in replacing MPs. Since Lesotho's general election of May 2002, which cost about R70 million (US$11.2 million), the country had held about eight by-elections by January 2005, each costing about one million rands (or US$ 143 601 at the rand rate on September 29, 2007).

At the time of this study, eight MPs had died, with seven of them having been elected through the FPTP system and one through the PR system.

3.2.3 Costs of replacing MPs in South Africa

Compared with those countries that operate the FPTP electoral system, in South Africa the replacement of MPs is relatively straightforward and less costly both financially and in terms of political power shifts in the legislature. Furthermore, the South African Parliament is unlikely to be dogged by the problem of reduced degree of political mandate due to low voter turnout that is often linked to by-elections relative to general and local government elections. In a study undertaken in 2001, Michael Sachs discovered that "on average 33% of registered voters cast their ballots in the 79 by-elections. Average turnout in the same wards in the December 2000 elections was 48% and in the 1999 General Election it was 86%" (2001: 2). Parliamentary data suggests that 227 MPs left Parliament between 1994 and 2006, with death causing 23 of the vacancies. No

evidence exists to suggest that the mortality trends correlate with those of HIV/AIDS attrition in the general population. The relatively low death rates have to do with the extent of medical cover extended to parliamentarians in South Africa.[8] Senior parliamentarians have been flown abroad for advanced medical attention when the need arose, indicating a disparity in the capacity and quality of medical care.[9] Though the loss of MPs due to death amounts to loss of political leadership in the topmost ranks of the party concerned, South Africa is not seriously financially affected by such losses, since the affected party merely reverts to its predetermined list to fill the vacancy. Neither does the PR system of replacement of MPs lead to shifts in the configuration of power among parties, since the party that loses an MP is the same party that fills the vacancy, with the seat not being open to contestation.

Figure 3.2: MP turnover in South Africa, 1994–2006

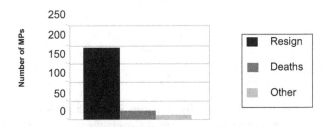

Source: South African Parliament, 2007.

3.3 Power shifts in legislature, reduced mandate of MPs

The trend depicted in figure 3.2 starkly contrasts with political developments in countries using the FPTP system. In some countries, the power shifts that are brought about by by-elections lead to such change in the legislature that the original election result changes mid-term.

Table 3.5 indicates that the results of the Zimbabwean 2000 general election were 62 elected seats for ZANU-PF, 57 elected seats for the opposition MDC and 1 elected seat for ZANU-Ndonga. That political power balance in the legislature is gradually changing, due to the by-elections held since Parliament was constituted. The trend suggests that the ruling party is gaining more political leverage out of the by-election, while that of the opposition is shrinking.

Between 2000-2004, five years after the country's most competitive parliamentary elections in history, 14 by-elections were held, with eight of them caused by deaths to illness. One was a suicide. The ruling ZANU-PF, by winning most by-elections, had increased its parliamentary strength during this period from 62 to 67 seats, amounting to an additional 5 seats. ZANU-PF's gain was MDC's loss. MDC was, accordingly, weakened, shrinking from 57 to 52 seats.

Table 3.5: Power shift in Zimbabwean Parliament due to by-elections since 2000				
Year	Number seats won by each party			
Elections	ZANU-PF	MDC	ZANU Ndonga	Total
2000 general election	62	57	1	120
By-elections since 2000[10]	67	52	1	120
Source: ZESN (Zimbabwe Election Support Network).				

3.5 Local government by-elections in South Africa

Local government by-elections in South Africa are governed by the 1998 Local Government Municipal Structures Act. Section 25 of the Act (1998) stipulates conditions that call for a by-election:

- If the IEC does not declare the result of the local government election within a period specified in the Electoral Act;
- If a court sets aside the election of a local government structure;
- If a council is dissolved; or
- If a vacancy in a ward occurs.

The electoral system used for local government elections and by-elections requires:

- for local councils (Category A) and municipal councils (Category B), 50% of ward councillors are elected directly through the FPTP system and the other 50% through the PR model to achieve overall political proportionality;
- at district (Category C) level, 40% of the councillors are directly elected by eligible district residents, while 60% of the councillors are indirectly elected, being appointed representatives of local and municipal councils (Department of Local Government and Housing, 2004).

Most local government by-elections since 1999 have been due to a vacancy at ward level caused by a number of factors, ranging from resignations, dismissals and floor-crossings to the death of the councillors concerned. Due to South Africa mixing FPTP and list PR in its local government elections, replacing councillors costs much more than does replacing MPs at the national level.

The total cost of the 1994 general election in South Africa was R912 132 326 (about U$250 million), while the 1999 election cost is estimated at R529 210 483 (IEC Election Report, 1994; IEC Election Report, 1999). According to the IEC, each ward by-election costs about R30 000. Given this estimate, the 2001 by-elections cost R2.3 million, while the 2002 by-elections cost about R2.2 million, with the 2003 by-elections costing about R2.5 million. The South African local government system comprises 312 metropolitan councils, 215 district councils and 1 711 local councils, so that about 3 754 wards exist (Department of Local Government, 2004).

Table 3.6: Local government by-elections, 2001–04				
Province	Size*	2001	2002	2003
Eastern Cape	601	12 (2%)	6 (1%)	12 (2%)
Free State	291	2 (0.69%)	4 (1.37%)	8 (2.75%)
Gauteng	446	9 (2.02%)	6 (1.35%)	8 (2.75%)
KwaZulu-Natal	748	27 (3.61%)	22 (2.94%)	21 (2.81%)
Limpopo	402	2 (2.24%)	5 (1.75%)	4 (1.5%)
Northern Cape	173	3 (1.73%)	9 (5.2%)	9 (5.2%)
North West	327	7 (2.14%)	8 (2.45%)	6 (1.83%)
Western Cape	340	8 (2.35%)	6 (1.76%)	9 (2.65%)
Total	3 729	79 (2.23%)	73 (1.96%)	83 (2.12%)
* Total number of ward councillors. Source: Independent Electoral Commission.				

In 2001, 79 by-elections were held, of which 27 took place in KwaZulu-Natal and 9 in Gauteng. In 2002, 73 local government by-elections (6 or 0.27% less than in 2001) were organised, with KwaZulu-

Natal again having the most (22), followed by the Northern Cape (9). In 2003, the number of local government by-elections soared to 83 (an increase of 10 or 0.16% from the previous year), with most by-elections again being held in KwaZulu-Natal (21), followed by the Northern Cape (9), the Western Cape (9), Gauteng (8) and the Free State (8). By May 2004, 60 by-elections had been held. The causes for the by-elections ranged from resignations to floor-crossings, dismissals and deaths of councillors.

Figure 3.3: Reasons for by-elections held in 2001

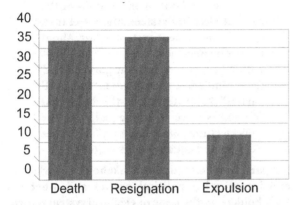

Though the HIV/AIDS epidemic adds to the mortality rate of councillors, the cause of death is a range of sometimes unknown factors. Sachs (2001: 1) argues that out of the 79 by-elections in 2001, "34 were precipitated by a councillor's resignation from his or her post, 33 resulted from the death of a councillor and 12 were a result of the expulsion of a councillor either from the party or the council concerned."

3.5.1 Increasing costs of by-elections

Though the information available did not show why individuals left their seats in local government, many have (see table 3.7).

The IEC has reported that each by-election cost roughly R20 000–R30 000 in 2004 (Personal communication, Mr M Mosery, IEC, 3 June 2004). The KwaZulu-Natal office of the IEC reported their concern about the high number of by-elections in their province: 70 in a three-year period (Personal communication, Mr M Mosery, IEC, 3 June 2004). The average cost of a by-election was confirmed by the IEC national office, who estimated it, on average, to be R30 000 (Personal communication, Mr M Hendrickse, IEC, June 2004).

3.6 South African electoral system reform debate

Few democracies regularly review their electoral models and reform where necessary. Reynolds and Reilly (2002: 9–13) recommend that states should review and design electoral systems that suit their own conditions in order to affirm their commitment to democratic governance by:

• Ensuring a representative Parliament;

• Making elections accessible and meaningful;

• Providing incentives for conciliation;

• Facilitating stable and efficient government;

• Holding the government and representatives accountable;

• Encouraging "cross-cutting" political parties;

Table 3.7: Number of by-elections for directly elected local councillors

Region	Size*	2001		2002		2003	
		Actual	%	Actual	%	Actual	%
Eastern Cape	601	12	2.00	6	1.00	12	2.00
Free State	291	2	0.69	4	1.37	8	2.75
Gauteng	446	9	2.02	6	1.35	8	2.75
KwaZulu-Natal	748	27	3.61	22	2.94	21	2.81
Limpopo	402	2	2.24	5	1.75	4	1.50
Northern Cape	173	3	1.73	9	5.20	9	5.20
North West	327	7	2.14	8	2.45	6	1.83
Western Cape	340	8	2.35	6	1.76	9	2.65
Total	3729	79	2.23	73	1.96	83	2.12

Source: Electoral Commission. *Represents the percentage of the total number of counsellors who left during the year.

- Promoting parliamentary opposition; and
- Enhancing cost and administrative capacity.

While such considerations suffice for consideration of electoral reform, the implications of HIV/AIDS demand attention.

The PR electoral model that South Africa has used since 1994 has served the country fairly well in several respects, by:

- helping to ensure the broad representation of key political forces in the legislature;
- catalysing gender balance and female participation in both Parliament and the executive branch of government;
- facilitating reconciliation and peace after a protracted violent conflict, acting not only as a conflict management instrument, but also as a guarantor for political stability;
- enhancing the participation of the electorate, by cutting wastage of votes, as all valid votes cast count towards the calculation of election results, with parties earning their legislative seats in proportion to their electoral strength.

The PR model applied in South Africa (see De Ville and Steytler, 1996) has been subjected to much questioning, especially after the country's second democratic election in 1999 (see Konrad Adenauer Foundation, 2003). Such general debate prompted the government to appoint an advisory task force on electoral reform, the Electoral Task Team (ETT) (2002: 3),[11] which was granted a fairly broad mandate to:

- Draft the electoral legislation required by the Constitution; and
- Formulate and draft the parameters of electoral legislation.

The ETT (2002: 4) had to:

- Identify the controlling constitutional parameters;
- Identify the salient and relevant aspects of, as well as the list of options available in, the South African context;
- Canvass the preferences and views of relevant role-players and stakeholders with special regard to political parties in respect of the list of identified options;
- Develop specific proposals identifying the preferable electoral system to be canvassed with such role-players and stakeholders; and
- Formulate a draft Bill for submission to Minister M. Buthelezi.

An international conference was organised jointly by the ETT, Konrad Adenauer Foundation and the Electoral Institute of Southern Africa (EISA) in Cape Town from 9 to 10 September 2002 to debate regional and international perspectives and experiences. However, opinion was divided on whether to adopt the MMP system, or whether to retain the full list PR system. Nevertheless, public opinion on electoral reform was overwhelmingly in favour of the latter.

The HSRC undertook a public opinion survey of 2760 randomly selected South African citizens of voting age. According to Southall and Mattes (2002):

> the survey asked … respondents a series of questions about their opinions of the current electoral system. Many feel that, overall, the present system is fair. About three-quarters say they are "satisfied" with "the way we elect our government" (74%) and agree the system is "fair to all parties" (72%). About two-thirds feel that "all voters were treated equally" in the 1999 elections (68%) and that "all parties were treated equally" in 1999 (63%).

Apart from conducting stakeholder workshops and interviewing political parties and other key stakeholders on the issue of electoral system reform, the Slabbert Commission engaged experts in the field to survey public opinion about such reform. The result was inconclusive, as members of the task force were divided into two schools of thought:

- A majority view, in favour of an MMP representation system, which led to the introduction of 69 multimember constituencies, from which 300 MPs would be elected by FPTP, and 100 MPs elected on the basis of a closed party list; and
- A minority view, eager to retain the current system, arguing that its strengths outweighed its perceived weaknesses.

Due to the divergence of opinion within the commission, two reports were produced: the main report, advocated change of the model, and a minority report, calling for the retention of the PR system.

After the ETT submitted both reports to the Minister of Home Affairs, they were presented to Cabinet. According to Faure and Venter (2003: 8), "the government's reaction to the ETT report was that the status quo would be maintained and that the newly elected government in 2004 would review the report and make a decision in preparation for the 2009 poll". The ANC government had still to revisit the two reports and promulgate floor-crossing legislation (see Southall, 2004).

Various factors influenced the government decision not to undertake electoral reforms in line with the majority position of the ETT (Southall, 2004):

- The challenges posed for civic and voter education by introducing a model just before the 2004 election;

- The perceived fairness and representativeness of the PR, especially its inherent benefits for a post-conflict South Africa;

- The familiarity and relative simplicity of the system for voters, in comparison with the proposed MMP model;

- The proven conduciveness of the system to gender equality in the political governance realm; and

- The fact that the commission itself had not formed a solidified and unanimous opinion on the reform imperatives.

The majority report urged the need for electoral system reform due to PR being insufficiently accountable. However, the problem of accountability could as well be addressed and redressed by adopting measures that require neither refinement nor change of the electoral model. The minority report confirmed the existence of popular support for the PR and that political parties had indicated that they would prefer to retain the model, so that the system required no change. It also argued that the fairness, inclusivity and simplicity of the list PR system suited South Africa.

The debate that was triggered by the ETT, though enriching for both policy and academic discourse on electoral models, failed to deal with the impact of HIV/AIDS on the electoral system, especially regarding by-election costs. Broad observations in this regard are that:

- Much as the FPTP electoral model is reputed for its accountability, it tends to be costly financially, administratively and politically, especially when it comes to replacing MPs through by-elections;

- While the PR system is reputed for broadening representation, it is less costly financially and administratively (though still costly politically) when it comes to replacing MPs through party lists; and

- The experience of Lesotho, which only recently adopted the MMP electoral model, shows that the system fails adequately to address the financial, administrative and political cost of replacing MPs.

As the HIV/AIDS epidemic takes its toll, the political elite are bound to be affected. South Africa needs to engineer its electoral machinery to ensure minimal impact of the pandemic on elected representatives in the National Assembly. South Africa should retain its current PR system, yet institutionalise accountability mechanisms.

Only Parliament can trigger electoral reform, though Graham states that the political leadership does not support such reform:

> However, the last thing that we can expect from MPs is to have the nerve to question and critique the system that earned them parliamentary seats. Let us recall that the British Prime Minister, Tony Blair, promised to prioritise the issue of electoral reforms when he assumed power. It is now eight years and the Blair government has never tabled the issue before Parliament.[12]

3.7 Conclusion

This section emphasised the significance of elections and electoral systems for vibrant and robust democratic governance. After introducing the FPTP in other sections of this book, our discussion on the MMP and PR electoral systems in this chapter, has shown that, on average, those countries using the former system are harder hit by the adverse effects of HIV/AIDS than those using the PR (especially the list PR).

Whereas, at the national and provincial levels, the list PR system might have strengthened the electoral position of the country regarding the impact of HIV/AIDS, the MMP electoral system used at local government has not protected it from the devastating effects of the epidemic.

4. Electoral administration and management

Democratic elections are generally managed by a specialised administrative structure within the public service, since the overall integrity of the electoral process should be guaranteed by the state above partisan interests. Weaknesses in the electoral process indicate a lack of commitment to democracy itself by the state and/or the incumbent government

(Olaleye, 2003). Electoral commissions need to develop an understanding of the nature and extent of the challenges posed by the HIV/AIDS epidemic to the effective administration of elections, or else, a lack of understanding might lead to limited intervention, which might undermine the effective administration of free and fair elections. The legitimacy of the electoral process and all efforts to develop a sustainable democracy would then be undermined.

Exploring how the HIV/AIDS epidemic might affect the effective fulfilment of the mandate given to the South African IEC should enable one to find out whether the IEC has already started to experience some effects of the epidemic. The IEC should be aware of and prepared for how such effects might increase over the next few years, as the epidemic moves into a phase when its consequences will be increasingly felt in AIDS-related illness and mortality. The IEC should develop a strategy for coping with the epidemic, so that it will not too severely affect future national elections.

After describing the legislative and institutional framework for the IEC's administration and regulating of elections in South Africa, on the basis of the findings and hypotheses presented in the existing research, an investigation will be undertaken into how the IEC might be directly affected by the epidemic and what the commission is doing to counter such negative effects.

4.1 Structures, staff, legislative framework of IEC

In the transition from apartheid to democracy, the negotiating parties recognised the need to set up an independent body to manage the elections to ensure that they would be free and fair (Asmal and De Ville, 1994). Two authorities, which had their independence enshrined in the Constitution, were accordingly created: the IEC and an independent authority to regulate broadcasting, the Independent Communication Authority of South Africa (Icasa).[13] The IEC was first set up by the Independent Electoral Commission Act, No. 150 of 1993 as an interim body with the mandate to organise and rule on the "freeness and fairness" of the first democratic elections held in April 1994. The Electoral Commission Act, No. 51 of 1996, later made it permanent, with the mission to strengthen, promote and safeguard constitutional democracy through the delivery of free and fair elections in which all voters are able to make informed choices.[14]

4.1.1 Structures and staff

With its head office in Pretoria and provincial offices in each of the nine provinces, the IEC has a multilevel structure (see figure 4.1), which is headed by five commissioners, appointed in terms of paragraph 6 of the Electoral Act. The commission is headed by a chief electoral officer, who has a deputy. A provincial electoral officer heads each of the nine provincial offices. In June 2004 the IEC had 116 fulltime staff at its national office and 7 to 13 staff at each of the nine provincial offices, amounting to a total of 92 provincial staff.[15] All provincial offices use local government municipal electoral officers (MEOs), who are employed by local governments, but seem to work under the direction of the provincial IEC office.[16] Temporary staff help the IEC during periods of national and provincial elections, with, during the 2004 elections, 224 such staff being employed, together with 215 460 electoral officials appointed in terms of section 74 of the Electoral Act (IEC, June 2004). The IEC has a formal arrangement with the Department of Education that 98% of the presiding officers and deputy presiding officers be drawn from the ranks of teachers.[17] The temporary staff fall into three categories:

- Casuals, who tend to be teachers employed at schools used as polling stations, are employed to work in the voting station on election days.

- Presiding officers and deputy presiding officers, who are usually teachers, are responsible for managing each voting station.

- Area supervisors are generally municipal staff who manage a number of voting districts.

Figure 4.1: The multilevel structure of the Independent Electoral Commission

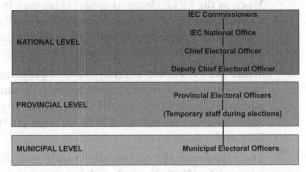

4.1.2 Legislative framework

Six state institutions are mandated in terms of chapter nine of the Constitution to support the constitutional democracy.[18] All such bodies must be impartial and act without fear, favour or prejudice (section 181[2]). All other organs of the state and government departments are, according to section 181(3), obliged to "assist and protect" the "chapter nine" institutions, without intruding on their autonomy.

The IEC's three core functions, set out in section 190 (1) of the Constitution, are:

- To manage elections of national, provincial and municipal legislative bodies in line with national legislation;

- To ensure that the elections are free and fair; and

- To declare the results of such elections within the shortest possible time.

The primary obligations imposed by sections 19(2) and (3)[19] of the Constitution appear to be positive, as they require that the state (through the IEC) ensure the right of every adult citizen to vote (De Waal, 2003). The Constitutional Court has confirmed this interpretation of the Constitution (through its decisions in *New National Party of South Africa versus Government of the Republic of South Africa*, paragraph 118, and *August and Another versus Electoral Commission*, paragraph 16). When the IEC decides where to place voting stations, sets the voting hours and describes the requirements for proof of identity, both the legislature and the IEC should promote democratic principles (*New National Party* case, paragraph 122).

The Electoral Commission Act (No. 51 of 1996) describes the constitutional provisions for the IEC in more detail, providing for the setting up of the Electoral Commission to "manage elections for national, provincial and local legislative bodies and referenda". The Act states that the IEC is an independent body, which is subject only to the Constitution and the law (section 3 [1]). Its aims are to "strengthen constitutional democracy and promote democratic electoral processes" (section 4). The powers, duties and functions of the IEC, as set out in section 5 of the Act, include:

- Managing elections;

- Ensuring that elections are free and fair;

- Promoting conditions conducive to free and fair elections;

- Compiling and maintaining voters' rolls by registering eligible voters, utilising government-sources data;

- Undertaking and promoting election-related research;

- Continually reviewing electoral legislation and proposing electoral legislation, making recommendations based thereon; and

- Appointing appropriate public administration in any sphere of government to conduct elections, when necessary.

The IEC clearly has a complex dual role: that of being both a manager and a regulator of elections, with the way in which the IEC should undertake such core functions being set out in the Electoral Act, No. 73 of 1998, and in the Electoral Laws Amendment Act, No. 34 of 2003. These Acts work with the Local Government Municipal Electoral Act, No. 27 of 2000, which regulates local government elections.

The core functions of the IEC, as defined by these Acts, include:

- *Maintaining a voters' roll.* Section 5 of the Electoral Act obliges the chief electoral officer to compile and maintain a national common voters' roll. Sections 5 and 6 of the Local Government Municipal Electoral Act requires that the national common voters' roll be split up for each municipality and used during the local government elections.

- *Organising voter registration.* Section 6 (1) of the Electoral Act provides that, to register as a voter, a person must be a South African citizen with a valid identity document. To vote, every citizen must register in the prescribed manner in the voting district in which they ordinarily reside (section 7 [1]), which the IEC describes as the place where they live and to which they return after temporary absences.[20] If a voter leaves the place of ordinary residence, they must apply to the IEC to change their voter registration details (section 9 [1]).

- *Organising voting.* Section 36 (1) of the Electoral Act requires the IEC to prescribe the voting hours of the election day, which the chief electoral officer is duty-bound to ensure are publicised in the media (section 36 [3]). Section 60 (1) of the Electoral Act requires the IEC to set up voting districts, in which the polling will take place. The Act also prescribes which criteria should be used to make such determinations (section 61). The criteria stated include the number and distribution of eligible voters; the accessibility of voting stations; the availability of transport; and the geographic or physical features that might impede access to voting. Within each voting district the IEC has to set up voting stations. Section 64 (2) refers to the factors that should be taken into account in deciding where to place such voting stations, including an assessment of the "general facilities at these venues". No specific mention is made of the need to ensure facilities for the disabled or sick. However, a registered voter may apply for a special vote if they are unable to vote at a voting station within the district where they are registered due to physical infirmity, disability or pregnancy (section 33 [1]) and a physically disabled voter may be helped to vote at a voting station (sections 39 [2] and 48). The Local Government Municipal Electoral Act states that, unless the IEC determines otherwise, the voting hours will be from 7.30am until 9pm (section 45). On a local level, the law does not provide for special votes.

• *Observing the elections.* Section 84 (3) of the Electoral Act provides that certain people may be accredited by the IEC as observers of the election, while section 41 of the Local Government Municipal Electoral Act states that people may apply to be observers of a local government election.

4.2 Internal impact of HIV/AIDS

4.2.1 Review of the literature

After a preliminary literature review, the way in which the epidemic is hypothesised to affect the staff within electoral institutions, being the internal impact of HIV/AIDS, is discussed,. The way in which the services provided by electoral institutions might be affected by the epidemic, being the external impact of HIV/AIDS, will be discussed in subsection 5.3. In the absence of literature that specifically addresses the internal impact on electoral commissions, literature will be considered that discusses the possible effects on state bureaucracies more broadly. The next subsection applies the more generally formulated impacts in the literature to the specific circumstances of the IEC, providing a basis for informed discussion of how the epidemic risk is likely to affect the commission negatively in future.

The literature identifies in which ways that the epidemic is likely to affect the internal functioning of workplaces, such as state bureaucracies. Since most assume that HIV-positive employees lack access to effective and comprehensive treatment, the scenarios sketched in this section should decrease in impact if such treatment becomes available for most infected employees in the near future.

4.2.1.1 Increased levels of morbidity

As more infected employees fall ill, they will tend to take more sick leave, which disrupts effective functioning.[21] The effects of such disruptions are amplified when more qualified and experienced employees are absent, since they are more difficult to replace temporarily (Whiteside, 2000). The public service is likely to be seriously affected by such developments. A report commissioned by the Department of Public Service and Administration, entitled the *Impact and Action Report* (2000), projected that, by 2011, 27% of skilled civil servants in South Africa will be PLWHAs (see table 4.1).

Table 4.1: Projected percentage of HIV infection levels by employment category

	1997	2005	2011
Low skilled	3	14	17
Skilled	4	20	27
Highly skilled	2	15	22
Supervisory	2	7	11
Managers	2	7	12
Senior managers	1	7	10
Source: DPSA, 2000.			

Table 4.2 shows the possible impact on morbidity if no measures are introduced to lessen the impact of HIV. As electoral commissions require a pool of skilled people for the effective management of elections, the loss of such personnel, particularly highly skilled staff, directly threatens the competence of commissions.

Table 4.2 Non-intervention scenario projections, based on the metropolitan Doyle model

	2001	2005	2010
% of SA workforce (16-59) HIV+	18.02	22.35	24.08
% of SA workforce AIDS sick	0.93	1.98	2.91
New AIDS cases a year	235 000	397 000	541 000
Life expectancy: females	52	43	37
Life expectancy: males	49	43	38
Source: George, 2003.			

Actual increases in AIDS-related illnesses approximating these estimates inevitably lead to corresponding increases in costs for employment benefits, such as medical schemes (George, 2003).

4.2.1.2 Cause of mortality or early retirement

The *Impact and Action Report* also projected that AIDS would have become the leading cause of death among civil servants by the end of 2002, resulting in 250 000 deaths by 2012 or 23% of the current 1.1 million strong workforce. Table 4.3 shows the projected annual AIDS deaths in the public service, as detailed in the *Impact and Action Report*.

Table 4.3: Projected percentage of annual AIDS deaths within government departments[22]			
Government department	1997	2005	2011
Water/Forestry	1	1.5	2.7
Government administration	1	1.5	2.6
National government	1	1.4	2.4
Justice	1	1.4	2.5
Home Affairs	1	1.4	2.4
Foreign Affairs	1	0.9	1.7
Labour	1	1.3	2.6
Source: DPSA, 2000.			

Teachers are particularly at risk of infection with HIV. A recent study undertaken in KwaZulu-Natal estimated an increase in AIDS-related deaths among educators from 0.64% in 1999 to about 5% by 2010.[23] The IEC is especially negatively affected by this, due to its reliance on the help of teachers on election day. High rates of infection, leading to higher than average rates of mortality, potentially threatens effective election administration by increasing loss of the particular skills and experiences of those who have worked for the IEC in previous elections (Chirambo and Caesar, 2003; Mattes, 2003). The loss of such employees requires an appropriate replacement to be selected and trained, which implies an extra cost to the organisation. For highly qualified staff, such replacement is often difficult, particularly in developing economies with skill shortages.[24]

An additional impact is the process of mentoring and skills transfer which must take place when staff are brought into the organisation (Barrett Grant, Strode and Smart, 2002). Manning (2003) reports

an interview with the Durban Fire Department, in which the Department noted that, though it only takes three months to train replacement fire officers, fire-fighters take years to gain enough experience to convey key skills and knowledge to younger staff members through informal training and mentoring. PLWHAs leave their jobs and might die with little warning because of the stigma that HIV carries and the discrimination to which they fear being subjected, complicating skills transfer.

Mattes (2003) warns of the resulting problems for election authorities: "The loss of non-partisan supervisory officials, combined with the complicated voter registration procedures of southern Africa's multi-party systems, will increase opportunities for voter fraud."

4.2.1.3 Increased absenteeism

As the HIV/AIDS epidemic advances, increases in AIDS-related illnesses and deaths will lead to increased absenteeism, as employees grow too sick to come to work; they attend funerals for family members, friends and colleagues; or take time off to care for sick family members (Whiteside, 2000).

4.2.1.4 Decreased staff morale

A fear of infection and death might lead to increased suspicion of others, as well as resistance to accepting the additional responsibilities for colleagues who are off sick, away from work or newly recruited and not yet fully functional. An eThekwini Municipality case study noted that human resource staff were burdened with the emotional impact of dealing with many young staff members dying and leaving behind children and families (Manning, 2003).

4.2.1.5 Employment equity profile

As African women are most affected by the HIV epidemic, probably the negative impacts of the epidemic on the workplace will also affect the employment equity profile of organisations negatively.

4.2.2 Internal impact of HIV/AIDS on IEC

Every workplace needs to respond to the impact that HIV/AIDS is likely to have on their employees and on the services that they provide. The literature review indicates the nature of the impact, which is explored in terms of the IEC staff profile and turnover.

All workplaces are only as vulnerable to the effects of HIV/AIDS as the degree to which their individual employees engage in behaviours that put them at risk of infection. Some workplaces are more vulnerable than others, due to the extent that their staff profile overlaps with the groups in the population that have a higher rate of infection than others. IEC staff comprise:

- More than 50% women, the gender most affected by the epidemic; 85% in the age group that is most vulnerable to HIV infection; and teachers, an occupation known to be hard hit by the epidemic, in almost all temporary posts.

Due to the IEC's permanent staff comprising four staff between the ages of 18 and 24 years, 178 staff aged between 25 and 49 years, and 28 staff aged between 50 and 60 years, it is vulnerable to the much higher HIV prevalence and effects of AIDS among the young and middle-aged. Such vulnerability is aggravated by most temporary staff falling within the same age brackets, which is likely to reduce the IEC's ability to rely on the same temporary staff to apply experience and skills gained in administrating previous elections to future elections.

In the four years leading upto 2003, four IEC permanent staff died, with three of such deaths occurring in 2003, roughly 1.44% of its permanent staff that year. The figure corresponds with the estimated number of deaths in government departments (see table 4.4).[25]

Table 4.4: Independent Electoral Commission staff turnover

Year	Number of staff leaving the IEC	Death*	Resignation	Other/ unknown
2001	153	1	3	149
2002	10	0	10	0
2003	15	3	12	0
Total	178	4	25	149

Source: IEC, 2004. *This represents the percentage of staff who died while still in service.

The data that was made available to us from the IEC provides us with no real basis from which to comment conclusively on what impact AIDS might have had on its internal structures in loss of staff. Information is needed on:

- *Temporary staff.* The impact of HIV on temporary

IEC election staff is uncertain. The commission uses the electoral staff system, which captures the details of all temporary election officers to allow the IEC to approach the same individuals to help with each election. The system does not, however, keep records of how many were not available for subsequent elections.[26]

- *Specialist staff.* How many of the staff who left the IEC or died over the last few years were specialists in a key section – information technology, electoral logistics, voters' roll management and electoral training – and what this implied for the effective functioning of such sections.

- *Staff absenteeism.* No information was available on staff absenteeism. More comprehensive research into the internal effects of the epidemic on the functioning of the IEC will have to take into account such additional information.

4.2.3 IEC's response to internal impact

The IEC developed and adopted an HIV/AIDS policy in May 2002. A review of the policy is still underway. The IEC is also busy developing a skills succession plan for dealing with the possible loss of highly skilled employees.[27] Such policy development has undergone a consultative process limited to the provincial offices. Mr Mawetu Mosery, KwaZulu-Natal provincial electoral officer, commented on the process: "Most staff did not see it as relevant to them, as they did not believe that they are at risk for infection with HIV. Resultantly, there has been very little buy-in from staff."[28]

The IEC's vision, as stated in its policy, which excludes temporary staff and MEOs., entails mobilising its staff to participate in:

- Prevention programmes;
- The counselling and supporting of infected and affected colleagues and their families;
- HIV/AIDS-related education;
- Providing resources and leadership to implement HIV/AIDS and associated workplace wellness programmes;
- The creation of a non-discriminatory environment, conducive to sensitivity and humanity within the working environment; and
- The protection of confidentiality within the workplace for staff who are known to be PLWHAs.

As, in developing the policy, the IEC assumed that all local governments have their own HIV/AIDS policies for MEOs,[29] no programmes or policies have been set in place to manage the impact of HIV on such staff. The policy neither addresses costs, nor ensures staff the right to antiretroviral treatment. However, with the rollout of the DoH's National Treatment Plan and the availability of antiretrovirals through medical aid schemes, all staff should be able to access treatment on an individual basis through either the private or public sector.

The IEC also has limited HIV/AIDS programmes in place, which are coordinated by an HIV/AIDS focal point employee in each office, who ensures the availability of condoms and HIV/AIDS information. Mosery said that such interventions only attracted attention around World AIDS Day. According to Mosery,[30] the IEC has neither promoted voluntary testing and counselling nor created a stigma-reducing environment to any extent.

4.3 External impact of HIV/AIDS

The HIV epidemic could negatively affect electoral commissions' service delivery due to the number of infected employees who are unable to work at their full capacity, as well as the increased demand for certain services. Such services in remote areas and disadvantaged communities might be particularly vulnerable to absenteeism or deaths among staff, because of shortages of skilled staff and resource constraints (Barrett Grant, Strode and Smart, 2002). Furthermore, planning for future service demands is complicated by the rapidly changing demographics of HIV/AIDS and uncertainty about how service needs will be affected.

4.3.1 Pre-election phase

Sharp increases in mortality due to AIDS complicate the correct and timely compilation and maintenance of the voters' roll, allowing for inaccuracies and facilitating electoral fraud. An effective and efficient public service is required (Olaleye, 2003).

Bedridden PLWHAs might be unable to register for elections if they have to travel to do so. Registering might also be difficult for AIDS orphans, since they often lack proper birth certificates, which they need to get the necessary identification documents for registration on the voters' roll. Furthermore, impoverished families affected by the epidemic might be unable to afford the travel costs involved in getting an identity document and registering as a voter.

Registration rates might also decrease, due to voter apathy resulting from the epidemic, which appears to have been the case in the most recent Zambian election (Chirambo, 2003: Chirambo and Caesar, 2003; Mattes, 2003). The effect on registration of such factors becomes even more problematic where the law or a shortage of resources prevents electoral commission officers from registering people in home visits. PLWHAs often have to move to get home-based care, having to reregister to cast their votes in their new residence.

4.3.2 Polling phase

During the polling phase, those who failed to register for AIDS-related reasons are lost to the electoral process. Registered voters might also choose not to vote, or not do so due to:

- The voting stations only being open for a few days, so that lack of transport, especially in the rural areas, might prevent people reaching them on time.

- Special provisions must be made to ensure that those voters who are pregnant, sick or disabled can quickly cast their votes, with the help of an electoral officer or trusted friend, if necessary.

- The need for voters to enter the public space of voting station to cast their votes might be problematic due to the stigma attached to the epidemic.

Electoral commissions must consider how to convince PLWHAs that staff at the voting stations will counter any prejudice and maltreatment that might be directed at them while at the voting station.

4.3.3 External impact on IEC

The recent Constitutional Court judgment (*Minister of Home Affairs v NICRO and Others*, paragraph 71) recognised the importance of an accurate voters' roll in protecting the legitimacy of elections. Before any election in South Africa, the IEC has to certify the details on the voters' roll, verifying any deaths, migrations or citizenship changes. All marked as deceased on the national population register,[31] on being identified as invalid on the voters' roll, are electronically removed from the roll.[32]

The registration process in South Africa for the 2004 elections went relatively smoothly, with all major political parties expressing satisfaction with its outcome.[33] The IEC established 17 000 registration points, staffed by 50 271 staff, made voter registration accessible to all registered voters. Furthermore, MEOs had to ensure that the hospitalised and bed-ridden were visited to enable them to register as voters.[34] The IEC has recommended that, to facilitate registration, voters should be able to register electronically. Political parties have, however, opposed such a move, arguing that it would increase the possibility of voter fraud.[35]

The 16 966 voting stations throughout the country were generally accessible, with the average distance between the boundary of a voting district and the voting station being between 7.5 and 8 km in urban areas and between 12.5 and 13 km in rural areas. Voters with special needs were able to cast their votes a day before election day, thus avoiding having to queue for long. Michael Hendrickse,[36] senior manager of the Electoral Democracy, Training and Legal Services Division of the IEC, elaborated on other measures taken to help people with special needs to cast their votes:

> As a rule, disabled and sick persons are given preference and moved to the front of the queue, if there is one. A person with a physical disability may be assisted to cast their ballot inside the voting station by another person at the request of that voter. Braille ballot papers are made available at each voting station to allow a blind person to vote without assistance if he or she so wishes. Accessibility of the voting station by a person in a wheelchair is highlighted when deciding on a venue and each voting station has at least one voting compartment/booth that is accessible to a person in a wheelchair.

The IEC ensured that water was available at all voting stations and encouraged the DoH to deploy staff at polling stations to help those with special medical needs, though the department resisted such deployment, arguing that medical personnel could not vote on a separate day, unlike some military and police personnel, who were so authorised by the Electoral Act.[37]

4.3.4 The special vote

The most constructive institutional device that the IEC had for countering the potential effects of the epidemic was the "special vote". The Electoral Act (33 [1]) (a) allows the IEC to arrange for the physically

disabled, infirm or pregnant, as well as those absent from South Africa due to government service holiday, business or tertiary education commitments, and election staff to cast special votes. Applications had to be lodged by 8 April 2004, with the casting of special votes being allowed between 9am and 5pm on 12 and 13 April 2004, while all other voters could visit the polls on April 14. A total of 651 438 special votes were cast during the 2004 general election (see table 4.5).

Table 4.5 Special votes cast in 2004			
	Total number of special votes	Special votes / registered (%)	Special votes / actual votes (%)
Western Cape	26 976	1.2	1.7
Eastern Cape	103 046	3.6	4.5
Northern Cape	15 544	3.6	4.7
Free State	49 526	3.7	4.8
KwaZulu-Natal	59 471	1.6	2.1
North West	103 302	5.9	7.6
Gauteng	130 835	2.8	3.7
Mpumalanga	76 293	5.3	6.6
Limpopo	80 278	3.7	4.6
National	651 438	3.2	4.1
Source: Independent Electoral Commission 2004.			

The IEC has not researched the reasons given by applicants for asking for a special vote.[38] The special vote does not seem to have been widely used in the provinces with higher estimates of HIV infection or increased projections of AIDS-related illnesses. The special vote was expensive and abused by some who did not qualify for such a privilege. Problems regarding maintaining the secrecy of the ballot and ensuring that no pressure was placed on voters were also encountered. Political parties frequently disputed special votes, due to such concerns.[39]

The existence of the special vote and its delivery to more than 650 000 voters in the last election show the commitment of the South African authorities to making voting as inclusive as possible.

Hendrickse argued: "There is thus a growing awareness that the IEC needs to factor in the various impacts of the epidemic into its strategic planning for how to best fulfil its mandate in future elections."[40] Such awareness seems not to have materialised in strategic planning about how IEC policies, budgets, training and research require adjusting.

4.4 Conclusion

Though HIV/AIDS will definitely affect the administration of elections in South Africa, determining the exact nature of, and finding ways to mitigate, this impact is more difficult. Unless the IEC commits itself to addressing the internal and external impact of HIV/AIDS, little progress will be made: The IEC must ensure that as many as possible can vote through deliberate campaigns to draw marginalised persons into the public arena and raise awareness on stigma and discrimination.

5. Impact on parties, policy proposals

5.1 Introduction

During the election process, politicians ask for the mandate to represent constituencies on the basis of certain policies, and the voter decides which candidate or party to entrust with their vote after carefully considering the alternatives, with the exchange sometimes comprising direct one–on–one communication between the elite and grassroots.

Arguably the most striking feature of the 2004 election campaign was how President Mbeki re-connected with ordinary people during his electioneering walk-abouts. Had one of those journeys taken him to a township AIDS clinic he would most certainly have been able to skilfully deflect any criticism by pointing to the international praise his government's overall policy programme on HIV and AIDS has received. Had anyone questioned his leadership he would have cited the many thousands of AIDS sufferers who will receive treatment through the government's ambitious roll-out plan. Every question would have had an answer, every demand would have been promised a supply. This is democracy in electioneering mode.

Our point here is not to single out President Mbeki in this regard; no other politician would have acted differently. The imagined encounter at the township AIDS clinic is rather meant to highlight what happened when the issue of HIV/AIDS was simplified and given a party-political "spin", often denying voters a reasonably informed and relevant basis for judging the parties' different proposals on how to address the epidemic. That a nationwide public debate on HIV/AIDS did not occur is largely due to the deep distrust existing between parties and party leaders on the HIV/AIDS issue resulting from the various policies and institutional arrangements set in place by the government since 1994.

5.2 Developing policies and institutions

The more critical junctures in this process[41] started with the ANC and pre-transition National Party government's DoH jointly convening a conference in 1992, which was attended by several actors from the health sector, academic institutions and civil society. The conference entailed mobilising a political response to HIV/AIDS and adopting a humanitarian and human rights-based approach to PLWHAs. The conference resulted in the setting up of the National AIDS Committee of South Africa (Nacosa), an umbrella organisation tasked with coordinating responses from the state and civil society. However, after publishing an "AIDS Plan", which was well received by stakeholders, the momentum was lost in the political turmoil of the time: "[Whatever] the reason," notes Nattrass (2004: 43), "it is clear that the transitional period of the early 1990s was not a conducive environment for addressing AIDS and contributed to the rapid spread of HIV".

When the ANC-led government of national unity (GNU) took office after the 1994 elections, it based its policy on the Nacosa plan, though further development and effective implementation of the plan was delayed. A severe shortage of skilled personnel in provincial level government and administration left available funding unused, and the positioning of HIV/AIDS policy within the DoH meant that the epidemic was regarded merely as a medical problem.

The financial mismanagement and controversial content of the musical Sarafina II undermined HIV/AIDS-directed efforts. Political support was given to Virodene, a product developed by South African researchers that was said to provide the cure against AIDS. For the politicians, Virodene seemed to provide a quick-fix solution to the epidemic. Both cases represented government efforts to bypass central principles and institutional checks, in the party as well as in the state, aimed at ensuring good governance. As well as the associated government loss of credibility, such scandals also severely disrupted efforts to counter HIV/AIDS within civil society.

Calling on South Africans to take personal responsibility to remain uninfected, then Deputy President Thabo Mbeki (cited in Shisana and Zungu-Dirwayi, 2003: 173) said in 1998:

> For many years, we have allowed the HIV virus [sic] to spread ... [and now] we face the danger that half of our youth will not reach adulthood. Their education will be wasted. The economy will shrink. There will be a large number of sick people whom the healthy will not be able to maintain. Our dreams as a people will be shattered.

However, in 1999, the government vowed that HIV did not cause AIDS and that antiretroviral treatment, consequently, was both ineffective and harmful. President Mbeki defended this position in a letter (cited in Shisana and Zungu-Dirwayi, 2003: 182-183) addressed to international political leaders and organisations in April 2000:

> We are now being asked to do precisely the same thing that the racist apartheid tyranny we opposed did, because, it is said, there exists a scientific view that is supported by the majority, against which dissent is prohibited. ... The day may not be far off when we will, once again, see books burnt and their authors immolated by fire by those who believe that they have a duty to conduct a holy crusade against the infidels.

In direct opposition to the stance taken by the national government, the two provincial non-ANC governments, run by the Democratic Alliance (DA) in the Western Cape and the IFP in KwaZulu-Natal, both announced their intention to start providing free antiretroviral treatment to pregnant women to prevent their children from being infected at birth. Such initiatives also had political ramifications within the ANC. Though the ANC, as such, did not run the Western Cape provincial government at the time, two of the ANC's most senior political figureheads in the province responsible for developing and implementing ANC health policy, were deeply involved in initiating and running the treatment initiative, for which they received much criticism from certain ANC leaders.[42]

Launched in 1998 to campaign for free antiretroviral treatment through the public health care system, the Treatment Action Campaign (TAC) laid a charge against the government with the Constitutional Court, arguing that the government failed to live up to its constitutional commitments by not providing treatment. Its greatest victory against the government came when the Court ordered the government to start providing Nevirapine to pregnant women to reduce the risk of MTCT at birth. The implementation of the order was still not fully realised when, in July 2004, the government stated it would no longer recommend Nevirapine as a single-therapy medication.

In January 2000 the South African government launched its institutional initiative to focus and coordinate interventions against the epidemic. On the one hand, the South African National AIDS Council (Sanac) showed government commitment to fighting the epidemic by addressing it as a comprehensive developmental problem beyond the scope of the health ministry, and by making the Deputy President its chair. However, on the other hand, it soon became obvious that the council would not engineer effective political intervention against the epidemic, as had been intended. Later evaluations of Sanac found it unrepresentative, inefficient and lacking in transparency and accountability (Strode and Barrett Grant, 2004),

In early 2000, President Mbeki announced the creation of an advisory panel of 33 controversial international AIDS experts, which was briefed with identifying the cause of AIDS. While the mainstream researchers argued that the evidence was already clear, the dissident researchers rejected such claims (Schoofs, 2000). The work of the panel culminated, in April 2001, in the presentation of a report that contained two separate and contradictory lists of recommendations, one from each group of researchers. In responding to the report, Health Minister Tshabalala-Msimang said that the government's approach would remain "rooted in the premise that HIV causes AIDS" (cited in Van der Vliet, 2004: 62). The panel appeared to be a waste of time and resources, causing widespread confusion, which undermined much of the HIV/AIDS awareness that had been generated by grassroots activists and non-governmental organisations (NGOs).

Details of the comprehensive overall policy framework, on which the government had been working since July 1999, were presented in the policy document, *HIV/AIDS & STD: Strategic Plan for South Africa 2000–2005*, launched in early 2000. Much praised by many world leaders for being one of the best in the developing world, not only did the framework elevate the fight against HIV/AIDS institutionally in government and state structures through Sanac, but it also included civil society in a partnership aimed at pooling resources in the fight against HIV/AIDS. However, the human resources and skills in the public health care system were inadequate. The government, despite having positioned its overall policy within the paradigm of mainstream research, continuously undermined its own efforts (Van der Vliet, 2004).

In November 2003 the government declared that it would launch a large-scale rollout of free antiretroviral treatment through the public health care system, despite previously having declared that such an ambitious programme would be too expensive or unwieldy. The government explained its shift in policy had been made possible by a sharp drop in the price of medication and the adoption of a phasing-in approach to the treatment, where capacity existed. Though the government had set itself to deliver treatment to 53 000 people by March 2004, by October of that year only about 11 200 South Africans were receiving such treatment.[43] The delays and the way in which the treatment programme was announced fuelled distrust of the government's intentions from some of its parliamentary critics.

5.3 Political parties on HIV/AIDS and elections

5.3.1 Integrity of elections

The integrity and legitimacy of elections might be undermined if the epidemic reduces the capacity of the electoral commission and the accuracy of the voters' roll. With the dominance of the ANC, the effect of HIV/AIDS was negligible on the 2004 election outcome. Almost unanimously, the IEC was though to have mobilised all necessary staff and that the voters' roll was as accurate as it possibly could have been.

The IFP's Rabinowitz criticised the IEC for failing to ensure enough fully equipped and that staffed voting stations had been in place to guarantee people the chance of voting in more distant rural areas. The IFP also noted that the "special vote" was not effectively employed in KwaZulu-Natal.[44] The ANC's Saadiq Kariem also spoke of the many hospitalised voters who had not been properly told about the special vote: "It did not work well in hospitals. It could have been much better."[45] The special vote, argued Kariem, is necessary to protect the right to vote of those who are ill, but many more resources and efforts are needed to realise its potential.

5.3.2 Party capacity to campaign

Political parties rely heavily on their many supporters around the time of elections. The level of mass support for a Party does not matter in the least if it does not transfer into the active casting of votes for the party on the day of elections. But the other instance when a strong and well-mobilised support base is necessary is when launching and sustenance of an effective election campaign. Such an ability largely hinges on the strong and active mobilisation of party cadres, including those in the many local branches, their reduced capacity to work in the campaign resulting from the impact of AIDS will aggregate into a weakening the campaign overall.

The IFP spoke of an increased need to replace party cadres due to AIDS-related illnesses or death. While the need to replace some party cadres, due to AIDS-related illnesses or death, constrained the ability of party structures to campaign, the regular processes for such replacements were still functioning on the whole. The party did not experience any "gaps" in its organisational structures. The loss of seniority and experience only somewhat reduced the party's capacity (interview, Rabinowitz).[46]

The ANC spoke in the same vein about the negative impact on the party of the loss of unique individuals: 'we have lost quite a lot of corporate and intellectual memory of the organisation, of its functioning and policies, to AIDS' (interview, Kariem). A more indirect effect of AIDS on party capacity in the campaign was reported by the ACDP. As a party explicitly based on Christian principles, the ACDP has many pastors in leadership positions throughout its national and provincial structures, who were unable to participate in many regular Saturday election rallies, as they were called on to officiate over an unprecedented number of funerals in their respective congregations.[47] However, such an effect on party capacity will be reduced as antiretroviral treatment becomes more readily available. Not all local-level representatives and party workers have the full access to comprehensive medical schemes that party leaders and representatives at national and provincial levels do. For the ANC, however, this had not merely been an issue of internal capacity. Saadiq Kariem, in an interview, stated that "quite a number of parliamentarians are [HIV] positive and are on treatment," saying that all the medical schemes that the ANC offers its employees provide full coverage antiretroviral treatment:

> I think that's also why so many of the grassroots, the ordinary membership, felt

so strongly about anti-retrovirals because if treatment was good for some in the organisation, obviously that same policy has to be good for everybody else. That is why there was so much anger at the dithering of everybody on the policy issue.

While no party reported that the epidemic had prevented it from campaigning effectively, such effects are beginning to be felt by some. The strength of negative impact on a party largely depends on the extent of its support in the population, as well as on whether its main constituency overlaps with the groups in the population that are particularly affected by the epidemic. The effect can partially be reduced by the practices that the party has institutionalised in response to the epidemic.

5.3.3 Party practice

In the community-oriented political party culture originating in Western Europe, political parties form an integral part of the web of political associations that continually inform, shape and help formulate people's social and political priorities, identities and interactions. The close ties between Social Democratic parties and trade unions, and between Christian Democratic parties and religious congregations, are perhaps the clearest examples of how such parties are woven into the social fabric of communities. According to such an interpretation, political parties should be "schools of democracy" with internal structures, practices and values mirroring those it would like to see throughout society.

As a "school of democracy", a political party would be expected to reflect the caring community that it wishes to create for the whole of society as a means of combating the epidemic. As such, the party would provide or facilitate access to counselling and treatment and its leaders would actively seek to break down stigma through various public initiatives that challenge the prejudices around the epidemic. The credibility of the party's promised HIV/AIDS policies for the nation would be undermined if the party did not have a track record of living by those policies on a small scale within its own "party-community".

South African political parties all are, or seek to become, community-oriented, with some, very ambitiously, wishing to permeate civil society. A party that seeks to be a "school of democracy" needs to implement democratic governance on HIV/AIDS within its own structures to be a fully credible political force for a progressive and comprehensive political response to the epidemic.

Most parties have not identified a process whereby members can get support when learning that they are HIV-positive. Party colleagues experiencing an HIV-related crisis are given support on an *ad hoc* basis, with the nature of the support partly depending on the seniority and/or well-connectedness of the party colleague. No spokesperson on HIV/AIDS for their respective parties was identified by their party as the person to whom party members should turn with personal concerns relating to the epidemic.

Apart from the ID, no party leadership had spearheaded a campaign for members to take an HIV test by publicly taking one themselves. Cheryllyn Dudley (ACDP) had done a test in the morning of our interview and spoke of how doing so had opened her eyes to the stigma that is attached to the test itself. She, as well as the DA's Mike Waters, said they naturally included their various personal experiences and reflections upon taking the test in their respective campaign speeches, thus personalising the issue with the intention of breaking down prejudiced perceptions of the test. The NNP's Kobus Gous said he too would do the same when he was convinced it served an actual purpose and was not only a form of political rhetoric. Saadiq Kariem of the ANC elaborated on the fact that the positions held by party leadership about taking the test and the epidemic more generally did not accurately represent the party:

> I get approached regularly by ordinary party members, and some Parliament members who are HIV-positive and need treatment or some form of advice. I think there is a lot more acceptance among rank and file, and there is a lot more awareness and openness. It is unfortunate that some of the leaders have come out so strongly publicly by saying that they are not aware of people with HIV/AIDS. But among the rank and file there is a lot more acceptance. The perception that the public get by statements that the leadership make are actually different from what is happening among rank and file membership.[48]

It is not our intention here to pass moral judgement in any way on any individual, be it a political leader or not, for what she decides in terms of publicly announcing an HIV test. There are, naturally, immensely highly personal considerations have to be respected in whether an individual publicly announces an HIV test.

Our comment though is that the epidemic places new demands of a more personal nature on a person who wants to be a constructive role-model in the fight against the epidemic by her very own actions – political leadership in the context of the epidemic is as difficult as that!

The resignation from the government of the leader of the IFP, Mangosuthu Buthelezi, after the April 2004 election seems to have enabled him to be more outspoken and critical on the issue of HIV/AIDS. While he has tried to raise awareness about the epidemic in his KwaZulu-Natal constituency for a number of years,[49] the decision to speak critically on the national scene was triggered by the tragic loss of two of his children to AIDS-related illnesses shortly after the April elections. The mere public recognition by Buthelezi of the true cause of death of his children was important as it seems to have been the first time that a South African politician of that stature personalised the effects of the epidemic so dramatically.

Though no doubt the most painful, these deaths in his family were not the first time Dr Buthelezi came into direct contact with AIDS. In a thinly veiled criticism of President Mbeki's statement that he knows of no one who has died from AIDS, the IFP's Ruth Rabinowitz said: "Buthelezi knows many HIV-positive people and many who have died from AIDS."[50] The dual leadership mandate held by Buthelezi – as the leader of a "modern" political party and as a traditional leader of Zulu loyalists – places a special responsibility on him to address the hardships of his community in a personal capacity. Even more important and impressive, Buthelezi's leadership profile on HIV/AIDS seems to have been translated into the adoption of an institutionalised programme in his party.

In mid-October 2004 the DA adopted a proposal by its spokesperson on health, MP Ryan Coetzee,[51] which has the potential to address the shortcomings in the DA's internal response to the epidemic. The policy, *Leading by example – a DA HIV/AIDS campaign*, sets out what "strong leadership" should mean for the DA in the context of the epidemic. The proposal holds that every DA representative must show stronger leadership by leading by example, not only talking openly about the epidemic, but also by publicly undergoing testing for HIV. On 12 November 2004, the media reported how most of the DA's national leadership had undergone such testing as part of the party's HIV/AIDS awareness campaign.

The ID, like the IFP, stands out as one of the parties that has done the most work on how to build a party, that in itself – in its structures, policies and internal party culture – seeks to address the epidemic in various ways. Unlike other parliamentary parties, the ID did not have to incrementally adjust its policies in strengthening its established constituency to face the worsening epidemic. Unlike other parties, for whom the resulting policies are sustainable compromises between competing moral and human right-based paradigms, as well as between contending representatives for alternative budget posts, the ID could formulate its policies and decide on strategies afresh. Though ID members and leaders have debated, and sometimes differed on, policies and strategies,[52] it has been less concerned with doing so than have other parties.

Before the November 2004 DA initiative, the leader of the ID, Patricia de Lille, was the only party leader to have openly said that she had taken an HIV test, though her example was later followed by the ID's nine provincial leaders. The party has also decided to nominate at least one openly HIV-positive member for a parliamentary seat. Well aware of the risks of such a person becoming merely a "token" for the issue, Greyling spoke about the need for the individual to be a strong member of the party with all the right qualifications for taking a parliamentary seat, over and above being able to speak out on HIV/AIDS from a immediate personal standpoint. At the time seats won in the 2004 elections were distributed to members on the party list, one of the candidates was so qualified. However, on medical advice, the member did not take up the seat, due to the stress that would have been imposed by the workload attached.[53]

Partly due to the different initiatives to provide leadership and representation in addressing the epidemic, members speak openly and without fear of stigma within the party about how the epidemic is affecting their lives. However, the party has not institutionalised a channel of support to ensure privacy when this is preferred by a party member. Nominations to parliamentary seats should, at least in part, receive the necessary backup, both from the party and from Parliament itself. While other infected MPs might be able to hide their potential problems in fulfilling all aspects of the workload behind various explanations, any such deficiency in an openly positive MP is likely to be blamed on the individual's HIV status. For a person to function effectively as an MP despite being openly HIV-positive, Parliament should recognise the infection as a disability, allowing the MP whatever she needs to enable her to function effectively throughout the various stages of her disease.

The previous Secretary of Parliament, S. Mfenyana, stated that Parliament lacks knowledge of the HIV status of MPs. However, if an MP decided to disclose his/her HIV-positive status, Parliament would provide professional counselling and advice on medical matters. As Parliament does not provide MPs with their own medical aid scheme, MPs are required to choose the scheme that best suits their needs. Mfenyana continues:

> Parliament's Human Resources Section is currently drafting a policy on HIV and AIDS in the workplace. The Policy will address issues of labour relations and conditions of service with regard to employees affected by HIV and AIDS, infected with HIV and/or suffering from AIDS-related diseases.[54]

Though Parliament is addressing the implications of the epidemic for its employed staff, it is not yet considering what institutional and other arrangements are necessary to enable HIV-positive MPs to work effectively in the political legislature after publicly announcing their HIV status.

5.3.4 Policy proposals

Much pre-election news commentary on the various parties' policy proposals in the election campaign noted their many similarities on most issues, including HIV/AIDS in particular. All parties suggested a combination of political interventions to prevent further infections, to treat PLWHAs and ensure that they are not discriminated against, and to care for those affected by the epidemic, especially orphans. Though the parties balance the different interventions somewhat differently in their overall response, what the parties offered the voters differed widely. The political representatives interviewed for this study concur with this observation. "The difficulty I had in pre-election debates where I was pitted against a DA person," says the ANC's Saadiq Kariem, "was that we were saying the same things".[55] The NNP's Kobus Gous agreed: "Parties are in agreement on 95% on what should be the political response to the epidemic, so it should disappear as a political issue. It should – but it will not."[56]

The inescapable reality of its presence is why political parties should focus their campaigning on the remaining 5% of policy differences to see whether so doing this could win them additional votes. Despite the many similarities in the policies of different parties, principles differ widely. The dis-

cussion is based on the main election manifestos and any other party-generated material aimed at telling the public, as part of the election campaign, about their HIV/AIDS-related policies, as well as on interviews conducted with party representatives.[57]

Analysing the various parties' policy positions on HIV/AIDS along two dimensions can be done on the level of principle: the first dimension is whether the political response should be based within a human rights approach, while the second is whether the political response should be directed at the infected individual or the affected community. The four different possible policy options that this analytical scheme generates are presented in table 5.1 with an interpretation of how the different parties should be placed along the two dimensions.[58]

Table 5.1: Two dimensions to HIV/AIDS policy		
Focus of policy	Human rights approach focus of policy	
Individual	Yes	No
	ANC, DA, ID	NNP
Community	IFP	ACDP

To take a human rights approach to HIV/AIDS is to argue that the political intervention against the epidemic should be based on a commitment to the respect for, and the realisation of human rights, regardless of public sentimentality or political expediency (Heywood, 2000). The South African Constitution provides unusually strong support for the relevance of wide-ranging human rights, as well as making socioeconomic rights legally binding on the state. The ANC, DA, ID and IFP are clear in their commitments to these rights, though the latter is focused more on the community than on the individual, seeking to create caring communities in which individuals who are known to be HIV-positive are cared for and respected. The human rights approach to dealing with the epidemic must shift from focusing on the individual's right to privacy and integrity to her right to non-discrimination from the community.[59]

The ACDP strongly opposes the human rights approach, arguing for a political intervention based on its understanding of Christian values. Cheryllyn Dudley of the ACDP criticised the ANC for treating HIV/AIDS:

> ...purely as a human rights issue and not as a contagious disease. Our understanding is that if it is going to be contained

and dealt with it is going to have to be treated as a contagious disease. We can't just wish it away. With the best will in the world, lighting candles and wearing ribbons until we are blue in the face will just not do it.[60]

Accordingly, the ACDP proposes making HIV testing compulsory and HIV infection notifiable, with the human rights of the individual not being allowed to obstruct effective political interventions to combat the epidemic.

The NNP's Kobus Gous agrees that the human rights approach is problematic:

By emphasising the HR approach to the epidemic, we have emphasised the stigma that we inherited from Western Europe and the US, where it was primarily a homosexual disease. In Africa, where the epidemic is not linked to homosexuality, we are perpetuating this "homosexual agenda" by elevating the disease as a human rights issue; whereas, if you treat it as simply another disease the stigma would have disappeared by now, as it did in relation to TB and other diseases. We are actually perpetuating the stigma by emphasising the HR aspects of the epidemic. Such rights are guaranteed anyway on an individual basis, so why make such an issue out of it?[61]

The NNP argues that making HIV or AIDS notifiable would be ineffective and counterproductive.[62] Whereas the NNP argues pragmatically that the human rights agenda "perpetuates the stigma", the ACDP's objection to such an agenda is based on the party's moral convictions. Its election manifesto states that inappropriately explicit sex education for children, coupled with the availability of contraceptives, represents "moral degeneration" in South Africa, which has already direct affected the epidemic. The party programme argues that "the unprecedented moral degeneration in the country over the past ten years of democracy has resulted in dysfunctional families, widespread crime and corruption and the spread of the HIV/AIDS pandemic" (ACDP, 2004). The proposed link between homosexuality and the human rights approach was elaborated on in Dudley's criticism of the DA's policies for being even more problematic in their human rights approach:

They [the DA] are "big talk" now about various issues, but when it comes down to it, nothing will get done because of their "super-liberal" policies. ... For a

long time we have realised that the DA are strongly motivated in terms of the gay agenda.[63]

The ACDP's policy argues that, to effectively combat the epidemic, political intervention is needed that infringes on individual right to privacy, integrity and sexual preference, for the sake of those in the community who are, as yet, uninfected by the disease. Such policies would reinvigorate the ACDP's moralistic stance.

The parties, therefore, can be seen to offer the same policy proposals, with only the details differing. The human rights dimension created a particularly clear dividing line between some of the parties. Parties embracing the same principles still had many grounds for disagreement and mistrust.

5.3.5 HIV/AIDS as a 2004 campaign issue

When HIV/AIDS becomes an electioneering issue, particularly in the context of a developing country in the grip of the epidemic, the democratic system becomes vulnerable to the populism of political entrepreneurs, who promise quick and simple solutions to complex problems. The alternative would be to form a "policy accord" between all or the largest parties contesting the elections; Botswana and Tanzania are good examples of countries where the parliamentary parties have institutionalised a common response to the epidemic.[64] Such a strategy would reduce the risk of populism taking hold, thereby ensuring some stability and long-term vision on the agreed upon political intervention against the epidemic. All party representatives interviewed for this study argued that ideally they would have preferred not to campaign on HIV/AIDS, but wished instead that all parties had agreed to a comprehensive policy accord certain to be effective against the epidemic. However, such an agreement would only be sound and constructive if the policy on which the parties agreed was strong enough to have a realistic chance of tackling the epidemic. The ACDP's Dudley elaborated on the importance of politicising the issue in the election campaign:

The government's u-turn would not have happened without pressure from opposition parties, but civil society lobby groups, such as the TAC, as well as the court cases, must also get credit; all of this has been continuing for some time. However, nothing will work like the election time. It would, therefore, have been cruel and wicked for us to have negotiated to keep it off the election agenda, leaving people behind, instead of pressuring government to do the right thing.[65]

By removing the issue from the election campaign, the parties would have made it much more difficult for the voters to hold the parties accountable for poorly devised or ineffectively implemented policy interventions. If the ANC had not changed its policy in November 2003 to launch a treatment rollout, the party would have been vulnerable to critique on this point in the campaign (Willan, 2004). The change in policy, and the timing of that change, can be explained by the success of ANC election strategists in convincing the party leadership that such change would be necessary to stop a haemorrhaging of party support at the polls. The argument was made most strongly by Dudley:

> I think in this last year they have realised the seriously negative impact that their behaviour has had and so the rollout has been held back purposely to be a gift from 'ANC-God' at this hour, and because it is such a life and death thing that is so close to people's hearts I really think that they may well have succeeded with that strategy It is sad.[66]

Mike Waters of the DA agreed that the issue was no longer as clear-cut as before November 2003, but argued that, since announcing the turnaround, the ANC had aroused doubt about its commitment to the programme:

> The first promise was that at end of March, 53 000 would be on ARV treatment. They announced in Parliament yesterday [25 February] that this is not going to happen, and they were not prepared to give a date for when it is going to happen. Now, if they are prepared to break their first promise on the eve of a general election, I shudder to think what they are going to do after the election, because they have got nothing to lose after that.[67]

The opposition strategy was therefore to question the ANC's and especially the Minister of Health's (and thereby implicitly the President's) commitment to the rollout.

The ANC's Kariem agreed that HIV/AIDS was problematic for the ANC in the election, as it was an issue on which the opposition could score points: "if anything the epidemic enhanced their ability to campaign because it was our Achilles heel ... our soft

spot."[68] Such a rallying point became even clearer to the party leadership, after a survey among ANC members was conducted in early 2003, during which ANC's policy on treatment was challenged.[69] He strongly opposed the interpretation, however, that the policy u-turn in November was based on anything less than a full commitment from the ANC, or that it had been timed strategically for maximum effect in the election campaign. While the ANC's internal policy survey would have provided important information that would have been useful for strategic purposes, he argued that:

> the policy u-turn, if you want to call it that, was more a result of sustained internal pressure over a long time. If the survey hadn't happened [the ANC] would still have gone down the same route. If anything, the survey would have added support to what we had been saying for the last four years. It's been a long battle.[70]

The "we" in the quote above refers to those members of the ANC National Health Committee who, since 1999, had been advising the ANC political leadership to strengthen and mainstream its approach to the epidemic. "The policy change in November 2003 on ARVs," continued Kariem, "came about as a result of sustained pressure from 1999 to change the mindset, which took several years to get to the point where politically we can now say that we have turned the corner." Kariem's insider analysis facilitates understanding recent developments and shifts in ANC policy on this issue, as he offers insights into the political dynamics that are internal to the ANC, a dynamic that comments by opposition representatives fail to include in the analysis. Though Kariem's analysis suggests a relatively complex process of policy-making and multidimensional reasons for policy change, he agrees with government critics that it took "sustained pressure" to change the minds of the ANC's top political leadership on HIV/AIDS.

5.4 Conclusion

Our analysis of the way in which the HIV/AIDS epidemic has impacted on the parliamentary parties in South Africa has presented a basic normative position that, to some degree, applies to all parties to lead by example within their own party-community if they want to ensure democratic governance on HIV/AIDS for the whole country. Most parties fell far short of what can be expected in this regard, though the IFP and the ID has already provided such leadership and the DA is planning to do the same. Interparty distrust hampers unifying the parliamentary parties in their approach to the epidemic. Competitive democratic elections are likely to encourage improving the political response to the epidemic.

6. Political opinion and participation

The Afrobarometer surveys of South Africans' political opinions and degree of political activism permit comparison of countries in sub-Saharan Africa and beyond. The survey data gleaned for this study enables investigation of how people prioritise epidemic-related issues and exploration of why some feel that they are key. How the epidemic affects people's ability to participate in political activities in civil society will also be examined.

6.1 Opinion and HIV/AIDS

The first round of the Afrobarometer survey, which contained a few questions that explored people's

HIV/AIDS-related opinions and experiences, was conducted in nine countries in southern Africa during the course of 1999 and 2000. Whiteside *et al* report that the attitudinal data from the survey corroborates the epidemiological data; both sources of information indicate that many in South and southern Africa are so ill that they are dying in increasing numbers. However, a surprising pattern emerges when they probe how people's political priorities relate to the epidemic:

> [Even] where HIV/AIDS has reached severe levels and people are dying in large and rising numbers, and even where people recognise those deaths as the result of HIV infection, very few of them place HIV/AIDS high on the agenda for government intervention. Rather, the epidemic is superseded in most countries by demands for government action to create jobs, expand the economy, and improve crime and security, or is masked by demands for overall improvements in health-related services (Whiteside et al., 2002: 26).

The authors conclude that this might indeed be a rational response, since the health of most in the region is threatened by poverty, which is more direct

Table 6.1: Opinions and experiences of the epidemic in sub-Saharan Africa

	AIDS most important problem[A]		Prioritisation of AIDS[B]	Personal loss from AIDS[C]		Adult HIV prevalence[D]
	2002–03	1999–2000	2002–03	2002–03	1999–2000	End of 2003
Botswana	30	24	47	36	32	37.3
Cape Verde	2	–	53	12	–	–
Ghana	3	–	35	19	–	3.1
Kenya	10	–	36	66	–	6.7
Lesotho	5	0.5	57	18	11	28.9
Malawi	3	2	47	57	65	14.2
Mali	1	0	46	17	12	1.9
Mozambique	16	–	53	27	–	12.2
Namibia	28	14	35	71	40	21.3
Nigeria	4	–	44	11	–	5.4
Senegal	1	–	44	14	–	0.8
South Africa	26	13	40	18	16	21.5
Tanzania	14	0.5	47	61	60	8.8
Uganda	7	0.5	52	85	–	4.1
Zambia	3	0	33	74	65	16.5

A) Percentage of people who regard AIDS to be the most serious problem facing their country. B) Percentage of people who think the government should spend more resources on AIDS, even at the expense of other development issues. C) Percentage of people who have lost at least one friend or relative to AIDS. Source: A–C) Mattes,[71] 2004. D) UNAIDS, 2004.

Table 6.2: Political opinions of those affected by personal loss

	Disapprove of President's job performance in last 12 months		Do not feel close to any political party		Would not vote in election tomorrow	
	No loss (%)	Loss (%)	No loss (%)	Loss (%)	No loss (%)	Loss (%)
All South Africans	42.1	39.8	36.1	26.1	23.6	18.6
Black	32.3	38.1	24.5	25.2	15.5	18.6
Black male	30.5	31.9	20.5	20.8	10.6	16.7
Black female	34.4	43.1	29.8	28.6	22.0	20.3
Black urban	35.2	41.3	25.1	25.4	14.7	18.2
Black rural	29.5	34.5	23.9	24.5	16.3	19.1

Source: Afrobarometer survey, South Africa, 2002. The numbers indicate percentages of people who disapprove of President Mbeki's job performance over the last twelve months; who do not feel close to any political party; and who would not vote in the next election. A difference in percentage is noted as "substantial" only if it exceeds the survey's 2.1% margin of error.

and visible than is the threat of HIV infection, or even illness and death from AIDS.

A second round of the Afrobarometer survey was conducted in 15 countries in the subcontinent during 2002 and 2003. Table 6.1 shows the percentages of people who thought AIDS was the most important problem facing their government; who thought the government should prioritise the fight against the epidemic, even at the expense of other development-related issues, such as education; and who had experienced personal loss in having had a close friend or family member die from an AIDS-related illness.

With a few exceptions, the epidemic was found to be experienced as a problem by larger sections of the populations than two or three years before. In some instances, the increase in public awareness was found to be considerable: twice as many South Africans and Namibians considered it as the most important problem, with the percentage of those who admitted having experienced an AIDS-related personal loss, apart from Malawians, increasing by about 70%.[72] Few other consistent patterns exist between these and other more political variables across southern Africa.

6.1.1 Political opinion on the epidemic

What people profess to think of the government's performance on the issue of HIV/AIDS, and whether they would like the government to prioritise spending resources on fighting HIV/AIDS, even if this implies less money for education and other development-oriented political goals, can potentially have many different explanations, which are in themselves linked to the epidemic. The only probable explanation, however, was that people had suffered the loss of a family member or a close friend to the epidemic, an experience that had a stronger correlation to the second question than to the first (*Pearson's r* = .195 at .01 level of significance). When the data was broken down according to race groups, gender and urban or rural setting, some correlations were even stronger.[73] However, to assess the strength of these correlations even further, a test was undertaken to see whether they would remain as strong and significant even after controlling for a person's level of education and household income, which required checking that the statistical pattern observed was caused by neither levels of education nor income. The experience of personal loss was a relatively good predictor of a person's opinion on the question, even when the two alternative explanations were taken into account.[74]

Assuming that this prioritisation by people who have suffered personal loss led them to be more critical of the government is contentious. When the same statistical analyses were made on the hypothesis that personal loss explains a person's opinion of whether the government had effectively dealt with the epidemic, the statistical correlations were weaker and less significant across the board. The result seemed to indicate that people's frustration with the government's priorities does not necessarily transform into outright criticism of the government's handling of the epidemic. Advocates for a stronger political response have, therefore, to consider a complex mix of political and personal considerations in mobilising such criticism.

The generation of greater criticism of politics in general, and of the government in particular, by "personal loss" could be perceived in response to the three questions (see table 6.2):

- Do you disapprove of how President Thabo Mbeki

has performed his job over the last 12 months?
- Do you feel close to any particular political party?
- Would you vote if there were elections for national government tomorrow?

The opinions held by those who have, and those who have not, experienced a personal loss to AIDS differ widely only in the five instances indicated, which shows that experiencing personal loss might cause people to be more critical in such instances.

Though the epidemic has begun to shape public opinion, the pattern of opinions is not uniform across all countries surveyed. A person's experience of personal loss is, nevertheless, a moderately strong predictor of a desire for the government to prioritise development resources to fight the epidemic.

Given that the South African epidemic has started to experience a sharp increase in the number of AIDS-related deaths, stronger response to the epidemic is expected from within the ANC's main support base, even at the cost of other development-related policy issues. However, the more direct and, for the government, potentially more difficult effect on people's political criticism of its performance is more limited. The 2002 Afrobarometer survey indicated a link between peoples' opinions on these two questions, in the sense that those who want to prioritise more resources for AIDS are also more likely to be critical of the president's job performance during the previous 12 months (*Pearson's r* = .103 at .01 level of significance). If the immediacy and effectiveness of the political response is seen to not correspond with people's harsh experiences of the epidemic, it might transform into a political issue that can shape electoral outcomes.

6.2 Political participation

Though the epidemic appears to have remobilised civic activism (such as that of TAC) in fighting for social justice in the form of medication against AIDS and the prevention and destigmatisation of HIV, some seem to have been demobilised by the epidemic, either because they have lost hope of an effective political response or because they are too busy with providing home-based care for their own or someone else's AIDS-related illness or AIDS orphans to engage politically. Both these experiences exist, simultaneously shaping society's joint response to the epidemic.

The Afrobarometer survey includes two sets of questions that will be used as proxies for the direct

and indirect effects of the epidemic: one relating to the home-based care that a person provides for orphans, sick family members or own illness, and the other relating to the person's physical and mental health. People were asked whether they provide home-based care for orphans, family or household members, or for their own illness, and, if they did for how many hours a day.[75] To allow for a more generalised and powerful test of the effect on the participation of those who provide home-based care, a scale was created by collapsing the three questions on such care.[76] Table 6.3 details how the levels of such care vary between those countries included in the Afrobarometer surveys, with the numbers representing the mean value for the different countries, though the values can only be roughly translated in actual hours spent. The value .33 signifies that the average person spends less than one hour a day on home-based care, while the highest possible value (4.0) would indicate that a person spends virtually all day providing all three kinds of home-based care. The values between .33 and 4.0 imply either that a person spends much time providing one type of care, or that the time is spent providing two or three different types of care. The numbers should be thought of as relative indicators of the amount of time spent by people each day, with 0.0 meaning no time at all, and 4.0 meaning that the full day is spent on providing home-based care.

Table 6.3: Average amount of daily individual home-based care	
Botswana	1.57
Namibia	0.32
Zambia	1.97
Ghana	1.08
Nigeria	1.43
Cape Verde	1.19
Lesotho	2.02
South Africa	0.83
Kenya	1.22
Malawi	2.43
Tanzania	1.18
Mozambique	1.93
Mali	1.23
Uganda	2.17
Senegal	1.21
Source: Afrobarometer surveys, 2002–03. For interpretation, see the paragraph above.	

The South African mean value is the second lowest, so that the "average" South African seems not to be particularly busy with home-based care. Figure 6.1 indicates how time profiles of home-based care vary. Many (41.3 %) South Africans spend no time at all on home-based care, with a decreasing number of people doing so as the amount of time increases.

Figure 6.1: The time profile of home-based care in selected countries

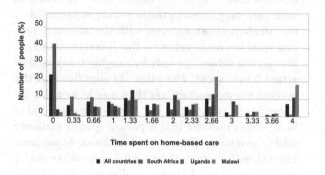

Source: Afrobarometer surveys 2002–03. Calculations by authors.

The relatively low numbers of people who provide home-based care in South Africa can be explained by a better than average health care system and an epidemic that, in 2002, had only recently entered the phase when increasing numbers of people needed care due to AIDS-related illnesses. The profiles of vulnerable groups only marginally differed from those for all South Africans (see figure 6.2).

Figure 6.2: The time profile of different groups of South Africans

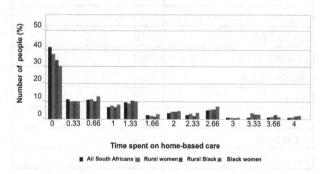

Source: Afrobarometer, South Africa survey, 2002. Calculations by authors.

Correlation analyses tested whether the degree to which a person provided home-based care was linked to the degree of activism in civil society (see table 6.4).[77]

In 2002, a person's responsibility for providing home-based care was found to be a poor predictor of the degree of participation in civil society activism.[78] However, home-based care providers were found to be somewhat more likely to be members of local development organisations and a great deal more likely to attend community meetings, though somewhat less likely to discuss politics with friends. While rural women carry heavy responsibilities, they were found to do so in a context of a relatively strong social capital that enabled them to act collectively to ease their plight.

A related set of hypotheses predicts what home-based care implies for a person's willingness or ability to get the relevant identity document and to register to vote. Either a person's motivation to do so is reduced by having to provide home-based care, or such hardships generate an awareness and mobilise a determination to ensure that as many votes as possible are cast in favour of a political programme that people hope will help them in their harsh situation.[79] A related variable was included to test whether the burdens of home-based care affect people's levels of general satisfaction with the South African democracy.[80]

The results indicated clearly that, in 2002, the responsibility for providing home-based care did not hinder people's ability or willingness to perform critical civic duties. A few significant positive coefficients suggested that those involved with home-based care were more likely to ensure their active participation in the electoral process. The many frustrations and hardships of home-based care also did not generate general dissatisfaction with the South African democracy.

6.3 Conclusion

Though those who have experienced an AIDS-related personal loss would like the government to prioritise its spending to avoid further losses, such sentiment does not translate into criticism of the government or of the president more specifically, nor into a change of choice of political party as a result of their dissatisfaction.

Table 6.4: Membership and activism in civil society and home-based care

	Membership				Activity			
	Religious group	Trade union or farmers' organisation	Profess-ional or business organisa-tion	Comm-unity/ dev-elopment self-help group	Discuss politics with friends	Attend commu-nity meetings	Meet with others to raise an issue	Attend demon-strations or protest marches
All	.075*	.022	-.024	.112**	-.041*	.192**	.121**	.049*
Black	.076**	.028	-.013	.074**	-.091**	.115**	.039	-.022
Black rural	.025	.046	-.015	.086*	-.084*	.116**	.075*	.001
Black women	.048	.027	-.040	.054	-.077*	.115**	.049	.010
Rural women	.008	-.007	-.038	.061	-.061	.198**	.130**	.041

Source: Afrobarometer survey: South Africa, 2002.Correlation coefficients (Pearson's r) between, on the one hand, different forms of membership and activity in civil society, and, on the other, the burden of providing home-based care. * indicates statistical signifi-cance on .05 level, and ** indicates statistical significance on .01 level.

Table 6.5: Effect of home-based care on civic duties and opinions of South Africa's democracy

	Easy to get identity document	Easy to reg-ister to vote	Satisfaction with democracy
All	.071*	.061*	.028
Black	.039	.024	.005
Black rural	.086*	.065	-.027
Black women	.047	.065	-.020
Rural women	.044	.111*	-.070

Source: Afrobarometer survey, South Africa, 2002. Correlation coefficients (Pearson's r) between, on the one hand, two differ-ent civic duties and an opinion about democracy, and, on the other, the burden of providing home-based care. * indicates statistical significance on .05 level, and ** indicates statistical significance on .01 level.

7. Registration levels, voter turnout

7.1 Introduction

The general elections of 2004 experienced a relative-ly low voter turn out considering the increase in the Voting Age Population(VAP). Part of the explanation would be the reluctance of voters to spend limited resources on participating in a collective action that would suffer only very marginally if they abstained.

The question of low participation has occupied academic inquiry for decades. But to simply rely on voter turnout as an indicator of low or high participa-tion could be misleading. Researchers should hence always include the VAP in the analysis to expose the disenfranchisement of an otherwise "invincible" sec-tion of the population (Norris, 2004: 40). Statistics SA, authorised to provide official statistics in South Africa, published its 2004 midyear estimate of the South African population at the end of July, only a few months after the elections. Since the population estimates in the report included residents who were not citizens – and who therefore did not have the vote – the VAP for the 2004 elections was generated by multiplying the numbers by the factor .9851817, which was the percent of residents in South Africa in the 2001 Census who were South African citizens. This calculation was done on the estimates provided by Statistics SA to generate the percentages of elec-toral participation for the different age cohorts and provinces presented in table 7.2.

The provincial figures differed substantially from the national average. Wide differences exist among the youngest voters between the sexes and the prov-inces, with the ratio dropping from 74.2% for the whole electorate, to 69.2% for those between 18 and 49, to a very low 52.1% for first-time voters.

The Statistics SA report details its estimate of the South African population in an "actual" estimate as well as in a "counterfactual" estimate, which

Table 7.1: Voter participation in South Africa's three national elections

Year	Voting age population (VAP)	Registered voters	Total votes	Vote/Reg. (%)	Vote/VAP (%)	Reg/VAP (%)
1994	22 709 152	–	19 533 498	–	86.0	–
1999	22 589 369	18 172 751	16 228 462	89.3	71.8	80.4
2004	27 865 537[A]	20 674 926[B]	15 863 554[B]	76.7	56.9	74.2

Source: Figures from Independent Electoral Commission for the 1994 and 1999 elections, as reported in Reynolds, 1994 and 1999b, respectively. A) Statistics SA (2004) mid-2004 estimates, see endnote for further details. B) Independent Electoral Commission (total votes including spoilt ballot papers).

Table 7.2: Electoral participation across provinces and gender, 2004

	Reg./VAP			Vote/Reg.	Vote/VAP
	Male	Female	Total	Total	Total
Western Cape	70.4	78.8	74.7	71.3	53.2
Eastern Cape	66.9	77.1	72.5	79.3	57.5
Northern Cape	74.3	80.7	77.5	74.7	57.9
Free State	68.8	75.9	72.5	77.8	56.4
KwaZulu-Natal	63.4	73.7	68.9	72.8	50.2
North West	69.6	80.8	75.1	75.6	56.7
Gauteng	73.2	80.3	76.6	74.2	56.9
Mpumalanga	74.4	81.6	78.1	78.3	61.2
Limpopo	65.3	90.4	78.5	74.8	58.7
National	68.9	79.2	74.2	76.7	56.9

Source: Independent Electoral Commission; Statistics SA, 2004.

presents what the population estimate should have been if the HIV/AIDS epidemic had not reduced the population. Given that the age 18 falls within one of the age cohorts, the assumption has had to be made that the estimated numbers within the cohort 15–19 are distributed equally across the five years, with the number being doubled, according to the formula (estimate/5) x 2. Such calculations generate the greatest reduction in VAP within the age cohort 18 to 49 years, which is most severely affected by the epidemic (see table 7.4). The differences in prevalence between the racial groups, as well as between men and women, are reflected in the statistics.

7.2 Formulating, contextualising hypotheses

The following three general hypotheses guide the statistical tests for correlation between electoral and epidemiological data:

- PLWHAs might choose not to participate in elec-

tions if they are frustrated and disillusioned by the weak political response of the formal political system.

- PLWHAs are prevented from participating in elections by the effort that such participation requires.
- Those who provide home-based care for AIDS orphans, or for family or friends who are PLWHAs, or who have to care for their own AIDS-related illness, either choose to not participate for the same reason as in (1) above, or are too busy to do so.

To test these hypotheses, some of the electoral data was compared to the DoH provincial percentages of HIV estimates, and the Actuarial Society of South Africa (ASSA) projections of the provincial percentage of PLWHAs. However, the assumption cannot be made that estimated infection rates are automatically reflected in levels of non-participation. The proxy questions for HIV/AIDS, as well as the precise questions for providing home-based care, also had little, if any, effect on the relative ease of obtaining an identity documents or registering to vote.

Table 7.3: Ratio between registered voters and voting age population, by age cohort, sex and province

| | Registered voters as percent of voting age population for different age cohorts | | | | | | | | |
| | 18 years and older | | | 18–49 years | | | 18–22 years | | |
Province	Male	Female	Total	Male	Female	Total	Male	Female	Total
Western Cape	70.4	78.8	74.7	66.3	74.4	70.4	52.6	59.7	56.2
Eastern Cape	66.9	77.1	72.5	61.1	70.7	66.2	40.2	46.8	43.5
Northern Cape	74.3	80.7	77.5	71.7	77.8	74.7	57.3	62.7	59.9
Free State	68.8	75.9	72.5	65.8	70.9	68.4	48.7	53.9	51.3
KwaZulu-Natal	63.4	73.7	68.9	59.2	67.3	63.4	42.7	48.0	45.3
North West	69.6	80.8	75.1	65.9	75.5	70.5	53.2	59.4	56.2
Gauteng	73.2	80.3	76.6	69.8	76.2	72.8	64.3	66.0	65.2
Mpumalanga	74.4	81.6	78.1	70.8	76.3	73.6	51.9	57.4	54.7
Limpopo	65.3	90.4	78.5	61.0	79.9	70.8	43.3	54.1	48.7
National	68.9	79.2	74.2	64.9	73.4	69.2	49.2	55.0	52.1

Source: Independent Electoral Commission. Calculations by authors.

Table 7.4: Estimated reduction of the voting age population due to AIDS

| Racial group | Gender | 18–29 years | | 18–49 years | | 18 years+ | |
		Estimate	%	Estimate	%	Estimate	%
Black		236 643	2.6	968 057	5.3	1 088 582	4.9
	Male	68 089	1.5	466 325	5.1	552 450	5.1
	Female	168 554	3.7	501 732	5.5	536 132	4.7
Coloured		8 740	1.0	42 795	2.0	48 279	1.8
	Male	2 363	0.5	20 399	2.0	24 232	1.9
	Female	6 377	1.4	22 396	2.1	24 047	1.8
Asian		907	0.4	4 370	0.8	5 213	0.7
	Male	236	0.2	2 068	0.7	2 660	0.7
	Female	671	0.5	2 302	0.8	2 553	0.6
White		6 845	1.0	41 500	2.0	51 947	1.5
	Male	1 634	0.5	19 552	1.9	26 618	1.6
	Female	5 211	1.5	21 948	2.1	25 329	1.5
SA total		181 135	2.3	1 056 723	4.6	1 194 082	4.1
	Male	72 323	1.3	508 344	4.5	606 021	4.3
	Female	180 812	3.3	548 379	4.7	588 061	3.9

Source: Statistics SA, 2004. Numbers calculated by authors. "Estimate" refers to the difference between the estimates in the "no AIDS" and "AIDS" scenarios, which is then given as the percentage of the total of that age cohort.

When the Afrobarometer findings are combined with the HSRC findings, electoral participation does not seem to have been much affected by the epidemic (see table 7.5).

While three of the four hypotheses regarding non-registration by eligible voters were confirmed, the result was somewhat more diverse for the hypotheses about non-voting by registered voters.

Table 7.5: Tests of hypotheses about the impact of HIV/AIDS on participation in 2004 election (N=9)

Observations	Non-registration by eligible voters	Non-voting by registered voters
Hypotheses	(1) Voters who are directly or indirectly affected by HIV/AIDS are disillusioned by the political response to AIDS or exhausted by the burdens they carry withdraw completely from participation, rather than vote for another party. (2) The dynamic of (1) should apply even more to adult women (15–49 years), who have higher prevalence levels than men. (3) In the case of young women, who are known to be particularly affected by the virus, the effect of disillusionment is increased still further. (4) AIDS-sick voters fail to re-register, as they move to live with their extended families to get "home-based" care.	(1) HIV-positive voters are so disillusioned by government policy on HIV/AIDS that they withdraw completely, rather than vote for another party. (2) AIDS-sick voters are too ill to visit a voting station. (3) The special vote was not effective in helping PLWHAs. (4) The voters' roll is inaccurate, due to unrecorded AIDS-related deaths.
Expectations	(1) A positive correlation exists between levels of non-registration and estimates of HIV prevalence. (2) A stronger positive correlation exists than in (1). (3) A considerable positive correlation exists between levels of non- and estimates of HIV prevalence among young women. (4) A positive correlation exists between levels of non-registration and projections of numbers of AIDS-sick.	(1) A positive correlation exists between levels of non-voting and estimates of HIV prevalence. (2) A positive correlation exists between levels of non-voting and projections of the numbers of AIDS-sick. (3) A negative correlation exists between the number of special votes as a percentage of the total vote and projections of the numbers of AIDS-sick. (4) A positive correlation exists between levels of non-voting and projections of numbers of AIDS deaths since the census in 2001 (ie projected numbers of AIDS deaths between 2001 and 2004).
Findings	(1) Confirmed: Pearson's r = .504 (2) Confirmed: Pearson's r = .590 (3) Rejected: Pearson's r = .346 (4) Confirmed: Pearson's r = .344	(1) Rejected for all provinces (Pearson's r = -.370). (2) Rejected for all provinces (Pearson's r = .368). (3) Confirmed, on the exclusion of outlier province WC (Pearson's r = -.142), but rejected on its inclusion (Pearson's r = .248).[81] (4) Rejected for all provinces (Pearson's r = -.267), but confirmed on the exclusion of outlier province WC (Pearson's r = .102).

Source: Electoral data from the IEC; epidemiological data from DoH and ASSA model, as detailed previously. Calculations by authors.

Most of the tests for non-registration were confirmed, indicating some support for the argument that the higher the impact of HIV prevalence in a province, the more likely it is that those of more vulnerable age (18–49 years) will not bother to register to vote, indicating female voter alienation from the democratic process by the women who arguably need it the most. The confirmation of the third hypothesis, albeit not very strongly, in relation to non-voting by registered voters suggests widespread problems with that there is a more general relevance to the complaints about the delivery of the special vote, and that this insufficiency did disenfranchise PLWHAs.

7.3 Conclusion

The analysis in this chapter generated additional information on the VAP in the 2004 South African election. This is not to deny that the numbers we present are ambiguous due to uncertainties about the reliability of the basic demographic data, the 2001 Census. We argued however that the VAP is an important part of any analysis of electoral participation, especially when the focus of the analysis is the risk of systematic non-participation by one or more groups in the population. Tests of the hypotheses to explain variations in participation indicated a link between non-participation and the HIV/AIDS epidemic.

8. Analysing levels, profiles of mortality on voters' roll

8.1 Introduction

Up to this point in our report we have used electoral data from the Independent Electoral Commission (IEC) to detail levels of registration and turn-out in the 2004 election, and we have consulted various estimates of HIV prevalence and projections of AIDS-related mortality to detail the effects of the epidemic. In this chapter we shall attempt to merge electoral and epidemiological data in an analysis of the impact of the HIV/AIDS on the electoral process in South Africa, which merges electoral and epide-

miological data, that is based on a unique set of data provided by the IEC, which shows that the epidemic has so affected the South African electorate that intervention is urgently required.

Rian Malan argued in *The Sunday Times* of 3 October 2004 that AIDS experts exaggerate the devastation brought by the epidemic, expounding his deep mistrust of the experts who generate the estimates. He views such experts, as well as most journalists in the uncritical media, as representing an alarmist AIDS establishment. The data details mortality among the South African electorate, as reflected directly on the South African voters' roll via the population register, with each number representing a deceased person. Our analysis below will show that South African voters are indeed dying in numbers and according to an age profile that, arguably, defies any other explanation than AIDS. While critics are free to question our motivations for presenting this data and challenge our analysis, we expect that all will trust the validity and reliability of the information.[82]

8.2 Data from South African voters' roll

The data reveals:

- The number of registered voters at the end of 1999, 2000, 2001, 2002 and 2003;

- The total number of deceased registered voters for 1999, 2000, 2001, 2002 and 2003, per gender and per age cohort (18–19; 20–29; 30–39: 40–49; 50–59; 60–69; 70–79; 80+);

- The number of registered voters at the end of 1999, 2000, 2001, 2002 and 2003, per gender, per age cohort (as above), per province and per municipality; and

- The total number of deceased registered voters for 1999, 2000, 2001, 2002 and 2003, per gender, per age cohort (as above), per province and per municipality.

This information is highly relevant for a number of analytical purposes. Demographers can use such information to check the validity of the assumptions about mortality that they use in their models for estimation, while political scientists can learn much about how levels of electoral registration vary between ages, genders and municipalities countrywide. If the data is used in combination with other sources of information the number of possible usages is multiplied and only limited by the availability of such information at the relevant level of analysis.

However, the data from the voters' roll cannot be assumed to be representative of all South African residents aged 18 or older. This report analyses the implications of the epidemic for the South African electorate, the part of the population who, at some stage, were registered on the voters' roll.

8.2.1 Research methodology

We realise that the analysis we will present below might be considered controversial and contestable on some grounds. In this section we will therefore try to be very clear and explicit about what factors and circumstances have to be considered when inter-pretation of the data considers:

- As the data contains no information on the caus-es of death, it is impossible to say with certainty how many of the deceased registered voters died from an AIDS-related disease.

- An increase in levels of mortality from one year to another – measured as a ratio between deceased and registered voters in the respective years (see below) – might to some extent be explained by an increased efficiency in the reporting and accounting of deaths by the relevant authorities, primarily the Department of Home Affairs;

- The data does not detail the total level of mortal-ity in South Africa but only the reported deaths of citizens who were registered to vote. Therefore, any analytical inferences made on the basis of the data excludes population groups such as citizens who are below the age of 18, adult citizens who had not registered to vote and non-citizens who reside in South Africa.

While our analysis will consider these caveats, they will not hinder us from making the argument that AIDS is the main cause behind the problematic "mortality profiles", based on the research reviewed briefly later in this chapter.

The absolute numbers in the dataset indicate an abnormal distribution of deaths among regis-tered voters. Absolute numbers refer to the actual number of deaths, as they are recorded by the IEC in the dataset. However, since an increase in absolute numbers might partly be explained by a correspond-ing increase in the number of registered voters, the relative number of deaths, which is the number of deaths as a percentage of the total number of registered voters during a particular year, is most

relevant. Having established the relative number of deaths, the increase in the relative number of deaths between 1999 and 2003 will be worked out, calcu-lated according to the formula:

$$\frac{(\% \text{ deaths } 2003 - \% \text{ deaths } 1999)}{\% \text{ deaths } 1999} = \begin{array}{c} \% \text{ increase in} \\ \text{relative number of} \\ \text{deaths from 1999} \\ \text{to 2003} \end{array}$$

</> deaths imply the relative number of deaths, as explained.

Greater precision is obtained by finding out varia-tions in the dynamic trend of how many voters, of a defined number of registered voters, died.

8.2.2 Research into HIV/AIDS and mortality

Two research publications are particularly relevant as points of comparison for data from the voters' roll. In 2001 Rob Dorrington *et al* published an extensive report – *The Impact of HIV/AIDS on Adult Mortality in South Africa* – that was based on death statistics from the Department of Home Affairs' population register. This information was processed through the ASSA model to generate estimates of AIDS-related mortality among different ages and racial population groups as well as between men and women for South Africa and the nine provinces (Dorrington, 2001). The result that the researchers emphasise is how mortality had increased sharply among young adults, and among young women in particular, peaking at about 30 to 35 years. In his foreword to the report, the then president of the Medical Research Council, Malegepuru Makgoba, also highlighted the fact that:

> the pattern of mortality from natu-ral causes in South Africa has shifted from the old to the young over the last decade particularly for young women – this is a unique phenomenon in biology (Dorrington, 2001: 4).

In a brief update of this analysis, Bradshaw et al (2004) analyses the trends in the actual number of deaths as reported in the population register between 1998 and 2003. The increase in mortality among women is also highlighted in this report:

> In the case of women 20–49 years, there has been an increase of 190% in the deaths registered which corresponds to a real increase in mortality of more than 150% once population growth and possible improvement in registration

are taken into account (Bradshaw *et al.*, 2004: 3).

Bradshaw *et al.* (2004: 4) concludes with:

> The uncertainty about the precise number of AIDS deaths should not allow people to dismiss the impact of HIV/AIDS on mortality. There has been a massive rise in the total number of adult deaths in the last 6 years. Given the ages at which these additional deaths occurred and the change in the cause of death profile, they can largely be attributed to HIV/AIDS.

The analysis of the IEC data shows the same general profiles and tendencies as the data and analyses presented by Dorrington and Bradshaw. The data largely corroborates the findings of South Africa's foremost analysts in the field.

8.3 General trends in the data

This subsection starts by clarifying some national trends in the data that are clear causes for concern as they, arguably, corroborate the hypotheses that AIDS mortality is affecting the level and distribution of mortality among the South African electorate. The analysis is then expanded by clarifying how these trends vary between the different South African provinces and municipalities.

8.3.1 National trends

Between November 1998 and the end of 2003 a total of 1 488 242 – or roughly 1.5 million – voters were removed from the voters' roll due to death. From 1999 to 2003 the absolute number of deaths among the total South African electorate increased by 66% (from 215 583 in 1999 to 358 486 in 2003). The number of deceased voters per year is detailed in figure 8.1 in both absolute and relative numbers.

The graph reveals that voters also died at an increasing rate in relative numbers. However, before we explore the relative numbers further, much important information is still hidden from us as to the absolute numbers of death since we are here looking at an aggregate number for all registered voters. Distinguishing between the eight different age cohorts in figure 8.2 shows that the rate of mortality differs between age cohorts.

Figure 8.2: Number of deceased voters by age group and year

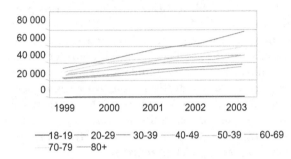

Source: IEC, 2004e. Calculations by authors.

Mortality within the two age cohorts 30 to 39 and 40 to 49-year-olds appears to increase at a higher rate than in the other age cohorts, in line with the general expectation among demographers working on the epidemic that it is within this age span that AIDS mortality becomes most clearly visible. A different way of clarifying the extent to which the increase in mortality is concentrated in some age cohorts more than others entails calculating the percentages of which the different age cohorts contribute to the overall increase in mortality. Figure 8.3 clarifies that the increase in mortality within the age cohort 30 to 39 years accounts for 29% of the total increase in mortality among registered voters.

Figure 8.1: Absolute and relative numbers of deceased voters by year

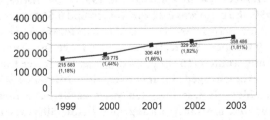

Source: IEC, 2004e. Calculations by authors.

Figure 8.3: Percentage share of increase in mortality by age group, 1999–2003

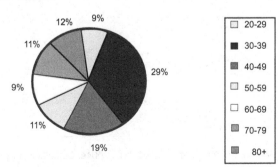

Source: IEC, 2004e. Calculations by authors.

The next distinction we shall explore is that between men and women. We start by presenting the mortality profiles for women and men separately. In figures 8.4 and 8.5 we will compare the absolute numbers of deceased men and women in age cohorts 20 years and older for the years 1999 and 2003. However, each graph also compares these profiles on the basis of two datasets. Data from the voters' roll is here compared with the profiles that Bradshaw *et al* (2004) generated on the basis of the population register, with the numbers of deaths in the data from the population register enabling working out of the numbers of deaths from the graphs. The comparison provides a valuable test as to how the mortality profile of the South African electorate differs from that of the population in general. Since more people are registered in the population register than on the voters' roll, the lines for the population register indicate a higher number of deaths for the two years, respectively, for both women and men. The particularly sharp increase in mortality for some age cohorts in the IEC data is almost identically reflected in the data from the population register.

According to predictions of AIDS mortality, women would be expected to die at a higher rate than men, since they are more vulnerable to the virus. However, the normal demographic "pattern" of mortality for South Africa is that higher numbers of men die at a younger age than do women, with women having a higher average age than men. However, only in 1999, in the data covered in this research, did more men than women die in the six younger age cohorts, and mortality among women only surpassed that among men in the age cohort 70 to 79 years. As figure 8.6 details, in 2000 this pattern shifted quite dramatically, with mortality among 20 to 29-year-old women being higher than that among men. The major thrust of the increase in the age cohort 30 to 39 is caused by a sharp increase in mortality among women, an increase in which mortality among women surpassed that among men in 2003.

Figure 8.6: Number of deceased voters among 20 to 29 and 30 to 39-year-old women and men

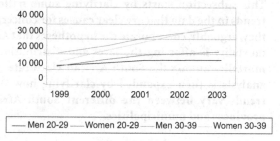

Source: IEC, 2004e. Calculations by authors.

Figure 8.4: Comparing mortality profiles of women for each age cohort, 1999 and 2003

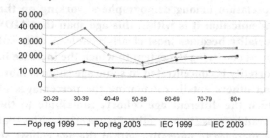

Source: Bradshaw et al., 2004; IEC, 2004e. Calculations by authors.

Figure 8.5: Comparing mortality profiles of men for each age cohort, 1999 and 2003

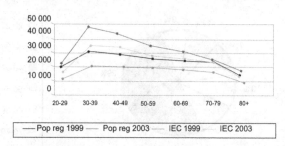

Source: Bradshaw et al., 2004; IEC, 2004e. Calculations by authors.

Yet another way of analysing trends in the mortality statistics is to investigate what share, or what ratio, mortality in one group represents compared with another group, measured in absolute numbers of death. In a "healthy" population, mortality among the younger sections of the population should, naturally, be lower compared with that of the older section of the population, showing a ratio far below 1. The South African mortality statistics, however, display a worrying trend in this regard. In their report from 2001, Dorrington *et al* show that the ratio of mortality between those who were 15 to 49 years old and those who were 50 years and older increased steadily from 1990 to 1999/2000. While, in 1990, the ratio was 0.31 for women and 0.66 for men, but ten years later it increased to 0.78 for women and 1.00 for men. While, in 1999/2000, mortality among young women (15–49 years old) was still lower than for women aged 50 and over, this difference was considerably less than ten years earlier. For men, however, mortality among men below 50 years in 1999/2000 equalled that of men 50 years and older.

Table 8.1: Ratio of deaths for different age cohorts to deaths among those aged 50+, by year and sex

Year	Ratio							
	Female				Male			
	20–29	30–39	40–49	20–49	20–29	30–39	40–49	20–49
1999	0.21	0.27	0.21	0.69	0.20	0.32	0.31	0.83
2000	0.23	0.31	0.22	0.76	0.20	0.35	0.33	0.87
2001	0.24	0.34	0.23	0.81	0.19	0.36	0.34	0.89
2002	0.25	0.39	0.26	0.90	0.19	0.40	0.35	0.94
2003	0.24	0.43	0.28	0.94	0.18	0.42	0.38	0.97

Source: IEC, 2004e. Calculations by authors.

Table 8.1 details the results from the same analysis of the mortality statistics from the voters' roll.

The ratios generated from the voters' roll are generally slightly lower than the figures presented by Dorrington, due to the groups that the IEC data excludes (as stated above). The similarities are more striking, however. The IEC data shows that the mortality ratio for the younger population increasingly approximates that of the older population, a development that is more pronounced among women, with an increase from 0.69 to 0.94 over the five years. As shown in figures 8.4 to 8.6, such an increase mainly occurs in the 30 to 39 age cohort, particularly among women.

So far into the analysis we have clarified what appears to be some worrying trends on the basis of absolute numbers of death among the South African electorate. But we get a better understanding of the different trends that we described above in considering whether one of two possible changes in the numbers of registered voters occurred simultaneously with the changes in the absolute number of mortality:

- *The number of registered voters has increased.* If an increase corresponds with a decrease in mortality, the conclusion can be drawn that the South African electorate is becoming healthier.

- *The number of registered voters has decreased.* A decrease in the numbers of registered voters corresponding with an increase in mortality among the voters would potentially be particularly problematic, as such a correspondence would indicate that the rate of mortality increases among a smaller group.

The data from the voters' roll clearly indicates that the number of registered voters has increased in all but the two youngest age cohorts. Registration campaigns that reportedly were particularly success-

ful in convincing youth to register to vote continued into 2004.

Table 8.2 details the national figures for the changes in numbers of registered voters that occurred between the end of 1999 and the end of 2003, by age and sex. The number of registered voters increased with an increase in age, especially when the age cohorts 50 to 59, 60 to 69, 70 to 79 and 80+ were looked at separately, with an almost 50% increase for the oldest voters. A strong downward trend has occurred in registration among younger voters, with the number of registered 18 to 19-year-old men more than halving in four years.

Table 8.2: Change in numbers of registered voters, 1999– 2003

Change	Age cohorts (%)				
	18-19	20-29	30-39	40-49	50+
Women	-49.0	-10.5	+12.7	+22.5	+23.5
Men	-54.7	-1.2	+13.3	+18.3	+26.8

Source: IEC, 2004e. Calculations by authors.

Taken as a whole, the number of registered voters increased by 8% over the four years, or by a total of 1 441 977 (from 18 011 064 to 19 453 041). However, as seen in figure 8.1, the *relative* number of deaths increased by 53% during the same period, an increase from 1.18% in 1999 to 1.81% in 2003 of the total number of registered voters. The increase in absolute numbers of deaths cannot be explained as "normal" levels of mortality among a higher number of people; the clear trend is that South Africa's voters died at a higher rate in the year preceding the 2004 elections than they did at the time of the 1999 elections. However, such an increase also varied significantly between age groups and between men and women. Figure 8.6 shows that women between 20 and 49 years of age were particularly affected, with an increase of 129% in the relative number of deaths for women 30 to 39 years old.

Figure 8.7: Increase (in %) in relative numbers of deaths among registered voters for each age cohort and sex, 1999 and 2003

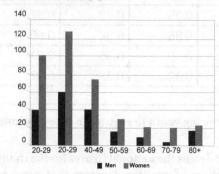

Source: IEC, 2004e. Calculations by authors.

The mortality profiles emerging from our analysis of the IEC data from the voters' roll in broad terms match the analyses that Dorrington *et al.* (2001) and Bradshaw *et al.* (2004) present on the basis of the ASSA model and data from the population register respectively:

- The level of mortality among the South African electorate increased more between 1999 and 2003 than a higher number of registered voters can explain.

- The "mortality profile" is heavily skewed against younger women, with particularly high levels of mortality among women who are 30-39 years old.

- In 2000 and 2003 the demographic aberration occurred that more women than men died in the 20-29 and 30-39 age cohorts respectively.

- In 2003 mortality among women and men in the age cohort 20-49 had increased to a level where it almost equalled that among those aged 50 years and older (with ratios of .94 and .97 respectively).

Such trends seem to indicate that AIDS is the only possible explanation for the increase in mortality according to the "profiles" we have been able to identify, but we shall put that hypothesis to some further tests in section 9 before we formulate any more definite conclusions. First we shall explore a geographic breakdown of the information.

8.3.2 Provincial and municipal variations

The three methods for establishing a national estimate of HIV prevalence, as well as the projections

of AIDS mortality based on the ASSA model, all identify a great, albeit somewhat different, variation in the impact of the epidemic in South Africa's nine provinces. If the increase in mortality on the voters' roll described above to some degree is caused by AIDS, some correlation should exist between the estimates and the provincial "profiles" of mortality in the South African electorate.

While most of South Africa's municipalities fall in one of the nine provinces, some municipalities lie cross provincial boundaries. The complexity of which is, however, not reflected in the IEC dataset, which identifies all municipalities as falling inside the boundaries of only one province. Where municipalities cross provincial boundaries, the change in relative number of deaths is then seen as falling within that particular province alone. However, while this is important to note for further and more detailed analysis of the data, it should not significantly alter the general trends in the data. The focus of attention is on the age cohorts of women, where particularly high levels and increases in mortality were noticed: 20-29-year-olds, 30-39-year-olds and 40-49-year-olds. The corresponding information for other ages and also for men is, in some instances, available in the appendices.

Figure 8.8: Relative numbers (in %) of deaths among women by age cohorts and province, 1999

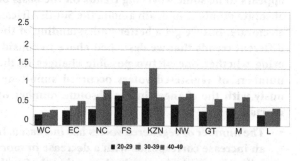

Source: IEC, 2004e. Calculations by the authors.

Figure 8.9: Relative numbers (in %) of deaths among women by age cohorts and province, 2003

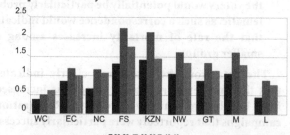

Source: IEC, 2004e. Calculations by the authors.

The relative number of deaths per province in 1999 placed KwaZulu-Natal clearly at the top of the list, a position it also held on the basis of absolute numbers of deaths (3 502 deaths among 30-39-year-old women). Figure 8.8 also showed that, with the exception of KwaZulu-Natal and the Free State, mortality was higher among older women than among younger women. By 2003 the pattern had changed quite dramatically (see figure 8.9). Not only had the relative numbers of deaths increased in four years, but the "profile" had changed in two important respects. In 2003, Free State had the highest relative number of deaths among women aged 30-39 and 40-49 years old, though KwaZulu-Natal, with 11 065 deaths among 30-39-year-old women, still led in absolute numbers (see appendix C). By 2003 mortality among 30-39-year old women had surpassed that of 40-49-year-old women, with the Western Cape being the sole exception.

While much can be learnt from the two mortality profiles for 1999 and 2003 that figures 8.8 and 8.9 present respectively, the mortality profiles seem to be changing. One such dynamic aspect concerns the rate at which mortality increased between 1999 and 2003 in the different provinces.

Figure 8.10: Increase (in %) in relative number of deaths among women by age cohort and province, 1999–2003

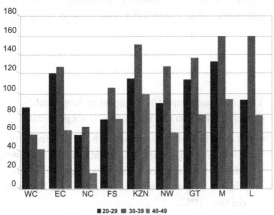

Source: IEC, 2004e. Calculations by authors.

Figure 8.10 shows that it is not in the provinces with the highest mortality in absolute or relative numbers of deaths that mortality is experiencing the sharpest increases among registered voters, but in Limpopo and Mpumalanga.

The description of the mortality profile at a municipal level will focus on registered voters between the ages of 20 and 49. To present the different municipal level profiles effectively, maps generated of South

Africa's municipalities have been coloured in accordance with a legend that identifies how the relative number of deaths differs between municipalities. The four relevant maps (included at the end of the book) all show the increase in the relative number of deaths from 1999 to 2003.[83]

Some features in the municipal profiles are particularly striking:

• The rates of increase in mortality are, in some instances, alarmingly high. While Limpopo was the province with the highest rate of increase in relative number of deaths between 1999 and 2003 (160% for women 30-39 years old), such provincial figures contain considerable municipal variations, with some increases being more than double that.[84]

• The rates of increase in mortality are, in some instances, surprisingly low. Even in provinces and areas where adjoining municipalities show high levels of increase in mortality, certain there are single municipalities that appear to have been spared this problematic trend.[85] A good example is the Letsemeng Local Municipality (Koffiefontein) in the Free State. While the province in itself has the highest relative number of deaths among women (30-39 years), an increase that exceeds 250% in the neighbouring Tokologo Local Municipality, the relative number of deaths decreased in the Letsemeng municipality.

• In some municipalities, the increase in mortality is higher among men than among women. Though the general pattern is the opposite, men are particularly vulnerable in some municipalities.[86]

• In most municipalities, the increase in mortality among women is considerably higher than among men.[87]

The four features highlighted above of the municipal level mortality profiles of the South African electorate exemplify the mass and complexity of the information that the maps and the original dataset contain. No one factor explains such variations between the municipalities or provinces. Exploring some of the most likely "suspects" enables one to see what causes such patterns in mortality on the South African voters' roll (see maps in the appendices).

8.3.2.1 A preliminary explanation of the variations

Statistical analysis might allow for determining whether any grounds exist for arguing that two possible and probable causes to the patterns observed, HIV/AIDS and poverty, contributed to their explanation. If either or both of the factors have anything to do with the explanation, correlations should be found between the rate of increase in the relative number of deaths, on the one hand, and levels of poverty and/or the various estimates and projections of HIV/AIDS, on the other.[88]

8.3.3.1 HIV/AIDS as explanation of increased mortality

AIDS is largely the explanation for the sharp increases in mortality among registered voters between the ages of 20-49, and particularly among 30-39-year-old women, due to the strong correspondence between the "profiles" generated and those described by expert demographers in the field of HIV/AIDS analysis. Since all HIV estimates and AIDS projections are only done on a provincial level, the mortality data has to be aggregated to the same level, with the cautions noted in the first section of this chapter also applying here. Such an aggregation results in loss of information about municipal variances.

Before we discuss the results of the tests we should clarify some of our assumptions that motivate this analysis. The logic of our thinking is as follows. While we do not know the cause of death for any of the deceased individuals who were taken off the voters' roll between 1999 and 2003, our argument that the problematic nature of the mortality profiles among 20-49 year old voters caused by AIDS-related deaths would be strengthened:

- If the provincial variations in estimates of HIV prevalence by different agencies correlated positively with provincial variations in increases in the relative number of deaths, the higher the estimated prevalence of HIV, the higher the number of actual deaths would be from AIDS.

- If provincial variations in the projections of the number of PLWHAs correlate positively with the provincial variations in increases in the relative number of deaths, the higher the projected number of people sick with AIDS, the higher the number of actual deaths would be from AIDS;

- If provincial variations in projections of numbers of AIDS-related deaths correlate positively with the provincial variations in increases in the relative number of deaths, the higher the number of deaths projected to be caused by AIDS, the higher would be the number of actual deaths from AIDS.

Table 8.3 details the results of tests for correlation, in which:

- **All correlations are positive. The general relationship holds that higher levels of estimated and**

projected impact of the epidemic correlate with larger increases in mortality, with some of the correlations being exceptionally strong.

- Some correlations are highly significant. In these cases the "fit" between the estimates and/or projections on the one hand and the increases in mortality on the other is very good.[89]

- Some correlations are weaker and not significant. As should be expected, since the various estimates and projections are done for adults up to the age of 49, with the correlations being weaker and not significant for older adults. The estimates and projections also do not provide as strong a basis for explanation for women 20-29 years old, perhaps because the actual increase in mortality exceeds expectations.

Of the three agencies, the HIV estimates provided by the HSRC through its household survey generate weaker correlations with the actual increases in mortality.

The statistical tests validated still further the argument that the profiles of mortality described were caused by the HIV/AIDS epidemic. These tests do not allow us to say anything of the strength of that relation, nor about how it should be understood to interact with other factors that have an impact on levels of mortality. We leave this to be explored in future research publications. In the next section we present a similar explorative analysis of our second plausible and potentially complementary explanation – poverty.

8.3.4 Poverty

The data confirms the understanding that poverty is closely linked to the impact of the epidemic:

- If provincial variations in the HPI correlate positively with provincial variations in the increase of relative numbers of deaths, people die at a higher rate in provinces that have a higher score on the HPI.

- If provincial variations in the HDI correlate negatively with provincial variations in the increases of relative numbers of deaths, people die at a lesser rate in provinces that have a higher score on the HDI.

- If provincial variations in income poverty correlate positively with provincial variations in the increase of relative numbers of deaths, people die at a higher rate in provinces with a higher percentage of people earning below the poverty line.

Table 8.3: Correlating increases in relative number of deaths with HIV/AIDS estimates and projections (N=9)

HIV/AIDS estimates and projections		Age cohort, by gender							
		20–29		30–39		40–49		50+	
		Female	Male	Female	Male	Female	Male	Female	Male
ASSA model	HIV estimate	.514	.948**	.817**	.887**	.830**	.834**	.459	.418
	Sick from AIDS	.285	.890**	.538	.790*	.725*	.691*	.228	.426
	Death from AIDS	.548	.919**	.719*	.845**	.840**	.836**	.492	.569
Department of Health		.581	.908**	.644	.771*	.751*	.808**	.435	.616
HSRC		.411	.719*	.359	.709*	.641	.687*	.058	.580

Sources: DoH, 2003; Dorrington et al., 2001; IEC, 2004e; Shisana, 2002. The table details the correlation coefficients (Pearson's r) between the increases in relative number of deaths between 1999 and 2003 for each gender and age cohort and three different estimates of HIV infection (ASSA model, DOH and HSRC), one projection of AIDS-related sickness (stage 4 of the disease) and one projection of AIDS-related death (ASSA model). All data and estimates are on the level of provinces. * Indicates significance at 0.05 level; ** indicates significance at 0.01 level.

The results of the statistical analysis are somewhat less striking than those for HIV/AIDS. Of the three poverty indicators, the more complex HPI provides the best basis for an explanation of the variations in mortality. The combination of the four poverty indicators that make up the HPI, namely, the probability at birth of not surviving to age 40; the adult literacy rate; the percentages of people not using improved water sources; and children under five who are underweight, provide a basis for arguing that poverty can partly explain the variation in the increase in mortality for the three age cohorts within the age span 20-49. The exception, yet again, is the youngest group of women. While the HDI generates the negative correlations expected, they are all weaker than the HPI and none is significant. The somewhat simplistic indicator "income poverty" was even more unsuccessful.

The statistical tests showed that both the HIV/AIDS epidemic and poverty help to explain interprovincial increases in the number of deaths.[90]

8.4 Conclusion

The profiles of mortality among the South African electorate establishes beyond doubt that South Africans are dying according to a pattern that clearly deviates from what should be normal for such a population. While young men should die at a higher rate than young women, and old people should die at a considerably higher rate than young people, such is not the case in South Africa: in 2003, female voters 20-39 years of age died in higher numbers than did their male counterparts and voters below 50 years of age died at almost the same rate as those 50 years of age and older. The rate of the increase in mortality between 1999 and 2003 among 30-39-year-old women is a particular cause for concern. With increases of about 160% in two provinces and municipal increases more than twice as high, South Africa is looking at a trend in mortality that should be a cause for the utmost alarm, mobilising a strong response from the whole of society and its political representatives.

Table 8.4: Correlating increases in relative numbers of deaths with poverty indicators (N=9)

Poverty indicators	Age cohorts, by gender							
	20–29		30–39		40–49		50+	
	Female	Male	Female	Male	Female	Male	Female	Male
Human poverty index	.538	.823**	.829**	.755*	.694*	.762*	.530	.256
Human development index	-.223	-.401	-.674*	-.430	-.352	-.393	-.423	.214
Income poverty	-.039	.210	.305	.124	.024	.089	.147	-.404

Source: IEC, 2004e; UNDP, 2003. The table details the correlation coefficients (Pearson's r) between the increases in relative number of deaths between 1999 and 2003 for each gender and age cohort and three different indicators of poverty. All data and estimates are on the level of provinces. * indicates significance at 0.05 level, ** indicates significance at 0.01 level.

Analyses suggest that such abnormal mortality profiles are largely caused by AIDS. Projections from computer modelling and from "straightforward" analyses of actual deaths on the population register show that mortality on the voters' roll display the same general features. The variations in increases in mortality on the provincial level correlated with the variations within various estimates and projections of HIV prevalence, as well as sickness and deaths from AIDS. The HIV/AIDS epidemic can therefore be seen to be causing the abnormal mortality profiles to some degree. We could show that poverty – when measured as the HPI – might also provide some explanation. Further statistical analyses and more elaborate theoretical work will explore how the two factors interact more precisely.

When we take a step back from the findings in this chapter we are reminded of the Kenyan nurse and her pessimistic premonition: Forget about elections. All the voters will be dead! While we have established here that South African voters die according to patterns that should not be, we are not raising the same banner as the nurse. Instead, the issue can be addressed through strong social and political interventions. Voters can participate in democratic elections by either putting pressure on the governments to adjust their policies to address people's concerns, or by exercising their right to select alternative policies by entrusting new mandates to fresh representatives.

9. Stigma and discrimination in elections

…even though we are suffering from this disease, we know that life is still continuing … and if we take good care of ourselves, we can live for a long time…

Rural African male,18-24 years, Nongoma.

9.1 Introduction

Public opinion data from the Afrobarometer survey has provided insight into generalised public perceptions on the effects of the pandemic and the political dynamic introduced by it. This section, in many

ways, adds a human face to the analysis. Put another way, it is the embodiment of our critical awareness of the limitations and impersonal nature of statistics in general. The use of multiple sources of data allows the triangulation of research. FGDs lend themselves to deeper qualitative analysis. Appraisal of those who have had practical experience of the problem studied constitutes a fundamental component of the research, enabling an understanding of the inter-relationship between those affected by the pandemic and their capacity to participate in elections.

The examination of HIV/AIDS and electoral data has been instructive in determining the unit of analysis. Evidently, the people most affected by the pandemic, for reasons cited earlier, are black registered voters who are living with HIV/AIDS or their care-givers who are not only the hardest hit by HIV/AIDS, but also comprise the largest segment of the voting population in South Africa. As a consequence of the legacy of apartheid, they also form the most economically disadvantaged group in the country. Focusing on the personal experiences of registered voters affected and infected by HIV/AIDS in South African society presents valuable insight into some of the realities of HIV/AIDS, as experienced by HIV-positive voters and their care-givers. We are also mindful of the danger of unwittingly contributing to the stigma and discrimination of certain parts of the South African citizenry by alluding to "high risk populations". We argue, however, that generalising the research would by itself dilute the gravity of the problem and drown the need for marginalised groups to access much-required support.

Extending the analysis of the impact of HIV/AIDS on political participation to the care-givers enables consideration of those potentially associated with the same vector of discrimination. Studies by South Africa's DoH not only confirm that there is indeed a social stigma directed at PLWHAs who have disclosed their status, but that AIDS discrimination is also aimed at those who associate with people who are known to carry the disease (Jennings et al., 2002).

9.1.1 Designing the focus groups

A total of 68 participants were selected from among care-givers and PLWHAs, all of whom were registered voters. The preponderance of HIV-positive individuals was allowed in the ratio 6:4, with the PLWHAs being the main interest. Eliciting participation from PLWHAs was more difficult in the rural areas and Citizen Surveys, conductors of the fieldwork for Idasa-GAP, solicited the help of health workers and counsellors to reach a reasonable ratio of participation. While 39 of the participants were PLWHAs, 29 were care-givers. Groups were disaggregated along gender lines and in relation to age cohorts, considering that different age groups might have different values and aspirations, and to allow more transparent debate. At least 50% of the group participated as voters in the 2004 elections. The central research question was to what extent, if at all, the HIV/AIDS pandemic contributed to the participation or non-participation of citizens in electoral processes. Participants were asked to discuss certain themes:

- Their reason for participation/non-participation in the 2004 elections;
- Whether they knew of the special vote;
- Their perception of change agents/political actors; and
- Their perception of the IEC and elections.

Six focus groups were held, in the urban areas of the city of Durban, Inanda and KwaMashu, and in the rural enclaves of Nongoma. The groups were selected from among the urban and rural populations in high prevalence areas, with KwaZulu-Natal being ideal for this purpose, as it is one of the areas worst hit by the pandemic. In addition, the geographical information system (GIS) used to map the mortality rates among registered voters in the study suggested a higher-than-average number of deaths among both male and female voters in the region.

9.2 Discriminatory attitudes

The DoH reports in its 2002 study that levels of discrimination are "quite high and widespread" in the country (Jennings *et al.*, 2002): "It would appear that human rights are not widely appreciated or respected. Furthermore, it appears that it is the level of education of a respondent that most seems to influence their attitudes" (Jennings *et al.*, 2002).

Table 9.1: Focus group composition

	Project Gap							
	AIDS sufferers			Caregivers				
	Total no respondents	Total AIDS sufferers	Age group AIDS sufferers	Total care-givers	Age group of care-givers			
					18-24	25-34	35-49	50+
Group 1								
Urban females - Inanda	12	7	18-24	5			3	2
Group 2								
Urban males - KwaMashu	12	7	25-34	5		2	2	1
Group 3								
Urban males	11	6	35-49	5		1	4	
Urban total	35	20		15	0	3	9	3
Group 4								
Rural females - Nongoma	11	6	25-34	5		2	1	2
Group 5								
Rural females - Nongoma	12	7	35-49	5	2	3		
Group 6								
Rural males - Nongoma	10	6	18-24	4		2	1	1
Rural total	33	19		14	2	7	2	3
Total	68	39	0	29	2	10	11	6

The departmental FGDs were homogeneous in age, race and gender, with participants being drawn from both metropolitan and rural areas. The survey focused on interviews with African populations in the East Rand metropolitan municipality of Gauteng and the Nongoma area of KwaZulu-Natal. Of the 501 respondents, 343 were female. Opinions were sought on a range of statements requiring individual responses on whether there must be compulsory pre-employment testing and whether PLWHAs should:

- be entitled to have children;
- have separate hospital facilities;
- be portrayed in the media as leading normal lives;
- have their names publicised;
- be restricted in any way, or not allowed to work; and
- be separated from others.

Many supported compulsory testing (22%), separate hospital facilities for PLWHAs (26%) and the prohibition of child-bearing among PLWHAs (84%) (see table 9.2).

9.2.1 Levels of discrimination

A higher degree of discrimination was found among rural than urban dwellers. The level of education and awareness of HIV/AIDS might have explained such variance:

> While one in five (20%) urban residents displayed a high level of discrimination, this proportion was far higher at one in three (34%) rural residents. One could surmise that the differences reflect the differential access to campaigns and resources dealing with HIV/AIDS (Jennings *et al.*, 2002: 27).

The study shows how discriminatory statements might affect would-be voters. The fact that 47% of the respondents said they would not disclose their status to colleagues shows the apprehension that accompanies the knowledge of one's status. Of the respondents, 37% chose not to tell their friends, while only 17% said that they would withhold their status from other family members. Many (55%) respondents feared contracting the disease, with 65% in the medium-risk category believing that HIV/AIDS was due to deviant behaviour. Lower levels of fear were found to decrease discrimination.

Table 9.2: Level of discrimination by age, employment status, dwelling area

	Low (%)	Medium (%)	High (%)
All respondents	37	36	27
Age			
18-35	42	35	23
36-55	31	38	31
56+	33	33	33
Employment status			
Employed	51	32	17
Unemployed	34	38	28
Area of dwelling			
Urban	48	31	20
Rural	25	40	34

Source: Jennings *et al.*, 2002.

9.3 Findings

The reflections of PLWHAs and care-givers in this Idasa-GAP study merely provide insight into how PLWHAs and their care-givers interact with electoral processes. As the analysis is subjective, it might not show how much voting is hampered within local communities, but rather indicates the nature and some of the causes of disconnection from, or connection to, political activity.

9.3.1 Principle of universal adult suffrage

The election process allows the greatest possible number of adult citizens to select their choice of policy (including HIV/AIDS policy) through the ballot. Such processes must be free and without fear, intimidation, violence and discrimination. The full participation of all citizens in electoral processes is an underlying principle embraced by all Africa in its goal of fulfilling universal adult suffrage and sustaining democracy. Nation-states must maximise the expression of the will of all eligible voters on public affairs.

Such principles are endorsed by the African Union (AU) in its Election Guidelines, the SADC in its Mauritius Charter of 2004, and the SADC Parliamentary Forum in its election norms and standards.[91] Universal adult suffrage prioritises realising full political rights over narrow political considerations. PLWHAs may access the special vote, as stipulated in the Electoral Act 33 (1) (a) of South Africa (EISA, 2004).

9.3.1.1 Knowledge of the special vote

One of the key determinants of participation in elections is the availability of information on civic and voting rights. Most participants in all six groups in this study had heard of the IEC-run voter education campaigns, including information on the special vote. Media coverage in South Africa is quite extensive, with private, public and community broadcasting services being available in addition to multilingual print products.[92] In the Afrobarometer October 2000 comparative study entitled *Views of Democracy in South Africa and the Region: Trends and Comparisons*, South Africans were described as having "the highest levels of access to political information through various forms of news media" (Mattes, 2000).

9.3.1.2 IEC information outreach

The IEC has the primary responsibility, in terms of the Electoral Commission Act (EISA, 2004), for voter education and information in South Africa. Based on its assessment of competences and the capacity to comply to its standards, the IEC might assign voter education and information outreach functions to accredited voter educators. Political parties and NGOs are also permitted to perform additional voter education functions. Election observer reports indicate that the IEC closely cooperated with media outlets to relay election information via live debates, special articles, news items and voter education drama series through the electronic and print media. NGOs, such as EISA and Idasa, also produced targeted voter education material with the IEC (EISA, 2004).

In KwaZulu-Natal, a fairly elaborate information outreach programme was discerned. FGD participants reported that radio and television, as well as newspapers reinforced by posters and loudhailers, were the chief sources of information accessed. However, while the IEC was the originator of the messages, the carry-on effect, participants say, was achieved by other agents, particularly political parties and traditional leaders. Most importantly, the rounds conducted by councillors, *indunas* and kingships to educate the masses appear to have reached constituencies in the locations of this study.[93]

School systems and home visits by IEC officials and party loyalists were valued as sources of infor-

mation on the special vote. However, none of the participants heard the IEC specifically refer to the eligibility of PLWHAs for the special vote, nor had they used it. The participants seemed uncertain as to whether PLWHAs could motivate their use of the special vote.[94] It is likely that the participants would use the special vote if it were explicitly stated that they were eligible to do so. Informed members of the groups strongly felt that the IEC does not specifically target PLWHAs and care-givers, but that it should do so to promote their participation in political life. The widespread fear among participants of stigma and discrimination in interactions with the wider community in an electoral environment combined with minority sentiments reflect the despair and resignation that comes with infection.[95]

9.3.1.3 Whether elections hold any value for people living with HIV/AIDS and care-givers

There was no variance between younger (18-24) and older (25-49) participants in respect of their desire to be involved in political activities, including elections: HIV/AIDS did not of itself seem to dampen the political enthusiasm of PLWHAs. Rather, the environmental factors within a community played a major role, particularly in the extent of stigma and discrimination. The extent of illness predetermined the degree of enthusiasm to override any perceived prejudice among the community and publicly vote.

Some of the reasons expressed by the participants for non-participation in elections echo the sentiments of citizens who are not infected. The younger group (18-24) more emphatically related non-participation to broken political promises. Such expressions would not differ from those of an uninfected ordinary citizen of the same voting age.[96]

PLWHAs were more likely to take part in elections if they had not publicly declared their status or if they did not exhibit any symptoms of AIDS, largely depending on whether they were in an urban or rural setting. The rural-based groups referred to stigma and discrimination more consistently and strongly than did their urban counterparts. Other studies on stigma and discrimination, such as the DOH research of 2002, which places rural-based South Africans at the receiving end of most AIDS-related discrimination, strongly corroborate such findings.

Some participants claimed to be involved in local rallies and campaign activities, or at least expressed an interest in being politically active. Care-givers tended to find political activities time-consuming, while some of the PLWHAs thought that they posed the danger of undermining their social standing by exposing their HIV-positive status beyond the family circle.

The most dominant opinion among the PLWHAs and care-givers interviewed in this study suggests that elections are viewed with utmost importance by most infected and affected people. That the respondents are African or black, perhaps, is of critical importance as this is the section of the population that had been denied rights before 1994, and they tend to have a more intense need to vote.

Among the larger pool of participants, voting was closely related to change, or high expectations of such, in personal and societal circumstances. Participants explained why they voted or wanted to vote by their wish tangibly to improve their quality of life, as well as to gain:

- Relatively more job opportunities and access to pension funds generated by a democratically elected government;

- Improved access to water and sanitation;

- An improved road and housing infrastructure; and

- Greater availability of health services, electricity and other social welfare benefits.

However, there were also negative factors that made some participants want to participate in elections. The supposed strides in improvements to social welfare since the advent of democracy in 1994 must be measured against the perceived failures, such as the alleged inability to arrest the spread of corruption in high places. Voting, they said, empowered ordinary citizens to elect a political party favouring the disadvantaged.

9.3.1.4 Why people living with HIV/AIDs and care-givers might not vote

That all groups hold some relative regard for elections seems to be a well expressed opinion. However, the flip-side of this explains why persons who should have voted opted out. Because there was a more emotive discussion on this topic by participants it is necessary to divide the factors that cause people not to vote into two: 1) attitudinal and 2) structural.

Attitudinal factors are those that might lead PLWHAs and care-givers not to participate in elections due to the negative predispositions of the community toward them, while structural factors relate to logistical arrangements to facilitate the processing of electors.

Attitudinal factors

Attitudinal factors include:

- Stigma and discrimination;
- Political disillusionment;
- Reacting to physical health circumstances; and
- Contending priorities (care for orphans versus elections).

Stigma and discrimination was the single most dominant determinant of lack of participation in elections. PLWHAs feared that communities would ostracise or marginalise them further if they attended major public events. Some described their status as "a serious issue", the knowledge of which is better confined to family and close relatives.

The participants' opinions correlate with the findings of studies on stigma and discrimination, particularly that of the DOH, that HIV/AIDS remains a taboo among South African communities, especially in the rural enclaves. The sense of stigma is strongest among those who are symptomatic, with respondents arguing that most community members would not stand in the same queue with someone with visible signs of the disease. Worse still, some suggested weight loss from any kind of disease was readily construed to be AIDS-related and therefore even those who were unaware of their status might eschew participation for fear of being mistaken for a PLWHA.

Some care-givers tending to sick relatives or to AIDS orphans were similarly apprehensive of participation in public affairs, arguing that merely associating with AIDS sick or AIDS orphans might cause them to become targets of discrimination.

The younger group, particularly urban males in the 18-24 age cohort, urged that PLWHAs should be given special job considerations to motivate them to participate in politics. Of the six groups, all 12 participants in the 18-24 groups of urban males had voted. Assuming that AIDS-related mortality has generally occurred in the age cohorts 30-39 years, then the 18-24 group is possibly the healthier and more energetic group, hence their optimism. The younger urban respondents are more critical, but also aspire for greater change. Being urbanites, they might also have greater access to information on campaign issues, including the availability of treatment programmes and government responsibilities in that regard.[97] This group seemed to demand more services for PLWHAs from the government, including education; larger budget allocations for treatment, care and support; and special employment considerations. Generally, all groups agreed that HIV/AIDS is primarily "a government problem" but that communities and families were also partly responsible for helping PLWHAs and orphans.

Personal illness and care-giving were important determinants of participation in elections. Male participants in the 18-24 cohort and females in the 25-49 age bands emphasised their personal state of physical health, and attendance to sick relatives or orphans as major impediments to participation. People with AIDS-related complexes were least likely to expose themselves at public events, such as elections. Several participants considered voting stations as "places of gossip".

Chores associated with care-giving, such as drawing water, finding food for the ill and orphaned children, and gardening, occupy more importance in the hierarchy of their priorities, according to care-givers in the 35-49 age band, who called for the voting period to be longer than two days to allow them to participate.

Some participants reported that, because most political rallies took place on Sundays, their favoured day of prayer, they chose to attend religious events, rather than political activities. PLWHAs expressed trust in church ministers and clerics, who often provide much needed counselling services.

Structural factors

In addition to societal attitudes, respondents blamed logistical or structural factors contributing to non-participation:

- Lack of ablution facilities;
- Lack of seating facilities;
- Long queues; and
- Lack of transport.
- Lack of ablution facilities. Many focus groups blamed PLWHA failure to participate in elections was worsened by the limited (or lack of) ablution facilities at polling stations, especially among the 24-49-year-olds in rural areas. PLWHAs tended to be afflicted by diarrhoeal diseases, requiring regular visits to such facilities. In the absence of running water, such regularity is likely to generate embarrassment, gossip and discrimination.
- Transport and seating facilities. To a lesser extent, transport and lack of chairs were also cited as problematic for PLWHAs. Though the average distance between homesteads and voting stations was 7.5-8km in urban, and 12.5-13km in rural, areas, according to the IEC, some participants felt that those afflicted by debilitating illnesses

should be transported for free to the polls. Some felt discouraged by the lack of seating, because they could not stand for long. Alternatively, it was suggested by a few that the sick should be allowed to vote from home. The younger voters (aged 18–24) found distance not to be a problem and that queues were processed relatively expeditiously in the 2004 general elections. Some cited misplaced identity cards, ignorance of the special vote and power relations between the sexes in households as predetermining involvement in the polls.

9.3.2 Stigma and discrimination as barriers to political participation

Depending on the levels of discrimination in their communities, PLWHAs are less inclined to vote if they have publicly disclosed their HIV status. Rural participants especially expressed profound fears of isolation and rejection. The generalised comments from respondents point to the possibilities that people with visible marks of illness or who had openly disclosed their status were prime targets of discrimination or even violence. Even those who suffer from weight loss from malaria might be assumed to have HIV/AIDS by ignorant members of especially rural communities. Concerns about stigma were more glaring among rural participants than among their urban counterparts. Most of the voters in the focus groups were comfortable with voting, as they had not yet publicly disclosed their status.

9.3.2.1 Likely change agents

While the situation of PLWHAs and care-givers, from their own accounts, does not amount to desperation, it does in a way expose the gulf between them and their elected representatives. Apart from attributing the acquisition of knowledge of the special vote to party agents in some cases, there is no mention of political leaders as "saviours" or the main change agents in regard to the situation of PLWHAs and care givers. When the respondents were asked directly who they thought was most likely to give them a voice in the political arena and respond favourably to their dire circumstances religious leaders and television stars, followed by community leaders and counsellors, were regarded as pivotal figures by all apart from 18-24-year-old urban males, who prioritised politicians and were also the keenest voters. Overall, politicians were viewed as potentially pivotal in dealing with stigma and discrimination, but usually unfulfilling of their electioneering promises.

Much comfort for ostracised people has been sought from the churches. Though some clerics are guilty of projecting HIV/AIDS as a form of punishment from God, the sick and rejected do tend to seek and find solace in prayer extended by local religious groups. Similarly, in close-knit rural communities, community leaders might play a key role in educating citizens about their rights and help to reduce the levels of stigma and discrimination against PLWHAs.

Participants also said that the media outreach encouraged their compassion and solidarity. Further, the government as an institution is seen to be a strong change agent in its capacity to reach all citizens, using medical professionals to educate them on the consequences of stigma and discrimination. Traditional healers occupy the lowest rating, presumably due to their inadequate outreach.

9.3.3 Visibility of PLWHAs in the political arena: a motivating factor

PLWHAs' involvement in political campaigning, in community forums and rallies, and in the government are regular forms of participation that should complement their electoral engagement. The public declaration of their HIV status by political leaders would alert the general electorate to HIV/AIDS not only being the disease of a condemned few, who are often poor and African. A few participants suggested that South Africa would go a long way to moderating stigma and discrimination if they allowed the HIV-positive to be elected or appointed to high office. Bridging the gulf perceived between elected officials and PLWHAs ensures that political dividends trickle down to all sections of society, including those infected and affected by the pandemic. PLWHAs value the dividends of democracy and, given the right conditions, would tend to express their will in the electoral arena.

9.3.4 Contextualising democratic dividends: Human development indicators

Human development indicators help explain the perception of progress, or lack of it, since South Africa became a democracy. Some of the voting participants of the FGDs use employment and improved health care, water and sanitation as motivators of participation, despite their status, while others want much more rapid change. Generally, the optimism

expressed by PLWHAs about the role of elections to their lives can be correlated with the UNDP's 2003 Human Development Report (HDR).

9.3.5 Improvements in education since 1994

According to the HDR for South Africa, the delivery of basic services has clearly improved in several areas since 1994:

- The number of schools without telephones decreased from 59% (1996) to 36.4% (2000).
- The percentage of schools without running water decreased from 34% to 27%.
- The percentage of students without access to proper toilet facilities declined from 55% (affecting 6.6 million students in 1996) to 16% (affecting 1.9 million students in 2000).
- Access to electricity improved from 40% to 54.9% in all schools.
- The number of schools with computers increased from 2 241 to 6 581.

The transformation of the education system since 1994 has brought several achievements, including:

- The creation of a single national Department of Education out of 19 racially, ethnically and regionally divided "departments of education";
- The creation of non-discriminatory school environments, with access based on criteria other than race or religion.
- The delivery of certain basic services has clearly improved and remains at high levels.

KwaZulu-Natal, like all other provinces, has benefited from such developments, as indicated in table 9.3, which gives a breakdown by province, with Kwazulu-Natal having improved from 31% to 97%.

9.3.6 Improvements in health care

South Africa's HDR (pp. 28–31) also illustrates headway in the health sector since the democratically elected government assumed power in 1994. The government consolidated the 14 health authorities under apartheid South Africa under one umbrella body, the national DoH. The restructuring of the apartheid health system introduced primary health care through the district health system. A strong focus on rural health programmes under the Reconstruction and Development Programme (RDP) brought services or made commitments to bring health facilities to rural areas, informal settlements and unserviced areas. Of 4 000 clinics, 2 298 have been upgraded since 2001 through programmes like the Clinic Upgrading and Building Programme (CUBP). Primary capital allocations to health, provided under the Hospital Facilities Revitalisation Grant, also made additional funds available for the construction of three major hospitals.

Table 9.3: Performance of provincial departments in stationery delivery, 2001-02

	2001	2002
	% stationery delivered*	% stationery delivered**
Eastern Cape	53%	varied, 45-88%
Free State	98%	100%
Gauteng	98%	varied, 45-88%
KwaZulu-Natal	31%	97% (all schools covered)
Mpumalanga	100%	100% (all schools covered)
Northern Cape	90%	100% (all schools covered)
Limpopo	95%	90% (95% of schools covered)
North West	98%	100%
Western Cape	89%	85.90%

Source: UNDP, 2003: 23. *% delivered per order. **Varies according to school district.

9.3.7 Housing delivery

Quoting the Department of Housing (2003), the HDR reports that about 1.5 million houses were completed between 1994 and 2003. Between 28% and 54% of all housing subsidies approved were awarded to women-headed households, depending on the province. At 256 542 units, KwaZulu-Natal is the second highest beneficiary after Gauteng (356 556) in the total number of housing units developed between 1994 and 2003.

9.3.8 Reliance on employment

The HDR further tells us that data from household surveys in 1995 and 2001, reflected in income quintiles, shows that 87% of the bottom 40% of South African households either had none or only one working family member and relied heavily on pensions or remittances in 2001. About 45% of African households in the lowest two income quintiles had no income earners at all in 2001, while 45% of African households in the bottom two quintiles relied heavily on one income earner. Such households are extremely vulnerable to the loss of an income or pension, with the long-term effect of the apartheid legacy continuing to skew the labour market. Some of the FGD respondents said that they felt that the government had not done enough to overcome unemployment, with HDR data indicating high levels of unemployment in present-day South Africa.

The high rate of unemployment can be blamed on dependence on a single breadwinner. When this individual dies, the family drops into the unemployment category. The employment category accounts neither for those who are employed in "low quality jobs", nor for those in part-time employment, who are largely women.

It is not certain from this study what course of action failure on the part of government is likely to provoke. However, there are theoretical perspectives and emergent social phenomena that might lend themselves to further analysis as we move into the next section of this report.

9.3.9 Stigma and discrimination as political and social processes

Responses to the pandemic will only be effective in the long term if there is understanding of the political and social dynamic generated by stigma and discrimination. Social and political theory emphasises that stigma and discrimination are neither isolated phenomena nor simply individual attitudinal expressions, but are social processes that are manipulated to generate and sustain social control and to produce and reproduce social inequality (Parker and Aggleton, 2002).

Parker and Aggleton (2002) consolidate this argument by highlighting concepts of symbolic violence and hegemony,[98] suggesting that societies achieve conformity by discriminating against those who are "different", in this way perpetuating social control. HIV/AIDS, they argue, exacerbates the marginalisation of social groups that are already sidelined, such as blacks, women, gay and bisexual communities and injection-drug users.

Table 9.4: Number of houses completed, 1994–2003

	1994-96	1997	1998	1999	2000	2001	2002	2003	Total
Eastern Cape	6511	32223	24659	20345	34021	10816	58662	7449	194686
Free State	13042	18001	17391	7177	16088	7005	9155	3371	91230
Gauteng	56239	70924	58170	45384	38547	46723	23344	15225	356556
KwaZulu-Natal	17553	78468	53105	28997	28547	14584	12077	11008	256542
Mpumalanga	11108	15743	22899	12401	20996	16667	14953	2722	117489
Northern Cape	19884	10873	16838	4808	16457	14584	21649	14919	120012
Limpopo	6666	4768	2387	2600	4148	2588	6056	2923	32136
North West	21287	20977	18367	12944	14109	13885	23784	6201	131554
Western Cape	25321	43834	34575	26916	17730	16634	20500	4795	190305
South Africa	177611	295811	248391	161572	190643	143281	203588	68613	1489510

Source: UNDP, 2003: 34.

Table 9.5: Employment and unemployment, 1995–2002

	Total	Gender		Type of area		Population group	
		Male	Female	Urban	Non-urban	African	Other
1995							
Employed (official, million)	9186	5244	3941	6047	3139	5882	3303
Unemployed (official, million)	1806	781	1026	1107	700	1495	312
Unemployed (expanded, million)	3799	1523	2276	1961	1838	3330	469
Unemployed rate (official) %	16.4	13.0	20.7	15.5	18.2	20.3	8.0
Unemployed rate (expanded) %	29.3	22.5	36.6	24.5	36.9	36.1	12.4
Labour market participation rate (official) %	45.2	51.0	39.8	54.9	34.0	40.8	58.2
Labour market participation rate (expanded) %	53.4	57.3	49.8	61.5	44.1	50.9	60.8
Labour absorption rate %	37.8	44.4	31.5	46.4	27.8	32.5	53.2
2002							
Employed (official, million)	11029	6184	4841	7431	3598	7239	3789
Unemployed (official, million)	4837	2259	2577	3186	1652	4213	624
Unemployed (expanded, million)	7925	3423	4501	4389	3536	7034	891
Unemployed rate (official) %	30.5	26.8	34.7	30.0	31.5	36.8	14.1
Unemployed rate (expanded) %	41.8	35.6	48.2	37.1	49.6	49.3	19.0
Labour market participation rate (official) %	56.7	63.3	50.7	64.8	45.2	53.8	65.8
Labour market participation rate (expanded) %	67.7	72.0	63.8	72.2	61.5	67.1	69.7
Labour absorption rate %	39.4	46.4	33.1	45.4	31.0	34.0	56.5

Certain races or so-called "high risk" groups are selected for HIV testing when they visit clinics or apply for bank loans, insurance, bonds or employment. Those found positive will not usually access the above benefits, and so will be marginalised from economic life. A life of poverty and isolation might result, depending on whether one is in a rural or urban environment.

The HDR report reaffirms that household incomes fall, due to the loss of wage earners and rising spending, particularly on medical care and funerals. In both Thailand and Tanzania, households are reported to spend up to 50% more on funerals than on medical care.

> Not only do household outputs and incomes decline, but household members, particularly women, have to make hard choices on the allocation of their time between production, meeting household needs, child care and care of the sick. In a recent study of 700 South African households affected by HIV/AIDS, more than half of the affected families did not have enough food to stave off starvation. Two-thirds of the households reported a loss of income as a result of the disease and larger proportions of household income being spent on health care and funerals.

Stigmatisation might play a critical function in transforming divergence, based on class, race, ethnicity or sexuality, into social inequality. It is posited that a process of legitimisation is instituted, causing those discriminated against to internalise their secondary status and accept existing social hierarchies that endure beyond a single generation.

9.3.10 Resisting the established order

Such hegemony constrains the ability of the marginalised to respond effectively. Currency for such arguments is sought in the identity theory, which suggests that those stigmatised are capable of resisting the forces that discriminate against them by:

- generating "resistance identities";
- utilising them to assume alternate identities;
- redefining their position in society; and
- seeking overall transformation of social structures.

Social mobilisation at all levels, including community, national and international, could result.[99]

Bearing this socio-political dimension in mind, we contextualise the analysis of the outcomes of focus group discussions by relating to how the varied threads of opinion from participants resonate with an emerging global, and certainly national, movement around treatment, care and support for PLWHAs.

The emergence of the Treatment Action Campaign and its Pan-African sibling (the Pan-African Treatment Campaign) confirms this thinking, and could be a precursor of things to come if urgency in

dealing with HIV/AIDS is consigned to the routines of government bureaucracies.

9.4 General comment

We conclude, given the extent of the discourse, that people infected and affected by HIV/AIDS generally still have a desire to participate in politics provided environmental and structural factors are addressed by authorities. The systematic reduction in the extent of stigma and discrimination and the availability of information on treatment, care and support would greatly boost the confidence levels of such people and encourage them to empathise with the rest of society.

The increasing pressure on grandparents to care and provide for growing numbers of orphaned children is placing a heavy burden on citizens who are already vulnerable. Care-givers themselves can be positive and therefore face the multiple threat of stigma, discrimination, loss of employment and income.[100]

HIV/AIDS is a potential threat to governance processes, as it not only dislocates the economic base by decimating productive members of society, but, by doing so, generates further poverty, creating fissures in societies, based on forms of discrimination and stigma. Such fissures might have political consequences in the long term if left unattended, judging by the capacity to mobilise across sectors already shown by social movements throughout Africa.

South Africa has launched possibly the largest treatment programme in the world. Such programmes are complex, requiring well-trained personnel, infrastructure and monitoring mechanisms. Experts from the World Food Programme (WFP) indicate that treatment programmes are most effective when accompanied by food and nutrition strategies, as PLWHAs only require medication on developing AIDS.

10. Conclusions and recommendations

We have already cautioned our readers about the potency of disease as a potential destabilising factor in politics; the history of Europe and its great plagues speak for themselves. We have illustrated the extent to which the pandemic has interacted with the political institutions and processes of the South

African democratic project and we are hopeful that the information, which has been tabled before the government, should assist it and its agencies to interrogate these new perspectives further and develop appropriate future strategies.

10.1 Recommendations

The concept of democratic governance carries much normative weight and can be a powerful advocacy tool for a strong political response to the epidemic, provided that it is used within a critical and politically forthright analytical framework that recognises the many previous governance failures on the continent.

10.1.1 Institutional/Structural reform

1. Given that an electoral system is the main instrument for translating votes cast in an election into seats for elected representatives, the impact of HIV/AIDS on the system has a direct bearing on the functioning of the two most important representative institutions, Parliament and local government authorities. Discovering the impact of the epidemic on electoral systems is a critical part of the broader electoral reform agenda.

2. Electoral reform should consider that both the financial and political costs of the HIV/AIDS pandemic are more onerous in countries that operate the FPTP, rather than the PR, electoral system. South Africa would, therefore, benefit from retaining its PR model at national level.

3. As the legislation does not allow for a special vote for people who are unable to travel to polling stations during local government elections, many people infected with HIV or affected by the epidemic are unable to vote in such elections. The IEC should advocate to the Justice Portfolio Committee in Parliament that the Local Government Municipal Electoral Act, No. 24 of 2000, be amended to ensure a special vote for such people in local government elections.

10.1.2 Strategic interventions

4. Political leaders, especially MPs and councillors, should participate in public education campaigns to reduce stigma and discrimination, which is one of the most compelling factors to impact on voter turnout and registration.

5. Traditional leaders should be empowered to redress the problems of stigma and discrimination in rural enclaves to allow for greater participation of PLWHAs in political, social and economic life. Traditional leaders are viewed as some of the key change agents of stigma and discrimination.[101] The participation of kings, councillors and religious leaders in HIV/AIDS-related community radio broadcasts and public forums is recommended, owing to the high degree of esteem they seem to command, particularly in rural settings.

6. The IEC should build HIV/AIDS awareness into its voter education programmes to reduce the extent of HIV/AIDS stigma and discrimination in communities. Establishing links with HIV/AIDS service providers and civic education groups should help to develop context-specific approaches to overcome misconceptions about HIV/AIDS and improve or sustain high participation levels. Apart from emphasising all aspects of HIV/AIDS, including prevention, treatment and nutrition, the human/political rights of all individuals in the IEC and civic group public communication programmes should be emphasised.

7. South Africa has launched possibly the largest treatment programme in the world. Although the mechanics of it are yet to be lubricated, we see potential in this programme to contribute significantly to efforts to reduce HIV/AIDS-related stigma and discrimination.

8. Monitoring PLWHA participation rates. Election monitoring and observation projects should build into their programmes mechanisms for gauging the participation of PLWHAs in political processes. Registration of orphans should be ensured to encourage their full integration into society.

9. The special vote could be an effective mechanism for increasing participation in electoral processes. However, it is recommended that specific details on people afflicted by chronic illnesses and those infected and affected by life-threatening diseases such as HIV/AIDS needs should be included in voter campaign messages to generate higher turnouts. Exploring possibilities of introducing or extending mobile voting might also be helpful.

10. South Africa should reassess structural aspects of the electoral process. Where necessary, polling stations and transport facilities should be placed within reasonable reach of all people to facilitate greater participation of citizens, especially PLWHAs. Availability of functional ablution facilities within the vicinity of the stations should also be considered.

Appendices

Appendix A

"Sad electoral roll deletions", Natal Witness
13 April 2004

We have now had 10 years of democracy behind us and we can all judge what has been achieved by those parties in power. The sadness for me has been the increasing number of deaths I have had to record in my "tidying up" of the voters' roll which we use in our election monitoring.

One of the tasks we have done in order to remove the names of those who have died since the voters' roll was last corrected. Unless one is completely insensitive, one can't but help notice the ages of those who have died. Just look at the first two numbers of the person's ID and it will tell you the year they were born in. When you delete an entry for someone with an ID starting 15 or 25, one can be philosophical and say they have had a good innings. But when one deletes IDs starting with the numbers 84 or even 74, then one realises that these South Africans died in their 20s and 30s. The names of the youngsters in the eThekwini area are predominantly Zulu and Xhosa.

The "deceased lists" do not indicate the causes of the death, so one doesn't know for certain whether these young people have died from an HIV/AIDS-related complications. Our president has said he knows no-one with AIDS so you can bet he has never had to do this job. It is really depressing.

Please go out and vote. Do so for all those young South Africans who didn't live long enough to cast their own democratic votes.

GDA PULLMAN

Tongaat (e-mail, shortened)

Appendix B. Change (in %) in numbers of registered voters between 1999 and 2003, for each age, gender and province						
Province	Gender	Age cohort				
		18–19	20–29	30–39	40–49	50+
Eastern Cape	Women	-52.7	2.1	13.8	26.8	22.7
	Men	-52.1	7.7	15.0	20.8	24.6
Free State	Women	-47.6	-17.4	6.9	16.8	20.7
	Men	-52.9	-15.4	3.2	16.1	23.3
Gauteng	Women	-55.3	-22.0	9.7	21.4	27.8
	Men	-59.3	-26.0	12.1	18.2	31.3
KwaZulu-Natal	Women	-53.7	-14.2	10.6	18.8	20.4
	Men	-58.6	-11.1	14.0	12.4	24.9
Mpumalanga	Women	-32.8	-8.1	13.1	18.9	23.6
	Men	-48.0	-8.3	9.3	16.0	27.9
Northern Cape	Women	-45.1	-3.1	16.5	22.9	22.4
	Men	-51.8	-3.3	18.2	20.5	22.0
Limpopo	Women	-25.8	8.8	16.7	26.1	21.2
	Men	-42.4	12.6	20.8	19.0	26.3
North West	Women	-45.9	-7.4	12.8	25.6	23.4
	Men	-51.2	-9.4	8.7	22.2	26.3
Western Cape	Women	-65.5	-14.0	21.6	27.7	28.4
	Men	-69.8	-16.2	21.3	25.2	27.7
National	Women	-49.0	-10.5	12.7	22.5	23.5
	Men	-54.7	-11.2	13.3	18.3	26.8
Source: IEC, 2004. Calculations by authors.						

Appendix C. Absolute numbers of deaths, by age, sex and province, for 1999 and 2003

Province	Gender	Age cohort									
		18–19		20–29		30–39		40–49		50+	
		1999	2003	1999	2003	1999	2003	1999	2003	1999	2003
Eastern Cape	Women	72	20	1.340	2.998	1.628	4.263	1.517	3.172	10.335	16.818
	Men	108	16	1.365	2.043	2.127	3.560	2.398	3.938	11.028	15.322
Free State	Women	48	6	1.323	1.909	1.757	3.889	1.225	2.502	4.536	6.756
	Men	37	4	957	1.199	2.064	3.542	2.075	3.383	5.068	6.885
Gauteng	Women	71	11	2.562	4.188	3.527	9.030	2.722	6.009	9.490	15.227
	Men	153	8	3.376	3.645	5.421	10.524	4.882	8.642	11.758	17.470
KwaZulu-Natal	Women	112	21	3.502	6.411	3.986	11.065	2.498	5.960	12.031	20.890
	Men	146	21	3.416	4.487	5.242	9.738	4.761	7.802	12.778	18.358
Mpumalanga	Women	43	6	1.001	2.127	1.170	3.439	934	2.137	4.060	6.733
	Men	55	8	972	1.356	1.596	3.132	1.568	2.936	4.805	6.934
Northern Cape	Women	17	4	255	386	373	731	392	562	1.589	2.341
	Men	22	4	300	339	487	776	529	808	2.129	2.740
Limpopo	Women	31	8	679	1.421	810	2.461	758	1.704	5.451	8.818
	Men	62	8	585	878	915	1.778	1.135	1.844	5.534	7.487
North West	Women	30	7	965	1.710	1.211	3.120	974	1.945	4.277	6.619
	Men	34	4	843	1.054	1.528	2.875	1.497	2.840	5.249	7.221
Western Cape	Women	31	4	549	891	758	1.454	729	1.335	4.727	7.823
	Men	80	8	1.098	1.035	1.351	1.998	1.364	2.063	6.206	8.882
National	Women	455	87	12.176	22.041	15.220	39.452	11.749	25.326	56.879	91.985
	Men	697	81	12.912	16.036	20.731	37.923	20.209	34.256	64.555	91.299

Source: IEC, 2004. Calculations by authors.

Appendix D

Government's response to Idasa study on HIV and AIDS and Governance

25 November 2004

Government has noted the release by Idasa of their report "HIV/AIDS and Democratic Governance in South Africa". It welcomes the dedication of research effort to issues of public importance and notes the practical nature of the recommendations being made to enhance participation in the electoral process.

At the same time caution needs to be exercised with regard to a number of aspects of the report and it is hoped that media and others will take note of the many caveats and qualifications contained in the report itself, so that the important issues raised are not obscured by sensational responses.

In assessing the implications of the report a number of considerations should be borne in mind.

In assuring the integrity of our institutions and systems there is a myriad of social dynamics that require ongoing attention and we should ensure that all elements of policy – social, economic, and those pertaining to governance as well as safety and security – are worked on taking into account major demographic realities.

These realities include: migration, population growth rate and trends in fertility, changes in household size, and changes in the structure of the economy. AIDS is one such matter, and a very critical one at that, and we welcome the research on this specific dynamic.

The proposal by Idasa that there should be consideration of the findings with regard to HIV and AIDS in electoral planning and other election-related decisions is appreciated. In the same measure, the impact of the other dynamics, such as the ones outlined above, should be factored into such planning.

The same challenge applies to promoting the participation of citizens in the electoral process: the need to take account of the conditions as well as the rights of people living with HIV, generally people with disability, and workers including in particular farm workers. Further, the current under-representation, proportionally, of young people on the electoral roll constitutes another critical challenge for our democratic system.

In other words, electoral planning should seek to incorporate all dimensions of the challenges we face.

The report brings to light interesting data and correctly reminds us that HIV and AIDS affect all sectors of the population. However, by positing worst-case scenarios and projections it then makes the exaggerated conclusion that democracy in South Africa is in danger, that there is a major political risk on the horizon. The report does not bring evidence that the trend in the pandemic has had a fundamental impact on the integrity of political systems anywhere in Southern Africa, including, say Botswana which is supposed to have the highest rate of infection, beyond suggesting that this might have been the case. Related to this is the fact that the populations of countries such as Botswana and Uganda have been growing at the rate of about 2% per annum during the 1990s.

While there is consensus that trends in mortality statistics are reflecting the impact of AIDS in particular amongst young people, the projections cited (from the UNDP and others) regarding population growth and life expectancy are not substantiated and do not appear to be consistent with population growth in our country and other Southern African countries at various stages of the pandemic.

Such worst-case scenarios with the most negative assumptions serve to heighten a sense of crisis. And in discounting the impact of programmes to counter HIV and AIDS, including levels of awareness, reduction in incidence among the youth, impact of treatment programme, the impact of anti-stigma campaigns, the report may serve its purpose in alerting all of society to an issue that requires attention; but it is less valuable in the detail, as a guide to action.

For further information please contact: Dr Lindi Makhubalo on (012)321 0775

Issued by: Government Communication and Information System (GCIS)

Endnotes

1   This discussion of the epidemic focuses on the theme for the report, so that omissions made on that basis are uncontroversial. However, the many children who are orphaned due to AIDS could and should be analysed from a governance perspective. With no or little parental guidance and community support, orphans will not be encouraged to participate meaningfully in the democratic society and its electoral processes (see Richter *et al.* [2004] and Bray [2003]).

2   At the stage of the final editing of the manuscript for this publication, Professor Rob Dorrington and his colleagues published a report based on the ASSA2000 model that estimated the national HIV prevalence in South Africa to be 5 million, slightly lower than the 2004 UNAIDS report. For reasons of timing, the most recent report from Dorrington *et al.* has not been worked into this document to the extent that it should. However, since the report does not present updated estimates and projections for the different provinces (which would have been useful for the correlation analyses), their previous report is used (Dorrington, 2002) for these purposes.

3   The HDI has a negative correlation with AIDS deaths (*Pearson's* $r = .36$) and with AIDS sickness (*Pearson's* $r = .28$). The HPI has a positive correlation with AIDS deaths (*Pearson's* $r = .81$) and AIDS sickness (*Pearson's* $r = .70$).

4   Data was not provided for the other categories.

5   HIV estimates correlate negatively with HDI, since prevalence should be higher where indicators of development are lower. The correlation with HPI is significant, at a .01 level. When plotted, the nine cases are clearly centred on the regression line. The very strong correlations between poverty indicators and the ASSA model are, in parts, explained by the fact that the model builds on such poverty data in generating its estimates.

6   Interview with Paul Graham, director of Idasa, Pretoria, on 19 August 2004.

7   Additional source: Gender Links website, 2004.

8   Mattes, R. and Strand, P., 2007. AIDS Impact Research at DARU: HIV/AIDS and Society: Building a Community of Practice. Cape Town.

9   In 2005, the speaker of the National Assembly of Malawi was flown to South Africa for further medical treatment. Similarly, leading politicians from Zambia often access medical aid from South Africa or in Europe.

11 Established on 20 March 2002, under the leadership of Dr Van Zyl Slabbert.

12 Interview with Paul Graham on 19 August 2004.

13 While the regulation of public broadcasting in a fair and non-partisan way is very important during the period leading up to elections, the structure and mandate of Icasa fall outside the primary scope of this report.

14 Independent Electoral Commission (IEC), 2004a. Fact sheet:: Vision and Mission, available at http://www.elections.org.za/Vision.asp, 16 February.

15 According to the IEC, in June 2004 its KwaZulu-Natal office comprised 13 staff members; its Gauteng office 11; its Western Cape office 9; its Limpopo office 10; its Eastern Cape office 11; its Free State office 9; its Northern Cape office 10; its North West office 10; and its Mpumalanga office 9.

16 For example, KwaZulu-Natal has 51 municipal offices and 102 MEOs. Mr Mosery of the IEC's KwaZulu-Natal office said, in an interview, that this point was the subject of a legal dispute at the Commission on Conciliation, Mediation and Arbitration (CCMA).

17 Interview with Mawetu Mosery, provincial electoral officer in KwaZulu-Natal, Durban, on 3 June 2004.

18 The other Chapter Nine institutions are the public protector; the Human Rights Commission; the Commission for the Promotion and Protection of the Rights of Cultural, Religious and Linguistic Communities; the Commission for Gender Equality; and the auditor-general.

19 The right to vote in free and fair elections.

20 Independent Electoral Commission (IEC), 2004c. Fact sheet 'Why and How Do I Register?' available at http://www.elections.org.za/Vision.asp, 16 February.

21 For example, the human resources department at eTekwini Municipality reported that its Parks, Recreation and Culture Department had a 32% turnover of staff over a period of six months (Manning, 2003), costing it a great deal, both financially and in terms of productivity.

22 The government departments were selected due to their staffing profile in some respects being similar to that of the IEC.

23 Badcock-Walters, P., Desmond, C., Wilson, D. and Heard, W., 2003. Educator Mortality in Service in KwaZulu-Natal, HEARD available at http://www.heard.org.za.

24 Smart (1999) predicts that this will sharply increase the remuneration budgets of organisations and state departments.

25 This observation in no way implies that any of the three permanent staff at the IEC who died during 2003 died from AIDS. The point is merely to highlight a correspondence between estimates of the impact of AIDS and actual occurrences on a more general level (see table 4.3).

26 Interview with Michael Hendrickse, senior manager in the Electoral Democracy, Training and Legal Services Division of the IEC, Pretoria, on 7 June 2004.

27 Ibid.

28 Interview with Mosery.

29 Ibid.

30 Ibid.

31 The national population register is managed by the Department of Home Affairs.

32 Interview with D. Mzaidume of the IEC on 3 August 2004. A letter to the Natal Witness regretted that, in the task of "tidying up" the voters' roll, the authors had observed that most whose names were removed were between the ages of 18 and 30. See appendix A for the full text of the letter.

33 The Star, 26 January 2004.

34 Independent Electoral Commission (IEC), 2004b. "Frequently Asked Questions", available at http://www.elections.org.za/FAQ.asp 15 January.

35 Interview with Mosery.

36 Interview with Hendrickse.

37 Interview with Mosery.

38 Ibid.

39 Ibid.

40 Interview with C. Sampson, provincial electoral officer in the Western Cape, on 28 May 2004.

41 The outline is based on Kauffman, 2004; Nattrass, 2004; Shisana and Zungu-Dirwayi, 2003; Sparks, 2003; and Van der Vliet, 2004.

42 Interview with Saadiq Kariem, secretary of the Health Committee for the African National Congress, Cape Town, on 4 June 2004.

43 Business Day, 28 October 2004.

44 Telephonic interview with Ruth Rabinowitz, spokesperson on HIV/AIDS for the Inkatha Freedom Party, on 23 April 2004.

45 Interview with Kariem.

46 Interview with Rabinowitz.

47 Interview with Cherryllyn Dudley, spokesperson on HIV/AIDS for the African Christian Democratic Party. Cape Town, on 15 March 2004.

48 Interview with Kariem.

49 Interview with Rabinowitz.

50 Ibid.

51 Coetzee, Ryan. E-mail communication with PS, policy proposal attached, 19 October 2004.

52 Interview with Lance Greyling, spokesperson on HIV/AIDS for the Independent Democrats, Cape Town, on 11 September 2004.

53 Ibid.

54 Letter from S. Mfenyana, Secretary of Parliament. dated 1 April 2004, in response to request for information from Dr P. Strand, Cape Town, 1 April.

55 Interview with Kariem.

56 Interview with Gous.

57 See list of party electioneering material in the list of references. To increase the flow of the text, citations will be taken from one or more of the respective documents detailed here as the different parties are discussed, without further notation in the text.

58 Though any such analysis is an over-simplification, it clarifies certain aspects.

59 As argued by the IFP's Ruth Rabinowitz.

60 Interview with Dudley.

61 Interview with Gous.

62 Ibid.

63 Interview with Dudley.

64 A policy accord between the main parties in Botswana has presented the population with a unified political establishment working together against prejudice and for effective implementation of a very ambitious overall response to the epidemic (Tlou, 2004). The parliamentary parties in Tanzania have created the Tanzania Parliamentarians AIDS Coalition (TAPAC). Launched in August 2001 by MPs from different parties, TAPAC seeks to mobilise parliamentarians, so they are more effective in implementing various aspects of the national response to the epidemic in their respective constituencies (see http://www.tapac.org).

65 Interview with Dudley.

66 Ibid.

67 Interview with Mike Waters, spokesperson on HIV/AIDS for the Democratic Alliance, Cape Town, on 26 February 2004.

68 Interview with Kariem.

69 Our various efforts to learn more from the ANC about this survey came to nothing. Saadiq Kariem referred to the survey more generally and was unsure whether the results had ever even been reported on in a comprehensive manner within the ANC.

70 Interview with Kariem.

71 Mattes, B., 2004. "Public Opinion and HIV/AIDS: Facing Up to the Future?" *Afrobarometer Briefing Paper*, No. 12, April, available at http://www.afrobarometer.org.

72 The increase tended to exceed the margin of error of about +/- 2%.

73 Correlations (*Pearson's r*) were .233 and .252 for "men" and "urban" respectively, both at .01 level, and between .097 to .166 for other categories. Only the black racial group had an "N" large enough to uphold these statistical analyses, with a correlation of .195.

74 The unstandardised regression coefficients were considerable in all categories – all South Africans (.219); black (.155); male (.270); female (.188); black women (.167); urban (.289) and rural (.115) – with them all being statistically significant at .01 level, except for "rural" which was significant at .05 level.

75 The questions also captured home-based care that was not AIDS-related, which should be taken into account in data interpretation and analysis.

76 In a factor analysis, the three variables loaded .921 (household member), .713 (self) and .454. We decided to keep all three variables in the scale, since a reliability analysis gave Alpha .7280 for the three variables.

77 The degree of activism in civil society was captured in two sets of questions. In the first, respondents were asked whether they were "not a member", an "inactive member", an "active member", or an "official leader" of four different kinds of civil society organisations (see table 6.4), all with a political agenda. In the second set of questions, respondents were asked to say whether, during the preceding year, they had done any of the four "activities" listed in table 6.4. The response alternatives were "no, would never do this", "no, but would do it if had the chance", "yes, once or twice", "yes, several times", and "yes, often". The fifth "activity" in survey – "used force or violence for a political cause" – has been omitted, since it yielded no statistically significant correlations at all. The response option "Don't know" (roughly 1% to 4% of responses for the different questions) was recoded as a missing value. The hypothesis that providers of home-based care become inactive in civil society would be confirmed if these tests generate negative coefficients that are statistically significant, signifying that the more a person is busy with providing home-based care, the less active she is in civil society. The opposite hypothesis would be confirmed if positive coefficients are statistically significant, and the null-hypothesis, that providing home-based care is not a predictor of civil society activism at all, would be "confirmed" by weak coefficients that are not statistically significant.

78 The results indicated that the null-hypothesis dominated, since most coefficients were too weak to be statistically significant

79 The null-hypothesis would indicate that home-based care had little or no effect on people's willingness or ability to perform these critical civic duties.

80 The question read: "Overall, how satisfied are you with the way democracy works in South Africa?" The response options were "South Africa is no democracy", "not at all satisfied", "not very satisfied", "fairly satisfied", and "very satisfied". "Don't know" responses had been recoded as missing values.

81 When the correlation tests were plotted, the Western Cape fell outside the general picture. Some correlation analyses were, therefore, conducted without the WC, as reported above.

82 The release of the data was an example of the IEC's commitment to their willingness to help with research, as expressed in a letter from the IEC's Chief Electoral Officer, Advocate Pansy Tlakula. Before the material was handed over, its release was also sanctioned by IEC commissioners.

83 Though the provincial level mortality profiles reflect AIDS mortality in South Africa, the same general claim cannot be made for the municipal-level profiles. The maps require further scrutinising to establish to what extent the variations in mortality are consistent with the HIV/AIDS hypothesis. For instance, while the data contained in the municipal-level maps for the KwaZulu-Natal province suggest no apparent challenge to the hypothesis, as an explanation of the variations in the Northern Cape province, such an hypothesis is more problematic. The presentation describes the variations in mortality profiles on the municipal level.

84. In 1999, a total of 11 women (30–39 years) out of 4 721 registered voters in Lephalale municipality (Ellisras) in Limpopo died, while

57 dead out of 5 240 voters in 2003, amounting to an increase of 367% in the relative number of deaths

85 A good example is the Letsemeng Local Municipality (Koffiefontein) in the Free State. While the province had the highest relative number of deaths among women in the age cohort 30 to 39 years, an increase exceeding by 250% neighbouring Tokologo Local Municipality, the relative number of deaths decreased in the Letsemeng municipality.

86 The Thaba Chewu municipality in Mpumalanga is a good example. An increase in the relative number of deaths among women (30-39 years) of 135% between 1999 and 2003 was surpassed by an increase of 241% among registered men of the same age.

87 In Utrecht municipality in KwaZulu-Natal, for example, the relative number of deaths of men (30-39 years) increased by 28% between 1999 and 2003 (seven more deaths among an additional 16 registered voters), while the increase for women of the same age was 343% (21 more deaths among an additional 22 registered voters).

88 The analysis can be taken much further through regression analyses under different assumptions.

89 This becomes clear when the correlation is plotted on the regression line.

90 The results from a series of partial correlations introduce much complexity into the general picture described through the correlations in tables 8.3 and 8.4. First, the tests for correlation between the increases in mortality and the various estimates and projections of the epidemic, were "controlled for" the effect of the variations in the HPI. The scale of human poverty in the provinces did not influence the strength and significance of the correlation between the epidemic and mortality in the provinces. After that, the correlation between poverty and mortality was tested while controlling, one by one, for the different estimates and projections of the epidemic. The full table of correlation coefficients and their significance is provided in appendix C. The theoretical suggestions that both the epidemic and poverty are valid predictors of the increase in mortality are borne out by the analysis to some extent in the bivariate correlation analyses.

91 According to the SADC Principles and Guidelines governing democratic elections, "the SADC Guidelines are not only informed by the SADC legal and policy instruments, but also by the major principles and guidelines emanating from the OAU/AU Declaration on the Principles Governing Democratic Elections in Africa – AHG/DECL.1 (XXXVIII) and the AU Guidelines for AU Electoral Observation and Monitoring Missions – EX/CL/35 (III) Annex II".

92 The major television channels are the government-controlled SABC 1, 2 and 3 and SABC Africa; E-TV, and the pay channels, MNET and DSTV, which has over 100 satellite channels. The 38 commercial radio stations use both local languages and English as a medium of communication. The 70 or more community stations are supplemented by 16 daily newspapers and 25 weeklies.

93 However, a few respondents confused the IEC with the government. This confusion manifested itself through continuous reference to the IEC's supposed responsibility for the treatment of PLWHAs. At least one respondent expressed total ignorance of what the IEC was.

94 One respondent said that he waited for an IEC official to come to help an ill family member to vote, but when the official did not comes, neither he nor his relative voted.

95 An urban African male aged between 18 and 24 years old, stated in KwaMashu: "…when a person finds out they are HIV positive, they can't see anything else in front of their eyes other than death. So even voting becomes pointless because why should I bother if I am dying anyway…?"

96 See the Afrobarometer study 2002: *Views of Democracy in South Africa and the Region: Trends and Comparisons.* Opinions of ordinary people sampled in Botswana, Zimbabwe, Zambia, Malawi, Namibia and South Africa place job creation, the economy, education, crime and security, health and poverty among the highest priorities for government.

97 The HSRC's 2002 joint study with the Nelson Mandela Foundation asserts that, while South Africans are generally well exposed to media messages, and while radio provides the widest multilingual diversity, African languages tend to be marginalised. The study notes that regular exposure to broadcast media is low in rural areas and poorer households. The most pervasive messages on HIV/AIDS related to condom use, with other slogans aired about fidelity and abstinence, with an emphasis on religious or cultural values and care for PLWHAs and their rights.

98 *Ibid*, citing Bordieu, 1977 and 1984: Symbolic violence is a process in which words, images and practices promote the interests of the dominant group, with hegemony being achieved through the use of political, social and cultural forces to promote the dominant meanings and values that legitimise unequal structures (Foucault, 1977; Gramsci, 1970; Williams, 1977; Williams, 1982).

99 Ibid.

100 UNDP HDR 2003 reports that the number of households whose primary care-givers are under the age of 18 years is also increasing, with the knock-on result of decreasing school attendance and retarding efforts at building human capital. Other social implications include the abandonment and abuse of PLWHAs, as well as their stigmatisation, poor morale and stress.

101 The potential of traditional governance systems to enhance service delivery and ensure that rural populations are not marginalised from development was also underlined and acknowledged by the ADF 1V, cohosted at Addis Ababa, Ethiopia by the Economic Commission for Africa, the AU and the African Development Bank in October 2004.

References

Literature

Arndt, C. and Lewis, J., 2000. "The Macro Implications of HIV/AIDS in South Africa: A Preliminary Assessment", *South African Journal of Economics*, August.

Asmal, K. and De Ville, J., 1994. "An Electoral System for South Africa", in Steytler, N., Murphy, J., De Vos, P. and Rwelamira, M. (eds) *Free and Fair Elections*, Kenwyn: Juta.

Barrett Grant, C.J., Strode, A. and Smart, R., 2002. *HIV/AIDS in the Workplace: A Guide for Government Departments*, Pretoria: Department of Public Service and Administration.

Baylies, C. and Bujra. J., 1997. "Social Science Research on AIDS in Africa: Questions of Content" Review of African Political Economy Vol 24 N0 73.

Bourne, D., 2003. "Wither the AIDS Epidemic – Or Lies, Damned Lies and Statistics?", Editorial in *South African Medical Journal*, 93 (12): 916.

Bradshaw, D., Laubscher, R., Dorrington, R., Bourne, D. and Timaeus, I., 2004. "Unabated Rise in Number of Adult Deaths in South Africa", *South African Medical Journal*, April.

Bratton, M. and Van de Walle, N., 1997. *Democratic Experiments in Africa: Regime Transitions in Comparative Perspective*, Cambridge: Cambridge University Press.

Bray, R., 2003. "Predicting the Social Consequences of Orphanhood in South Africa", CSSR Working Paper No. 29, Centre for Social Science Research, University of Cape Town, Cape Town.

Butler, A., 2004. *Contemporary South Africa*, Hampshire: Palgrave Macmillan.

Campbell, C., 2003. *"Letting Them Die": How HIV/AIDS Prevention Programmes Often Fail*, Cape Town: Double Storey.

Cherry, J., 2004. "Elections 2004: The Party Lists and Issues of Identity", *Electionsynopsis*, 1 (3): 6-9.

Chirambo K., 2003. "Impact of HIV/AIDS on Electoral Processes in Southern Africa", presentation at the UNDP/IDASA Satellite Conference on AIDS and Governance held at the 13th Icasa Conference, Nairobi, September 2003.

Chirambo, K. and Caesar, M. (eds) 2003. *AIDS and Governance in Southern Africa: Emerging Theories and Perspectives*, Pretoria: IDASA.

Chirambo, K., 2004. "AIDS and Electoral Democracy: Implications for Participation, Political Stability and Accountability in Southern Africa", IDASA, mimeo.

De Ville, J., 1996. "Proportional Representation: Formulae for the Translation of Votes into Seats", in De Ville, J. and Steytler, N. (eds) *Voting in 1999: Choosing an Electoral System*, 19-27.

De Ville, J. and Steytler, N. (eds) 1996. *Voting in 1999: Choosing an Electoral System*, Durban: Butterworths.

De Waal, A., 2003. "How Will HIV/AIDS Transform African Governance?", *African Affairs* (102): 1-23.

De Waal, J., Currie, I. and Erasmus, G., 2001. *The Bill of Rights Handbook*, Cape Town: Juta.

Dorrington, R., Bourne, D., Bradshaw, D., Laubscher, R. and Timæus, I.M., 2001. *The Impact of HIV/AIDS on Adult Mortality in South Africa*. Medical Research Council Technical Report, Burden of Disease Unit, Cape Town: MRC.

Dorrington, R., Bradshaw, D. and Budlender, D., 2002. *HIV/AIDS Profile in the Provinces of South Africa: Indicators for 2002*, Cape Town: Centre for Actuarial Research, Medical Research Council and the Actuarial Society of South Africa.

Dorrington, R., Bradshaw, D., Johnson, L. and Budlender, D., 2004. *The Demographic Impact of HIV/AIDS in South Africa: National Indicators for 2004*, Cape Town: Centre for Actuarial Research, South African Medical Research Council and Actuarial Society of South Africa.

Dwivedi, D., 2002. "On Common Good and Good Governance: An Alternative Approach", in Olowu, D. and Sako, S. (eds) 2002. *Better Governance and Public Policy: Capacity Building and Democratic Renewal in Africa*. Bloomfield: Kumarian Press.

EISA Election Observer Mission Report, 2004. *South Africa National and Provincial Elections, 12-14 April 2004*, Electoral Institute of Southern Africa.

EISA "Mauritius: political party funding" 2006 http://www.eisa.org.za/WEP/mauparties2.htm.

Elbe, S., 2002. "HIV/AIDS and the Changing Landscape of War in Africa", *International Security*, 27 (2): 159-177.

Elklit, J., 2002. "Lesotho 2002: Africa's First MMP Elections", *Journal of African Elections*, 1 (2): 1-10.

The Encyclopedia of Democracy, 1995. London: Routledge.

Epstein, S., 1996. *Impure Science: AIDS, Activism and the Politics of Knowledge*, Berkeley: University of California Press.

Evian, C., 2003. *Primary HIV/AIDS Care*, 4th ed., Durban: Jacana Media.

Faure, M. and Venter, A., 2003. "Electoral Reform in South Africa", University of South Africa/Rand Afrikaans University, South Africa, mimeo.

Fortin, A. J., 1990. "AIDS, Development, and the Limitation of the African State", in Misztal, B.A. and Moss, D. (eds) *Action on Aids: National Policies in Comparative Perspective*, New York: Greenwood Press.

Fox, R. and Southall, R., 2003. "Adapting to Electoral System Change: Voters in Lesotho, 2002", *Journal of African Elections*, 2 (2), December, 86-96.

Fredland, R., 1998. "AIDS and Development: An Inverse Correlation?", *Journal of Modern African Studies*, 36 (4): 547-568.

George, G., 2003. "Company Practices on HIV/AIDS in the Durban Metropolitan Area", HEARD, University of Natal.

Harris, P. and Reilly, B. (eds) 1998. *Democracy in Deep-Rooted Conflict: Options for Negotiators*. IDEA Handbook Series, Stockholm: IDEA.

Heywood, M., 2000. "HIV and AIDS: From the Perspective of Human Rights and Legal Protection", in Sisask, A. (ed.) *One Step Further: Response to HIV/AIDS*, Stockholm: Sida.

Heywood, M., 2000. in Jennings, R. *et al.*, 2002. *Discrimination and HIV/AIDS*, researched and written for the Department of Health.

Hope, K. R. (ed.) 1999. *AIDS and Development in Africa: A Social Science Perspective*, Binghampton: Haworth Press.

Hsu, L.-N., 2004. *Building Dynamic Democratic Governance and HIV/AIDS Resilient Societies*, Geneva: UNAIDS and UNDP.

Hunter, S., 2003. *Who Cares? AIDS in Africa*, New York: Palgrave Macmillan.

Hyden, G., 1992. "Governance and the Study of Politics", in Hyden, G. and Bratton, M. (eds) *Governance and Politics in Africa*, Boulder: Lynne Rienner, 1-26.

Hyden, G. and Court, J., 2002. "Comparing Governance Across Countries and Over Time: Conceptual Challenges", in Olowu, D. and Sako, S. (eds) *Better Governance and Public Policy: Capacity Building and Democratic Renewal in Africa*, Bloomfield: Kumarian Press.

Jennings R. *et al.*, 2002. *Discrimination and HIV/AIDS: S&T/ALP Research into the Nature and extent of HIV/AIDS discrimination*. Department of Health, South Africa.

Karume, S., 2004. "Party Systems in the SADC Region: In Defence of the Dominant Party System", EISA Occasional Papers Series No. 16, January.

Kauffman, K. D., 2004. "Why is South Africa the HIV Capital of the World? An Institutional Analysis of the Spread of a Virus", in Kauffman, K. D. and Lindauer, D. L. (eds) *AIDS and South Africa: The Social Expressions of a Pandemic*, New York: Palgrave Macmillan.

Kelly, K., Parker, W. and Gelb, S. (eds) 2002. "HIV/AIDS, Economics and Governance in South Africa: Key Issues in Understanding the Response", USAID, South Africa, mimeo.

Konrad Adenauer Foundation. 2003. "Electoral Models for South Africa: Reflections and Options", Johannesburg, mimeo.

Krennerich, M. and Nohlen, D., 1998. "Local Electoral Systems: Options for Reform in South Africa", in Atkinson, D. and Reitzes, M. (eds) *From a Tier to a Sphere: Local Government in the New South African Constitutional Order*, Sandton: Heinemann.

Lewis, J. D., 2004. "Assessing the Demographic and Economic Impact of HIV/AIDS", in Kauffman, K. D. and Lindauer, D. L. (eds) *AIDS and South Africa: The Social Expression of a Pandemic*, New York: Palgrave Macmillan.

Lodge, T., 2004. "The ANC and the Development of Party Politics in Modern South Africa", *Journal of Modern African Studies*, 42 (2).

Manning, R., 2003. "The Impact of HIV/AIDS on Local-Level Democracy: A Case Study of the eThekwini Municipality, KwaZulu Natal, South Africa", CSSR Working Paper No. 35.

Matlosa, K., 2003a. "Electoral System Reform, Democracy and Stability in the SADC region: A Comparative Analysis", Electoral Institute of Southern Africa (EISA) Research Report No. 1.

Matlosa, K., 2003b. "Survey of Electoral Systems and Reform Imperatives in the SADC region", Electoral Institute of Southern Africa (EISA), Occasional Paper No. 12.

Matlosa, K., 2004. "Democratic Governance and the Role of Political Parties in Parliament: the Case of Lesotho", paper prepared for a conference on Government and Opposition Roles, Rights and Responsibilities, jointly hosted by

Commonwealth Parliamentary Association, SADC Parliamentary Forum and FECIV, Maputo, Mozambique, 26-30 January.

Matlosa, K, 2004 "Electoral Systems, Constitutionalism and Conflict Management", African Journal on Conflict Resolution Vol.4, No.2

Mattes R. et al., 2000. Views of Democracy in South Africa and the Region: Trends and Comparisons, IDASA/CDD/UM.

Mattes, R., 2003. "Healthy Democracies? The Potential Impact of AIDS on Democracy in Southern Africa", Institute for Security Studies, Paper 71, April.

Mbali, M., 2004. "HIV/AIDS Policy-Making in Post-Apartheid South Africa", in Daniel, D., Habib, A. and Southall, R. (eds) State of the Nation: South Africa 2003-2004, Pretoria: HSRC Press.

Morna, C., 2004. Ringing up the Changes: Gender in Southern Africa Politics, Johannesburg: Gender Links.

Nattrass, N., 2004. The Moral Economy of AIDS in South Africa, Cambridge: Cambridge University Press.

Ngwembe, N., 2003. "Southern African Development Community Electoral Commissions' Forum: The Role of SADC-ECF in Mitigating the Impact of HIV and AIDS on Elections and Electoral Processes", in Chirambo, K. and Caesar, M. (eds) AIDS and Governance in Southern Africa: Emerging Theories and Perspectives, Pretoria: IDASA.

Nohlen, D., 1984. Elections and Electoral Systems, Bonn: Friederich Ebert Foundation.

Norris, P., 2002. Democratic Phoenix: Reinventing Political Activism, Cambridge: Cambridge University Press.

Olaleye, W., 2003. "Impact of AIDS on Participatory Democracy: Elections, Electorate and Electoral Systems", in Chirambo, K. and Caesar, M. (eds) AIDS and Governance in Southern Africa Emerging Theories and Perspectives, Pretoria: IDASA.

Olowu, D. and Sako, S., 2002. (eds) Better Governance and Public Policy: Capacity Building and Democratic Renewal in Africa, Bloomfield: Kumarian Press.

Ostergard, Robert L. Jr., 2002. "Politics in the Hot Zone: AIDS and National Security in Africa", Third World Quarterly, 23 (2): 333-350.

Panos/Unicef, 2001. "Stigma, HIV/AIDS and Prevention of Mother-to Child Transmission: A Pilot Study in Zambia, India, Ukraine and Burkina Faso".

Parker R. and Aggleton, P., 2002. HIV/AIDS Related Stigma and Discrimination, Population Council.

Reynolds, A. (ed.) 1994. Election '94 South Africa: The Campaigns, Results and Future Prospects, Cape Town: David Philip.

Reynolds, A. (ed.) 1999a. Election '99 South Africa: From Mandela to Mbeki, Cape Town: David Philip.

Reynolds, A. and Reilly, B., 1997. The International Idea Handbook of Electoral System Design, Stockholm.

Richter, L., Manegold, J. and Pather, R., 2004. Family and Community Interventions for Children Affected by AIDS, Cape Town: HSRC.

Sachs, M, 2001 " By-elections in 2001: a statistical review"

http://www.anc.org.za/ancdocs/pubs/umrabulo/umrabulo14/elections.html

Sachs, M., 2004. "Voting Patterns in the 1999 and 2004 Elections Compared", Electionsynopsis, 1 (4): 8-12.

Schönteich, M. and Pharaoh, R., 2003. AIDS, Security and Governance in Southern Africa: Exploring the Impact, Pretoria: Institute for Security Studies.

Schoofs, M., 2000. "Debating the Obvious: Inside the South African Government's Controversial AIDS Panel", Village Voice, July, 5–11.

Shilts, R., 1987. And the Band Played On: Politics, People and the AIDS Epidemic, New York: Penguin Books.

Shisana, O. (ed.) 2002. Nelson Mandela/HSRC Study of HIV/AIDS: South African National HIV Prevalence, Behavioural Risks and Mass Media, Cape Town: Human Sciences Research Council, Medical Research Council, Centre for AIDS Development Research and Evaluation, Agence Nationale de Recherches sur le Sida (ANRS).

Shisana, O. and Zungu-Dirwayi, N., 2003. "Government's Changing Responses to HIV/AIDS", in Everatt, D. and Mphai, V. (eds) The Real State of the Nation: South Africa After 1990, Johannesburg: Interfund.

Sisk, T. and Reynolds, A. (eds) 1998. Elections and Conflict Management in Africa, Washington D.C., United States Institute of Peace.

Smart, R., 1999. "HIV/AIDS in the Workplace:

Principles, Planning, Policy, Programmes and Project Participation", *AIDS Analysis Africa*, 10 (1): 5.

Southall, R. and Mattes, R. 2002. "Popular Attitudes Towards the South African Electoral System", CSSR Working Paper, No. 16, November, Centre for Social Science Research, University of Cape Town.

Southall, R., 2004. "Containing Accountability", *Election Synoposis*, 1 (1): 6-8.

Sparks, A., 2003. *Beyond the Miracle: Inside the New South Africa*, Johannesburg: Jonathan Ball.

Strode, A. and Grant, K. 2004. "Understanding the institutional dynamics of South Africa's response to the HIV/AIDS pandemic." Institute for Democracy In South Africa

UNAIDS, 2006. "Report on the global AIDS Epidemic 2006".

Van de Walle, N., 2001. *African Economies and the Politics of Permanent Crisis, 1979-1999*, Cambridge: Cambridge University Press.

Van der Vliet, V., 2004. "South Africa Divided Against AIDS: A Crisis of Leadership", in Kauffman K. D. and Lindauer, D. L. (eds) *AIDS and South Africa: The Social Expression of a Pandemic*, New York: Palgrave Macmillan.

Whiteside, A., 2000. "AIDS and the Private Sector", *AIDS Analysis Africa*, 10: 5.

Whiteside, A., 2002. "Poverty and HIV/AIDS in Africa", *Third World Quarterly*, 23 (2): 313-332.

Whiteside, A. and Barnett, T., 2002. *AIDS in the Twenty-First Century: Disease and Globalization*, Basingstoke: Palgrave MacMillan.

Whiteside, A., Mattes, R., Willan, S. and Manning, R., 2002. "Examining HIV/AIDS in Southern Africa Through the Eyes of Ordinary Southern Africans", *Afrobarometer Paper*, No. 12, August 2002.

Whiteside, A. and Sunter, C., 2000. *AIDS: The Challenge for South Africa*, Cape Town: Human & Rousseau and Tafelberg Publishers.

Willan, S., 2000. "Will HIV/AIDS Undermine Democracy in South Africa?", *AIDS Analysis Africa*, 11 (1): 14.

Willan, S., 2004. "Briefing: Recent Changes in the South African Government's HIV/AIDS Policy and its Implementation", *African Affairs*, 103: 109-117.

Wisten, Anne, forthcoming. "Does HIV/AIDS Generate Corruption? Testing a Link Between the Epidemic and Good Governance in Africa",

mini-thesis presented to the Department of Government at Uppsala University, Sweden.

Youde, J., 2001. "HIV/AIDS and Democratic Legitimacy and Stability in Africa", in Ostergaard, R. Jr (ed.) *HIV/AIDS and the Threat to National and International Security*, Hampshire: Palgrave Macmillan.

Zimbabwe Elections Support Network (ZESN) 2005 "By-elections in Zimbabwe, since the 2000 general election"

Election Manifestos and Policy Statements

African Christian Democratic Party (ACDP), 2004. *Election Manifesto.*

ANC, 2004. *Election Manifesto: A People's Contract to Create Work and Fight Poverty.*

Azanian Peoples' Organisation. *Azanian Peoples' Organisation Policy Positions.*

Democratic Alliance, 2004. *Election Manifesto: A Better South Africa; Solutions that Work: the DA's Solutions for HIV/AIDS: A Programme of Hope.*

Freedom Front+, 2004. *Election Manifesto.*

Independent Democrats (ID), 2004. *Election Manifesto: Bridging the Divides – Uniting South Africa behind a Common Vision; Health Policy of the Independent Democrats.*

Inkatha Freedom Party (IFP), 2004. *Election Manifesto: Real Development Now: Let's Make a Difference – Together; IFP AIDS Manifesto: an African and Immediate Response.*

New National Party (NNP), 2003. *Election Manifesto Nationally; Election Manifesto Western Cape: Cape Plan 2010 HIV and AIDS; Latest Developments on Comprehensive Treatment Plan, 19 November 2003; NNP's HIV/AIDS Perspective, statement by Dr Kobus Gous, NNP Spokesperson on Health, 13 February 2003.*

Pan African Congress of Azania (PAC), 2004. *Election Manifesto.*

United Christian Democratic Party. *Election Manifesto: Ready to Govern Where Others Have Failed.*

United Democratic Movement, 2004. *Election Manifesto: UDM Health Policy Proposals.*

Official sources

August and Another v Electoral Commission and Others (1999 (3) SA 1 (CC)).

Certification of the Constitution of the Republic of South Africa (10) BCLR 1253 (CC).

Constitution of the Republic of South Africa, Act No. 108 of 1996.

Department of Health (DoH), 2003. *National HIV and Syphilis Antenatal Sero-Prevalence Survey in South Africa: Summary Report*, Pretoria.

Department of Local Government and Housing 2004 HIV/AIDS framework document for the Department of Housing (Provincial Government of the Western Cape).

Department of Public Service and Administration (DPSA), 2000. *Impact and Action Report: Impact of HIV/AIDS on the Public Service.* November. Pretoria.

Economic Commission for Africa, 2004. *Striving for Good Governance in Africa: Synopsis of the 2005 African Governance Report Prepared for the African Development Forum IV*, Economic Commission for Africa.

EISA Election Observer Mission Report, 2004. South Africa National and Provincial Elections, 12-14 April, ISBN: 1-91981461-2, Electoral Institute of Southern Africa.

Electoral Commission Act, No. 51 of 1996.

Electoral Commission of Southern Africa, 2004. *Election Update*, No. 1, February.

Electoral Task Team, 2002. Report, 3.

Independent Electoral Commission (IEC), 1994. *Report on the National and Provincial Elections*, April.

Independent Electoral Commission (IEC), 1999. *Report on the National and Provincial Elections*, 2 June.

Independent Electoral Commission (IEC), 2004. Dataset from the voters' roll, detailing registered and deceased voters for the five years 1999 to 2003, for each gender, for each age cohort and for each municipality, Pretoria: IEC.

Independent Electoral Commission Act, No. 150 of 1993.

Local Government Municipal Structures Act, No. 117 of 1998.

Local Government Municipal Electoral Act, No. 27 of 2000.

Minister of Home Affairs v NICRO and Others CCT ¾.

New National Party of South Africa v Government of the RSA (1999 (3) SA 191 (CC)).

SADC Principles and Guidelines Governing Democratic Elections, 2004.

South African Government, 2003. *Towards a Ten-Year Review*, Pretoria.

Statistics SA, 2001. *Advanced Release of Recorded Deaths, 1997-2000: Statistical Release P0309.1, Statistics South Africa, Pretoria, December.*

Statistics SA, 2004. *Mid-year population estimates, South Africa.* Statistical release P0302. Pretoria: Statistics South Africa.

UNAIDS, 2002. *Report on the Global HIV/AIDS Epidemic,* July.

UNAIDS, 2003. *Epidemiological Update.* Geneva: UNAIDS.

UNAIDS, 2004. *Report on the Global AIDS Epidemic.* Geneva: UNAIDS.

UNDP, 2002a. *Human Development Report*, Oxford: Oxford University Press.

UNDP, 2002b. *Assessment of UNDP Assistance for a Multi-Sectoral National Response to HIV/AIDS in Tanzania.* Pretoria: UNDP.

UNDP, 2003. *South Africa Human Development Report 2003: The Challenge of Sustainable Development in South Africa: Unlocking People's Creativity*, Geneva: UNDP.

World Bank, 2000. *Intensifying Action Against HIV/AIDS in Africa: Responding to a Development Crisis*, Washington: The World Bank.

Abbreviations

AU	African Union
AIDS	Acquired Immune Deficiency Syndrome
ACDP	African Christian Democratic Party
ARV	antiretroviral
ASSA	Actuarial Society of South Africa
CARE	Centre for Actuarial Research
CBO	community-based organisation
CUBP	Clinic Upgrading and Building Programme
DA	Democratic Alliance
DoH	Department of Health
EC	Eastern Cape province
EISA	Electoral Institute of Southern Africa
ETT	Electoral Task Team

FGD	focus group discussion
FPTP	First Past The Post
GDP	gross domestic product
GIS	geographical information system
GNU	government of national unity
HDI	Human Development Index
HDR	Human Development Report
HPI	Human Poverty Index
HSRC	Human Sciences Research Council
ICASA	Independent Communication Authority of South Africa
ID	Independent Democrats
IDASA	Institute for Democracy in South Africa
IEC	Independent Electoral Commission
IFP	Inkatha Freedom Party
HDI	Human Development Index
HPI	Human Poverty Index
HSRC	Human Sciences Research Council
MEO	municipal electoral officer
MMP	mixed member proportional
MP	Member of Parliament
MTCT	mother–to–child transmission
Nacosa	National AIDS Committee of South Africa
NGO	non-governmental organisation
NNP	New National Party
PLWHA	people living with HIV/AIDS
PR	Proportional Representation
RDP	Reconstruction and Development Programme
SADC	Southern African Development Community
Sanac	South African National AIDS Council
STI	sexually transmitted infection
TAC	Treatment Action Campaign
UDM	United Democratic Movement
UNAIDS	Joint United Nations Programme on AIDS
UNDP	United Nations Development Programme
VAP	voting age population
WFP	World Food Programme

Tanzania

Flora Kessy, Ernest Mallya, Oswald Mashindano

1. Introduction

HIV/AIDS, which is a serious health and socio-economic problem in Tanzania, is considered to be a major development impediment that threatens all socioeconomic sectors. Accordingly, the government, in collaboration with different stakeholders, has committed several interventions, policies and strategies to forming specific institutions for coordinating its response to the epidemic.

The cost of operating electoral systems in Tanzania is likely to soar unless the government takes practical steps to prioritise disease management. The increasing number of deaths at leadership level and among the electorate might undermine the value of elections as a pillar of democracy. Little empirical evidence shows how exactly HIV/AIDS is likely to affect politics and what type of interventions can best counter it. Therefore, the Economic and Social Research Foundation (ESRF), jointly with Research and Education for Democracy in Tanzania (Redet), and supported by Idasa, undertook a study of the effect of HIV /AIDS on Tanzanian electoral processes.

2. Methodology

Four different data collection methods were employed in the study; document review; structured interviews; a public opinion survey and focus group discussions (FGDs).

2.1 Document review

The review analysed the legal and constitutional framework governing the conduct of elections; political manifestos; the status of the voters' roll (in relation to the size of the electorate and the availability of voter tracking and purging mechanisms); parliamentary records on the morbidity/mortality of MPs and Electoral Commission (EC) staff; the administrative capacities of the EC; and election results and voter turnout at the most recent elections. Research findings on HIV/AIDS-related issues were also explored.

2.2 Structured interviews

Structured interviews were conducted with National Assembly and EC representatives, as well as with members of political parties, which were represented in Parliament, as well as of political parties which, though not in Parliament, had nominated Presidential candidates for the October 2005 national elections. With regard to the National Assembly, the study focused on both the Social Services Parliamentary Committee and the Tanzania Parliamentarians' AIDS Coalition (Tapac), which is a non-governmental organisation (NGO) within the Parliament that is involved with HIV/AIDS-related issues. In Zanzibar, interviews were held with two House of Representatives members. Five members from the EC, consisting of three from the mainland and two from the Isles, were interviewed.

At the time of the 2005 general elections, 17 political parties existed in Tanzania. The five represented by Members of Parliament (MPs) in the current Parliament were sampled (see Table 2.1). As the sample represents more than 30% of the total number of political parties on the Tanzanian mainland, it is deemed statistically representative. Before embarking on the interviews, the research team investigated whether their political manifesto contained an HIV/AIDS-related agenda.

Interviews were held with the two major political parties of Zanzibar, the *Chama cha Mapinduzi* (CCM) and the Civic United Front (Cuf), as well as with a promising political party (Jahazi Asilia). The current HIV prevalence rate in Zanzibar is 0.87%,[1] so that little might yet have been done at political party level, as HIV/AIDS is regarded as a future threat only.

Table 2.1: Number of respondents from political parties		
Sn.	Name of political party	Number of leaders interviewed
Tanzanian mainland		
1.	Chama cha Mapinduzi (CCM)	3
2.	Civic United Front (Cuf)	3
3.	Chama cha Demokrasia na Maendeleo (Chadema)	3
4.	United Democratic Party (UDP)	3
5.	Tanzania Labour Party (TLP)	3
Zanzibar		
1.	*Chama cha Mapinduzi* (CCM)	3
2.	Civic United Front (Cuf)	3
3.	Jahazi Asilia	3

Parliament-related details were obtained from both Parliament and the EC offices. Interviews with parliamentary and political party representatives examined the extent to which HIV/AIDS had affected both their membership and leadership, as well as the ability of political parties to participate in democratic processes. The organisational policies of Parliament, political parties and the EC, as well as their contribution to national policy, were researched.

2.3 Public opinion survey

A brief analysis of public opinion survey data from the Idasa-driven Afrobarometer project was undertaken to understand the concept of public participation in politics and the perceptions of HIV/AIDS response. Round I (2001), round II (2003) and round III (2005) data were used.[2] The Afrobarometer is an independent, non-partisan research instrument that measures the social, political and economic atmosphere in Africa.

2.4 Focus group discussions

FGDs were used to collect data relating to citizen perceptions, particularly those of people infected and affected by HIV/AIDS and their ability to participate in the elections and the effect of HIV/AIDS on the electoral process, voter registration and the HIV/AIDS response. A total of 16 FGDs were conducted in two regions in Tanzania, one representing rural and another urban settings. While Dar es Salaam was sampled mainly because of its urban orientation and high prevalence rate (11%), Makete District in Iringa region (23% at the time of survey) was sampled not only because of its rural orientation and high HIV/AIDS prevalence rate, but also because the District has received significant attention from the media and from politicians. Section 10.1 in Chapter 10 provides the profile of FGD members.

3. HIV/AIDS in Tanzania

3.1 Demographic and epidemiological data

3.1.1 Mainland Tanzania[3]

The first cases of AIDS in Tanzania were reported in 1983 in the Kagera region in the North West. Since then, the number of cases has continued to rise at an increasingly faster rate, with, by 1986, just three years later, all regions of the Tanzanian mainland reporting AIDS cases. By the end of 1999, only a decade later, 118 713 AIDS cases were reported, with a comparable number of orphans. By 2004, the cumulative number of reported cases had risen to 192 532 (URT, 2005b). Figure 3.1 depicts the trend in reported AIDS cases from 1983 to 2004. So few cases were reported to the National AIDS Control Programme (NACP) from 1983 to 1986 that they were not characterised in terms of age group. Overall, the number of reported cases increased only gradually from 1983 to 2004, with a significant increase in the number of reported cases occurring between 1990 and 1993. However, the peak detected merely reflects aggressive data collection during the period and not a peak in AIDS morbidity as such.

According to two rounds of data collected by NACP, the infection rate among pregnant mothers attending antenatal clinics (ANCs) has declined (see Table 3.1). The 2003/2004 HIV surveillance results, when compared with those of the first ANC survey conducted in 2001/2002, show a decrease in preva-

Figure 3.1: Trend in reported number of AIDS cases in Tanzania (1983-2004)

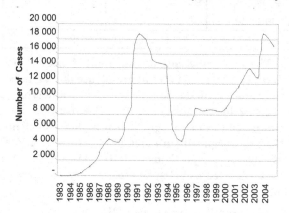

Source: URT (2005b).

lence in the Dar es Salaam and Mtwara regions, with the other regions experiencing negligible change. The HIV prevalence among women attending border clinics also fell from 17.3% to 15.3%. However, such changes are relatively minor, probably resulting from random variation in the different regions and sites.

Table 3.1: HIV prevalence levels found in ANC surveillance studies

Region	ANC surveillance 2001/02 HIV prevalence (%)	ANC surveillance 2003/04 HIV prevalence (%)
Dar es Salaam	12.8	10.8
Dodoma	6.1	7.8
Kagera	5.6	4.7
Kilimanjaro	6.3	5.7
Mbeya	16	5.7
Mtwara	7.1	5.1
Kigoma	ND	5.1
Lindi	ND	7.1
Morogoro	ND	9.0
Tanga	ND	9.2
Residence		
Urban	12.1	11.2
Semi-urban	3.7	4.7
Roadside	10.3	9.1
Border	17.3	15.3
Rural	4.1	3.7
Peak age	25–34	25–34
Overall prevalence	9.6	8.7

Source: URT (2003a); URT (2005b); ND = no data.

The HIV prevalence among blood donors is also declining. The 2002 overall prevalence of HIV infection among blood donors was 9.7%, reflecting a decrease of 1.3% from the 2001 11%, while women continued to show a significantly higher prevalence (12.3%) compared with men (9.1%). In 2002 a total of 1 894 160 people living with HIV/AIDS (PLWHAs) were reported as being between 15 and 49 years of age.

The overall prevalence of HIV infection among blood donors during 2003 was 8.8%, which is a decrease of 0.9% from the 2002 prevalence of 9.7%.

The sex-specific prevalence was recorded as higher among females at 11.9%, compared with that of 8.2% among males. In terms of such figures, in 2003 1 810 000 people (840 000 males and 960 000 females) were estimated to be PLWHAs.

The overall prevalence of HIV infection among blood donors during 2004 was 7.7%, which was a decrease of 1.1% from the 2003 prevalence rate of 8.8%. Such a decrease in prevalence has been noted for three years running among blood donors, with the decrease first being noted in 2002, when the sex-specific prevalence was higher among women at 10.7% compared with that among men of 7.2%. In terms of such figures, it is estimated that, in 2004 1 840 000 people were living with HIV (860 000 males and 980 000 females) on the Tanzanian mainland.

The sensitivity of HIV/AIDS to social context means that its prevalence varies strongly in terms of demography and regional pattern across Tanzania. The Tanzania HIV/AIDS Indicator Survey (This) 2005, a population-based survey shows, in contrast to the NACP figures, which are based on the number of blood donors and attendance at ANCs, that HIV/AIDS prevalence is higher in urban areas (12% for women and 9.6% for men), compared with rural areas, where it was found to be 5.8% for women and 4.8% for men (see Table 3.2). This 2005 further indicates that, overall, the regions with highest HIV prevalence rates are Mbeya (14%), followed by Iringa (13%) and Dar es Salaam (11%). Regions with the lowest (2% each) HIV prevalence levels are Manyara and Kigoma. Overall, seven regions had HIV prevalence levels below 5% (URT, 2005a). Again, in many regions, women have a higher degree of prevalence of HIV infection than do the men. In Pwani region, the prevalence of HIV infection among women is almost three times that of men, and the prevalence among women is twice that of men for Tanga, Singida and Tabora.

The predominant mode of HIV transmission has remained heterosexual, amounting to 78.1% of all reported AIDS cases in 2004, with mother-to-child transmission constituting 4.6% and blood transfusion 0.5%. In about 17% of the cases, the mode of acquisition of infection was not stated (URT, 2005b).

HIV prevalence is related to marital status, with formally married individuals having a higher prevalence rate (18%) than other groups. Single people who have never been in a relationship have a relatively low prevalence (3%), while those in a marital union were found to have intermediate HIV prevalence levels: 7% for men and 8% for women. Women

Table 3.2: HIV prevalence by residence and region

Residence	HIV prevalence (15–49 years)		
	Women (%)	Men (%)	Total (%)
Urban	12.0	9.6	10.9
Rural	5.8	4.8	5.3
Region			
Dodoma	4.2	5.7	4.9
Arusha	5.7	4.8	5.3
Kilimanjaro	7.3	7.4	7.3
Tanga	7.4	3.2	5.7
Morogoro	6.7	4.1	5.4
Pwani	10.5	3.9	7.3
Dar es Salaam	12.2	9.4	10.9
Lindi	3.5	3.6	3.6
Mtwara	7.1	7.7	7.4
Ruvuma	6.4	7.4	6.8
Iringa	13.4	13.3	13.4
Mbeya	15.2	11.5	13.5
Singida	4.2	2.1	3.2
Tabora	9.5	4.7	7.2
Rukwa	6.4	5.5	6.0
Kigoma	2.1	1.9	2.0
Shinyanga	7.6	5.3	6.5
Kagera	3.5	3.9	3.7
Mwanza	7.0	7.5	7.2
Mara	4.3	2.4	3.5
Manyara	2.0	1.9	2.0

Source: URT (2005a).

in polygamous unions are 10% more likely to be HIV-positive. HIV prevalence is sensitive to sexually risky behaviour, such as the number of sexual partners, the age of initial intercourse, condom use during sex, and other HIV risk-related characteristics, such as alcoholism and a recent history of sexually transmitted infections (STIs) (URT, 2005a).

Figure 3.2 shows the age and sex-specific cumulative case rates for 2004. The figure shows that females generally have a higher case rate than do males in the age group 15 to 39 years, though males have especially high case rates for the age group 40 years and above. The age group 25–44 years has a high case rate for both sexes.

Likewise, This 2003–2004 indicates that 7% of Tanzanian mainland adults were found to be infected with HIV, with the prevalence being higher among

Figure 3.2: Age and sex-specific distribution of reported AIDS cases, January-December 2004

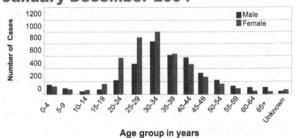

Source: URT (2005b).

women (8%) than men (6%). The findings, just like in the other studies, imply that women tend to be affected at a younger age than men, except among 15 to 19 year olds, for which the prevalence for both men and women was 2.1%, with the prevalence for women being higher than that for men between the ages of 20 to 39, while, between the ages of 40 and 49, the pattern reverses, with the prevalence being higher among men than women. The prevalence for both men and women increases with age until it reaches a peak, which for women is attained between the ages of 30 and 34 (13%) and for men between the ages of 40 and 44 (12%).

3.1.2 Zanzibar Islands

The trends of HIV infection in Zanzibar are increasing, albeit for some population subgroups. The total number of cases diagnosed has increased from 3 in 1986 to 3 926 in 2004 (see Table 3.3 and Figure 3.3). Newly reported HIV-positive patients among specific groups also support the general increase in the epidemic.

Research has shown that the HIV/AIDS epidemic in Zanzibar is concentrated in high-risk groups in three different population sectors: substance users (SUs), especially injecting drug users (IDUs); sex workers (both male and female) and their clients; and men who have sex with men (MSM). Studies carried out in 2005 showed that the HIV prevalence was 13% among SUs, and 26% among IDUs (Dahoma, Salim, Abdool, Othman and Abdullah, 2005). The vulnerable groups in the population are equally affected by the epidemic, given the likelihood that they will engage in unsafe sex.

Infection rates among voluntary counselling and testing (VCT) attendees also increased sharply from 0.6% in 2002 to 5.6% in 2003, but declined to 4.3% in 2004. HIV screening of donated blood doubled over the three-year period from 1996 (0.7%) to 1998 (1.5%), with a consequent decline to 0.5% in 2004. A much higher proportion of HIV-positive patients has been recorded among patients with STIs (5.6%) and tuberculosis (TB) (25.5%).

HIV/AIDS among pregnant women at ANCs has doubled from 0.3% during the mid-1980s, to 0.6% in 1997, to 1% in 2002. In general, women show infection rates that are five times higher than those of their male counterparts (0.9% and 0.2% respectively) (RGoZ, 2002). Accordingly, despite the low levels of infection among the general population, the rate of infection in certain subgroups is high.

Table 3.3: HIV infection rate in Zanzibar, 1986–2004

Year	Screened	Positive	HIV+ as % of screened
1986	83	3	3.6
1987	1 896	18	0.9
1988	3 294	51	1.5
1989	6 612	80	1.2
1990	7 248	110	1.5
1991	2 962	92	3.1
1992	3 862	84	2.2
1993	5 590	290	5.2
1994	3 293	174	5.3
1995	4 276	234	5.5
1996	4 453	161	3.6
1997	3 848	166	4.3
1998	4 951	163	3.3
1999	6 301	179	2.8
2000	5 002	108	2.2
2001	5 174	284	5.5
2002	6 833	497	7.3
2003	9 871	598	6.0
2004	13 577	634	4.7

Source: RGoZ (2005a).

Figure 3.3: Cumulative frequency of HIV infection in Zanzibar

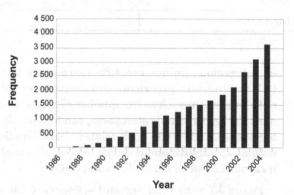

Source: RGoZ (2005a).

With prevalence estimates of less than 1%, the 20-year-old HIV/AIDS epidemic in Zanzibar has progressed relatively slowly, compared with the mainland (7% in 2004) or other neighbouring countries. Unprotected sex in heterosexual relations is the main route of transmission. Sexual intercourse, especially heterosexual, accounts for more than 90% of the transmission that occurs in Zanzibar. HIV transmission through body fluids and blood products in hospital settings is controlled/minimised through standard screening and the stringent application of sterilisation procedures for any invasive equipment used. HIV transmission through piercing and other surgical invasive equipment accounts for the remaining percentage. Guidelines and directives aimed at ensuring the following of aseptic techniques are now strictly followed in all health facilities. The Zanzibar AIDS Control Programme (ZACP) estimates that about 4% of HIV transmission is of a vertical nature, consisting of mother-to-child transmission, inclusive of the breastfeeding period.

In Zanzibar HIV has affected all age categories. Disregarding the age categories, due to the small sample taken, the overall HIV prevalence is nevertheless high in the age category >45 years in general, as well as more specifically for males, though it is also high in the age category 35–44 years for women. The infection rate has increased among 15 to 24-year-olds, compared with that experienced in the preceding year, though all other age categories indicate a declining trend.

3.2 Factors contributing to the spread of HIV/AIDS

Several factors contribute to the spread of HIV/AIDS in Tanzania, with community-based lifestyle, social and behavioural patterns being largely affected by cultural factors. For this study, contributory factors are grouped into conventional/societal factors and economic factors.

3.2.1 Conventional and societal factors

HIV/AIDS in Tanzania is predominantly transmitted through heterosexual contact (78%) due to ignorance and culturally affected social behaviours, exacerbated by alcoholism, infidelity, ignorance and carelessness (Kessy, Tax and Aiko, 2004). While especially children are not well informed about preventive measures, in some cultures sex among children is considered normal social behaviour for those as young as 10 years old, and is encouraged by parents. During the farming season, parents migrate from home to farm, leaving the children unsupervised and, thus, free to do as they wish. Living together and partner sharing (*kuazima*) is common. The "*mafiga matatu* culture" encourages brides to cultivate three sexual partners: her husband; her material provider and one to satisfy her sexual desire. Social gatherings at which people become intoxicated facilitate unplanned and unprotected sexual intercourse.

Condom promotion is thought to contribute to the spread of HIV/AIDS, as it is considered to lead to sexual risk-taking (Kessy *et al.*, 2004). However, even those who initially might have intended to use condoms do not do so due to anxiety, cultural barriers, and carelessness. Some are also unfamiliar with how to use them. The unavailability of protection and the stigma associated with requesting condoms from health facilities have led many to use plastic bags as protection.

The silence surrounding the HIV/AIDS epidemic has led to the families of PLWHAs risking contracting the virus through their care-giving.

In Zanzibar, substance abuse is increasing among the young. Needle-sharing between IDUs is com-

Table 3.4: HIV prevalence by age and gender among VCT attendees, 2004								
Age group	Tested			HIV-positive			Total	
	Males	Females	Not indicated	Males	Females	Not indicated	Total tested	HIV-positive
0–4	61	60	–	11.5	15.0	–	123	13.0
5–9	18	24	–	5.5	33.3	–	42	21.4
10–14	12	19	–	0.0	5.3	–	31	3.2
15–24	979	1 038	1	2.2	3.6	0	2 018	3.0
25–34	2 006	882	1	3.2	12.0	0	2 889	6.1
35–44	837	289	–	6.7	17.0	–	1 126	9.3
>45	504	243	11	8.0	12.7	1	758	9.5
Not indicated	1 841	1 563	2	2.0	4.7	0	3 404	3.3
Total	6 258	4 118	15	3.6	7.7	1	10 391	5.2
Source: RGoZ (2005a).								

mon, as is unprotected penetrative sex, rape and domestic violence due to drug abuse. Gender-related constraints induced by the patriarchal culture prevalent on both the Tanzanian mainland and Zanzibar empowers men to make all major decisions. Some of the sociocultural norms and values embodied in national policies and legislation regarding sexual practices lead to the setting of unattainable dowries, early and forced marriages, multiple partners, premature sexual relations, a high rate of teenage pregnancy, induced abortions, a high rate of STD infection, and the transmission of HIV/AIDS.

3.2.2 Economic factors

Due to poverty, women might become engaged in high-risk sex as a means of earning a living due to lack of alternatives. Their inability to negotiate for safer sex due to gender imbalances puts them at high risk. The so-called "mobile populations", which comprise those who work and stay away from home for some time, are both exposed to infection and, simultaneously, contribute to spreading the virus.

3.3 Impact of the epidemic[4]

A study by ESRF (2003) has identified the following economic and social variables for how the HIV/AIDS epidemic affects infected households, sectoral economic performance, and macroeconomic variables.

3.3.1 Impact on labour supply

HIV/AIDS-related mortalities and morbidities have shrunk the size of the workforce. Most PLWHAs were found to be in their economically and socially productive years, between the ages of 30 and 40. About 57% of those that experienced a death in the household in the year preceding the survey gave HIV/AIDS as the cause of death. HIV/AIDS also accounted for most deaths of teachers in that year, with the reported proportion of such deaths at district level for 2001 ranging from 40% to 100%. The total number of teachers' deaths per district due to HIV/AIDS-related illness ranged from 2 to 16 in 2002. The companies surveyed reported losing a yearly average of 6 employees.

3.3.2 Impact on productivity

The loss of productivity was examined in terms

of rate of absenteeism, total years of experience lost, and paid sick leave. All PLWHAs interviewed reported losing between 1 and 183 workdays, with an average of 43 days lost during the six months preceding the survey. About 26% of the PLWHAs attending the health facilities surveyed were granted paid sick leave during the same period, with the average sick leave lasting 3.6 months, within a range of 1 to 9 months.

Only 7 out of 27 teachers who died due to the effects of HIV/AIDS had fewer than 10 years experience, with the average being 15, with a minimum of 2 years and a maximum of 27 years. Their replacements were found, on average, to have only 3 years teaching experience. In the health sector, the mean for years of service of deceased employees ranged from 7 to 18 years. The companies surveyed reported losing employees with between 2 years to 29 years of experience, with an average of 6 years, in 2001. They also had an average of 6 employees on paid sick leave, losing between 60 to 1 530 workdays, with an average of 598 workdays per company, in 2002.

3.3.3 Impact on time allocation

HIV/AIDS was found to have affected the time allocation of both infected and affected households. About 8% of the individuals interviewed at household level indicated that they had attended to an HIV/AIDS patient in or outside the household during the 14 days preceding the survey, with most spending fewer than 5, or more than 20, hours. More than 43% of the female respondents and 36% of the men reported spending more than 20 hours during the fortnight preceding the survey caring for PLWHAs. Most of the respondents said that they spent at least 3 hours visiting PLWHAs during the same period. The household survey results further show that about 13% of the respondents reported attending a funeral, lasting from one to 280 hours, of someone who had died from HIV/AIDS-related complications during that period. Health care providers generally reported taking longer with PLWHAs than with patients suffering from other diseases, with, on average, each attending clinician seeing 32 patients per day, with an average 31 minutes spent with PLWHAs, in comparison to the fewer than 13 minutes spent with other patients.

3.3.4 Impact on financial resources

The medical treatment of opportunist infections results in increased expenditure on testing, drugs to cure both AIDS-related opportunistic infections and HIV/AIDS-related STIs, and both out- and in-patient care. The costs are borne by the PLWHAs, household members, extended family members and friends, employers, the private sector, the donor community and the government.

HIV/AIDS treatment, on average, costs more than that of any other health problem reported as affecting people at household level. Though PLWHAs did not report the highest expenditures, on average, the respondents incurred more expenses, with a mean in Tanzanian shilling (TZS) of 79 000 (US$63.25) and a median of TZS28 000 (US$22.42).[5] Workplace findings reveal that 21% of the companies surveyed provided specific medical support to employees living with HIV/AIDS. On average, about TZS11.76 million (US$9 419.30) a company were spent on providing such services in 2002, with a minimum of TZS80 250 (US$64.27) and maximum of TZS65 million (US$52 062.47). The rate at the time of writing is 1US$ = TZS1 248.5 .

Family support, terminal benefits, replacement costs and expenditure on preventive programmes have all increased due to the epidemic. An average cost of TZS158 000 per funeral was reported at household level, ranging from TZS2 000 (US$1.60) to TZS2 million (US$1 601.92). Individual households members' contribution to such costs ranged from TZS100 (US$0.80) to TZS300 000 (US$240.28), with a mean contribution of about TZS11 797 (US$9.44). The average household reported spending more on a funeral than their members contributed towards it, implying that households received funeral support from relatives, friends, employers, neighbours and other sources.

Most (86%) of the surveyed companies provided funeral support for the deceased. On average, TZS1.8 million (US$1 441.73) was provided in 2002, ranging from TZS60 000 (US$48.05) to TZS4.6 million (US$3 684.42). Transport and burial costs for teachers who died from AIDS-related illness constituted a large proportion of the total transport and burial costs (from 45% to 84% in 2002).

The companies surveyed reported spent an average of TZS7.22 million (US$5 782.93), ranging from TZS100 000 to TZS14 million (US$11 213.45) on 12 families of deceased employees in 2002. Only 10% of the companies surveyed had employees to whom they had to pay premature retirement benefits due to the employees experiencing HIV/AIDS-related problems. The total benefits paid ranged from TZS1.3 million (US$1 041.24) to TZS16.5 million (US$13 215.85), with an average of TZS10.3 million (US$8 249.89) in 2002.

3.3.5 Impact on delivery of social services

AIDS is also affecting the delivery of social services in both the educational and health sectors in staff attrition; decreased productivity, due to illness and absenteeism; and depletion of resources, which detracts from the delivery of quality education. The health sector is experiencing increased costs, loss of work hours and increased demands placed on health care staff. Antiretrovirals and the drugs needed for HIV testing and to cure opportunistic infections are exceptionally expensive.

3.3.6 Impact on demographic and macro-economic variables

The annual cumulative number of AIDS-related deaths is increasing, with most AIDS deaths being expected to fall in the 15 to 49 year age group, of which the members are most sexually active and at the height of their productivity. AIDS-related deaths are also projected to increase annually from about 99 000 deaths in 2000 to about 175 000 deaths in 2015, with the number of AIDS-related deaths a day increasing from 252 in 2000 to 480 in 2015. Population growth will tend to be 18% below what it would have been without HIV/AIDS, while the active workforce is likely to be 9% lower than it might otherwise have been, with women being worse affected than men.

The ESRF (2003) study found that, by 2015, 22% of the health budget is likely to be required for spending on HIV/AIDS-related patients. By 2015, 50% of hospital beds are likely to be occupied by HIV/AIDS patients, despite the economy shrinking by 8.3% due to the epidemic, with a drop in gross domestic product (GDP) of 4%.

3.3.7 The plight of orphans and the elderly

Orphans increased in number, as well as in school dropout rate, over the four-year period covered by the survey, with the consequent projection of 2.7 million by 2015, of whom 1.45 million are likely to be HIV/AIDS orphans. The dropout rate for orphans far exceeds that for other students, with that for girl dropouts being higher than that for boys.

Grandparents were caring for 34% of the orphans interviewed, of whom 51% said that their grandparents were also caring for other orphans. About 71% of the grandparents were caring for between one and three other orphans, while the remaining 29% were taking caring for up to seven other orphans. Most grandparents cannot afford to meet all the basic needs of the orphans, so that 15% were forced to earn their own keep.

3.4 Multisectoral response

3.4.1 Government policies and strategic efforts

3.4.1.1 Mainland Tanzania

History of government response to HIV/AIDS

In 1985, the Ministry of Health (MoH) formulated the NACP, consisting of a short-term plan (1985–1986), and three five-year medium-term plans (MTPs); MTP-1 (1987–1991), MTP-11 (1992–1996) and MTP-111 (1998–2002). Initially, HIV/AIDS was perceived purely as a health problem, with the national response developing strategies aimed at preventing, controlling and mitigating the impact of the HIV/AIDS pandemic by means of health education and community participation. HIV/AIDS was declared a national disaster in December 1999, resulting in the demand for a multisectoral approach (URT, 2001). In December 2000, Tanzania Commission for AIDS (Tacaids) was launched to spearhead the response, which was followed by the inauguration of a National Policy on HIV/AIDS in November 2001, and, in May 2003, a National Multisectoral Strategic Framework (NMSF) on HIV/AIDS 2003/07 (URT, 2003b). The NMSF is responsible for translating the National Policy for HIV/AIDS.

Government HIV/AIDS policy

The National Policy for HIV/AIDS aims to provide a framework for the leadership and coordination of the national multisectoral response to the HIV/AIDS pandemic. The policy emphasises the formulation, by all sectors, of appropriate interventions aimed at effectively preventing the transmission of HIV/AIDS and other STIs. In terms of the policy, vulnerable groups are protected and supported, while the socioeconomic impact of HIV/AIDS is mitigated.

The national policy maintains that HIV/AIDS is a social, cultural and economic problem, so that its prevention and control largely depend on effective community-based prevention, care and support

interventions. In strengthening the capacity of institutions, communities and individuals in all sectors to arrest the spread of HIV/AIDS, the policy uses local government councils to coordinate both the public and private sector, NGOs, faith-based organisations (FBOs) and other groups in planning and implementing HIV/AIDS interventions (URT, 2001).

The policy aims to:

- Prevent HIV/AIDS transmission;
- Promote HIV testing;
- Ensure the provision of care for PLWHAs;
- Mobilise adequate financial resources for HIV/AIDS-related activities;
- Provide a framework for promoting and coordinating multisectoral and multidisciplinary research into HIV/AIDS, as well as for disseminating and applying the research findings;
- Create a legal framework by enacting HIV/AIDS-related legislation;
- Monitor community mobilisation in support of living positively with HIV/AIDS;
- Safeguard the rights of PLWHAs by improving their quality of life and minimising stigma;
- Provide appropriate treatment for opportunistic infections throughout the health care system;
- Fight against substance abuse, which increases the risk of HIV transmission; and
- Prohibit misleading advertising of products meant to prevent, treat and cure HIV/AIDS.

HIV/AIDS programmes fall into the following NMSF categories (URT, 2003b):

Crosscutting issues

- Advocacy;
- Resistance to stigma and discrimination;
- District and community responses;
- Mainstreaming of HIV/AIDS; and
- HIV/AIDS and development/poverty reduction.

Prevention

- STI control and case management;
- Condom promotion and distribution;
- VCT;
- Prevention of mother-to-child transmission (PMTCT);
- Health promotion among specific vulnerable groups;

- School-based prevention at primary and secondary level;
- Workplace interventions;
- Safety of blood products; and
- Universal precautions.

Care and support

- Medical and nursing care;
- Psychosocial support; and
- Food and other material support.

Impact mitigation

Structures and institutions for implementing government programmes

Mechanisms have been instituted to facilitate the coordination, management, and implementation of the national response.

Roles and functions at national level

The NMSF translated into specific plans, programmes, projects and interventions. Tacaids has been responsible for the following (URT, 2003a):

- Compiling policy guidelines for the response to the HIV/AIDS epidemic and the management of its consequences on mainland Tanzania;
- Developing a strategic framework for all HIV/AIDS control programmes and activities falling within the overall national strategy;
- Fostering national and international linkages among all stakeholders through coordination of all HIV/AIDS control programmes and activities within the overall national strategy;
- Mobilising, disbursing and monitoring, and ensuring the equitable distribution of resources;
- Sharing HIV/AIDS-related information;
- Promoting the high-level advocacy of, and education on, HIV/AIDS prevention and control;
- Monitoring and evaluating all continuing HIV/AIDS activities;
- Coordinating HIV/AIDS management;
- Facilitating efforts to find a cure, to promote access to treatment and care, and to develop a vaccine;
- Protecting the human rights of PLWHAs; and
- Advising the government on all HIV/AIDS-related matters.

The MoH and NACP are responsible for service delivery, especially in regard to prevention and care intervention; blood safety and VCT; the distribution of HIV/AIDS-related products and health education materials and research, and may exert technical jurisdiction over related policy-making. Other ministries are also responsible for instituting HIV/AIDS plans, policies and activities in their respective sectors (URT, 2003c).

Roles and functions at regional level

At the regional level, the regional administrative secretary (RAS) and regional technical entities play an intermediate role in planning, implementing and monitoring activities, by:

- Compiling district HIV/AIDS operational plans and reports and forwarding them to the Prime Minister's Office, Regional Administration and Local Government (PMO – RALG) and Tacaids;
- Providing technical help to districts and communities;
- Forming a regional consultative committee and a regional forum for discussing and documenting multisectoral HIV/AIDS responses at regional level.

Roles and functions at district and village levels

Local government councils are responsible for coordinating all HIV/AIDS-related activities in the respective districts. Local government councils are focuses for involving and coordinating both the public and private sector, NGOs and FBOs in planning and implementing HIV/AIDS interventions through the council, ward (WMACs) and village multisectoral AIDS committees (VMACs). They also ensure the mainstreaming of HIV/AIDS in council plans and budgets from hamlet level up, with all levels of local government being charged with policy-making, budgets, decision-making and service delivery.

3.4.1.2 Zanzibar Islands

The history of the national response

Shortly after the first three cases of HIV/AIDS were detected in 1986, the Zanzibar government formulated a short-term plan (1987–1988) aimed at creating public awareness and training health personnel. In 1987, ZACP was set up under the Ministry of Health and Social Welfare (MoHSW). MTPs I

(1989–1991) and II (1992–1996) consolidated and expanded the initial interventions and motivated behaviour change, ensuring blood safety, health counselling and care. MTP II involved the community in providing HIV/AIDS-related education and counselling. MTP III (1998–2000) provided a framework for multisectoral response in the setting up of the autonomous Zanzibar AIDS Commission (ZAC) in line with the realisation by the government of the need for a national legislative focus with defined mandates for coordinating the national response, mobilisation and advocacy, including monitoring and evaluation.

The Zanzibar AIDS Commission

In September 2002, the Zanzibar government set up ZAC under the Chief Minister's Office to coordinate the national response to the HIV/AIDS pandemic. ZAC has three operational sections: Finance and Administration; Policy, Planning, National Response and Advocacy; and Information, Education and Communication (IEC). The commission is funded by the government to perform largely routine operations and to coordinate funding supplied by its development partners.

HIV/AIDS policy

Based on the findings of the situation and response analysis undertaken in 2003, the Zanzibar National HIV/AIDS Strategic Plan 2004/5–2008/9 was developed. The plan focuses on the prevention of HIV/AIDS transmission among vulnerable groups, including certain workers, such as the military and police; sex workers and their clients; substance abusers; mobile traders; and people with disabilities; as well as among the workforce as a whole. The health sector focuses on HIV/AIDS-related prevention, treatment, care and support. The plan is key to supporting impact mitigation and crosscutting issues, like coordination, advocacy, capacity-building and resource mobilisation (RGoZ, 2004).

The overall mission of the national HIV/AIDS policy implemented in Zanzibar in 2006 leads and coordinates the national multisectoral response aimed at reducing infection and related socioeconomic factors. It strives to enhance the capacity of key role-players to develop and implement relevant interventions sensitive to gender and human rights.

Coordination of the national response

ZAC coordinates the HIV/AIDS response through its

Board of Commissioners, its secretariat and various consultative boards. The district AIDS coordinating committees (Daccoms) coordinate response at district level, and there is a Shehia AIDS Coordinating Council (Shaccom).[6]

Coordination of the national response is achieved through:

- Quarterly meetings of ZAC commissioners;
- The Principal Secretaries Committee on HIV/AIDS;
- Public sector technical committee meetings;
- Consultative stakeholder meetings;
- A technical committee;
- A technical platform between various stakeholders, including UN agencies and international NGOs; and
- Zanzibar NGO Cluster for HIV/AIDS Prevention (ZANGOC) meetings and activities.

3.4.2 Non-state actors' response

3.4.2.1 Mainland Tanzania

The multisectoral Tanzanian responses to HIV/AIDS have involved the government, the private sector, development partners and civil society. While some such players provide sources of funding or act as intermediaries, others provide crosscutting services. The NMSF demands that Tacaids strive for a regular consultative forum with HIV/AIDS-related NGOs regarding participation and support at district and community levels (URT, 2003b).

Bilateral and multilateral aid for HIV/AIDS

Most national spending on HIV/AIDS is sourced from bilateral and multilateral foreign aid and international corporations. The total amount of aid has increased from TZS14 494 million in 2001/02, to TZS39 962 million in 2002/03, and from TZS53 200 million in 2003/04 to TZS66 103 million in 2004/5, while government funding increased from TZS2 296 million in 2001 to TZ7 050 million in 2002/03, flattening out in 2003/04 and 2004/05, at which time it was TZS14 500 million and TZS 14 582 million respectively (URT, 2005c).

According to its NMSF on HIV/AIDS, Tanzania encourages partnering with development partners in implementing NMSF through joint planning, management, resource mobilisation and allocation, as well as monitoring and evaluation. The conditions of such partnership are clearly set out in articles 3 and 4 of the Memorandum of Understanding between the United Republic of Tanzania (URT) (mainland) and Development Partners regarding the implementation of the NMSF on HIV/AIDS. Donors, therefore, largely determine how HIV/AIDS interventions occur.

The private sector

The private sector contributes substantially to the fight against HIV/AIDS in Tanzania by funding and providing services. Private hospitals and health centres, while providing curative and preventive services, also offer charitable support to PLWHAs and orphans. The private sector also funds prevention, advocacy, care and support programmes implemented by community-based organisations (CBOs), NGOs, FBOs and government departments and agencies. Most Tanzanian PLWHAs have spent out of pocket on HIV/AIDS.

Civil society

Civil societies (like CBOs, NGOs and FBOs), media institutions, as well as associations of PLWHAs play a key role in the fight against HIV/AIDS in Tanzania, intervening in several areas ranging from crosscutting issues, prevention, care and support to impact mitigation. In 2004, 142 organisations providing HIV/AIDS-related services were identified (Kessy, 2005).

Traditional healers

Over 60% of Tanzanians rely on traditional healing (URT, 2003d) to treat opportunistic infections. The Tanga AIDS Working Group has proved such healing to be effective in heightening the immunity of HIV/AIDS patients.[7] Though modern practitioners tend not to approve of such methods, the Tanzanian government recognises the role played by traditional and alternative healing in countering HIV/AIDS.

3.4.2.2 Zanzibar Islands

Partnership with development partners

The Zanzibar–UN programme focuses on four major operational areas: policy and planning; advocacy; monitoring and evaluation; and care and treatment. The commission, which cooperates with bilateral partners on capacity-building and resource mobilisation, holds joint forums with the Donor Group on HIV/AIDS, which meet on a quarterly basis. Development partners are involved with priority setting; policy-making and strategic planning, as well as with programme design, implementation, resource mobilisation and monitoring and evaluation.

The foreign financial sources which are the major source (more than 80%) of funding for HIV/AIDS activities in Zanzibar, consist of the World Bank, the Global Fund, the United States government and the United Nations (UN). Except for the latter two bodies, all other funds are channeled through ZAC.

Civil society organisations

Civil society organisations (CSOs) and networks have focused on prevention, awareness, support, impact mitigation and VCT. NGOs are clustered together in ZANGOC. FBOs are coordinated by the Zanzibar Association of Interfaith on AIDS and Development (ZAIDA). CSOs, through Zanzibar Against AIDS Infection and Drug Abuse (ZAAIDA), have also worked to counter HIV/AIDS-related substance abuse.

However, the participation of CSOs still largely depends on the funding available from development partners. As in the public sector, the NGO response is constrained by the lack of capacity to design, implement and mobilise resources, as well as to monitor and evaluate programmes.

The private sector

The involvement and participation of the private sector is poorly coordinated, depending on individual businesses. ZAC has recently started to involve the private sector in the planning and coordination of various programmes, as well as in the setting up of the AIDS Business Coalition in Zanzibar (ABCZ).

Religious organisations

As Zanzibar is predominantly Muslim, religious leaders need to be involved with the fight against HIV/AIDS. The FBO response to HIV/AIDS started with MTP III, which encouraged religious leaders through open meetings and sermons to ban extramarital sex and to insist on morally sound behaviour. ZACP and ZAC conducted sensitisation meetings to inform and obtain the cooperation of religious leaders in fighting the epidemic.

As their contribution to the fight, the Office of the

Mufti has spearheaded the HIV/AIDS Guidelines for the Zanzibar Muslim Community, which aims to provide user-friendly information on HIV/AIDS, consistent with the Islamic perception of mobilising and educating the Muslim community in Zanzibar in the fight against HIV/AIDS (Mufti's Office, 2004).

4. HIV/AIDS and democratic governance

4.1 Democratic governance: Historical perspective

4.1.1 Tanzanian mainland

URT comprises mainland Tanzania (Tanganyika) and Zanzibar. The mainland attained its independence under the leadership of the Tanganyika African National Union (Tanu) on 9 December 1961. The Afro-Shirazi Party (Asp) staged a revolution in Zanzibar on 12 January 1964, while the Union was created on 26 April 1964. Legally, Tanu was the sole political party on the mainland from 1965 while Asp remained the only political organisation in Zanzibar. On 5 February 1977, Tanu and Asp merged to form the ruling CCM.

The government of the United Republic has jurisdiction over all union matters throughout the Republic and over non-union matters on the mainland, while the Revolutionary Government of Zanzibar (RGoZ) has jurisdiction over all non-union matters in Tanzania and Zanzibar.

4.1.1.1 Political leadership

The Tanzanian system of political leadership is part presidential and part parliamentary, with the cabinet being chosen from among legislative representatives and the executive forming part of the legislative process. Upon electoral victory by his or her party, the prime minister becomes the chief executive and the leader of government business in the legislature, participating daily in the house. Often someone else will be the head of state, playing a background, arbitral stabilising role, with powers ranging from the almost purely ceremonial to ones that carry much more weight.

In presidential systems, the head of the government is mandated by popular vote as both the head of government and state. The president appoints a prime minister, often from the majority party that controls government business in the legislature. If the majority party in the legislature is not that of the president, the prime minister shares executive power with the president. Such power-sharing does not reduce the power of the president.

The executive president is empowered by combining the functions of the head of government and head of state, effectively eliminating any checks or balances within the executive. Moreover, the cabinet is often the sole preserve of the president in a presidential system. As the president is usually popularly elected, he/she is even more legitimate than the legislators due to his/her national constituency.

The parliamentary system may be regarded as fused, since members of the executive are also members of the legislature. Due to ready access to resources, such as information, the executive tends to dominate the legislature over time. Since the Tanzanian system is partially parliamentary, with members of the executive forming an active part of the legislature, the executive dominates the legislature as well as the presidency, the terms of which are included in both the Union and Zanzibar Constitutions.

4.1.1.2 The apportionment of power among branches of the government

The scheme of checks and balances of power spread out among the three major branches of the government was devised to prevent any one branch from becoming tyrannical, or from becoming so disjointed that it paralyses the government. The apportionment of governmental powers in Tanzania has changed over time, with each major change relating to an identifiable historical period.

The colonial and single-party legacy

Colonial rule was a command mode of governance in which the legislature and the judiciary were largely fused into the executive for most of the time. Towards the end, though, a paternalistic legislature, which was mostly appointive and numerically dominated by government officers, was instituted, and a relatively separate judiciary was created. Only as colonial officers were departing at decolonisation did they try to leave a balanced arrangement of power in place. For Tanganyika, then, Britain designed a parliamentary system in which the chief executive's power could be curtailed both within the executive branch by the presence of the governor-general and the cabinet, and among the different government branches by the Parliament through a motion of no confidence in the government. Its success depended on a formal constitutional arrangement and the existence of a vigorous opposition party. However, in 1962 the Constitution was changed to usher in the now familiar half-presidential, part-parliamentary system. In 1965 the opposition parties, consisting of the African National Congress and the All Muslim National Union of Tanganyika, which had effectively withered away by then, were formally abolished to bring in the single-party system.

Parliament, having immediately lost a great deal of its power, had to compete with the party organs for rule-making. Eventually the latter triumphed, with the legislature becoming subordinate to the executive through the latter's leadership of the party. Such an arrangement was entrenched in the permanent Constitution of 1977, so that only in 1984 was the status of the Tanzanian legislature enhanced by means of Act No. 15 of 1984, which was the fifth amendment to the 1977 Constitution. The said extensive Act also enshrined the Bill of Rights in the Constitution. In terms of the apportionment of power, the amendment provided for the separation of powers in article 4, which clearly defined the role of each branch of the government. However, checks and balances were few. All three branches – the legislature, the executive and the judiciary – were to operate with the understanding that the ultimate authority in the country was the CCM, as clearly stated in articles 3 and 10 of the Constitution.

The multiparty amendment

After the switch to a multiparty political system in 1992, a review of the Constitution to expunge the notion of the single party and its supremacy was undertaken, resulting in the passing of Act No. 4 of 1984 (the 8th Amendment). The amendment modified at least 40 of the 152 articles of the Constitution, with the most notable changes occurring in articles 3, 10, 37, 41, 44, 63, 66, 67, 72, 78, 80, 81 and 104, which had referred to the supremacy of the party and its monopoly on politics. Such change paved the way, at least in the formal constitutional sense, for a plural and competitive system. The amendment shared more power among the three branches. Article 37 (2) elevated the Speaker of Parliament to the status of a participant, and the Chief Justice to that of ultimate authority, as regards determining whether a president may be removed from office due to disability.

Previously, the ultimate authority rested with the Party's National Executive Committee, of which the Speaker was not a member. Similarly, article 44 (2) abolished the Party's role in approving a declaration of war by the president, assigning that to the Speaker and the Parliament.

Other constitutional amendments

The 9th Amendment, effected by Act No. 20 of 1992, not only gave Parliament the power to remove a prime minister through a vote of no confidence (articles 51 and 53A), but also the authority to prosecute and possibly remove a delinquent president by means of a 20% parliamentary vote in favour of impeachment (article 46A). Article 90 first came to delineate the conditions permitting the president to dissolve Parliament, as previously he/she had discretionary powers to do so.

The significance of the 13th constitutional amendment, which was enacted in 2000, as regards the apportionment of powers lies in three areas. First, the list of appointments, usually associated with executive presidents and enshrined in both the Tanzanian and Zanzibar Constitutions (articles 33 to 37 and 51 to 54 respectively), has now been shortened. Second, the judiciary has gained stature by requiring that the two top leaders of the all-important national EC, as well as those of the Commission for Human Rights and Good Governance, be judges of the court of appeal or high court, or qualified as such. The independence of the judiciary has been clearly affirmed (articles 107(A1) and 107(B1)). Third, the Constitution now authorises the president to appoint up to 10 people to Parliament, in this way clearly tilting the power relation between the Executive Branch and the Legislature (Mallya, 2000).

4.1.1.3 The status of the judiciary

The 1984 amendments gave the judiciary the constitutional power of judicial review (including, the authority to remove an unconstitutional Act). The judges of the high court and the court of appeal (the highest appellate court), though appointed by the president, enjoy tenure until retirement age, unless removed on the recommendation of a panel of peers appointed by the Commonwealth of Nations. The president alone appoints the Chief Justice, with whom he/she is constitutionally compelled to consult when appointing other judges of the court of appeal. Similarly, the president must also consult with the Judicial Service Commission (chaired by the Chief Justice) in the appointment of high court judges. With the multiparty constitutional changes, the Chief Justice enhanced his/her position by becoming the ultimate authority in determining the fate of a sick or debilitated president, and in chairing the special committee of inquiry into whether a president has committed impeachable offences.

4.1.1.4 The Bill of Rights

The Fifth Amendment introduced the Bill of Rights as a result of a protracted human rights lobby. Any existing laws that limit such rights were called "bad" by the Nyalali Commission, which recommended the adoption of a competitive plural system in 1991. One such "bad" law is the decree that a politically appointed district commissioner should authorise a political party to hold a rally.

The high court interprets the legally entrenched freedom of assembly to mean that a party needs to inform the police only so that security arrangements for the rally may be made. The police, however, have seen the law as authorising the barring of a rally if security is threatened. Rallies of the more militant or strongest opposition parties have so often been barred by the police that the latter appear to be ordered to do so by the ruling party.

4.1.2 Zanzibar

4.1.2.1 Formation of political parties

The Zanzibar Nationalist Party (ZNP) was founded in December 1955, while Asp was founded in February 1957 after the merger of two ethnic associations; the African Association, formed in 1934, and the Shirazi Association, formed in 1938. Intraparty conflict resulted in Asp members forming the breakaway Zanzibar and Pemba People's Party (ZPPP) in 1959. The smaller Communist Party of Zanzibar was founded in 1962, with some ex-ZNP members forming the Umma Party in 1963.

The setting up of one-party rule in Zanzibar followed a different trend to that on the mainland, where Tanu enjoyed the support of almost the entire population before independence. In Zanzibar, the two main political parties, Asp and ZNP, both had different interests and had a large number of supporters. When the ZPPP decided to form an alliance with the ZNP, the people of Zanzibar were virtually divided.

4.1.2.2 Political leadership

Zanzibar is part of the United Republic of Tanzania, which comprises a union between the State of Zanzibar, comprising the two main islands of Unguja and Pemba, and the Republic of Tanganyika. The two sovereign states united on 26 April 1964 to form URT in such a way that both governments retained a certain degree of power.

While the Tanganyikan government ended on union, with Tanganyikan domestic affairs being handled by the Union government, Zanzibar retained its own legislature, executive, and judiciary. The articles of union stipulated which affairs were to be treated as Union matters, thus falling under the Union government, and which remained under Zanzibar control. Zanzibar still maintains a separate foreign reserve and has the capacity to negotiate and enter into agreement with both local and foreign parties on all domestic matters.

Zanzibar has its own government within the United Republic of Tanzania, which is called the Revolutionary Government of Zanzibar (RGoZ), known in Kiswahili as *Serikali ya Mapinduzi ya Zanzibar* (SMZ). The government, which was set up under Chapter Four of the Constitution of Zanzibar of 1984 (Articles 26 to 62), is headed by a president and chief minister (*Waziri Kiongozi*). The cabinet is called the revolutionary council. The president is elected by all the people of Zanzibar for a term of five years, which may only be renewed once. The executive arm of the Zanzibar government is also provided for in Part I of Chapter Four of the Constitution of the United Republic of Tanzania of 1977 (articles 102 to 104). Article 105 of the same Constitution provides for the Zanzibar Revolutionary Council and its functions.

Article 106 of the Union Constitution provides for the Parliament for the RGoZ. The members of the house are a mixture of elected, appointed and *ex officio*. The Parliament of Zanzibar, which is called the Zanzibar House of Representatives (*Baraza la Wawakilishi*), is provided for in Chapter Five of the Constitution of Zanzibar of 1984 (articles 63 to 92). Parliamentary representatives are elected by means of a general election held every five years throughout the 50 constituencies in both Zanzibar and Pemba. Their main function is to enact laws for Zanzibar and to endorse other commitments.

4.1.2.3 The status of the judiciary

Zanzibar has its own judiciary under the chief justice of Zanzibar, with the highest court being the high court of Zanzibar, which gains its legitimacy from Chapter Six of the Tanzanian Constitution and articles 114 and 115 of the Constitution of the United Republic of Tanzania. The subordinate courts, consisting of the regional courts, district courts and primary courts, are set up under the Magistrates' Court Act of 1984.

Apart from sharing the court of appeal of the United Republic with mainland Tanzania, Zanzibar has a distinct and separate legal system. The URT Constitution clarifies that the high court of Zanzibar is not a Union matter. Article 114 of the Constitution of Tanzania expressly reserves the continuance of the high court of Zanzibar institutions with their jurisdiction. Similarly, the attorney-general's chambers of Zanzibar fall outside the purview of Union matters, as it is a department of the RGoZ, forming part of the portfolio of the Minister of State in the Chief Minister's Office.

The judicial system of Zanzibar comprises a high court, the subordinate kadhis' and magistrates' courts and tribunals. Appeal is made to the appeal court of the United Republic except for constitutional and religious court issues, which are settled by the high court. High court judges are appointed by the president in consultation with the Judicial Services Commission (Constitution of Zanzibar, 1984, articles 93, 94 and 99).

5. Impact of HIV/AIDS on electoral systems

5.1 Elections, electoral systems

We have already alluded to the creation, at least formally, of a permitting environment for enhanced electoral competition that was ushered in by the Multiparty Amendment. We also referred to its modification of qualifications for candidature. Here two results were produced. One was the removal of certain disabilities such as previous detention. The other was the retention of party membership as a requirement for candidature. The latter has been seen as a denial of constitutional rights of those people who want to participate in politics without being forced to become party members. The question asked is why should one be a party member in order to seek political office?

Among other recent amendments related to elections is the constitutional authorisation, now in place, that may have the Parliament, through an enactment, take away a citizen's right to vote because he/she has been convicted of electoral offences [Art. 5(2)]. This is apparently in response to increasing corrupt practices during elections. In addition, a Permanent Voters Register (PVR) was established in 2005, in response to many calls for such a register, and in view of the numerous complaints that accompany registration, as well as the escalating costs of fresh registration for every election.

There is a controversial amendment relating to when the term of a parliament ends. The constitution still maintains that the term ends with the dissolution of Parliament, but stipulates further that the duties and rights of a parliamentarian (including, most importantly, his/her financial benefits) end only when a new election has been completed. This obviously adds to the government bill, but also increases the advantage, financial or otherwise, of an incumbent Member of Parliament. In the 2000 election in particular, this may have favored the ruling party, CCM, which has many more incumbent parliamentarians than others.

Another recent amendment is the requirement that candidates, including presidential ones, should not have any unpaid legitimate taxes, otherwise they will be disqualified. The Constitution has also moved from requiring a majority (or absolute majority) to a plurality (or simple majority) of votes for a winning presidential candidate. This has raised concern over the possibility of getting a minority president, and even of a president essentially elected by a limited geographical zone or a single ethnic group.

The Constitution now requires a plurality (or simple majority) of votes for a winning presidential candidate, with the possibility of a minority president who is essentially elected by a limited geographical zone or a single ethnic group.

Though the PVR is electronic, its management faces:

- The lack of a reliable vital statistics database, resulting in reliance on ward and village leaders for details of the fluctuating population;
- The cost of hiring competent and incorruptible managers, especially at regional level;
- Difficulties in identifying Tanzanians in border regions, where people might have the same surname as others in neighbouring countries; and

- Given the prevailing political competition and culture of corruption, the names of some deceased might remain on the PVR, allowing for forgery.

On mainland Tanzania, the applicable law is the Elections Act No. 1 of 1985, which governs the election of the president and MPs of the United Republic of Tanzania. Local government and town council elections fall under the Local Authorities (Elections) Act, 1979 (Act No. 4 of 1979).

All elections in Zanzibar are governed by the Elections Act No. 11 of 1984, which governs the election of the president of Zanzibar, members of the House of Representatives and representatives to local councils. The Zanzibar Municipal Council Act No. 3 of 1995 is also important. Section 7 of the 1984 Zanzibar Constitution provides for the right to vote, while section 21 provides for the right of every Zanzibar resident to participate freely in all public affairs, including the right to participate in governing the country, either directly or through representatives who are elected voluntarily. Section 7 offers every Zanzibari the right and freedom to participate fully in deciding on which issues are pressing.

5.2 The electoral systems

Two common electoral systems shape and influence voting behaviour and election results in liberal democracies. First, the plurality or majority system, which is also referred to as the FPTP electoral system, can either be absolute or relative. At present the system is applied in many former British territories in Africa. The second type of electoral system is the PR system.

5.2.1 The First-Past-The-Post system

Since independence, the results of constituency elections in Tanzania have been determined by the Westminster principle of the FPTP electoral system. The 1977 Constitution provides for the country to be divided into a certain number of electoral districts, each to be represented by one representative (single-member constituencies). The parties participating in the election in a constituency nominate an election candidate, with the candidate with the most votes being seen as the winner (relative majority). Thus, most MPs and local councillors are elected by means of a single-district plurality system (URT, 1979). Candidates stand in parliamentary constituencies or local council wards, with the candidate who obtains the most votes winning the seat. The whole country has been demarcated into 231 constituencies, with each constituency electing one MP.

The system of FPTP benefits the large parties, so that the country might be ruled by one dominant party for a long time. Small parties, with relatively few supporters and sound national policies, might, accordingly, not be able to make it into Parliament and may even disappear if regulations deregistering political parties that do not garner a given percentage of votes, are enforced. In a multiparty political system, the concept of parliamentary democracy requires that the party securing more than half the total number of seats form the government (Nyalali Commission, 1991).

In the 1995 Tanzanian parliamentary election, for example, though the "opposition" parties polled a total of 36% of the votes, they won only 20% (46) of the seats, while the CCM, which polled 59% of the votes, won 80% (186) of the seats. Omitting Cuf, which won 22 seats with only 5% of the votes (due to the small size of the Zanzibar constituencies), the picture changes dramatically, as the remaining opposition parties polled 31% of the votes, while winning only 11% (24) of the seats (Bomani, 1996).

5.2.2 The Proportional Representation system

Women have special seats in Parliament and on the local councils. In both elections, every contesting political party is required to provide a list containing a given number of names. In the 2000 elections, the special seats were allocated to the political parties in proportion to the share of plurality seats obtained. In the 2005 elections, seats were allocated in proportion to the number of valid votes obtained by a political party, in accordance with the 14th Amendment of the Constitution of February of the same year (URT, 1977, Constitution, section 78 [1]).

5.2.3 The accessibility of suffrage

5.2.3.1 Entitlement to register

Any citizen aged 18 years or more has the right to register as a voter and to vote in any public election held in Tanzania. A citizen loses the right to vote if he/she is:

- Under a declaration of allegiance to some country other than Tanzania;

- Under a sentence of death imposed by any court in Tanzania;

- Under sentence of imprisonment for a term exceeding six months (short-term prisoners are allowed to register and vote, with special provisions being made for voting to take place outside prison buildings);

- Disqualified from registering as a voter by law; or

- Declared to be of unsound mind (URT, Elections Act, 1985, section 11 [1] a–d).

Before the PVR was introduced, registration was redone for each general election and by-election. The PVR, which was compiled from mid-2004 to April 2005, was used in the general elections of the same year. Nec, which has custody of the PVR, directs its updating (URT, 1985, Elections Act, section 15 [1]).

Such updating will involve deregistering those who are disqualified from the PVR and registering those who become qualified. Decentralisation of updating will involve each voting district in respect of its territorial area.

5.2.3.2 Registration process

Under the PVR system, persons qualified to vote register in the polling districts where they normally reside. Potential voters must personally complete an application form at the registration centre where their picture and fingerprints are taken, and be ready to answer any questions put to them by the registration assistants. A resident whose application is allowed is issued with a voter's card, bearing a picture of the holder, as well as a unique number. Copies of the records, which are stored centrally with the NEC in Dar es Salaam, are made for each polling district and are available in the districts.

5.2.3.3 Rejection of applications

If a person fails to qualify to register, his/her application is rejected, with the record of each rejection, and the reasons for it, being maintained by the registration assistant. A prescribed form is issued to the applicant, who is also informed of the right to appeal.

5.2.3.4 Appeal against a rejection of an application for registration

If a returning officer (RO) upholds the decision of a registration assistant, he/she is required to set out his/her grounds for dismissing the appeal. Any applicant aggrieved by the decision of the RO has the right of appeal against that decision to a court presided over by a resident magistrate. The appeal must be submitted within 21 days after the receipt of the RO's written statement. The resident magistrate must notify the parties concerned, stating details of the appeal, which must be heard by the resident magistrate in open court. If the appeal is successful, the resident magistrate who has determined the appeal is required to inform the RO of the name of the person to be registered (Election Act, 1985, section 15 [2]).

5.2.3.5 Objections against registration

At the end of the registration period, an RO is required to display the PVR prominently to enable registered voters, candidates and political parties to inspect the register of the polling district concerned. A registered voter may object to the retention in the PVR of his/her own name or the name of another person where such person is not, or is no longer, qualified to be registered as a voter or where such person has died. The RO has to send notices of objection to those whose inclusion in the roll has been objected to, stating the details regarding where and when their complaints will be heard. He/she also has to hold a public inquiry into all objections which have been made as soon as is practicable. Any person aggrieved by the RO's decision may appeal to a court presided by a resident magistrate. The resident magistrate's determination of appeal is final and conclusive (URT, Elections Act, 1985, sections 21–31).

5.2.3.6 Offences and penalties

No person may:

- Intentionally give any false statement with the aim of procuring a registration card for himself/herself or for another person;

- Present himself/herself for another registration as a voter;

- Present himself/herself for registration as a voter in a polling district while his/her earlier application in another district is pending investigation;

- Forge or fraudulently deface or fraudulently destroy any certificate of registration or duplicate certificate of registration or any official mark on such certificate of registration; and

- Upon conviction, such a person is liable to a fine of between TZS100 000 and TZS300 000 or to imprisonment for a period not exceeding two years or both (URT, Elections Act, 1985, section 88 [a–e]).

5.2.4 Composition of Parliament and House of Representatives

5.2.4.1 The Parliament (2000–2005)

The 2000–2005 Tanzanian Parliament had 295 members, composed of the following:

- 231 constituency members (181 from the mainland and 50 from Zanzibar);
- 48 special seats for women members (between 20% and 30% of all MPs);
- 10 MPs nominated by the president;
- Five members elected by the Zanzibar House of Representatives;
- The attorney-general of URT, who sits in Parliament as ex officio (Nec, 2001).

Only five political parties won constituency seats in the 2000 elections, with the breakdown being as follows at the time of dissolution of Parliament in August 2005: CCM (199); Cuf (17); *Chama cha Demokrasia na Maendeleo* (Chadema) (4); the Tanzania Labour Party (TLP) (4); and the United Democratic Party (UDP) (1). NEC declared 48 women elected to the special seats (CCM (41); Cuf (4); TLP (1); UDP (1) and Chadema (1).

According to the recent amendment of the Constitution (2005), (also referred to as the 14th Amendment), the 2005–2010 Parliament could comprise up to 324 MPs, with the number of special seats for women being raised to 30%. The number of women who are special seats members is now

75, with the other women MPs being elected by the constituencies. Since January 2000, the president has been authorised by constitutional amendment to appoint up to ten members who need not belong to parties and may be chosen for their expertise or their social representation (Constitution of the United Republic of Tanzania, 1977, article 66 [1]).

The current Parliament comprises 320 MPs, though it is supposed to have a grand total of 323 MPs,[8] consisting of 232 members elected by the constituencies, 75 special women's seats, five members elected by the Zanzibar House of Representatives, an attorney-general and six presidential appointees. The remaining three MPs have yet to be appointed by the president. In terms of party representation, CCM has 275 MPs; Cuf, 31; Chadema, 11; and TLP and UDP one each. The total number of woman in the house is 97, comprising 30.4% of all MPs, with 16 women MPs elected from the constituencies.

The House of Representatives in Zanzibar is composed of the members indicated in Table 5.1.

5.3 Impact of the epidemic on electoral systems

5.3.1 The economic costs of HIV/AIDS

Economic costs incurred due to the loss of elected representatives include those related to holding of by-elections, care for the ill and the dying, including direct and indirect funeral expenses. As the number of deaths increases, the costs to the treasury will rise, which has many implications for the resources required to deal with the FPTP system.

Tanzanian by-elections have largely resulted from MPs dying or being moved to other non-elec-

Table 5.1: Composition of the House of Representatives (2005–2010)

	Total	Current total	CCM (ruling party)	Cuf (opposition)	Male	Female
Elected members	50	50	31	19	48	2
Presidential nominees	10	6	6	–	5	1
Special seats – women	15	15	9	6	–	15
Registered commissioners	5	–	–	–	–	–
Attorney-general	01	1	1	–	1	–
Total	81	72	47	25	54	18
Percentage	100	96.29	77.78	18.51	71.6	24.7

NB: The statistics in this table were obtained from the Zanzibar Electoral Commission (ZEC) in mid-March 2006. More appointments might have been made since then to the vacant positions/seats existing at the time.

tive political positions. However, the advent of the multiparty system has given rise to by-elections from successful petitions against winners deemed to have assumed power fraudulently. More recently, by-elections have resulted from mismanaged elections. The 2000–2005 Parliament experienced 17 Pemba by-elections due to gross irregularities, with about six others arising from the deaths of MPs.

On mainland Tanzania, a manual by-election cost about TZS500 000 000 (about US$416 000) before the introduction of PVR. In Zanzibar, a by-election for an MP and nine councillors cost TZS54 000 000 (about US$45 000) in total.[9] By-elections cost much more on the mainland than they do in Zanzibar, as the former has electoral zones with more than 100 000 eligible voters, while the latter has constituencies with 2 000 voters.

MPs are being asked personally to donate to multiple AIDS-related funerals and attend burials for members of their constituencies. In November 2006 MPs were found to incur costs ranging from between TZS200 000 (about US$157) and TZS1 000 000 (about US$787) a year due to HIV/AIDS. Further, each MP interviewed claimed to have lost a close relative due to HIV/AIDS, with one maintaining a clinic to treat PLWHAs. Some people seek financial help from their MPs in Dodoma during parliamentary sessions.[10]

More by-elections have taken place since the reintroduction of multiparty politics than before, due to interparty competition. To curb settlement of issues procedures within party caucuses, the Elections Act was amended during the 2000–2005 parliament session, stating that anyone intending to file a petition had to pay about 5 million shillings (US$4 167) as a down payment to the court. The need for such payment raised concerns about how the rights of citizens were being restricted in respect of their democratic right of appeal, despite a legal challenge to such an amendment being successful, Parliament quickly amended the law again, so that the case could not be decided by the courts. The payment of 5 million shillings is still demanded. While taxes should be used for development activities rather than to finance "unnecessary" by-elections, while the amendment is considered to infringe on the right of citizens to access the courts.

5.3.2 The political costs

On the Tanzanian mainland, six constituencies had no MPs at the time of the December 2005 general elections, as the incumbents had died in the course of the 2000–2005 Parliament. The views and needs of citizens from these electorates have therefore not been represented for some time.

When an MP dies, the development of a constituency is halted before the calling of a by-election. Even after a by-election, the constituency might be governed by a new MP who does not honour the development efforts of the former MP due to differences in political ideology.

Hypothetically, the Parliament might also suffer due to the loss of expertise and experience of the deceased or those suffering from opportunistic infections, detracting from effective policy-making and the quality of debate in the house. MPs felt that new, young MPs have enlivened parliamentary debate, though one MP lamented:

> Kuna Waheshimiwa Wabunge ambao tunawamiss hasa wakati wa majadiliano Bungeni kama akina marehemu …. (Names withheld) … lakini hatujui chanzo cha vifo vyaomeaning (We are missing some of the deceased honourable MPs, particularly during parliamentary debates, for instance … [Names withheld] … however, we do not know the cause of their deaths.)

5.4 Electoral system reform debate

In early 1995, the government published a Bill which would have introduced PR into Tanzania's parliamentary elections, but it was withdrawn, "apparently due to misconceived allegations that those seats were meant as a gift to the new political parties or, cynically, that they were intended for some party bulwarks" (Bomani, 1996).

In terms of the 14th Amendment of the Constitution, the smaller parties in Tanzania could be represented in Parliament through the special seats for women which will be apportioned according to the votes gained by a political party, though the threshold will be 5% of all valid votes (URT, 1977, Constitution, section 78 [1]).

However, activists want the PR system to be applied to some constituency seats as well. Introducing PR seats alongside constituency representation might diminish the effects of the winner-take-all system connected to the simple majority electoral system. Parliament would then have two groups of legislators: one comprising those elected from the constituencies on a simple majority basis and a second selected on a proportional basis, with the entire country serving as one constituency and each party nominating MPs according to the number of votes it received.

If the PR system had been applied in Tanzania for the 1995 general elections, the opposition parties would have been allocated at least 83 of the 232 constituency seats, showing that the system tends to reflect the relation of seats to votes more accurately. The Nyalali report however, cautions that PR has its drawbacks. In a multiparty system, such drawbacks might prevent any single party from forming a viable government, due to the need to form coalition governments, which might lead to political instability. A combination of the two systems is preferable to switching from one system to another (Bomani, 1996; Fimbo Report, 1995).

While the opposition favours system change, the ruling party opposes it. During the single-party era one could have proposed that the candidate who came second at the polls accede to the seat once an MP died, but with multiparty democracy, the second in line would represent a different political party. The party losing an MP would want to contest the seat through the polls. One MP stated:

> You cannot eliminate and/or reduce the cost of electoral process by abolishing by-elections, because democracy is always very expensive. What is important is to campaign and work hard towards a war against the spread of the disease, rather than struggling to reduce and/or avoid costs such as those related to by-elections. We should work on the root cause rather than the outcome.

Given the current HIV prevalence rate of 7%, the probability is that, of every 100 individuals, seven are HIV-positive in the National Assembly. Given the debilitating nature of HIV/AIDS, the psychological suffering, stigma and illness resulting from opportunistic infections, efforts geared towards reducing infections among the members of the House are imperative.

6. Impact of HIV/AIDS on parliamentary configuration

Both Parliament as an institution and parliamentarians as individual leaders can play a significant role in contributing to the improvement of the quality of good governance in Tanzania at both the national and local level. The impact of HIV/AIDS might inhibit Parliament's legislating and enacting policies and programmes. The deaths and sickness of MPs might deprive Parliament of what might otherwise have been valuable contributions by the affected MP and representation of the constituency. HIV/AIDS might cause a rise in government expenditure through by-elections having to take place to fill vacancies left by deceased MPs. However, such loss can be avoided if Parliament acts appropriately to prevent the spread of HIV/AIDS among its members.

6.1 Parliament and HIV/AIDS

6.1.1 Mortality rates

HIV/AIDS could be one of the major causes of deaths of members of the National Assembly, as seen in the following quote from the Report on Assessment of the HIV/AIDS Impact on the National Assembly of URT in 2005 (URT, 2005d): "The impact of HIV/AIDS has started to show on Members of Parliament and their functioning. This is becoming evident in terms of the number of by-elections and increased demands from the constituencies to deal with the issue."

Since 1991, a total 31 MPs have died,[11] of whom four died from motor accidents and shooting incidents while the rest died of either short or long-term illnesses of which the nature was undisclosed. Mortality rates in the House of Representatives in Zanzibar are low. During the 1990–1995 Parliament two deaths (both of women) occurred, while during the 1995–2000 Parliament one death (of a woman) occurred. During the 2000–2005 Parliament, two deaths (both of men) occurred. Contrary to mainland Tanzania, where the HIV prevalence is high, the prevalence of HIV/AIDS in Zanzibar is low, so that the likelihood that these deaths were HIV/AIDS-related is also low. An increasing number of deaths and by-elections is envisioned (URT, 2005d).

MPs expressed a belief that Parliament had not lost expertise, experience and vibrancy in the house due to HIV/AIDS. The house is as active as ever and none of the deceased has been officially declared a casualty of the disease. Though MPs have admitted that sometimes the cause of death of a member has seemed to be HIV/AIDS, no official proof of such is available.

One participant during the research inception workshop referred to the loss of his MP:

> Our MP was sick for a long time and one day we were told that he got very sick while attending parliamentary sessions in Dodoma and he passed away. All his development efforts at our constituency were halted because it took two years before a by-election was called.

6.1.2 Parliamentary membership

Most (65%) MPs are in their 40s and 50s, with their average age being 52 years. About 8% of the MPs are younger than 40. Compared with the previous Parliament (2000–2005), age-wise, most (84%) previous MPs did not fall in the group (15–49 year olds) most at risk to HIV/AIDS, while those in the current Parliament are. As about 37% of the MPs fall in the age group with the highest risk level (as they tend to be younger than the previous parliamentarians), they are as susceptible to the virus as the general population (see Table 6.1). Apart from age, their risk is increased by other factors, such as the nature of their work and their enhanced liquidity. The risks to which MPs are exposed are shown in the following quote (URT, 2005d):

> HIV and AIDS is a problem of the entire society, of which MPs are a part. MPs are at high risk for several reasons: They come for sessions, which are sometimes very long, such as the budget session, but their spouses do not accompany them. Many visitors also come to Dodoma during the parliamentary sessions to take advantage of the increased money in circulation and to lobby for interventions and assistance from MPs and Ministers. Some of the visitors may be persons with high-risk sexual behaviour and in the interactions that take place MPs may become exposed or vice versa.

Table 6.1: Age of Tanzania's parliamentary membership		
Age (years)	Proportion in 2000-05 Parliament*	Proportion in 2006-10 Parliament**[12]
<30	–	1.07
30–39	2	7.14
40–49	14	28.93
50–59	40	46.07
60–69	36	15.00
70+	8	1.78
Note: *Adapted form URT (2005d); **Own calculations		

6.2 Debates on HIV/AIDS in National Assembly[13]

6.2.1 Legislative debates

Little HIV/AIDS-related legislation has taken place, though the national HIV/AIDS policy provides for the formulation of HIV/AIDS-related law. Stakeholder input is usually sought when the committees are involved with lawmaking. Tanzania's legal framework is characterised by a pluralistic legal system, which is influenced by ancient traditions, Islamic law and the colonial heritage. Statutory law regulates both customary and Islamic law. The 2001 National Policy on HIV/AIDS is the only comprehensive instrument that provides a framework for leadership and coordination of the national multisectoral response. HIV/AIDS has been included as an internationally notifiable disease under the Infectious Diseases Ordinance, which is seen by human rights activists as infringing on the rights of PLWHAs.

The Review and Assessment of the Laws Affecting HIV/AIDS in Tanzania by the Tanzania Women Lawyers Association (Tawla) recommends the enactment of comprehensive legislation to support the national policy. Such law would also serve to address gaps in the national policy, including that pertaining to HIV/AIDS as it affects people with disabilities, refugees and VCT policy guidelines, which have not yet been promulgated. Some of the specific recommendations from Tawla on areas for HIV/AIDS-related law reform are:

- The state monitoring and enforcement of human rights;
- Media laws;

- Control of food quality, given the nutritional needs of PLWHAs;
- Harmful traditional practices;
- Women, children and other vulnerable populations;
- Criminal justice and correctional systems; and
- Protection of the rights of PLWHAs.

6.2.2 Other debates

During the past few years, the amount of HIV/AIDS-related discussion and debate has increased considerably. The URT (2005d) classified the HIV/AIDS-related discussions in terms of the contents of *Hansards*:

- *The Tacaids Bill*: Lengthy discussions and debates have taken place, especially in terms of the mandate and operational mechanisms. The location of Tacaids in the PMO was challenged and the removal of the coordination of HIV from the MoHSW was questioned. Tacaids has received much criticism relating to the embezzlement of funds, laxness, subjectivity and ineffectiveness. Tacaids has been able, through its criticism, to effect change and reform in institutional policies and strategic plans.

- *Rape and the deliberate transmission of HIV/AIDS*: A concern for many MPs over the years, the need for appropriate legislation bearing harsh penalties has been recognised.

- *Traditional and alternative medical practices*: MPs have asked the government to exert control over such practices so as to ensure the safety of their constituencies. False claims of HIV/AIDS cure and misleading advertisements are controlled by law.

- *TB and HIV/AIDS*: Members raised concerns about the increase in the number of TB cases, due to its link to HIV.

- *Orphans*: MPs expressed concern about the lack of service provision by the government for orphans, as it has left much of such work to NGOs.

- *Security*: The army wanted an increase in HIV/AIDS awareness campaigning in the military, which has not yet been penetrated by AIDS-based NGOs and CBOs. The Commission for Human Rights in Tanzania has noted serious violations of human rights in prisons, where conditions could fuel homosexual (men who have sex with men [MSM]) behaviour.

- *VCT*: MPs have been encouraging one another to take the HIV test.

- *Behaviour change*: MPs were concerned that while people know about HIV/AIDS, little behaviour change has occurred. Edutainment was suggested as a way of addressing such change.

- *Care and treatment*: MPs wanted to learn about the latest developments in care and treatment.

- *Budgetary allocations*: Concern about allocations and disbursement was expressed. MPs felt that lack of finances is a major impediment to their more active participation in the HIV/AIDS battle. Concern was also expressed about how funds earmarked for HIV/AIDS were used at all levels in relation to accountability and efficiency issues.

- *Culture*: The link between HIV/AIDS and culture was discussed and seen from the perspective of cause as well as prevention.

- *Homosexuality*: MPs feel that this phenomenon is growing in importance as a cause of HIV/AIDS and therefore must be adequately addressed.

- *Government response*: Parliamentarians are concerned about the role of Tacaids, as well as the effectiveness of current strategies and activities, such as workshops for town-based persons and officials.

- *AIDS and the economy*: Impacts on development efforts have been discussed and acknowledged.

- *Preventive methods*: Those who recommend condom use see them as an effective control method and recommend their use, while others see them as encouraging promiscuity and as a source of HIV infection.

6.3 Parliamentary response to HIV/AIDS

6.3.1 Parliament and HIV/AIDS

HIV/AIDS is frequently discussed in the Social Services Committee, which is directly responsible for the MoHSW, and the Constitutional, Legal Affairs and Administration Committee, which is directly responsible for the Prime Minister's Office where Tacaids is situated.[14] All such standing committees have an important role to play in dealing with HIV/AIDS and its linkages to specific sectoral issues, which the committee deals with as part of its normal business.

Though the Parliament Workplace Programme was developed in 2005, by the time of writing it had not yet been fully implemented. The programme has adopted the following strategies:

- Internalisation and adaptation of the HIV/AIDS national policy;

- Creation of a separate parliamentary budget to fight HIV/AIDS;

- Informed and educational prevention and positive living strategies;

- VCT; and

- Condom availability and proper use.

Parliamentary HIV/AIDS-related resources have been limited (URT, 2005d). MPs have expressed the need to work more on HIV/AIDS-related issues in their constituencies, but have cited lack of funds as a key issue. The report proposes an action plan for parliamentarians for HIV/AIDS-related interventions. With a parliamentary action plan in place, funding will become available from both the government and the donor community. With an increased budget and further elaboration of the role of MPs, the oversight role played in terms of spending priorities and budgets is bound to become more active.

The Tanzanian Parliament has linked up with relevant role-players both within and outside the country. Within Tanzania, the Parliament has links to government institutions dealing with HIV/AIDS, the donor community and development organisations. The Tanzanian Parliament is represented at the Southern Africa Development Community – Parliamentary Forum (SADC–PF). Many such links have been developed through Tapac.

6.3.2 Tanzania Parliamentarian AIDS Coalition (Tapac)

Formed in 2001, Tapac is the foremost HIV/AIDS organisation in the Tanzanian Parliament. Its origin stems from heightened appreciation by parliamentarians of the necessity to become more active on HIV/AIDS matters. Some of the organisation's key aims and objectives, according to its constitution, are:

- To act as a spokesbody for HIV/AIDS-related issues both inside and outside Parliament;

- To fight for the rights of HIV/AIDS-affected persons and to ensure that they are neither discriminated against, nor alienated by society;

- To foster and collaborate with other countries'

parliamentarians which share the same objectives in the fight against HIV/AIDS;

- To ensure that multisectoral national strategies and financial plans for combating HIV/AIDS that directly address the epidemic by confronting issues of stigma, silence, denial and gender, as well as the full participation of PLWHAs, those in vulnerable groups and people mostly at risk, are maximally resourced in terms of the national budget;

- To encourage and pressurise for legislation and government commitment to the protection of the basic rights and fundamental freedoms of the PLWHA and vulnerable groups, including women and youth;

- To generally raise AIDS awareness among parliamentarians and communities by way of media and constituencies;

- To ensure that the resources provided for the country's response to address HIV/AIDS are substantial, sustained and directed at achieving results;

- To ensure that there is are increased and prioritised national budgetary allocations for the HIV/AIDS programme; and

- To ensure that all ministries and other relevant stakeholders make sufficient budgetary allocations to reach grassroots level.

Membership of Tapac, which stands at about 180, is open to current and previous MPs from all parties. Since it is an NGO and not an integral part of the parliamentary system, it depends on donor funds and membership fees. Tapac organises activities to empower MPs and has been playing an advocacy role to ensure greater leadership commitment at parliamentary level. Most MPs have only been involved with HIV/AIDS-related activities through Tapac. While Tapac has placed HIV/AIDS issues on the agenda, it needs to play a greater role in mainstreaming such issues into the work of the standing committees. Only further capacity-building will ensure effective implementation of countermeasures. Tapac might lead the way for other countries to mobilise MPs around HIV/AIDS-related issues.

Tapac has made inputs into the amendment of the HIV/AIDS policy. Further, given the active role played by Tapac, Parliament has encouraged the government in deciding to provide care and antiretrovirals for PLWHAs. Efforts are under way to sensitise MPs to the importance of passing the HIV Bill.

6.3.3 House of Representatives

The House of Representatives in Zanzibar passed an HIV/AIDS policy in 2006. The House itself is aware of the threat that HIV/AIDS poses to Zanzibar. All members of the House belong to the non-profit NGO the House of Representatives Coalition against HIV/AIDS (which, in Kiswahili, is *Umoja wa Wawakilishi wa Kupambana na Ukimwi Zanzibar*) (UWAKUZA). UWAKUZA was set up by members of the House of Representatives in 2003 to educate, sensitise and mobilise society to participate in the fight against HIV/AIDS, and to encourage the positivity of PLWHAs. The NGO aims to check the spread of HIV among members and employees of the House and their families. UWAKUZA organises meetings at which members discuss HIV/AIDS-related strategies to be adopted in the constituencies, how to sensitise people about the impending pandemic, and how to forge connections with ZAC.

Employees of the House have a workplace Technical HIV/AIDS Committee (Tac), on which the office of the chief minister is represented by one person. The secretary of UWAKUZA is also an employee of the House. The House allocates only 10 million shillings, which is enough to cover only the costs of the meetings. The committee is unable to participate in other activities due to lack of funding. ZAC noted that it receives much cooperation from members of the House and UWAKUZA, as well as from individual members in their constituencies.

6.3.4 Other organisations in Parliament/ House of Representatives

Other relatively small organisations in the Parliament/House of Representatives that are gaining momentum include: the Tanzania Women's Parliamentary Group (TWPG) and the Tanzania Parliamentary Association for Population and Development (TPAPD) on the Tanzanian mainland and the House of Representatives Women's Association (which, in Kiswahili, is *Umoja wa Wawakilishi Wanawake Kupambana na Ukimwi Zanzibar*) (UWAWAZA) in Zanzibar. TWPG and TPAPD deal with HIV/AIDS issues as they arise. One of their key constraints is limited resources, especially in terms of doing more extra-parliamentary work. The women's organisation in the House of Representatives has not yet done any substantive work on HIV/AIDS, as it is still in its infancy.

6.3.5 Other parliamentary initiatives

Some MPs have had their sero status tested voluntarily. MPs have invited PLWHAs to share their experiences with Parliament in the hope of reducing the level of stigma. MPs also discuss the pandemic at meetings held in their constituencies, to which they have invited children infected with HIV/AIDS for meals. MPs have noted that they were not the only driving force in formulating and adopting the AIDS policy, but, nevertheless, recognise that they are key stakeholders and were frequently consulted in its formulation.

7. Electoral administration

7.1 Structures, staff, legal framework of Electoral Commission

7.1.1 Structures and staff

7.1.1.1 Tanzanian mainland

Appointed members

The commission, chaired by either a judge of the high court or of the court of appeal or a person who has been a judge or has qualifications to be appointed a judge, comprises seven members appointed by the president. The vice chairperson, who must be a judge of the high court or of the court of appeal, is appointed on the basis that he/she must come from another part of the Union to where the chairperson comes from.

The five other members of the commission are:

- One commissioner, appointed from among the members of the Tanganyika Law Society; and
- Four commissioners, who are required to be people experienced in the conduct and supervision of parliamentary elections or who have any other qualifications that the president may deem appropriate.

Persons disqualified from appointment as electoral commissioners, according to article 74, section 4 of the Constitutional and Elections Act of 1985, are:

- A minister or deputy minister;

- An MP or member of a local government council; and

- Any political party leader.

A commissioner stops being a member of the commission:

- Five years after appointment date, though terms of office are renewable;

- If anything happens which, had he/she not been a member of the commission, would have made him/her ineligible for appointment to be a member of the commission; or

- If the president removes a member from the commission for failing to discharge his/her functions (URT, 1977, article 75).

The chairperson of the commission presides over all meetings of the commission. In his/her absence, the vice chairperson does so. If the vice chairperson is also absent or unable, the members present may elect one among themselves to act as the chairperson. The quorum for a meeting of the commission comprises four commissioners. Decisions are made by majority vote. The chairperson, vice chairperson or temporary chairperson presiding over any meeting of the commission has a casting vote where votes are equal. The commission may continue to discharge its functions, notwithstanding any vacancy among its membership or the absence of some members, provided that there is a quorum.

The commission records its meetings and is allowed by electoral law to compile regulations, rules and directives to govern the electoral process (Elections Act, 1985, Section 4).

The Secretariat of the commission

The director of elections, who is the chief executive of the commission and the secretary to the commission, is not a member of the commission and does not have a vote. The president appoints the director of elections on the recommendation of the commission. The director of elections is in overall charge of the following sections and units:

- The Elections Section, headed by a principal elections officer (PEO), which deals with all matters concerning supervision, coordination and the conduct of all three elections;

- The Information, Research and Statistics Section, headed by a principal information officer (PIO), which deals with civic education, public relations, research, library management and statistics;

- The Legal Unit, headed by a principal state attorney (PSA), which is charged with advising the commission on legal matters;

- The Administration and Personnel Unit, headed by a principal administrative and personnel officer (PAPO), which deals with all administrative, personnel and supply-related matters;

- The Accounts Unit, headed by a senior treasurer accountant, which handles all financial matters; and

- The Internal Audit Unit, headed by a senior internal auditor, which handles all internal auditing.

The NEC comprises eight electoral committees: international organisations and observers; supplies and logistics; press and public relations; the government and political parties; civic education and NGOs; electoral authorities and electoral processes; and coordination. Of the seven NEC commissioners, only two are women. The law instituting the NEC does not refer to gender.

Political parties are represented on the seven committees created by the commission to create goodwill and confidence among the electorate. Members from public and private institutions, independent citizens and representatives from political parties form the committees.

Permanent and part-time employees

The NEC is staffed by 58 permanent employees, though, during elections, it draws 90 more staff members from other government departments to work on a temporary basis for the commission. About 100 other temporary employees deal with warehousing activities in the three shifts that operate around the clock.

During elections, the commission appoints a regional election coordinator (REC) for each region and a RO for each constituency. Before the 1995 general elections, and for the by-elections that followed, the posts of RECs, liaison officers, ROs and assistant returning officers (AROs) were advertised in the news media. Any person with the right qualifications, apart from those in government service, could apply. There were many shortcomings in the elections and, according to the amendments made to address these, both the 2000 and 2005 elections were staffed by central and local government officers, with the posts of ROs being occupied by city directors, municipal directors, town directors, and district executive directors (Elections Act, 1985, Section 7 (1)). Such officers are used because they tend to have a sound knowledge of the areas in which they work; they can salvage situations, due to local networks that they might have built up over the years; and they can be held accountable for any oversight.

The ROs are responsible in their constituencies for:

- Administrative matters;
- All matters relating to voter registration;
- Administering candidate nomination procedures in the parliamentary and local elections;
- Coordinating election campaigns;
- Preparing and setting up registration centres and polling stations;
- Issuing election notices;
- Totalling the election results forwarded from the polling stations;
- Announcing election results in the case of parliamentary and local authority elections; and
- Compiling presidential election results for the constituencies and submitting them to the EC.

The main duty of the REC is to coordinate the electoral process at regional level, specifically by ensuring that the required materials are available, and to attend to other matters necessary for the efficient conduct of elections in the constituencies within their respective regions.

7.1.1.2 Zanzibar

The Directorate of Elections in Zanzibar is composed of the following divisions:

- Elections suboffice Pemba;
- Elections;
- Administration and Planning;
- Legal matters;
- Communication and Information; and
- Finance, Budgeting and Audit.

During elections the commission employs temporary contractual workers. During the 2005 elections, a presiding officer, two assistants, and a police officer were allocated to each of the 1 600 polling stations. The total of about 6 500 temporary employees included the ROs and their assistants in the 50 constituencies.

The commission has 43 permanent employees, of whom 28 are stationed at the main office in Zanzibar (20 men and eight women) and 15 in the Pemba suboffice (13 men and two women).

7.1.2 Legislative/Constitutional framework

7.1.2.1 Tanzanian mainland

The first independent NEC in the recently set up multiparty system was appointed on 14 January 1993. In exercising its constitutional duties, it is not obliged to follow the orders issued by any person or government department, nor to follow the views of any political party (URT, 1977 Constitution, section 75). The duties of the commission are to:

- Supervise and coordinate the registration of voters in presidential and parliamentary elections in the United Republic;
- Supervise and coordinate the conduct of the presidential and parliamentary elections;
- Supervise and coordinate the registration of voters and the conduct of the elections of local councillors on the Tanzanian mainland (URT, 1977, Constitution, section 74);
- Provide voter education (URT, Elections Act, 1985, section 4 [c]); and
- Demarcate the United Republic into constituencies for parliamentary elections. Article 75 (3) and (4) of the URT Constitution empowers the NEC to review the delimitation of constituencies at least once every ten years. The same provisions prescribe three criteria for the delimitation of constituencies: the population density of an area; the availability of means of communication; and the geographical condition of the area intended for demarcation. However, the NEC included the following criteria in the delimitation exercise before the 1995 general elections: the extent of economic development in the area concerned, save in exceptional circumstances; that the constituencies which were split in 1990 should not split again; and that areas which used to consist of two different constituencies, but were merged into a single constituency, should be split back into two constituencies. In 1994, the EC tried to involve the registered political parties in the delimitation exercise. Members of the NEC also visited the regions, towns, municipal councils and district councils to seek the advice of various people about the exercise. The system of delimitation has been in use since 1965.

Article 74 (7) of the Constitution of the United Republic states: "In the exercise of its functions under this Constitution, the EC shall be an independent department, and its chief executive officer shall be the Director of Elections who shall be appointed and will discharge his duties as may be prescribed by an Act of Parliament."

Article 74 (11) states: "In the exercise of its duties under the provisions of this Constitution, the EC shall not be subject to the orders or directions of any person or department of government or the opinions of any political party."

Articles 74 (7) and (11) of the 1977 Constitution accord independent status to the EC of Tanzania. However, the commission is not, in effect, an independent institution for the following reasons:

1. Under article 74 (5) of the 1977 Constitution, the incumbent president appoints NEC members, who therefore lack security of tenure, as the former is empowered to remove them from office.

2. According to section 6 (1) of the Elections Act of 1995, the director of elections is also appointed by the president from among the senior civil servants recommended to him by the commission. The director, being a civil servant, can therefore also be dismissed by the president by virtue of the presidential powers granted under article 36 (1) of the 1977 Constitution to constitute and abolish public service officers.

3. The president is the chairperson of one of the parties contesting the elections and handpicks those required for the commission without consulting the other contestants, so that the elections are neither free nor fair.

4. Due to the one-party state legacy, all members of the NEC who are public officers are presumed by the opposition to be members of CCM (Fimbo, 1995; Temco, 1995).

5. Furthermore, the NEC lacks financial independence, as neither the Constitution nor the Elections Act secures funds for the commission. Fiscally, the commission operates as a department of the Prime Minister's Office. The lack of an independent budget subjugates the commission to government dictates.

7.1.2.2 Zanzibar

The Zanzibar Electoral Commission (ZEC) is set up under article 9 of the Zanzibar Constitution of 1984. Section 119 of the Constitution stipulates that the ZEC will consist of the following members:

- The chair of the commission, with whatever relevant qualities the president may feel are appropriate;

- Two members appointed by the president after consulting with, and hearing the recommendations of, the leader of government business in the House of Representatives;

- One member to be appointed by the president;

- One member appointed by the president from among the judges of the high court; and

- Two members to be appointed by the president after consultations with, and recommendation by, the leader of the opposition in the House of Representatives. If there is no official opposition in the house, then the two will be appointed after consultation with the political parties concerned.

The Constitution safeguards the rights of members of the commission, including their removal from office without valid reason and the denial of their benefits (security of tenure). A member of the commission may stop being a member due to:

- Death;

- Ending a five-year term;

- The occurrence of anything that would have stopped him/her from being appointed a member of the commission if he were not already a member of the commission; and

- Being dismissed by the president, which only happens when the member fails to do his/her duty. The president has then to institute a commission to conduct the appropriate investigation, on the basis of whose findings a recommendation may be made whether the member be removed from office.

The chief executive of the commission is the presidentially appointed director of elections, as well as the secretary of the commission and works in accordance with the electoral law of 1984.

The ZEC administers the conduct of elections for the following positions:

- The president of the RGoZ;

- Members of the House of Representatives; and

- Members of local councils.

Elections for the president of the Union and the members of the National Assembly from Zanzibar are conducted by the NEC.

The ZEC is independent in terms of the Constitution (Constitution of Zanzibar [1984], Section 119 [9]), though donor funding might make it less so, with donor intrusion reducing the independence of the commission when it comes to decision-making. The commission is funded by the Ministry of Finance and Economic Affairs (MoFEA). Some requisitions might be delayed or not honoured. The presence of party representatives in the commission has led to situations of impasse, with some commissioners putting party interests before the interests of the nation as a whole.

7.2 Internal impact of HIV/AIDS

HIV/AIDS is a major problem in the public sector in Tanzania. Young, trained and energetic human resources in all sectors – banking, insurance, education, health, police, and the army – have been affected.

Many HIV/AIDS-related deaths are not recorded as such on death certificates. Colleagues of the deceased can only surmise the cause of death from the HIV/AIDS symptoms, which they have seen. Activists have urged the government to enact a law which will require that certificates clearly indicate the cause of death, even in cases where HIV/AIDS-related illnesses are concerned. The public is largely exposed to indicative statistics on the extent of the epidemic. For instance, some regional medical officers have claimed that about half the hospital beds in their regions are occupied by PLWHAs.

NEC officials acknowledge the fact that, during elections, officers travel extensively, which poses a risk of HIV/AIDS infection. Officers also earn an extra income from the elections, which enables them to "misbehave" in a way that would have been otherwise unlikely. Risks tend to be field-based rather than present in the Dar es Salaam offices. One NEC officer declared: "If they are risk-prone, it is because of their independent lifestyles and not because of the electoral processes."

Despite such risks, the commission has no policy on HIV/AIDS. However, the general government directive that ministries, departments and agencies (MDAs) should have HIV/AIDS-related workplace programmes has led to the NEC initiating an HIV/AIDS-related internal programme aimed at prevention, VCT and the provision of medication for those already infected. The NEC provides condoms to its employees, especially when they travel, and antiretrovirals to HIV-positive staff and their families.

No external policy as yet targets part-time staff who, particularly at the regional, constituency and ward levels, tend to be government employees already involved with HIV/AIDS-related workplace interventions. As voters are also stakeholders in the electoral process, they tend to be directly concerned with HIV/AIDS-related issues, benefiting from the nationwide campaigns that encourage fighting the virus and avoiding infection.

7.3 External impact of HIV/AIDS

7.3.1 Pre-election and polling phase

The education and health sectors, in which many have been infected with HIV, supply temporary employees to the NEC during election periods, with veterinary and agricultural officers being used in some constituencies. The 2003 ESRF study has clearly shown that more teachers died between 1999 to 2002 from AIDS-related illnesses. The proportion, of teachers dying from AIDS-related illnesses as a percentage of the total number of teachers who died during the period ranged between 66% to 100%.

The fact that the sectors that provide part-time employees to the NEC have been affected does not appear to compromise NEC operations as such, as the NEC employs such personnel only briefly. The registration period lasts, on average, three weeks in each zone, with many part-time staff being employed for only five days (three days of training and work on election day and the day after). They are usually also posted in their own neighbourhoods. Teachers, nurses and other government employees are plentiful. Replacement of any part-time employees who die would be instant, with the NEC training reserve personnel to fill in any gaps. The NEC has not suffered significant pecuniary loss through losing those whom they have trained to participate in election activities.

The loss of many public workers, no matter whether part-time, to AIDS would lead to the loss of skills and experience. The ROs (mostly RASs) and AROs (mostly ward secretaries) are key employees, in that they gain experience whenever they supervise an election. Since election work is specialised and requires efficiency the NEC should strive to retain the details of experienced part-timers on a database as part of continuing capacity-building.

7.3.2 National and Zanzibar Electoral Commissions' response to external impact

Though the NEC has procedures in place to help the disabled to vote, PLWHAs are unaware of whether they qualify for such treatment. The presiding officer at a polling station is directed to allow the old, the sick and the disabled to vote immediately after arriving at a polling station. The 2005 elections allowed the blind to use a tactile ballot paper, which meant those who could read braille did not even have to ask for help.

The disabled had many organisations that fought for their interests even before HIV/AIDS became an issue in Tanzania. They have requested to be represented in nearly all forums, including those related to elections. PLWHAs have only now started to form organisations to voice their needs as regards policy. However, the Tanzanian interest groups related to PLWHAs are not yet aiding the infected to participate in the electoral process. However, members of political parties have clearly pointed out that PLWHAs have little hope of winning an election, as people tend to think that PLWHAs do not have long to live, and, as they are preoccupied with their own problems they will not have enough time to deal with the problems of their constituencies.

PLWHAs are not yet treated as a special case, as other sick people have not been treated as disadvantaged by the NEC. No hospital visits have yet taken place to register voters. A more deliberate campaign to enlist disadvantaged persons might be instituted. The Director of Elections has said that the society should help those who are disabled to "present themselves" to the polling assistant on the election day "as the law states":

> Every voter who wishes to vote shall present himself at the polling station allotted to him in the polling district for which he is registered ... if a voter is incapacitated by blindness or other physical cause or is unable to read he may ask a person of his own choice other than the presiding officer .... to assist such an incapacitated person to record his vote... (Elections Act, 1985, section 61 [a–b]).

No special transport facilities are available for the disabled, with the quality of polling station facilities depending on the location of the station. Polling stations set up at schools can make the school facilities available to voters. However, other polling stations are in areas where such facilities are not available. While, in rural areas, the average distance to a polling station is one kilometre, in urban areas the distance is about half a kilometre. To simplify the process and to utilise available buildings better, one place – such as a school – can host multiple polling stations, which might confuse some voters. However, such provision against inclement weather is preferable to losing voters. Registration then occurs in the same venue, as the compilation of the temporary register takes several weeks, while the PVR takes only three. On polling day all voters come together to vote in a single day, which implies that registration is much more accessible to the disabled than are the polls.

During the 2005 election campaigning, ZAC asked the political parties to sensitise the population about HIV/AIDS-related dangers and risks, underlining the island's determination to minimise infection rates in the face of increased tourism and fledgling foreign businesses. However, the ZEC feels that the scourge of AIDS will affect the electoral process and that there is a need to update the PVR regularly to cope with the number of HIV/AIDS-related deaths.

8. Impact on parties, policy proposals

Interparty democracy means the observance by political parties of the norms and processes which ensure that political competition in elections is exercised in a manner that exhibits political tolerance, rule of law, fairness, and enforcement of any self-imposed codes of conduct, all of which are aimed at securing free and fair elections. In the 2005 elections, 15 of the 17 participating political parties signed a code of conduct in which they agreed that some basic rules of engagement should be observed.[15] The code of conduct was a tripartite agreement between the parties themselves, the government and the NEC. The do's and don'ts were set out in a document of which the engagement between political parties constituted the major part, showing that political parties are central to elections, as well as that their actions or omissions can wreck an election. That so many parties signed the code of conduct which covers the entire election process from campaigning to the declaration of results shows that the parties wanted the three main stakeholders to engage in free and fair elections.

This study sampled five political parties which won parliamentary seats in the 2005 elections and one political party in Zanzibar with future potential. The parties were the CCM, CHADEMA, CUF, TLP and UDP on the mainland and the CCM, CUF and Jahazi Asilia in Zanzibar.

8.1 Political parties on the fight against the epidemic

8.1.1 HIV/AIDS and integrity of electoral process

The political parties of both sides in the Union believe that, though in the last elections HIV/AIDS did not appear to affect them, the epidemic will become a key political issue in future. Both Chadema and CCM see HIV/AIDS as a problem. The CCM's former President Benjamin Mpaka has a foundation in his name dedicated to dealing with the problem. CUF on the mainland noted the absence of data that might otherwise help in assessing the extent of the problem, the lack of openness and denial inherent in society. The political parties, including the UDP, saw the problem as one requiring strategic planning and further research.

All parties indicated that they had not capitalised on HIV/AIDS for electioneering purposes, but rather viewed it as a national problem that required cooperative handling.

8.1.2 HIV/AIDS political parties' capacity to campaign

Political parties in Tanzania face key financial challenges, as the government subsidises only parliamentary parties, with the subsidy being allocated relative to the number of MPs that a party has in the house. Due to such a method of subsidisation, Tanzanian political parties do not compete on level terms.

As the political parties are not institutionalised, they do not keep accurate records of their membership. Since multiparty politics was reinstated, the membership of all parties has been problematic to estimate, with even CCM not knowing its membership to the nearest thousand. The newer parties are even less aware of their membership figures, with their inability to track membership levels compromising their ability to determine to what extent – if at all – HIV/AIDS is depleting their support bases.

8.1.3 Party practices

Some parties have acted on behalf of the AIDS commissions in regards to campaigns and public education. TACAIDS, in collaboration with the NEC and UNAIDS, produced leaflets, such as that shown in Figure 8.1, on HIV/AIDS for distribution during

Figure 8.1: Leaflet produced by TACAIDS during 2005 elections

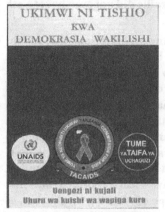

Source: TACAIDS (2005).

political campaigns. The cover conveys the message that HIV/AIDS is a threat to inclusive democracy and that leadership entails caring about voters' quality of life.

The collaboration between ZAC and political parties during the 2005 general elections is another example of best practice. ZAC produced leaflets, titled "2005 General Elections in Zanzibar without HIV", explaining the relationship between the electoral process and HIV/AIDS which referred to the intensified spreading of the virus during campaigns and when celebrating the results (see Figure 8.2).

HIV/AIDS risks in Zanzibar were particularly high during campaigning, because the youth tend to join in campaigns far from home, during which time they are more likely to engage in unanticipated, unsafe sex.

Figure 8.2: Leaflet produced by ZAC during 2005 elections

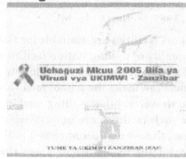

Source: RGoZ (2005b).

8.2 Policy proposals

All political parties address health issues, especially HIV/AIDS, in their election manifestos. CCM, in article 66 (f) of its electoral manifesto, for instance, pledges to strengthen the war against HIV/AIDS by making proper use of donor funding, and educating voters about stigma and discrimination. The party further vows to try harder to increase awareness of the disease and its effects on the economic, social and political spheres from street to village level, and to intensify provision of antiretrovirals to PLWHAs (CCM, 2005).

The National Convention for Construction and Reform–Mageuzi (NCCR–Mageuzi) seeks to set up participatory and sustainable programmes to prevent the spread of HIV/AIDS. According to article 5 (a) (3) of the party manifesto, NCCR pledges to improve the services dedicated to the care of PLWHAs to reduce the burden on family members, as well as to facilitate the buying and manufacturing of antiretrovirals within the country by making them cheaper. Research into HIV/AIDS-related treatment is addressed in the party manifesto (NCCR, 2005).

CUF also included the issue of HIV/AIDS in its electoral manifesto, emphasising its intention to devise a strategy focused on preventing HIV/AIDS (CUF, 2005), encouraging national dialogue as a basis for publicly declaring HIV status information, and publishing monthly updates on HIV/AIDS prevalence rates in each area, including announcements stemming from grassroots level. CUF also introduced an HIV/AIDS internal programme in 2001 to campaign for VCT among its members. Top party leaders, including the chairperson, the secretary-general, the vice-chairperson and the deputy secretary-general all took HIV tests and made their HIV-negative status public (Cuf, 2001).

CHADEMA maintains that entrenching HIV/AIDS-related education of communities in national policy would reduce stigma.

However, the manifestos have not been translated into action, especially when the political parties concerned are not in power. However, the parties are cooperative towards TACAIDS and ZAC on issues such as public awareness campaigns and the circulation of HIV/AIDS-related printed matter.

9. Political opinion, civic participation

During the first two rounds of the 2001 and 2003 Afrobarometer survey the sample was representative of the mainland and random, with a stratified prob-

ability of about 2 100 and 1 200 Tanzanians from the mainland alone. Round three of the data was collected by Research on Poverty Alleviation (REPOA), but, at the time of writing, had not yet been made public. The information presented here is only based on REPOA's preliminary analysis and presentations.[16]

9.1 Political opinion and HIV/AIDS

9.1.1 Participation in politics

Most citizens in 2001 indicated an interest in politics, with about 36% being very interested. In the second round in 2003, the question was recast to reflect an interest in public affairs, with only 34.5% of the respondents indicating an interest in public affairs (see Table 9.1).[17]

Though more men asserted an interest in politics and public affairs, the number of women interested in the same issues is also significant (33% and 30% in 2001 and 2003 respectively), due to the liberalisation of politics with the advent of multiparty democracy. Politics is also frequently discussed, as indicated by about 30% (in 2001) and 41% (in 2003) (see Table 9.2). A significant number (23% in 2001 and 31% in 2003) of women indicated that, when meeting with friends and family, they frequently discuss politics.

Despite the interest observed in politics in the 2001 and 2003 rounds, most respondents in rounds two (2003) and three (2005) agreed that politics and the government sometimes seem so complicated that they cannot fully be understood (see Table 9.3).[18] Such lack of comprehension can be blamed on the lack of civic education, of which most Tanzanians are in dire need, especially regarding electoral systems and policies (Mushi, Baregu and Mukundala, 2001).[19] Donor funding of voter education for all elections shows that wider civic education is needed. Despite such a lack, almost all respondents had registered after the introduction of the national PVR during the December 2005 general elections (see Table 9.4).

9.1.2 Explaining political opinion on HIV/AIDS

Of the respondents in the 2001 and 2003 Afrobarometer surveys, 60% and 61% respectively indicated having lost a close friend or relative due to AIDS. Despite such findings, only a negligible

Table 9.1: Interest in political/public affairs

Response	Afrobarometer (2001)			Afrobarometer (2003)		
	Male %	Female %	Total %	Male %	Female %	Total %
Not interested	13.5	19.4	16.5	10.8	15.1	13.0
Somewhat interested	46.5	46.5	46.4	47.3	50.5	48.9
Very interested	39.2	33.3	36.3	39.2	30.3	34.7
Don't know	0.8	0.8	0.8	2.4	4.1	3.3
N	1 069	1 065	2 134	609	614	1 223

Source: Own analysis using Afrobarometer rounds 1 and 2 data.

Table 9.2: Discussion of political matters

Response	Afrobarometer (2001)			Afrobarometer (2003)		
	Male %	Female %	Total %	Male %	Female %	Total %
Never	19.5	30.0	24.7	13.3	20.7	17.0
Occasionally/Sometimes	43.7	46.1	44.9	33.5	46.3	40
Frequently/Often	36.4	23.1	29.7	51.07	31.4	41.2
Don't know	0.4	0.8	0.6	2.1	1.6	1.9
N	1 069	1 065	2 134	609	614	1 223

Source: Own analysis using Afrobarometer rounds 1 and 2 data.

Table 9.3: Politics and government interface

	Repoa (2005)			Afrobarometer (2003)		
	Male %	Female %	Total %	Male %	Female %	Total %
Strongly agree	20	13	16	21.2	19.4	20.3
Agree	30	32	31	37.8	37.8	37.8
Neither agree nor disagree	11	13	12	12.3	14.0	13.2
Disagree	19	14	16	14.6	12.0	13.3
Strongly disagree	9	5	7	6.2	3.4	4.8
Don't know	11	24	17	7.9	13.4	10.63

Source: Own analysis using Afrobarometer round 2 data; Repoa (2005)

percentage of the 2 134 individuals surveyed in 2001 stated that they wished HIV/AIDS to receive immediate government attention, despite the HIV prevalence rate being higher then (11% among blood donors [URT, 2003a]) than now. Though the percentage of respondents perceiving HIV/AIDS to be a major problem increased in 2003, it was still seen as being less important than other development problems (see Figure 9.1). Due to the high national poverty levels, the epidemic is superceded by other major demands, such as those for access to social services, including water, education and overall health improvement. The respondents accordingly prioritised measures to increase the rate of economic growth, such as the provision of loans for purposes of investment and job creation, investment in farming, and the improvement of the transportation system.

Such findings supported those of the analysis conducted by Whiteside, Mattes, Willan and Manning (2002), who pointed out that, in areas where the level of HIV/AIDS infection is high, people are dying in increasing numbers. Even where people recognise such an increase as resulting from HIV infection, few prioritise HIV/AIDS for government intervention.

Table 9.5 summarises poverty status by regions as reported in the latest *Poverty and Human Development Report* (PHDR) (URT, 2005e). More than half of all the regions have a poverty status above the national average, with the national percentage of the population below the basic needs poverty line being 36.5. Singida and Lindi regions have the lowest poverty status indicators, with 55% and 53% of the population respectively being below the basic needs poverty line.

Table 9.4: Registration for the 2000 and 2005 general elections

Registration status	2000			2005		
	Males (%)	Females (%)	Total (%)	Males (%)	Females (%)	Total (%)
Were/Are registered as a voter	92	88	90.0	97	93	95
Did not want to register	2	3	3	1	1	1
Could not find a place to register/ Were prevented from registering/ Did not register for some other reason	6	9	7	2	6	4
Don't know	0	0	0	0	0	0
N	1 099	1 099	2 198	–	–	1 030

Source: Own analysis using Afrobarometer round 1 data; Repoa (2005).

Table 9.5: Poverty status by region

Region	% of households below basic needs poverty line
1. Dodoma	34
2. Arusha/Manyara	39
3. Kilimanjaro	31
4. Tanga	37
5. Morogoro	29
6. Pwani	46
7. Dar es Salaam	18
8. Lindi	53
9. Mtwara	38
10. Ruvuma	41
11. Iringa	29
12. Mbeya	21
13. Singida	55
14. Tabora	26
15. Rukwa	31
16. Kigoma	38
17. Shinyanga	42
18. Kagera	29
19. Mwanza	48
20. Mara	46

Source: URT (2005e).

Figure 9.1: Most important problem facing the country

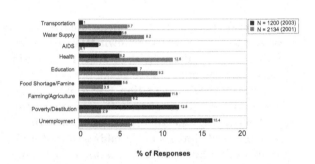

Source: Own analysis using Afrobarometer rounds 1 and 2 data.

Only 42% of the respondents said that they thought that the government was excelling in improving health services, while about 21% and 27% of the respondents thought that the government had done very badly and fairly badly, respectively. Tanzanian health services tend to be inaccessible, due to con-straints on physical access, quality of care, financial and social barriers. The mean distance to the nearest hospital for the poor is 25.6km, compared with 19.0km for the non-poor, with the mean distance for the poor to the nearest health centre/dispensary 4.45km, compared with 3.71km for the non-poor (Smithson, 2006). However, the difference might be due to the urban–rural divide, with the mean distance to a hospital in Dar es Salaam being just 2.8km and 25.7km in rural areas. Households living in some remote regions, such as Shinyanga, Dodoma, and Tanga, live more than 5km from a primary health facility. Nationally, 11% of rural households, or roughly 3.5 million people, live more than 10km from the nearest primary facility. Also, only 42% of rural and 85% of the urban population can access clean water within 30 minutes.

The responses received to a request for perceptions of how the government is doing in preventing the spread of HIV/AIDS and whether the government should devote more resources to combating the epidemic, in preference to solving other development problems, are shown in Table 9.6.

Table 9.6 shows that Tanzanians are generally satisfied with government efforts to prevent the spread of HIV/AIDS. Further, 47% of the respondents indicated that government should increase HIV/AIDS-related resources at the expense of developing sectors like education. Such findings are supported by the 43% agreement received on the follow-up question as to whether the government should focus on solving its many other problems, even if many are dying because of AIDS. Despite most people having lost at least one relative to AIDS, some still believe that PLWHAs should be blamed for contracting the virus through poor personal decision-making, and that the government budget should not be unduly depleted as a result.

9.2 Civic participation

For ethical reasons, Afrobarometer studies do not ask respondents about their own HIV sero status or the status of those in their care, rather using health-oriented questions to gauge the effect of the epidemic on civic participation. Five proxy variables have been used in this section: the amount of time spent on taking care of respondents' own illness; the amount of time spent on taking care of a sick member of the household; the amount of time taken to take care of orphans, and personal physical and mental health. Table 9.7 shows the amount of time spent on home-based care.

Most respondents reported not taking care of any orphan during the period under study (about 71%), with the rest of the respondents (about 27%) reporting spending time on caring for orphans. The analysis was disaggregated by gender on the understanding that women tend to take care of the sick and orphans more often than do men. About 70% of women reported not spending any time taking care of orphans, while 7% reported spending more than five hours a day on caring for orphans. Why most respondents reported that they did not spend time taking care of orphans, might be because orphans are usually integrated into the extended family system. Except for the small group of respondents which reported spending more than five hours a day taking care of orphans (6%), such care does not obstruct effective participation in civil activities.

The URT (2005f) assumed that 5.3% of the total population of children might be categorised as "most vulnerable" children, which translated into 968 439 MVC (5.3% of the population under 18 years of age in Tanzania in 2002). Data from the 2002 population and housing census for the Tanzanian mainland show that 2% of children have lost their mothers, but not their fathers; 6% have lost their fathers, but not their mothers; while 1% has lost both parents.

Only about 4% to 6% of orphans and vulnerable children live in households that reported receiving various types of external support. Given the poor economic conditions of most households, most orphans start to work at a very young age to provide for themselves. Many orphans live alone without a parent or guardian.[20]

Though some respondents reported spending

Table 9.6: Perceptions of government commitment to combat the epidemic		
Variable	2001 (N = 2134)	2003 (N = 1223)
How the government is doing in preventing HIV transmission		
Very badly	11.2	8.0
Fairly badly	15.1	11.5
Fairly well	44.1	48.0
Very well	28.0	30.1
The government should devote many more resources to combating AIDS, even if doing so entails spending less on education and other services.		
Agree very strongly	–	29.8
Agree	–	17.4
Many other problems face Tanzania besides AIDS – even if people are dying in large numbers, the government needs to keep its focus on solving the other problems.		
Agree very strongly	–	25.0
Agree	–	18.2
Source: Own analysis using Afrobarometer rounds 1 and 2 data.		

Table 9.7: Amount of time spent on home-based care

Response	% time spent on care of orphans	% time spent on sick household member	% time spent on own illness
Spend no time	70.8	44.6	27.9
Less than 1 hour	7.3	16.8	13.7
1–2 hours	8.9	18.1	22.2
3–5 hours	4.6	8.3	12.1
More than 5 hours	6.1	7.2	16.6
Do not know	2.3	5.0	7.6
N	1 223	1 223	1 223

Source: Own analysis using Afrobarometer round 2 data.

some time in taking care of the sick household members, many (about 45%) reported spending no time in doing so during the period under study. About 17% reported caring for their own illness, including HIV/AIDS, for more than five hours a day. Based on time use data, we cannot conclusively say that HIV/AIDS has impeded civic participation. A study by Strand et al. (2005) collapsed the findings on the three variables on home-based care (the percentage of time spent on caring for orphans, a sick household member or one's own illness).

The average Tanzanian spends little (1.18) time on home-based care.[21]

Most respondents reported being both physically and mentally well (see Table 9.8). About 14% of the respondents reported experiencing many episodes of physical problems, while 16% reported experiencing many episodes of mental problems. However, given that the question did not specifically refer to HIV/AIDS and the many other health conditions that can make a person sick, the conclusion cannot be drawn that HIV/AIDS impedes the capacity of citizens to participate in civic activities. Only about 2% of respondents reported suffering from permanent physical or mental conditions.

Table 9.8: Suffering inflicted by physical and mental conditions

Response	Physical condition	Mental condition
Never	52.0	54.5
Once or twice	29.9	24.4
Many times	13.9	16.3
Always	1.9	2.2
Don't know	2.3	2.4
N	1 223	1 223

Source: Own analysis using Afrobarometer round 2 data.

Over 90% of Tanzanians registered to vote in both the 2000 and 2005 elections, showing that the population is active in civil matters, despite the presence of HIV/AIDS.

10. Exploring impact on voter turnout

Tanzania started to use a PVR in the 2005 General Elections, in accordance with a 2000 constitutional amendment, as a way of reducing the costs of registering voters every time an election or by-election is due, as well as of expediting voter registration. Voter registration is now continuous, with the PVR being regularly updated.

Decentralising the registration process enables each constituency to update its own list of voters, which are then displayed in each hamlet, village/street and ward for stakeholders to verify, facilitating identification of the dead and those who have migrated to other areas. Political parties, through their agents, will be key players in this regard. HIV/AIDS is likely to decrease the size of the electorate, especially in communities with a high prevalence and high mortality rates.

10.1 HIV prevalence and voter turnout

Table 10.1 shows that the percentage of those registered relative to those who voted has remained relatively constant, with about 27%–30% of those registered not voting. HIV is not the culprit, as even in 2000, when the HIV prevalence was highest, about the same number of people voted. Other structural factors prevent people from voting, including:

• Rigorous registration campaigns conducted during the registration phase motivating people to register no longer provide sufficient impetus during the elections.

• The voter's card was, previously, used as an identity card for accessing important consumables, such as sugar from public stores, especially when such commodities were scarce. When the PVR was implemented in 2005 voters were given a permanent card which serves as an identity card

in the absence of an established citizen registration system which issues identity documents to citizens.

• Many people travelled on election day. Before the implementation of the PVR, special permission could be requested, within a specified period, to vote at another registration post, rather than at that where one had registered. Such a mechanism was discouraged, as it could be defrauded.

• Voter apathy might have prevailed.

Table 10.2 presents the total number of registered voters, total population and HIV prevalence by

Table 10.1: Voter participation

Year	Estimate	Registered	Voted	% voted	HIV prevalence
1995	11 017 429	8 929 969	6 440 913	72	8.6*
2000	10 303 891	10 088 484	7 099 636	70	12.3*
2005	16 000 000	16 401 694	11 900 000	73	7.0**

Source: *Nec (2005); **Various NACP HIV/AIDS surveillance reports (URT, 2005a).

Table 10.2: Registered voters, population and HIV prevalence by region

No.	Regions	Estimated voters	Actual registered voters (2005)	% registered	% HIV prevalence (2004)	Population (2002)[25]
1.	Mtwara	635 115	572 510	90.14	7.4	1 128 523
2.	Lindi	432 563	388 384	89.79	3.6	791 306
3.	Iringa	744 322	673 686	90.51	13.4	1 495 333
4.	Mbeya	1 046 970	951 011	90.83	13.5	2 070 046
5.	Rukwa	475 142	427 948	90.07	6.0	1 141 743
6.	Ruvuma	576 730	504 470	87.47	6.8	1 117 166
7.	Kigoma	643 942	600 872	93.31	2.0	1 679 109
8.	Singida	524 839	482 544	91.94	3.2	1 090 758
9.	Dodoma	847 259	759 251	89.61	4.9	1 698 996
10.	Tabora	816 867	723 319	88.55	7.2	1 717 908
11.	Mara	636 461	663 774	104.29	3.5	1 368 602
12.	Kagera	918 040	906 852	98.78	3.7	2 033 888
13.	Shinyanga	1 288 162	1 236 560	95.99	6.5	2 805 580
14.	Mwanza	1 407 356	1 397 673	99.31	7.2	2 942 148
15.	Arusha	650 756	650 199	99.91	5.3	1 292 973
16.	Manyara	501 516	484 230	96.55	2.0	1 040 461
17.	Kilimanjaro	705 549	661 288	93.73	7.3	1 381 149
18.	Tanga	824 225	789 244	95.76	5.7	1 642 015
19.	Dar es Salaam	1 503 494	1 680 831	111.79	10.9	2 497 940
20.	Pwani	477 940	469 924	98.32	7.3	889 154
21.	Morogoro	921 218	895 179	97.17	5.4	1 759 809

Sources: URT (2003e); URT (2005a); NEC (2006).

Table 10.3: Population, registered voters, selected regional HIV prevalence			
Region	Registered voters (2000)	% HIV prevalence (2002)[27]	Population (2002)
Dar es Salaam	768 482	12.8	2 497 940
Dodoma	445 805	6.1	1 698 996
Kagera	312 161	5.6	2 033 888
Kilimanjaro	472 567	6.3	1 381 149
Mbeya	519 046	16.0	2 070 046
Mtwara	359 756	7.1	1 128 523
Source: NEC (2000); URT (2003a); URT (2003e).			

region. The more people in a region, the larger the number of registered voters.[22] The finding that more people register in areas with a high HIV prevalence[23] might have occurred due to HIV not having substantially affected voter turnout – that is, with or without HIV/AIDS, the number of voters would increase, due to the growth in population – or HIV/AIDS intervention being seen as a chance to strengthen participation in the governance system and structures. The battle against HIV/AIDS will be won when the people and their government unite in the struggle. PLWHAs must approach their local representatives to secure easier access to prevention, care and support.[24]

Table 10.2 also shows the percentage of estimated number of voters in relation to those registered for the 2005 elections. Kigoma region, which has the lowest (2.0%) HIV prevalence, has a modest percentage of registered voters, whereas Dar es Salaam, which ranks third in terms of HIV prevalence (10.9%), has the highest percentage of registered voters. A higher HIV prevalence rate is indicated for Mbeya (13.5%) and Iringa (13.4%), which have about the same registration rates as Rukwa, for which HIV prevalence is less than the national average (6.0%). Thus, a number of factors are at play, apart from HIV/AIDS, which are determining the individual decision to register to vote.

Analysis of previous election data indicating high HIV prevalence also seems to show that HIV has not significantly affected voter turnout (see Table 10.3).[26]

11. Stigma and discrimination

Focus group discussions were used to collect data on the perceptions, mainly of PLWHAs, of:

- Their ability to participate in the elections;
- The effect of HIV/AIDS on the electoral process; and
- Voter registration, in line with the response to HIV/AIDS.

A total of 16 FGDs were conducted in one rural and one urban region of Tanzania. While Dar es Salaam was sampled mainly due to its urban orientation and high prevalence rate (11%), Makete district in the Iringa region was sampled not only because of its rural orientation and high HIV/AIDS prevalence rate (23% at the time of survey), but also because the district has received significant attention from the media and politicians, due to the devastation caused by the epidemic.

Participants in the FGDs were selected from the following registered HIV/AIDS organisations:

- Phaera (Promote HIV/AIDS Education in Rural Areas), Tayopa (Tanzania Youth Plan of Action), People Living with HIV/AIDS in Vingunguti Ward (PLWHAVW), and the Network for Young People Living with HIV/AIDS (NYP), based in Dar es Salaam;

- *Pima ili Uishi kwa Matumaini* (PIUMA), Makete Support to People with HIV/AIDS (MASUPHA), and Iringa Development of Youth, Disabled and Children Care (IDYDC), based in the Makete District; and

- the Zanzibar Association of People Living with HIV/AIDS (ZAPHA+) in Zanzibar.

The focus groups were stratified in terms of age and gender (see Table 11.1), with 139 individuals ultimately participating in the FGDs.[28]

11.1 Stigma and discrimination

Over 95% of all adults are aware of the HIV/AIDS pandemic, according to several state-sponsored studies. Much learning about ways in which to prevent HIV transmission has occurred since 1996. In 1996, 39% of Tanzanian women and 55% of Tanzanian men reported using condoms to prevent HIV transmission, with an increase to 56% for women and 71% for men in 1999 and a further increase to 68% for women and 75% for men in 2003/04 (see Table 11.2). Despite such high levels of understanding, increasingly, PLWHAs and AIDS orphans have been discriminated against and stigmatised in the household, the workplace, schools and the community. Due to the stigma associated with HIV/AIDS, the epidemic was found to directly affect the social relations of PLWHAs with family members, neighbours, close friends, relatives and coworkers. Discrimination, neglect and marital problems have also been observed (ESRF, 2003).

The Demographic and Health Survey (DHS) (NBS, 2005) indicates that in Zanzibar, while most respondents were willing to care for a family member with HIV at home (92.8%) and believe that an HIV-positive female teacher should be allowed to teach (80.2%), only about half of the respondents indicated that they would buy fresh food from a shopkeeper with AIDS (46.8%) and would want the

HIV-positive status of a family member to remain a secret. Only 22.1% of all respondents expressed acceptance on all four measures of stigma.[29]

This 2003–2004 survey shows the following high percentage of refusal of VCT among the individuals sampled: Shinyanga (31.8%); Dar es Salaam (30.2%); and Mara (24%). Such refusal is a result of the stigma attached to being HIV-positive.

11.2 Perceptions of people living with HIV/AIDS and care-givers

11.2.1 Participation in 2005 elections

In the Dar es Salaam region, discussions were held with 54 PLWHAs and 16 care-givers, who were organised into eight different focus groups. Most (91%) participants took part in the 2005 general elections. In the Makete rural district, discussions were held with 50 PLWHAs and 16 care-givers of PLWHAs.

Table 11.1: The focus group discussions sample

Age (years)	Dar es Salaam		Makete	
	Males	Females	Males	Females
People living with HIV/AIDS				
18–24	8	8	8	8
25–34	8	10	8	9
35–49	10	10	8	9
Care-givers				
25–49	8	8	8	8
Total	34	36	32	34

Table 11.2: Knowledge of AIDS and ways in which to avoid transmission

Data source	Knowledge of AIDS[30]		Knowledge of ways to avoid transmission	
	Males	Females	Males	Females
Demographic and Health Survey (DHS), 1997	98.8	97.0	62.9	62.3
Tanzania Child and Reproductive Health Survey (TCRHS), 1999	99.1	97.0	84.2	77.0
Tanzania HIV/AIDS Indicator Survey (This), 2005	99.8	99.1	88.4	86.6[31]
Demographic and Health Survey (DHS), 2005	99.1	98.9	85.1	87.4[32]

During the 2005 general elections, all 16 care-givers voted, while 15 of the PLWHAs (37.5%) had not. The majority who voted felt that participation in the election was a human right. The main reasons for not participating in the elections included:

- Being seriously ill and bedridden in hospital or at home during registration or on election day, without access to the "special vote";
- The stigma experienced by the sick and by other community members;
- Mourning recently deceased relatives;
- Excessive delays in voting queues;
- Inadequate campaigning on HIV/AIDS-related issues by political parties;
- Inadequate government response/performance on HIV/AIDS issues;
- Taking care of sick relatives; and
- The excessive distance required to be travelled to the polling stations.

Those PLWHAs who did not vote explained why they had not in terms of:

- Being seriously ill and bedridden in hospital or at home during voter registration or on election day, without access to the "special vote";
- The stigma attached to their physically deteriorated condition; and
- Mourning deaths of their relatives.

In rural Makete, a deceased is mourned for three consecutive days. Therefore, if a death of a relative occurred two days before elections, none of the household members would leave home to vote. A nurse at Makete District Hospital reported: "During the time of registration of voters and during the time of voting, our hospital wards were full of in-patients affected by HIV and AIDS. I can estimate that about 60% of PLHWAs did not vote."

Most participants in both urban and rural settings denied that people infected or affected by HIV/AIDS are less likely to participate in politics, with the few supporting the assertion doing so due to the poor condition of some PLWHAs. The study revealed that few PLWHAs participated either in IEC observation and monitoring activities, or in voter education. Those who did participate in this way attributed their being able to do so to their HIV sero status not being known to the public and therefore not allowing for stigma.

Many participants did not know the role and mandate of the EC, associating it with the provision

of antiretroviral services. Those who did pointed to the lack of mainstreaming of HIV/AIDS in election activities, stating that queues were long (in urban and rural areas alike), resulting in it taking a long time (four to seven hours) to vote. On humanitarian grounds, PLWHAs who had already publicly declared their status were allowed to vote first at some polling stations. However, such an arrangement was purely local, rather than nationally determined by the EC.

11.2.2 Participation in leadership and elections

Most participants thought that the participation of PLWHAs as leaders in the election process had positively affected the decisions made by voters, since infected leaders were felt likely to work hard to ensure that the needs of their fellow non-leaders, who are infected, are met. One participant lamented: "We PLWHAs, are supposed to eat special diets, including fish and vegetables. If a leader is a PLWHA, he/she can see to it that his fellow non-infected leaders understand our needs and mainstream them in the district budget."

PLWHAs tend to be poorly organised and without a special seat in Parliament, such as the disabled have. Though some MPs might be PLWHAs, they have not publicly disclosed their status.

Measures to increase the involvement of PLWHAs in leadership and elections have been called for. Most respondents suggested that voter education should be emphasised, as it is through such education that other PLWHAs might be attracted to participate in political issues. Equally important, such education can help to reduce the degree of stigma associated with them by the rest of society. Though a few respondents demanded access to the special vote, such a view was strongly opposed by their fellows on the basis that such a practice would both exacerbate their misery and perpetuate stigmatisation, resulting in PLWHAs not voting. Respondents have proposed the following measures:

- Making special arrangements for registering voters who are seriously ill at home or in hospital;
- Facilitating voting for such voters;
- Providing voter education to PLWHAs;
- Increasing the number of polling stations;
- Encouraging political campaigns to spread HIV/AIDS-related messages;
- Allowing registered voters to vote anywhere, not necessarily where they were registered, so that

those who are in hospital can cast ballots regardless of where they have been admitted; and

- Ensuring that every hospital has a mobile polling station, so that registered patients can easily vote.

PLWHAs see elections as forums that can be used to improve their quality of life, which is associated with the type of leaders elected. If HIV/AIDS issues are mainstreamed in the electoral process, then electorates can elect leaders who:

- Can reduce stigma;
- Will design and implement policies aimed at addressing concerns of PLWHAs;
- Will increase the availability and accessibility of antiretrovirals for PLWHAs;
- Will ensure that PLWHAs have access to food aid and other help; and
- Will innovatively introduce new or more services to PLWHAs.

Most respondents were involved with at least one CBO campaigning around HIV/AIDS issues. For instance, at the time of the survey, PIUMA CBO, which is based in Bulongwa village in the Makete district had 210 members living with HIV/AIDS, whereas Jiendeleze and Tupendane CBO in Ivalalila village had 197 members living with the virus. Reasons given for affiliation to CBOs were that they provided:

- A source of consolation;
- An environment conducive to the exchange of ideas;
- Easy access to PLWHAs; and
- Encouragement of HIV testing.

Apart from being members of HIV/AIDS-specific organisations, PLWHAs are involved with activities conducted by other social economic organisations prevalent in their communities. The activities include being members of savings and credit cooperative societies, members of political parties, leaders in village government and active participants in a number of CBOs not specifically concerned with HIV/AIDS issues.

11.2.3 Strongest change agent on HIV/AIDS issues

Most participants see themselves as the major agent of change, followed by religious leaders, with political leaders coming only fifth (see Table 11.3).

However, participants argued that religious leaders were not doing enough as change agents, because they consistently discouraged the use of condoms as one of the ways of protecting against HIV infection. In contrast, the participants thought that condoms should be promoted as preventive measures for those who are unable to abstain. Traditional leaders are distrusted for being "greedy" and therefore regarded as hindering the fight against HIV/AIDS. They were also accused of discouraging people from going to hospital, resulting in PLWHAs dying at a relatively young age.[33]

11.3 Approaches to reducing HIV/AIDS-related stigma

11.3.1 Educational approach

Stigma might be directly countered through education. FGDs support:

- Involving PLWHAs in voter education;
- Involving PLWHAs in conveying HIV/AIDS-related messages during campaigns; and
- Training of subvillage government leaders and primary school teachers to educate villagers concerning HIV/AIDS.

11.3.2 Palliative care

Palliative care is a "continuum of care" that begins from the time a person is diagnosed as HIV positive (ICRW, 2002). Apart from including psychosocial and spiritual support to help PLWHAs and their families cope with stigma and illness, such care also emphasises relieving the suffering of PLWHAs. A well-designed and implemented palliative care programme can include a complete package of services adapted to deal with the social context of stigma and to lessen the burden of caring for PLWHAs in the community.

Table 11.3: The role of change agents in combating HIV/AIDS

Change agents	Explanation for the comparative strength of the change agent
People living with HIV/AIDS	• Being examples of the effect of HIV/AIDS, they can provide testimony of how they acquired the virus and can warn healthy people to protect themselves from infection. • Due to the counselling that they have undergone, they can educate others in turn.
Religious leaders	• They can easily convey HIV messages to the many with whom they are in contact. • Their preaching against sin predisposes their followers to avoid risky behaviour. • They command respect and confidence.
Arts performers	• They can illustrate how people acquire HIV and the consequences of doing so. • Most performers are young and can reach out to others of the same age relatively easily.
Athletes	• Participating in sport occupies time that might otherwise be spent on risky activities. • Their physical exhaustion discourages engaging in risky activities.
Political leaders	• They campaign and call people together for meetings, which they can address with HIV/AIDS messages. • They can promote the availability and accessibility of antiretrovirals.
Community leaders	• As they are aware of the behaviour of community members, they can easily warn them against risky sexual behaviour. • They hold regular village and subvillage meetings at which they can disseminate HIV/AIDS-related information. • They can encourage the promulgation of by-laws aimed at halting transmission of the virus.
Home-based care-givers	• Apart from counselling PLWHAs, they also counsel other people and encourage them to undergo HIV testing.
Primary school teachers	• They educate learners on HIV/AIDS-related issues.
Non-governmental organisations	• They provide various types of support to PLWHAs.
Community-based organisations	• They provide various types of support to PLWHAs.
Mass media	• They educate people through the various forms of mass media.

12. Conclusion and recommendations

12.1 The electoral system

Due to the increase in the number of by-elections, a movement towards MP substitution in the FPTP system or a migration to the PR or MMP system is worth considering.

12.2 Electoral management bodies

The challenge of registering new voters and of removing the names of the deceased and emigrants from the PVR started in the 2005 elections is immense, given the poor record-keeping of the Immigration Department.

Due to the silence surrounding HIV/AIDS deaths and the small size of the NEC and ZEC, no conclusive results exist on the internal affect of HIV/AIDS on these bodies. The NEC does not consider it important to recall the same people it has trained over time for each new election. Since election work is specialised and requires efficiency; we would assume that it is in the interest of the NEC to retain experienced part-timers on a data base as part of continuing capacity-building. The loss of large numbers of public workers to AIDS might lead to a failure to retain skills and experience.

The NEC should consider including all categories of sick people in a framework that encourages and/or enables the participation of people infected or affected by HIV/AIDS in the electoral process. The EC should also indicate in information campaigns that PLWHAs are eligible to use special voting mechanisms.

12.3 Political institutions: Parliament, political parties

- MPs have been hit by the scourge just like any other member of the general population. Data on the number of deaths of MPs from 1990 show that few MPs have died and their deaths could not conclusively be linked to HIV/AIDS due to data limitations. The previous parliament in Tanzania had cohorts with the age above the risky age groups. However, about 37% of the current members of parliament are in the risky age group, being younger than previous MPs. Thus, the need to address HIV/AIDS issues in the Parliament is apparent.

- During the past few years (from 2000), debates on HIV/AIDS in the National Assembly have intensified with discussions on legal and other HIV/AIDS-related issues. These discussions affect the situation of HIV/AIDS orphans and people living with HIV/AIDS, condom use and culture and tradition as they relate to HIV/AIDS, care and treatment, VCT, among other things. However, the country (both Tanzania mainland and Zanzibar) has only managed to pass an HIV/AIDS policy. An HIV/AIDS Bill has not been deliberated on.

- A major response by the parliament in Tanzania mainland and the House of Representatives in Zanzibar includes formation of bodies such as TAPAC and UWAKUZA. While both TAPAC and UWAKUZA have placed HIV/AIDS on the agenda they need to play a greater role in mainstreaming HIV/AIDS into the workplace (the Parliament and House of Representatives) and into the work of Standing Committees. To do this they need further capacity building to ensure effective implementation. These two bodies have the potential to become examples for other countries to look

at in terms of mobilisation of political members around HIV/AIDS issues.

- Resources for HIV/AIDS for the Members of the Parliament and Members of the House of Representatives have been limited. MPs have expressed the need to do more work on HIV/AIDS issues in their constituencies but have cited lack of funds as a key issue. This calls for resource mobilisation for TAPAC and UWAKUZA so that they could scale up their activities to local council level/their constituencies.

- Political parties have started including HIV/AIDS in their election manifestos. This however needs to be amplified and facilitated to flow through the structures and membership of all political parties. This will then resonate in all governance structures of the country including Parliament.

- Tanzanian interest groups related to the PLWHAs have not really focused on elections yet. They are not encouraging any of the affected to participate in the electoral processes. However, members of political parties pointed out clearly that an individual living with HIV/AIDS has little opportunity of winning an election because of their perceived short life span which would allegedly not allow time to deal with the problems of their constituencies.

12.4 Voter turnout and participation

One weakness in relation to participation and representation of PLWHAs is in relation to formation of a strong organisation that can form an electorate. Contrary to the disabled who are organised and who have been able to get a special seat in Parliament due to the electorate they are representing, PLWHAs have not been able to do so. Nevertheless, only few PLHWAs seconded the idea of having representation/a special seat in the Parliament. The major reason is that such a practice would exacerbate their misery as it would perpetuate stigma.

The electoral process has been impacted in particular with relation to individual voters' participation. This has vividly been expressed in FGDs conducted in the rural area where it was estimated that about 60% of PLWHAs did not vote because they were bed-ridden at either the time of registration and/or the voting time. This calls for a special arrangement for registration/voting for PLWHAs who due to physical debilitation cannot get to the polling stations.

Endnotes

1   The figure is that for the general population (12–65 years) estimated from the ANC attendee data.

2   Data for round 3 have not yet been officially released so that the information used in this chapter has been extracted from the 2005 REPOA presentations.

3   Except when otherwise stated, data presented in this subsection are drawn from the HIV/AIDS/STIs Surveillance Reports produced by the National AIDS Control Programme (NACP).

4   This subsection draws heavily on the ESRF (2003) study on the socioeconomic impacts of HIV/AIDS on Tanzania.

5   The exchange rate was about $1 = Tanzanian shilling (TZS) 1300 in early 2007.

6   Shehia – the lowest administrative government structure at grassroots level in Zanzibar.

7   See Collaboration between Tanga AIDS Working Group and Traditional Healers in Tanga Region, Tanzania, a paper presented at the SADC Summit on HIV/AIDS in the session on Africa Knowledge and Learning Fair: Scaling Up Efforts in the Fight against HIV/AIDS held in Lesotho National Convention Centre, Maseru, from 1–4 July 2003.

8   Parliament has a maximum of 323 members instead of 324, because the Speaker is also a constituency-elected MP.

9   The figure represents an example of one election involving the election of one MP and nine councillors. This figure may/may not be representative of other constituencies, given the differences in sizes of constituencies and population.

10 Some MPs indicated having spent up to TZS20 000 000 per year on HIV/AIDS-related activities. However, such costs were not personal, but pragmatic, incurred under specific funded programmes.

11 Finding pre-1990 records has been extremely difficult, inhibiting detection of whether an increase in mortality among parliamentarians has occurred. If the relevant data had been available, it would have been insightful to compare MP mortality levels during the pre-HIV/AIDS era (before 1983) and the HIV/AIDS era (after 1983).

12 The analysis is based on the details supplied by only 280 MPs.

13 This section draws heavily on the Assessment of the HIV/AIDS Impact on the National Assembly of the United Republic of Tanzania, Final Report, submitted by the consultant in March 2005.

14 The Tanzanian Parliament has 14 standing committees, with each ministry being assigned to a committee. The committees are: the Finance and Economics Committee; the Public Accounts Committee; the Local Government Accounts Committee; the Social Services Committee; the Community Development Committee; the Agriculture and Land Committee; the Trade and Investment Committee; the Committee on Infrastructure; the Natural Resources and Environment Committee; the Defense and Security Committee; the Constitution, Legal Affairs and Administration Committee; the Foreign Affairs Committee; the Rights, Powers and Responsibilities Committee; and the Parliamentary Rules and Regulations Committee.

15 Two parties – the DP and the NCCR – Mageuzi refused to sign the code of conduct, claiming that the Constitution had first to be changed, and that a NEC elected by the President from the ruling party (CCM) cannot be impartial, thus, under its jurisdiction, elections can never be free and fair.

16 Face-to-face interviews were conducted by the Afrobarometer team based at REPOA. The sample was drawn by taking the smallest geographic units, census enumeration areas (EAs) and stratifying all EAs nationwide into separate lists according to region and urban/rural status. EAs were randomly selected from the lists with the probability proportionate to their size in the overall population, as represented in the 2001 Tanzanian census, which ensured that every eligible adult had an equal chance of being selected. A gender quota ensured that every other interviewee was female.

17 Though the sample sizes for different Afrobarometer rounds are different, the results have been presented inin percentages, rather than in absolute numbers.

18 In round 3, data were collected from 1 030 Tanzanians, with respondents providing their perceptions on the interface between the government and politics and on whether they registered to vote in the 2005 elections.

19 REDET's opinion polls show that Tanzanians generally are ignorant about basic political issues.

20 In 2002, a NORAD-commissioned study estimated the number of orphans to be 2 549 885, as well as that about 45% of orphans lacked a guardian. However, the study was regarded as biased and unrepresentative (NORAD, 2002). Anecdotal evidence from Makete shows the number of children-headed households to be insignificant (Kessy, Kweka, Makaramba and Kiria).

21 A value less than 1.0 signifies that the average person spends less than one hour a day on home-based care, while the highest possible value (4.0) indicates that a person spends virtually all day providing all three kinds of home-based care.

22 The correlation between the total number of voters registered and the total population is very high and positive (correlation coefficient = 0.92).

23 The correlation between the number of registered voters and HIV prevalence while controlling for the population is also positive (correlation coefficient = 0.41).

24 Another reason may have been that the correlation analysis failed to capture all other variables that affect voter registration, resulting in underestimation of the affect of HIV/AIDS on voter participation.

25 Adult population projections for 18 years and above by regions were not available at the time of this study, necessitating the use of 2002 figures. Nevertheless, assuming uniform population growth, the 2002 regional figures could suffice.

26 When an analysis is undertaken using a small segment of the data available from the 2000 election registration (see Table 10.3), the correlation between the population and number of registered voters and that between the number of registered voters and HIV prevalence are both high and positive (0.65 and 0.66 respectively).

27 The figures represent HIV prevalence among ANC attendees.

28 At ZAPHA+, two PLWHAs and one management team member were interviewed.

29 Different measures of stigma have been identified in DHS (2005): the willingness to provide home-based care for an HIV/AIDS-positive family member; whether an HIV-positive female teacher should be allowed to teach; the willingness to buy fresh food from a shopkeeper with AIDS; and wanting the HIV-positive status of a family member to remain secret.

30 Knowledge is assessed by asking the respondents on whether they have heard of HIV/AIDS.

31 The chances of contracting HIV can be reduced by limiting sex to one partner who is not infected and who has no other partners.

32 Average of three variables: using condoms; limiting sex to one uninfected partner; and abstaining from sex.

33 The traditional healers referred to here are witchdoctors, not herbalists. Herbalists have provided herbs that reduce signs of AIDS and the pain associated with some opportunistic infections.

References

Bomani, M., 1996. "Proposals for a New Constitution and Electoral Law", Paper presented at the Symposium on Constitution and Electoral Regimes, Dar es Salaam, 4–5 July.

Chama cha Mapinduzi (CCM), 2005. "CCM Electoral Manifesto for 2005 General Elections", National Executive Committee of CCM, Dodoma, Tanzania.

Cuf, 2001. "Report on HIV and AIDS Testing for Senior Leaders of Civic United Front", as reported in the media .

Cuf, 2005. "Party Elections Manifesto", Dar es Salaam: Cuf.

Dahoma, M., Salim, A. A., Abdool, R., Othman, A. A. and Abdullah, A, 2005. "Prevalence of HIV, Hepatitis B and C and Syphilis Infection in Substance Users in Zanzibar, Tanzania ". Paper presented at the XVI International AIDS Conference, Toronto, Canada, 2006.

Economic and Social Research Foundation (ESRF), 2003. "The Social and Economic Impacts of HIV in Tanzania", Research report submitted to SIDA, Dar es Salaam.

Fimbo, G. M., 1995. "Towards the Separation of Powers in a New Democracy in Tanzania", *The African Review*, 22 (1 and 2): 16–31.

Goffman, E., 1963. *Stigma: Notes on the Management of Spoiled Identity*, Englewood Cliffs, NJ: Prentice-Hall.

International Centre for Research on Women (ICRW), 2002. *Addressing HIV-Related Stigma and Resulting Discrimination in Africa: A Three-Country Study in Ethiopia, Tanzania and Zambia*, Washington D.C.: International Centre for Research on Women.

Kessy, F., Tax, S. and Aiko, R., 2004. "The Impact of HIV and AIDS on Agriculture: The Case of Kilombero and Ulanga Districts", Final draft submitted to Eastern Zone Client-oriented Research and Extension Program (EZCORE), October 2004.

Kessy, F., 2005. "Inventory of HIV and AIDS Service Providers in 2004", Report submitted to the Swedish Cooperative Center, Nairobi.

Kessy, F., Kweka, J., Makaramba, R. and Kiria, I., (ND) "Vulnerability and Property Rights of Widows and Orphans in the Era of HIV and AIDS Pandemic: The Case Study of Muleba and Makete Districts in Tanzania", Preliminary research findings submitted to FAO.

Mallya, E. T., 2000. "The State of Constitutional Development in Tanzania", in Issa Shivji (ed.), *Constitutional Development in East Africa for the Year 2000*, Dar es Salaam: E&D.

Maman, S., Mbwambo, J. and Hogan, N., 2001. "HIV and Partner Violence: Implications for HIV Voluntary Counseling and Testing Programs in Dar es Salaam, Tanzania", Washington D.C.: Population Council.

Man, J., 1987. Statement on Information Briefing on AIDS to the 42nd Session of the United Nations General Assembly, New York.

Mufti's Office, 2004. "HIV/AIDS Guideline for Zanzibar Muslim Community", Zanzibar: Mufti's Office.

Mushi S. S., Baregu, M. and Mukandala, R. (eds), 2001. *Tanzania Political Culture: A Baseline Survey*, Dar es Salaam: University of Dar es Salaam, Department of Political Science and Public Administration.

National Bureau of Statistics (NBS) (Tanzania) and Macro International, 1997. *Tanzania Demographic and Health Survey, 1997*, Dar es Salaam: National Bureau of Statistics; Calverton, Maryland: Macro International.

NBS (Tanzania) and Macro International, 2000. *Tanzania Reproductive and Child Health Survey, 1999*, Dar es Salaam: National Bureau of Statistics; Calverton, Maryland: Macro International.

NBS (Tanzania) and ORC Macro, 2005. *Tanzania Demographic and Health Survey, 2004–05*, Dar es Salaam: National Bureau of Statistics; Calverton, Maryland: ORC Macro.

National Electoral Commission (NEC), 2001. "The Report of the National Electoral Commission on the 2000 Presidential, Parliamentary and Councilors' Elections", Dar es Salaam: NEC.

NEC, 2006. "The Report of the National Electoral Commission on the 2005 Presidential, Parliamentary and Councilors' Elections", Dar es Salaam: NEC.

National Convention for Construction and Reform – Mageuzi (NCCR – Mageuzi), 2005. "The Electoral Manifesto of NCCR – Mageuzi for 2005 General Elections", Dar es Salaam: NCCR.

NORAD, 2002. "Children Neglected – HIV and AIDS Orphans Study: Identification and Needs Assessment", Report to NORAD by Eastern and Southern African Universities Research Programme (ESAURP).

Nyblade, L., Ponde, R., Mathur, S., Banteyerga, H. and Kidanu, A., 2003. "Disentangling HIV and AIDS Stigma in Ethiopia, Tanzania and Zambia", Washington D.C.: International Centre for Research on Women (ICRW).

Nyalali Commission, 1991. "Taarifa ya Mapendekezo ya Tume Kuhusu Mfumo wa Siasa Nchini Tanzania", Dar es Salaam: Nyalali Report.

Ogden, J, and Nyblade, L., 2005. *Common at its Core: HIV-Related Stigma across Contexts*, Washington D.C.: International Center for Research on Women.

Research on Poverty Alleviation (Repoa), 2005. "Afro Barometer: A Comparative Series of National Public Attitude Surveys on Democracy, Markets, and Civil Society in Africa." Dar es Salaam: Repoa.

Revolutionary Government of Zanzibar (RGoZ), 2002. "Zanzibar HIV Validation Study", Zanzibar: Zanzibar AIDS Control Programme.

RGoZ, 2004. "Zanzibar National HIV/AIDS Strategic Plan, 2004/5–2009/9", Zanzibar: Zanzibar AIDS Commission.

RGoZ, 2005a. "Report on Implementation of Planned Activities by the Zanzibar AIDS Control Program for the Year 2004–2005", Zanzibar: Zanzibar AIDS Control Programme.

RGoZ, 2005b. "Uchanguzi Mkuu 2005 Bila ya Virusi vya Ukimwi Zanzibar", Zanzibar: Zanzibar AIDS Control Programme.

RGoZ, 2006. "National HIV/AIDS Policy", Zanzibar: Zanzibar AIDS Commission.

Smithson, P., 2006. "Fair's Fair: Health Inequalities and Equity in Tanzania", Research report prepared on behalf of Ifakara Health Research and Development Centre and Women's Dignity Project.

Strand, P., Matlosa, K., Strode, A. and Chirambo, K., 2005. *HIV and AIDS and Democratic Governance in South Africa: Illustrating the Impact on Electoral Process*, Cape Town: IDASA.

Tanzania Election Monitoring Committee (Temco), 1995. "Report of the 1995 General Elections in Tanzania", Dar es Salaam: Temco.

United Republic of Tanzania (URT), 1977. *The Constitution of the United Republic of Tanzania*, Dar es Salaam: Government Printer.

URT, 1979. *Local Authorities Elections Act No. 4 of 1979*, Dar es Salaam: Government Printer.

URT, 1985. *The Elections Act No. 1 of 1985*, Dar es Salaam: Government Printer.

URT, 2001. "National HIV and AIDS Policy." Dar es Salaam: Prime Minister's Office.

URT, 2003a. "HIV/AIDs/STIs Surveillance Report, Report Number 17", Dar es Salaam: NACP.

URT, 2003b. "National HIV and AIDS Multi-Sectoral Strategic Framework", Dar es Salaam: Tacaids.

URT, 2003c. "National Health Policy", Dar es Salaam: Ministry of Health.

URT, 2003d. "Health Sector Strategy for HIV and AIDS (2003–2006)", Dar es Salaam: National AIDS Control Program.

URT, 2003e. "2002 Population and Housing Census", Dar es Salaam: National Bureau of Statistics.

URT, 2005a. "Tanzania HIV and AIDS Indicator Survey 2003-04", Dar es Salaam: Tacaids and National Bureau of Statistics; Calverton, Maryland: ORC Macro.

URT, 2005b. "HIV/AIDS/STIs Surveillance Report – Report Number 19", Dar es Salaam: NACP.

URT, 2005c. "Tanzania Public Expenditure Review Multi-Sectoral Review: HIV/AIDS 2005 Update", Dar es Salaam: Tacaids and Ministry of Finance.

URT, 2005d. "Assessment of the HIV and AIDS Impact on the National Assembly of the United Republic of Tanzania", Dar es Salaam: Parliament Secretariat.

URT, 2005e. *Poverty and Human Development Report 2005*, Dar es Salaam: Mkuki na Nyota.

URT, 2005f. "Plan of Action for MVC in Tanzania", Dar es Salaam: Ministry of Health and Social Welfare.

URT, Various years. "HIV/AIDs/STIs Surveillance Report", Dar es Salaam: National AIDS Control Program.

URT, Ministry of Health Tanzania Mainland, 2001-2002, 2003. National AIDS Control Programme Surveillance of HIV and Syphilis Among Antenatal Clinic Enrollees: Dar Es Salaam.

Whiteside, A., Mattes, R., Willan, S. and Manning, R., 2002. "Examining HIV/AIDS in Southern Africa Through the Eyes of Ordinary Southern Afrobarometer Paper No. 12, August.

Abbreviations

ABCZ	AIDS Business Coalition in Zanzibar
AIDS	acquired immune deficiency syndrome
ANC	antenatal clinic

ARO	assistant returning officer
ARV	antiretroviral
Asp	Afro-Shirazi Party
AU	African Union
CBO	community-based organisation
CCM	*Chama cha Mapinduzi*
CHADEMA	*Chama cha Demokrasia na Maendeleo*
CUF	Civic United Front
Daccom	district AIDS coordinating committee
EA	enumeration area
EC	Electoral Commission
ESAURP	Eastern and Southern African Universities Research Programme
ESRF	Economic and Social Research Foundation
FBO	faith-based organisation
FGD	focus group discussion
FPTP	First Past The Post
GDP	gross domestic product
ICRW	International Centre for Research on Women
IDASA	Institute for Democracy in South Africa
IDU	injecting drug user
IEC	Information, Education and Communication
MDAs	ministries, departments and agencies
MMP	mixed member proportional
MoH	Ministry of Health
MoHSW	Ministry of Health and Social Welfare
MP	Member of Parliament
MSM	men who have sex with men
MTP	medium-term plan
NACP	National AIDS Control Programme
NCCR – Mageuzi	National Convention for Construction and Reform – Mageuzi
NEC	National Electoral Commission
NGO	non-governmental organisation
NMSF	National Multisectoral Strategic Framework
NYP	Network for Young People Living with HIV/AIDS
PAPO	principal administration and personnel officer
PEO	principal elections officer
Phaera	Promote HIV/AIDS Education in Rural Areas
PIO	principal information officer
PLWHAs	People Living with HIV/AIDS
PLWHAVWs	People Living with HIV/AIDS in Vingunguti Ward
PMO	Prime Minister's Office
PMO–RALG	Prime Minister's Office, Regional Administration and Local Governance
PMTCT	prevention of mother-to-child transmission
PR	Proportional Representation

PSA	principal state attorney
PVR	permanent voters' register
RAS	regional administrative secretary
REC	regional election coordinator
Redet	Research and Education for Democracy in Tanzania
Repoa	Research on Poverty Alleviation
RGoZ	Revolutionary Government of Zanzibar
RO	returning officer
SADC	Southern Africa Development Community
SADC-PF	Southern Africa Development Community – Parliamentary Forum
Shaccom	Shehia AIDS Coordinating Council
SMZ	*Serikali ya Mapinduzi ya Zanzibar*
STI	sexually transmitted infection
SU	substance user
Tac	Technical HIV/AIDS Committee
Tacaids	Tanzania Commission for AIDS
Tanu	Tanganyika African National Union
Tapac	Tanzania Parliamentarians' AIDS Coalition
Tawla	Tanzania Women Lawyers Association
Tayopa	Tanzania Youth Plan of Action
TB	tuberculosis
Temco	Tanzania Election Monitoring Committee
This	Tanzania HIV/AIDS Indicator Survey
TLP	Tanzania Labour Party
TPAPD	Tanzania Parliamentary Association for Population and Development
TWPG	Tanzania Women's Parliamentary Group
TZS	Tanzanian shilling
UDP	United Democratic Party
UN	United Nations
URT	United Republic of Tanzania
UWAKUZA	*Umoja wa Wawakilishi wa Kupambana na Ukimwi Zanzibar*
UWAWAZA	*Umoja wa Wawakilishi Wanawake Kupambana na Ukimwi Zanzibar*
VCT	voluntary counselling and testing
VMAC	Village Multisectoral AIDS Committee
WMAC	Ward Multisectoral AIDS Committee
ZAAIDA	Zanzibar Against AIDS Infection and Drug Abuse
ZAC	Zanzibar AIDS Commission
ZACP	Zanzibar AIDS Control Programme
ZAIDA	Zanzibar Association of Interfaith on AIDS and Development
ZANGOC	Zanzibar NGO Cluster for HIV/AIDS Prevention
ZAPHA+	Zanzibar Association of People Living with HIV/AIDS
ZEC	Zanzibar Electoral Commission
ZNP	Zanzibar Nationalist Party
ZPPP	Zanzibar and Pemba People's Party

Zambia

Derrick Elemu, Elijah Rubvuta and Adrian Muunga

With contributions by Stella Mwase

1. Study overview

This report presents findings from a research project undertaken by the Foundation for Democratic Process (FODEP) between 1st September 2005 and 30th October 2006, with collegial from Idasa.

1.1 Hypotheses

The literature in the area of HIV/AIDS and governance is quite recent and conclusions still only tentative. Most contributions to this field of research have so far been based on conjecture, and have at best only generated a set of hypotheses for further investigation.

More recent contributions have however started to test such hypotheses through empirical research (Rugalema 2002; Chirambo, 2003; Strand, Strode, Matlosa and Chirambo, 2005). Evidence, which has played a significant role in guiding this research, already points to the fact that the HIV/AIDS epidemic could be exerting considerable stress on already strained African democracies. In conditions where democracy is generally weak and political institutions are inefficient due to either corruption or lack of human and financial resources, HIV/AIDS could further decrease both the responsiveness of governmental institutions and participation of the people in democratic processes.

Further, evidence points to the fact that HIV/AIDS is negatively affecting the effectiveness and integrity of the various institutions of the state and its democratic structures. As civil servants and elected officials are infected and affected by HIV/AIDS, institutions could see higher levels of staff turnover. This is likely to result in reduced productivity and lower levels of morale, as well as the loss of talent, skills, networks, and experience that enable institutions to function effectively. It could also make it increasingly difficult to replace experienced personnel in legislatures, political parties, government ministries and electoral management bodies (Patterson 2000; Rugalema 2002; Barnett and Whiteside 2002: Strand et al., 2005).

This study therefore hypothesises that the HIV/AIDS epidemic is negatively impacting on the electoral system, electoral processes and the various institutions involved in Zambia.

1.2 Methodology

The researchers took a very participatory approach to the collection of information for this report and a wide range of methods was employed. These included the following:

1.2.1 Document Review

Document review included analyses of the legal and constitutional framework governing the conduct of elections, the status of the voters' roll (size of electorate and availability of voter tracking and purging mechanisms), research findings on HIV/AIDS, and other relevant research documents, parliamentary records on deceased Members of Parliament (MPs), information on the administrative capacity of the Electoral Commission of Zambia (ECZ), delimitation reports, election results and voter turn-out of the most recent elections.

The review provided the much needed background information that informed both sampling of the respondents, development of research tools, and also helped the researchers to have a better appreciation of the subject at hand.

1.2.2 Study sites

The study was undertaken in a number of Zambian districts, incorporating both rural and urban areas. These included Mumbwa, Mansa, Ndola, Lusaka, Petauke and Livingstone.

1.2.3 In-depth Structured Interviews

Structured in-depth interviews were used to generate information from different categories of stakeholders, namely, national assembly representatives, the ECZ and members of political parties that are represented in parliament, local government administrators, members of HIV/AIDS-related civil society organisations (CSOs) and other government agencies. This methodology allowed for deeper and richer interaction with the informants. In all the cases, confidentiality of sources of information was emphasised to allow for discussion of more sensitive issues.

1.2.4 Public Opinion Survey data

A detailed analysis of public opinion survey data from the Idasa-driven Afrobarometer project of 2003 was undertaken to correlate public perceptions with government actions vis-à-vis HIV/AIDS and governance in the country.

1.2.5 Statistical analysis

Detailed analyses of epidemiological data as they relate to HIV prevalence and mortality among the voting age population in the country were undertaken.

1.2.6 Focus Group Discussion (FGDs)

This methodology was used during consultations with representatives of political parties, and people living with HIV/AIDS (PLWHAs) in the districts studied. This methodology allowed for the generation of a wide range of views on key research questions. FGDs further enriched the qualitative analyses of citizen perceptions, particularly with regard to people infected and/or affected by HIV/AIDS and their ability to participate in electoral processes. In addition, FGDs were used to test preliminary research results, upon which a final report was produced. Consultations with stakeholders during this process helped refine solutions to the deficits identified by the study. The FGD were very engaging.

1.3 Dissemination workshop

At the end of fieldwork and preliminary data analysis, a workshop was held with representatives from all stakeholders involved in HIV/AIDS and electoral processes in Zambia. The essence of the workshop was to share preliminary findings with all the stakeholders in order to receive feedback and reach consensus on key issues to establish whether there were links between the HIV/AIDS epidemic and the electoral process in Zambia. It is in this context that the workshop was a data collection tool for this report.

1.4 Structure of the report

The report is divided into eleven sections. To appreciate the context and magnitude of the challenges we are confronted with, immediately following this introductory section, we begin by mapping the extent of the epidemic and providing a response.

Thereafter, we analyse key electoral institutions and their role in democratic governance, focusing on the thematic areas: the electoral system, electoral management, political institutions and citizens' participation in the electoral process. Section 3 focuses specifically on the impact of HIV/AIDS on democratic governance. The chapter begins by describing governance in Zambia from a historical perspective. This is followed by an analysis of the implication of the HIV/AIDS epidemic for democratic governance and the impact HIV/AIDS could be having on the electoral processes more specifically. The impact of HIV/AIDS on electoral systems is then presented in section 4. We make a comparative analysis of the different electoral systems and their implications in the context of the HIV/AIDS epidemic. The chapter highlights the costs associated with the FPTP electoral system currently in place in Zambia and the surrounding electoral system reform debates.

The interactions of HIV/AIDS and electoral administration and management are presented in section 5. The section looks at the legal and institutional frameworks governing electoral administration and management and how these are affected by the epidemic. Parliament is then singled out in section 6, which looks at the impacts of HIV/AIDS on the configuration of Parliament in Zambia. The implications of high death rates and the ever-increasing occurrence of by-elections and how Parliament as an institution is responding to the epidemic are also highlighted. Section 7 then focuses on the impact of HIV/AIDS on political parties as critical players in governance and electoral processes. HIV/AIDS policy positions and debates within and among political parties are reviewed. This section closes by examining the impacts of the epidemic on political parties vis-à-vis their relevance and effectiveness in the electoral process.

The overall national public opinion is then captured in Section 8, which reviews public Afrobarometer opinion data and civic participation in the context of the HIV/AIDS epidemic. Section 9 then highlights the importance of mass participation and how the epidemic could be affecting citizens' ability to effectively participate in politics and electoral processes. Section 10 then ties up the discussions from focus group discussion with regard to attitudinal and structural HIV-related challenges that infected and/or affected persons face and how these challenges could be affecting their participation in politics and elections. The last section (11) highlights the major conclusions and points the way forward through a number of recommendations for further research, policy and specific interventions for improving the national response to HIV/AIDS in order to reduce the adverse impacts of the epidemic on governance and electoral processes in Zambia.

2. HIV/AIDS in Zambia

At national level, Zambia's case is just as alarming as the general SADC scenario illustrated in the first chapter of this book. The first case of HIV/AIDS in Zambia was reported in 1984. This was followed by a rapid rise in HIV prevalence (that is, the proportion of people who are living with HIV in the 15 to 49 year-olds age group). Doctors practising in the early 1980s recall being perplexed by a series of cases of compromised immunity at that time, which in retrospect they now identify as the beginning of the HIV epidemic (NAC, 2005: 12).

The HIV/AIDS epidemic continues to have devastating impacts on the social, economic, and political well-being of the country, draining the country of scarce resources and depleting institutions of workers and leaders necessary to sustain development. For a poor country such as Zambia, this period has been very difficult and the consequences of HIV/AIDS are going to be with us for decades.

2.1 HIV/AIDS prevalence

The population of Zambia now stands at approximately 10.3 million people with a growth rate of 2.9 per cent per year (CSO, 2000 Census). More than 50 per cent of the population is less than 20 years of age and constitutes the most susceptible group to HIV infection in Zambia. It has been acknowledged that HIV/AIDS appear to be underreported and poorly diagnosed in Zambia (NAC, 2004). Prevalence data on HIV come from testing pregnant women at antenatal clinics and population-based surveys in selected areas. Since 1990, Zambia established sentinel surveillance systems to detect and track changes in the epidemic in key communities over time. However, the survey only involved 36 sites and did not collect age data until 1993. Subsequently, Zambia undertook full sentinel surveys in 1994, 1998, and 2002 in which all sections of the country were represented. These surveys have become a major source of information

on prevalence and trends in the epidemic.

In addition, the University Teaching Hospital (UTH) in Lusaka serves as a referral health facility for more than 1.5 million people in greater Lusaka, and its data collection systems provide reliable information on disease trends and disease presentation. The hospital is the only tertiary hospital in Zambia, and it has provided the majority of clinical care for individuals with HIV/AIDS. Therefore, morbidity and mortality figures recorded at the hospital, with information from satellite clinics, are used to represent the national status of the disease (USAID, 2002: 2).

In spite of complications in determining the figures, HIV/AIDS prevalence in Zambia has been rising steadily since the first case in 1984. Both the total number of infected persons and deaths show a consistent rise, as is shown in the table below.

Table 2.1: HIV/AIDS Prevalence rates in Zambia, 1985-2005

Year	% of HIV prevalence	No. infected with HIV	No. AIDS deaths
1985	0.8	36,707	845
1990	10.4	293,581	10,594
1995	16.7	665,935	40,955
2000	15.8	877,040	76,715
2001	15.6	899,650	83,155
2002	15.2	910,704	87,659
2003	14.8	915,267	90,571
2004	14.4	917,718	93,670
2005	13.9	914,691	95,373
Source: NAC, 2005b			

2.2 Estimates of prevalence

Presently, about 16 per cent of the adult population aged 15-49, or around one in every six individuals in this age group, is HIV positive in Zambia. It has been observed that the majority of these people do not know their HIV-status. As indicated in the graph below, infection rates are much higher in women, pegged at 18 per cent, than in men, at 13%. It should be noted that infection rates also vary with age. While the HIV prevalence is 5% among 15-19-year-olds, it rises to 25% among individuals in the 30-34 age group, before falling to a level of 17% among individuals aged 45-49 (GRZ/NAC, 2004: 10). Figure 2.1 shows the distribution of HIV prevalence by age and sex:

Figure 2.1: Percentage of HIV-positive by age

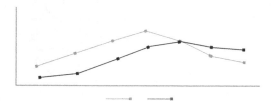

Source: NAC 2004

Furthermore, urban residents are more than twice as likely to be infected with the HIV virus as rural residents. Twenty-three percent of urban residents were HIV positive in 2002 compared to 11% of rural residents (ZDHS, 2002). The trend has not changed much since. Figure 2.2 shows the average prevalence rate by province:

Figure 2.2: HIV prevalence – ages 15-49 (2002)

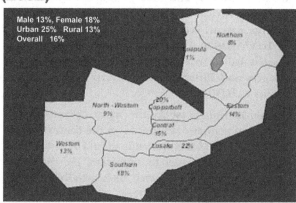

Source: NAC 2004

It is equally important to highlight here the other side of the picture because usually there is a tendency to focus on the negative side. In Zambia, about 84 of every 100 people aged 15-49 remain uninfected. All these women and men can actively take measures to protect themselves and help stop the spread of the virus. This is why a strong response to the epidemic from all sectors of the country makes a lot of sense.

2.3 Trends in prevalence

The epidemic is certainly not a new phenomenon in Zambia. Although HIV prevalence has remained

relatively lower in Zambia than in other Southern African countries, such as Botswana, South Africa, Swaziland, and Zimbabwe, evidence indicates that it was already at high levels by the early 1990s. The only comfort is that HIV-prevalence has remained quite stable at the current level for many years. With regard to the social, economic and other impacts of the epidemic, the consequences are going to be serious regardless of what happens to prevalence levels in the future.

Trend projections by the Central Statistical Office (CSO) as at 2004 revealed that the number of HIV-infected persons in the population (including children) would rise from 293 600 in 1990 to 877 000 in 2000 and 914 700 in 2005 and would then drop back to 881 100 by 2010. Over this period, large numbers of people will die from the disease and be removed from the HIV-infected population. This is why the number of infected persons does not grow at an even faster pace.

Alternatively, the number of PLWHAs will grow more rapidly if antiretroviral drugs (ARVs) are widely and effectively used to prolong life. Many projections in Zambia do not take into account expanded ARV use. The graph below presents a snapshot of the trends in infection rates:

Figure 2.3: Projected number of people infected with HIV, 1990 – 2010

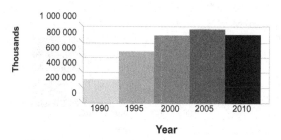

Source: NAC 2004

Full-blown AIDS is determined by how far the immune system has deteriorated, as defined by the presence of opportunistic infections and tumours. In 2003, approximately 10% of infected persons had developed AIDS (NAC 2004).

The number of new cases developing each year amongst PLWHAs is very important. Infected persons who develop AIDS place tremendous demands on the health sector until they die. NAC projections of new AIDS cases were about 13 700 in 1990 but this rose to 82 300 in 2000. This was projected to rise to 95 800 in 2005 before falling slightly to 93 100 in 2010.

In the period between 2000 and 2010, about 260 persons would be developing AIDS every day, even with the assumed decline in prevalence (NAC, 2004). The very large number of annual new AIDS cases would place severe pressure on the health sector, as well as households, to provide the added intensive care and support required by AIDS patients.

Figure 2.4: Projected annual new AIDS cases, 1990-2010

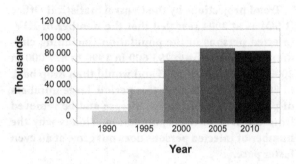

Source: NAC 2004

The death toll from AIDS has been high and it continues to rise. In 1990, about 10 600 persons died of AIDS. The annual death toll then soured to 76 700 in 2000, and it was projected to reach 95 400 in 2005 and 94 100 in 2010.

Figure 2.5: Annual AIDS deaths, 1990-2010

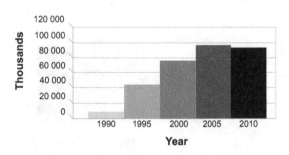

Source: NAC 2004

The devastating impacts of AIDS will continue well into the future even after prevalence has declined. This can be seen when one considers cumulative AIDS deaths over time. From 1983 when the epidemic started to 2000, the CSO reported that an estimated 482 000 Zambians had died of AIDS. In the following years between 2000 and 2010, another 928 000 Zambians are projected to die from the disease in the absence of widespread use of ARVs. This would result in an accumulated total death toll of about 1.4 million by 2010.

Figure 2.6: Cumulative AIDS deaths, 1990–2010

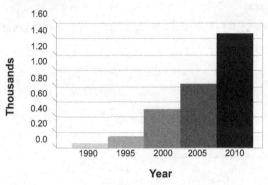

Source: NAC 2004

3. Factors that fuel spread of HIV

The HIV/AIDS epidemic emerged against a backdrop of many other problems, such as illiteracy, poverty, and in some cases, poor or inadequate governance structures. The nexus between HIV/AIDS, illiteracy, poverty and good/poor governance among Southern African countries is quite complex and to a large extent, self-reinforcing. The manifestation of HIV/AIDS and illiteracy among the citizens has usually led to increased poverty, while the state of poverty and illiteracy also directly creates vulnerability to HIV/AIDS.

This section presents the main theoretical and analytical frameworks that form the context within which the HIV/AIDS epidemic should be understood and analysed in order to appreciate the challenges facing the countries affected, be it socially, economically, politically or even in terms of good governance and electoral processes.

3.1 Poverty

The inter-relationship between the HIV/AIDS epidemic and poverty are complex. On a global scale, HIV appears to be clustered towards the poorer countries. Within these countries, the earliest victims were amongst the urban rich. However, it has now become clear that poverty creates vulnerability to HIV/AIDS, through lack of the essential human assets of education, autonomy, confidence and aspiration. Social-cultural beliefs, which deprive women of the same assets, can make them more vulnerable to HIV infection. Women have limited access to productive resources such as land, credit, skills, capital, technology and information. Because of this, most women are economically dependent on men, contributing to their inability to negotiate for safer sex and also leading them to engage in commercial or transactional sex in order to survive (NAC, 2005: 9). Girls from poor families are sometimes forced into early marriages, sexual arrangements in exchange for money, or school requisites and thus become vulnerable to HIV.

Further, not only does HIV/AIDS flourish in poverty, but it also accentuates it. AIDS largely eliminates the productive sector of society, the 15-45 year age group. It impoverishes households through expenditure on medical and care necessities, and impacts on household livelihoods as critical labour is lost. Long-term prospects for individuals, families, communities and the nation are damaged as poverty brings malnutrition, loss of education, emotional and psychological trauma and loss of a secure future (NAC, 2005: 10).

3.2 Mobility

Specific groups are more susceptible to HIV due to their mobility. These include refugees, long distance truckers, migrant workers, cross-border traders, fishmongers and uniformed security personnel. This workforce spends days and weeks away from their matrimonial homes, and consequently they find themselves establishing other sexual relationships during their stay away from home (NAC, 2005: 10).

3.3 Inadequate knowledge and beliefs

Even where basic knowledge about HIV/AIDS is universally high, many myths and misconceptions still exist that override what people have "learned" about prevention, treatment and care. These include beliefs about sex and abortions, bereavement, witchcraft, possible modes of transmission, and the framework of "sex-sin-punishment" that is emphasised by most churches (ibid). Furthermore, beliefs in witchcraft often lead people to seek traditional healers before or instead of western medicine for diagnosis and treatment, thereby delaying appropriate treatment in most cases.

3.4 Silence, stigma and discrimination

The continuing high prevalence in HIV/AIDS is also due to the "S-factor" – "Stigma", "Shame" and "Silence" (NAC, 2005: 10). The three Ss lead to discrimination, denial and blaming others, thereby delaying life-prolonging action. There are many people who have died without admitting to their conditions, even when their denial is directly responsible for the loss of several years of life. AIDS is widely seen as a consequence of "immoral" behaviour, and even as a just reward for wrong behaviour. This situation is not helped by the taboo that forbids open discussion on sexual matters between parents and their children, as parents often sit by and pretend it's not happening while young people engage in early, unprotected sexual activity (NAC, 2005: 10).

4. Impact on socio-economic spheres

The HIV/AIDS epidemic is a major challenge both to public health and the socio-economic development of the country. It is threatening to arrest, or even reverse, some of the important hard-won gains in various sectors such as health, education, agriculture and human development. The physical, psychological and emotional devastating effects of the HIV/AIDS epidemic have brought great suffering to the people of Zambia; poor productivity has been entrenched; mortality and morbidity rates for both infants and adults have worsened; and sectors such as health, education, agriculture, transport, the economy in general, has been adversely affected as the labour force is bogged down by the epidemic (NAC, 2005: 11).

What is even more significant is that, as AIDS kills people in the prime of life, the workforce is stripped of valuable skills and experience. The situation becomes yet worse as there are fewer people to teach the next generation. All of this means that production costs rise, while at the same time consumer spending falls because people affected by AIDS have less money to spare. To demonstrate the impacts of HIV/AIDS on the economy, empirical impacts on three sectors are hereby analysed.

4.1 Healthcare sector

In the health sector, HIV/AIDS has presented a massive demand for care and treatment of opportunistic infections and related illnesses. This has placed an unprecedented burden on the delivery of comprehensive health care, as government is unable to provide adequate resources to meet demand (NAC, 2005: 11). In major hospitals patients with AIDS-related illnesses occupy more than 50% of bed space. Not only has the epidemic increased the number of people seeking medical services, but it has also greatly increased costs as most AIDS-related conditions are especially expensive to treat (GRZ/NAC, 2004: 13). There is consequently less money available to treat other conditions.

Historically, Zambia's health system has suffered from years of under-investment, and is now on the brink of collapse. Almost all health facilities lack adequate personnel, drugs, and/or equipment, and the physical infrastructure is deplorable. Further, HIV/AIDS has also created high morbidity and mortality among health workers, with negative consequences for the health care offered. For example, mortality rates among nurses in Monze and Choma Districts were calculated for three periods, 1980-85; 1986-88; and 1989-91. The mortality rate during the second period showed a four-fold increase from the first period and by the third period, the increase was 13-fold. Information available from death certificates suggested AIDS to be the probable cause of the rise in mortality (NAC, 2005: 11). It is in such a context that health workers must struggle to cope with the rise in demand (due to increased morbidity in the country) - just as their own number is being depleted by illness and AIDS deaths (GRZ/NAC, 2004: 13).

4.2 Education sector

The education system has been adversely affected by the HIV/AIDS epidemic. This has manifested in the high mortality rates among teachers. Studies have reported an HIV prevalence of up to 40 per cent among teachers and a mortality rate of 6 per cent per annum (NAC, 2005: 11). The productivity of teachers has dropped in part because of absenteeism due to frequent illness. This in turn, has affected the quality of education in the country.

In 2001, a nationwide survey found that just two-thirds of primary-school-age children attended school, and less than a quarter of those aged 14-18 years attended secondary school. Twelve percent of all respondents said that a child in their own family did not attend school because a parent or guardian was suffering from AIDS or had died from AIDS (CSO, 2003). In 1999, the government launched a programme called BESSIP, which envisages education for all by 2015. However, it is acknowledged that, "the spread of HIV and AIDS may make the attainment of some of the BESSIP goals difficult if not impossible".

4.3 Agriculture, food production

Agriculture, from which the vast majority of Zambians make their living, is also affected adversely. In particular, the loss of a few workers at the crucial periods of planting and/or harvesting can significantly reduce the size of the harvest. AIDS is believed to have made a major contribution to the food shortages that hit Zambia in 2002, which were declared a national emergency (Noble, R., 2006).

Negative trends in the economy and food production fuel the epidemic that helped to create them. Poor nutrition makes HIV-positive people more vulnerable to infections, and hastens the progression of AIDS; and when people are poorer they are more likely to turn to risky occupations, and are less able to pay for medical care or school fees. As Zambia's Poverty Reduction Strategy Paper (PRSP) acknowledges, "the epidemic is as much likely to affect economic growth as it is [to be] affected by it" (GRZ, 2004).

5. HIV/AIDS and governance

Based on empirical evidence from different countries, the link between HIV/AIDS and socio-economic aspects of life has been clearly established (NAC, 2005: 11). For the most part however, the direct link between the HIV/AIDS epidemic and governance, and the electoral process in particular, has not been considered with the seriousness that it deserves. In most cases, HIV/AIDS has not been considered as a significant factor in electoral processes, and thus, such issues have mistakenly been confined to the health sector. Increasingly, however, the HIV/AIDS epidemic is being associated with the changing landscape in African politics and governance, so that serious empirical explorations into the impacts of HIV/AIDS on good governance and electoral processes are imperative in order to increase our understanding of these interlinkages (Strand, et al., 2005: 12).

Idasa's findings from its seminal work in this field were corroborated by representations from other stakeholders who attended a stakeholder workshop in Lusaka on 30th September, 2005. The Central Board of Health (CBoH) revealed that HIV/AIDS posed one of the greatest challenges to governance as it claimed some of the eligible voters, community and political leaders at various levels and a great number of employees at workplaces, including those involved in the management of electoral processes. Further, HIV/AIDS are impacting negatively on people's ability to exercise their choice and to participate in decision-making about issues that affect their lives.

All respondents who participated in this research project were unanimous on the view that the HIV/AIDS prevalence was high and worsening and that they were likely to have even more adverse impacts on governance and electoral processes in the not so distant future. Participants observed that with the worsening HIV/AIDS epidemic, it was almost inevitable that ultimately this will have significant impacts on elections and the electoral process in general. It was noted further that the impacts would vary in nature and extent, but that they would certainly be adverse. For example, the Network for Zambian People Living with HIV/AIDS (NZP+) highlighted only one aspect of this impact in their sharing of the general challenges that they face vis-à-vis voter registration and their participation in the electoral process both prior to and during the elections. It was revealed that as long as nothing was done to rectify such problems as long queuing time during registration and voting, long distances to polling station, only to mention a few, HIV/AIDS is definitely bound to have adverse impacts on the participation of PLWHAs and caregivers, which would ultimately affect elections and the electoral process in the country. This was especially so in that the numbers of people being infected was high and mostly in the age groups where most of the voting population is found.

6. Gender implications

In Zambia, women are disproportionately affected by HIV/AIDS epidemic (NAC, 2004: 38). Women are nearly 1.4 times more likely to be infected with the HIV/AIDS virus than men in similar circumstance (ZDH 2002).

The biological makeup of women may have contributed to this imbalanced sex ratio in HIV/AIDS incidences. Women are biologically more prone to HIV/AIDS infection during unprotected sexual intercourse than men. In the same vein, women are more vulnerable to other STIs, the presence of which greatly enhances the risk of HIV transmission. In addition to this, the tendency for older men to engage in sexual relations with younger women may have also contributed to the higher rates of HIV infection among young women (NAC, 2004: 38).

Further, inequality and power imbalances between women/girls and men/boys in Zambian society have heightened the vulnerability of females to HIV infection. In Zambia, women and girls are often taught from early childhood to be obedient and submissive to males. Sexual violence has been identified as the worst manifestation of women's subordination and unequal power relations between men and women. The ZDH Survey (2001-2002), revealed that 15% of women aged 15-19 have been forced to have sexual intercourse against their will at some time in their lives and this is generally accepted as normal in most Zambian cultures and traditions. About 8% of these women had such experiences within the 12 months prior to the survey. Thus, certain cultural and traditional practices and beliefs have increased the risk of HIV/AIDS transmission among women by contributing to their subordination. Women are therefore not usually empowered to negotiate for safe sex, such as demanding the use of condoms by men, and lack equal protection under statutory and customary law (NAC, 2004).

Other factors that are worth noting include widow inheritance and sexual cleansing after the death of a spouse. In addition, property grabbing from the widow can impoverish their households, causing them to use sex as a survival mechanism. Even under "normal" circumstances, more women than men are poor in Zambia. Exchange of sex for money or gifts is a coping strategy for dealing with poverty for many women. Involuntary and arranged early marriages between young girls and older men and formal and informal polygamous arrangements often increase the exposure of women to HIV/AIDS infection. Additionally, because of their low social and economic status, women and girls have more limited access to HIV/AIDS-related information, prevention, treatment, and care and support than men and boys.

At the same time, the burden of care for the sick and ailing family members falls disproportionately on females. As a result, women, especially those in rural areas, face competing demands upon their time - between reproduction and care and productive engagements in the fields. Because an HIV/AIDS death of an adult results in the loss of household labour and/or income, children are often required to leave school and remain home or go to work to compensate for the losses and avoid school fees. Usually, girls are more often than not likely to be sacrificed for social and cultural reasons. By necessity, women and older girls are also called upon to nurture the growing number of orphaned children, the majority of who are survivors of HIV/AIDS-affected households (NAC, 2004: 38).

Therefore, women and girls are a special group in all efforts to resolve the HIV/AIDS epidemic in Zambia. With regard to governance and electoral processes, this reality is very significant in that women form the majority (51%) of the Zambian population. Thus, by their sheer numbers, whatever impact the disease has on women would therefore invariably impact on governance and electoral process because democracy and elections in particular are a phenomenon of numbers.

Gender mainstreaming in HIV/AIDS issues is therefore a central element in the fight against the epidemic and ensuring good governance and legitimate electoral processes. In this context, any programmes that promote gender equality and HIV/AIDS control can also be seen as good governance enhancing and promoting effective and legitimate electoral systems.

7. Zambia's response to HIV/AIDS

The Zambian Government's response since the beginning of the HIV/AIDS epidemic has been through awareness raising and prevention measures, and care. Since then, communities, nongovernmental organisations (NGOs), the National AIDS Prevention and Control Programme (NACP), bilateral donors, the World Health Organisation (WHO), and other United Nations (UN) agencies have fostered a variety of activities to improve HIV/AIDS care and support to people infected and affected by HIV/AIDS (USAID, 2002: 5). Further, in the last decade or so, we have seen the introduction and expansion of antiretroviral therapy (ART) to PLWHAs.

7.1 Resources

Implementation of the national programme to address HIV/AIDS in Zambia has been expensive, and most likely to be even more expensive as more and more people access ART. The encouraging trend is that considerably more resources are now becoming available to fight HIV/AIDS than were available even only a few years ago. These resources come from the international community, government budgets, the private sector, and individual households. However, the ability to absorb these funds and the capacity to utilise them effectively remains a challenge. This is even more critical in that Zambia has not had a National HIV/AIDS Account (NHAA) to track the different financial inflows for HIV/AIDS interventions and the amounts spent on these different interventions. Nevertheless, the following graph provides the general allocation as was proposed in the National HIV/AIDS Intervention Strategic Plan of 2004.

Figure 7.1: Proposed distribution of resources in National HIV/AIDS Intervention Plan

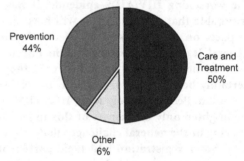

Prevention 44%

Care and Treatment 50%

Other 6%

Source: NAC 2004

7.2 Interventions

The NACP was established in 1986. The first medium-term plan (MTP I) for the 1988-1992 period focused on eight areas: TB; leprosy; information, education, and communication; laboratory support; epidemiology and research; STIs and clinical care; programme management; and home-based care. Support groups for PLWHA were established and received support, and many private sector activities were initiated (ibid).

The second medium-term plan (MTP II) for the 1994-1998 period focused on the development of a multi-sectoral approach. The goal was to foster continuous political commitment at the highest levels through an inter-sectoral committee of all ministries. The private sector, civil society, and many support groups of PLWHAs continued to play a major role. The plan also sought to increase access to STI care, control TB, strengthen condom promotion and distribution, voluntary counselling and testing (VCT), and home-based care; and develop strategies to mitigate the impact of AIDS (USAID, 2002: 5).

The follow-up plan to the MTP II is the Zambia HIV/AIDS/STD/TB Strategic Framework 2001-2003, emphasising even stronger multicultural responsibility and the establishment of a National AIDS Council (NAC) within the office of the Vice President.

Along with the policy work of the Ministry of Health (MoH), initiatives have been carried out through the CBoH and NGOs, supported by international agencies and cooperating partners. Through policy guidance from the MoH and technical guidance from the CBoH, and within the health reform framework, District Health Management Teams (DHMTs) are now responsible for HIV activities related to the health sector. These teams form District AIDS Task Forces (DATFs), in which public, NGO, and community representatives can partner to expand the public's access to sexually transmitted infection (STI) care; to control TB; to strengthen condom promotion and distribution, VCT, and home-based care; and to develop strategies to mitigate the impact of AIDS (USAID, 2002: 5).

The framework for the multi-sectoral approach was established under the NAC in 1999 with an interim committee. The NAC became operational at the end of 2000. The framework emphasised the need for VCT, facility- and home-based care, medication and supplies, and made special efforts to address stigma. The NAC coordinates the activities of 14 line ministries and others such as NGOs and community-based organisations (CBOs).

Many innovative HIV/AIDS care and support approaches have been developed in Zambia, and the country is recognised as a pioneer in this arena and as a global learning site. HIV care and support is promoted as a comprehensive package of inter-related interventions designed to meet psychosocial, social, spiritual, nutritional, and health needs. Comprehensive care is being promoted with a particular focus on VCT as an entry point to prevention, care and support services (USAID, 2002: 6).

As a consequence of health reforms, DHMTs and DATFs are promoting linkages between VCT provid-

ers; medical and home-based services; social support services; and support groups for PLWHA to create a continuum of comprehensive care and support.

The Zambia HIV/AIDS/STD/TB Strategy Framework for 2001-2003, which was subsumed into the 2002-2005 Framework, called for a further strengthening of prevention, care and support activities. The framework identified the following high-priority aspects of care and support (NAC, 2005).

• Behavioural change communication
• Condom promotion and availability
• More voluntary counselling and testing (VCT)
• Better care and support for people living with HIV/AIDS
• Better drugs supplies (ART)
• Preventing mother-to-child transmission (PMTCT).

7.2.1 Key elements of Zambia's response:

The promotion of condoms - the "C" in the ABCs of HIV/AIDS prevention – is not meant to undermine efforts to promote abstinence or being mutually faithful. But being faithful to one partner is sufficient to avoid infection only if (a) the other person is also being faithful, and (b) the other person is uninfected.

In any relationship where there is any doubt about the HIV/AIDS status or faithfulness of the partner, condoms should be used. Certainly in any casual relationship or in any relationship where the partner may have had other sexual engagements, correct and consistent condom use should be promoted (NAC, 2005).

7.2.2 How VCT works

VCT is a critical component of an effective HIV/AIDS intervention as it serves as an entry point for all efforts towards treatment. Before people could access treatment, they need to know their status first. Thus, VCT is a very critical first-line intervention in the multi-sectoral response to HIV/AIDS in Zambia (GRZ/NAC, 2004).

Before going for an HIV/AIDS antibody test, an individual spends some time with a counsellor, who will help him/her think about his/her issues and concerns.

The actual steps are represented in Figure 7.1:

Figure 7.1

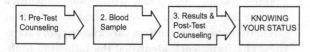

VCT has many benefits in that it facilitates behavioural change and prevention of HIV/AIDS transmission, improved health and medical treatment, informed decision-making, psychosocial support, reduced stigma and access to other services such as ART, TB treatment, and home-based care and support (GRZ/NAC, 2004).

However, in spite of these benefits, many people in Zambia still do not know their status. The graph below provides a sense of what is actually prevailing regarding testing for HIV/AIDS in Zambia.

Figure 7.2: Testing for HIV among 15 to 49 year-olds

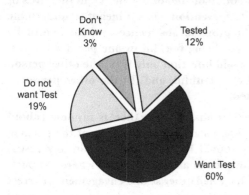

Source: NAC 2005

8. Care, support for those with HIV/AIDS

More than 900 000 Zambians are currently living with HIV. In the absence of effective and widespread use of ART, nearly all of these and their families – as well as those who get infected in the future – will eventually require some level of care and support to improve their quality of life and increase their survival prospects. The number of those in need of care and support is growing, and the basic support systems, which mainly depend on the family unit, are incapable of coping with increased numbers.

The overall goals for care and support activities are to improve the quality of life and survival of PLWHAs and to provide for those otherwise affected by the epidemic

8.1 Drugs supplies (ART)

ART can enable HIV-infected Zambians to live healthier and longer lives. The initiation and expansion of ART programmes in the public sector is therefore one of the more encouraging developments in the fight against HIV/AIDS in Zambia (GRZ/NAC, 2004).

It was a conventional belief only a few years ago that anti-retroviral drugs (ARVs) could not be used widely in poor African countries. The costs for ARVs alone were estimated to be about US$10 000 to $12 000 per person per year. However, due, in part, to intensive international pressure on governments, international organisations, and pharmaceutical companies, the costs have dropped dramatically. In Zambia, the cost of therapy for AIDS patients ranged from K40, 000 ($9.98) to K150 000 ($37.40) per month around 2000. While this meant that ART remained inaccessible for the majority of poor Zambians, it signals that ART could be made more readily accessible, especially where governments work hand-in-hand with international funding sources.

In Zambia today, free ARVs are now available. Government has been implementing the WHO 3 x 5 HIV/AIDS initiative that targeted 3 million people globally to be on ARVs by 2005. The number of people receiving ART increased from as low as 10 000 patients in 2003 to 45,000 patients by the end of 2005 (NAC, 2005). This figure has now come up to 60 000 in 2006. Zambians benefiting from ARVs have even formed what is called Network of ARV Users, which works to guide and advise ARV users on how to manage their ART (NAC, 2005).

However, this level of coverage is still very low. With about one in five sexually active Zambian adults infected, it means 1.6 million of the estimated national population of 10.3 million are infected. With only 60 000 PLWHA accessing ART, more needs to be done for this intervention to have significant impacts on the epidemic.

8.2 Preventing mother-to-child transmission

MTCT is an important mode of HIV transmission in Zambia. More than 20% of annual new infections are a result of MTCT. It has been estimated that approximately between 50 and 60 babies become infected with HIV each day in Zambia. WHO indicates also that the transmission rates are 5-10% during pregnancy; 10-20% during labour and delivery; and 10-20% during breastfeeding, where the child is breastfed for two years (GRZ/NAC, 2004).

This means that two-thirds of babies born to HIV-positive mothers are not infected with the virus. So, efforts aimed at preventing MTCT could have an important overall impact on the epidemic.

The current strategy framework as discussed above is meant to offer broad guidance to formulate policies for care and support activities. However, it does not provide detailed guidance or standards for programme planners and implementers. Further, as in many other countries, whereas the country has comprehensive guidelines for HIV/AIDS prevention and treatment, it is unfortunate that such guidelines often do not include aspects related to good governance and the electoral processes. In most aspects, the guidelines do not fully address the specific needs and protection of the PLWHAs and the general impacts of the epidemic on the electoral process (GRZ/NAC, 2004).

One of the general conclusions arising from this discussion is that Zambia is in a region that is most adversely affected by the HIV/AIDS epidemic, making the country and its population vulnerable to HIV/AIDS infection and the accompanying consequences. As such, although HIV/AIDS prevalence levels have been relatively lower in Zambia than in some neighbouring countries in the region, they have remained high from as early as 1994. This has huge implications for the extent of the impacts the epidemic has had on the country.

However, there are also positive signs in that although HIV prevalence rates have been relatively high, they have remained stable for quite a long time. Further, projections indicate that HIV prevalence, new AIDS cases, and AIDS deaths will remain stable and then begin to decline by 2010. The fact that these projections do not take into account expanded ARV use suggest an effective care and treatment programme could improve the situation even further.

Despite these somewhat benign projections, Zambia needs to continue and even expand its HIV/

AIDS response if the adverse impacts of the epidemic are to be contained within reasonable levels. This is important because the factors that have been noted as having fuelled the spread of HIV in the first place still exist.

9. Electoral system in Zambia

This section applies historical analyses of Zambia's progression to democracy and the significant developments that have affected the political and electoral systems. It proceeds to explore the linkage between the electoral system and democratic governance in Zambia over the "three republics" defined by a change from one-party to multiparty systems.

9.1 Democratic governance

9.1.2 Pre-independence

The first step towards the establishment of what has become the Zambian Parliament can be traced back to 1924, when the first Legislative Council and its Executive Council were set up immediately after the introduction of direct British Colonial Office rule in what was then Northern Rhodesia. The Governor of Northern Rhodesia, who was appointed by the British Crown, was the President/Chairman of the Legislative Council up to 1948, when the Speaker was introduced in the Ninth Legislative Council. The Executive Council (Cabinet) comprised colonial civil servants known as "officials" whose number varied between eight and ten from 1924 to 1954 (ERTC, 2006).

White settlers were represented in the Legislative Council from the time of the first Legislative Council in 1924, when five settler representatives known as "unofficial" members were nominated. In 1926, the nominated white settler representatives were replaced by the same number of elected white settler representatives, also known as "unofficial" members. In 1941, the number of elected settler representatives was increased to eight, plus one nominated. In 1945 the number of nominated unofficial members was increased from one to five. In 1932, in the Fourth Legislative Council, however, one European settler, Sir Stewart Gore Brown, an unofficial member, was nominated to represent African interests in the Legislative Council for the first time.

In 1945, three white unofficial members were nominated to represent African interests. Africans did not enter the Legislative Council until 1948. In response to African political pressure exerted through African Welfare Societies and the Northern Rhodesia African Congress founded that year, under the leadership of Godwin Mbikusita-Lewanika, two African members, namely, Henry Kasokolo and Nelson Nalumango, were elected to the Legislative Council by the African Representative Council. In addition, two white unofficial members were nominated to represent African interests (ERTC, 2006).

In 1953, the Federation of Rhodesia and Nyasaland was imposed on the three Central African Territories by the British Government against the wishes of the African majority. The result of this was increased African resistance to white rule. In 1954, in the Tenth Legislative Council, the number of Africans elected by the African Representative Council was increased from two to four. There were in addition to the four Africans, two white nominated unofficial members representing African interests.

The Northern Rhodesia African National Congress suffered a split in 1958 over, among other issues, the 1958 Northern Rhodesia Constitution. The militants wanted a boycott, while the moderates led by the then Party President, Harry Mwaanga Nkumbula, agreed to participate in the elections which were held subsequently. The splinter party was the Zambia African National Congress (ZANC), the forerunner to the United National Independence Party (UNIP) under the leadership of Kenneth D. Kaunda (ERTC, 2006).

The 1958 Northern Rhodesia Constitution

Following the 1958 Northern Rhodesia Constitution, representation in the Eleventh Legislative Council and subsequent Councils, was based on political parties winning seats in territorial elections. The majority of the indigenous Africans however, could not qualify to vote due to a franchise that was encumbered with qualifications based on education, property and income (ERTC, 2006).

The 1962 Territorial Elections – The ANC and UNIP Coalition Government

In the subsequent elections in 1962, UNIP won 14 seats, while the ANC won 7 seats. The predominantly European United Federal Party won 16 seats. The African National Congress and UNIP came togeth-

er in a coalition, to form the first ever predominantly African Government in Northern Rhodesia. Kenneth David Kaunda of UNIP became a member of the Legislative Council and the Executive Council as Minister of Local Government, while Harry Mwaanga Nkumbula of the ANC became the Minister of African Education (ERTC, 2006).

The January 1964 Territorial Elections

January 1964 ushered in self-rule and a 75-member Legislative Assembly. The January 1964 elections were held on universal adult suffrage for all Northern Rhodesia citizens aged 21 years and above. There were two electoral rolls. Sixty-five seats were on the predominantly African "Main Roll", while 10 seats were on the predominantly European, Asian and Euro-African "Reserved Roll". UNIP, with 24 unopposed seats, won a total of 55 seats, all on the Main Roll. The ANC won 10 seats, all on the Main Roll. The National Progressive Party (NPP), successor to the United Federal Party (UFP), won 10 seats, all on the Reserved Roll (ERTC, 2006).

The January 1964 elections had a 94% voter turnout, out of which UNIP won 69.02% of votes cast, and the ANC won 30.5% on the Main Roll. The NPP won 63.63% of votes cast on the Reserved Roll, while UNIP received 35.23% of the votes cast on the Reserved Roll. Kenneth David Kaunda of UNIP became the first Prime Minister of Northern Rhodesia. When Zambia attained independence and Republican status on 24th October 1964, no elections were held. It was provided in the Independence Constitution of 1964 that Kenneth David Kaunda was to be the first President and Head of State of the Republic (ERTC, 2006).

Like many other Southern African states, being a British colony, at independence Zambia just adopted the Westminster constitution and the political arrangements that go with it. Consequently, the British single-member plurality First-Past-The-Post (FPTP) electoral system became Zambia's electoral system. It is important to also note here that the adoption of the FPTP electoral system in Zambia, as is the case elsewhere in the region, was never a product of public debate or broad-based internal political consensus. As Molutsi has observed, "…the electoral systems in the region were hardly ever debated and carefully chosen on the basis of consensus among stakeholders" (Molutsi, 1999:9-10). Matlosa (1999) notes further that "…independent Southern African states … simply inherited these systems from the colonial rulers together with other constitutional frameworks."

9.2 First Republic 1964-1972

The Parliament elected in January 1964 was dissolved by President Kaunda on 2 November 1968. The 1968 elections were held under the Republican Independence Constitution. It was the first time that Zambia went to the polls to elect a President who is also the Head of State.

In 1968, the Constitution was amended to increase the number of constituencies from 75 to 105, with an addition of five seats for nomination by the President. In the general election, with a national poll of 82.47%, the ANC won 23 seats, while only one independent (pro-ANC) out of three independent candidates was successful. The United National Independence Party had a landslide victory, winning 81 seats, 30 of which were unopposed, scoring 73% of the poll (ERTC, 2006).

Under the 1964 Independence Constitution, a presidential candidate was deemed duly elected to the Office of President if she or he was unopposed at nomination. Where there were two or more presidential candidates, the candidate whose party won the highest number of votes cast in the parliamentary election, was deemed duly elected to the Office of President (ECZ, 2006). In the election contest for the Presidency in December, 1968, Kenneth David Kaunda of UNIP defeated Harry Mwaanga Nkumbula of ANC, when he polled 1 059 087 votes, as compared to Mr Nkumbula's 242 155 votes (ERTC, 2006).

In the 1968 elections, a voter was required to vote simultaneously for the parliamentary candidate of the voter's choice, and the presidential candidate supported by the parliamentary candidate, both on one ballot paper. Both the parliamentary candidate and the presidential candidate were deemed elected to their respective offices if unopposed at nomination. The Returning Officer for the presidential election was the Chief Justice, who was also given powers to determine any question relating to the presidential election (ECZ, 2006).

9.2.1 June 1969 referendum

The 1964 Constitution provided for a Referendum Clause and an Amendment Clause. The latter could not be amended without at least 50% plus one approval of eligible voters in a national referendum.

In April 1969, the government decided to change this provision. The government was of the view that the constitutional requirement for a two-thirds majority to be obtained in the National Assembly for any proposed amendment to the Constitution was sufficient. In the 17th June 1969 Referendum to remove the Referendum Clause, the government won 57.07% of the votes of registered voters, and 85% of the votes cast. Parliament was thus given power to amend the Constitution by a two-thirds majority of the House without resort to a referendum.

9.3 Second Republic 1973-1991

9.3.1 One-party state

In December 1972, the Republican Constitution was amended to enable the Republic of Zambia to become a one-party state. This ushered in the Second Republic. UNIP became the sole and only recognised political party under the law. The UNIP Constitution, which was annexed to the Republican Constitution, made the party supreme over all the institutions including government (ERTC, 2006).

The one-party Constitution, which was mostly based on the recommendations of the Chona Constitution Review Commission (CCRC), was however not enacted until August 1973. This meant that, although the ANC was outlawed through the Constitutional Amendment of December 1972, members elected to parliament on the ANC ticket in the December 1968 elections remained members of the House until new elections based on the new Constitution were held or until their full term of office was realised. Further, under the 1973 one-party Constitution, the composition of the National Assembly was increased from 105 to 125 elected members and 10 nominated members, and one elected Speaker (ERTC, 2006).

The electoral system under the one-party state was based on provisions of both the Republican and the UNIP Constitutions of 1973. Eligibility to contest the presidency and a parliamentary seat was confined to card-carrying members of UNIP. The contest was intra party, with several members of the party competing against each other. While the Electoral Commission, chaired by a Supreme Court Judge, conducted the elections, the party was in charge of the election campaign for all candidates. The party, which under the new Constitution received a government grant, was also funded for purposes of introducing candidates to the electorate and conducting election campaigns (ECZ, 2006).

Innovations were introduced in the recruitment of candidates for the parliamentary elections in the form of primary elections (abolished after the 1978 elections) and vetting by the Central Committee of UNIP. To qualify as a candidate in the presidential election, during the Second Republic, the Republican Constitution provided that only a person who was elected as the UNIP Party President by the Party General Conference could contest the Republican Presidency. Consequently, Dr Kenneth David Kaunda emerged as the sole candidate in all successive presidential elections (ERTC, 2006).

Further, to qualify as the Republican President, a presidential candidate was required to win at least 50% + 1 vote of the total votes cast in the presidential election. The electorate voted "Yes" if they supported Dr Kaunda, whose election symbol was always the "Eagle", while the symbol for the "No" vote varied each election year from "Kalulu" (Hare), to "Frog" to "Hyena". Dr Kaunda obtained the 50% + 1 vote threshold in all the four successive Presidential Elections during the Second Republic. It must be noted here, as has been shown in section four, that Zambia operated two separate systems at presidential and parliamentary levels until 1996. The Single Member Plurality (SMP) or FPTP system was used at parliamentary level while the Single Member Majority (SMM) or Absolute Majority system was used for the presidential elections whereby the winner was required to obtain 50% + 1 of the votes. Where no candidate achieved that, a run-off would be held between the two candidates with the highest votes in the first round of voting.

Generally, elections under the one-party state were trouble free and peaceful although the 1978 elections generated a lot of controversy, due to the fact that Simon Mwansa Kapwepwe, Harry M. Nkumbula and Robert Chiluwe intended to challenge Dr Kaunda for the presidency. Amendments which were suspected to have been tailored to make candidature in the presidential election impossible for Dr Kaunda's challengers were made to the party Constitution at the party general conference. Four successive presidential and parliamentary elections were held under the one-party state from 1973 to 1988. It can be said that generally all these elections were characterised by low voter turnout, registering 39% in 1973 and 59% in 1988. Dr Kaunda obtained the 50% + 1 vote in all the four successive presidential elections (ERTC, 2006).

9.4 Third Republic since 1991

9.4.1 Re-introduction of multi-party politics and the 1991 elections

By 1990, UNIP had come under increasing pressure to change the political system. This is demonstrated by the following events that occurred within the same year:

- The UNIP National Convention held in March;
- Food riots in Lusaka and the Copperbelt in June;
- The foiled *coup d'état* attempt in July; and
- The birth of the Movement for Multi-Party Democracy (MMD) in July.

Owing to increased pressure for political change agitated by the MMD and the foiled undemocratic attempts to topple the UNIP government, President Kenneth Kaunda's one-party state government yielded to demands for a new dispensation in 1990. Government decided to hold a referendum on whether Zambia should re-introduce a multi-party system or not. However, it abandoned the idea of a referendum and instead in December 1990 Article 4 of the Constitution was amended to provide for the formation of other political parties. The Mvunga Constitution Review Commission (MCRC) was then appointed to recommend a new Constitution for the Third Republic (ERTC, 2006).

A new Constitution was enacted on 24th August, 1991 and led to the holding of multi-party presidential and parliamentary elections on 31st October in the same year. Whereas the MMD and UNIP contested both the presidential and parliamentary elections, other political parties confined their participation to parliamentary elections only. Under the new Constitution, the number of elective seats in Parliament was increased from 125 to 150 and eight nominated MPs. The Movement for Multi-Party Democracy, led by Frederick Jacob Titus Chiluba, won the 1991 elections with an overwhelming majority, obtaining 125 seats out of 150.

9.4.2 The 1996 multi-party elections

The 1996 Constitutional changes reversed the requirement for an absolute majority that had been provided for in the 1973 one party state Constitution. The 1996 presidential and parliamentary elections were generally viewed as undemocratic due to the following events:

- The "state of emergency" was invoked and some top UNIP officials were charged with treason;

- The Constitution was amended by the introduction of Article 34(3)(b), which requires that a person shall be qualified to stand as President if both his parents are Zambians by birth or descent. Further, Article 129 was introduced and provides that "a person shall not, while remaining a Chief, join or participate in partisan politics". As a result, the opposition political party UNIP decided to boycott the 1996 elections; and

- Government contracted NIKUV Computers Limited of Israel, a foreign company, to design software for the compilation of a voters' register, without broad consultation with stakeholders. This led to suspicion by the public about the integrity of the resultant voters' register.

9.4.3 2001 elections

The 2001 elections were preceded by a controversy over the intentions to amend the Republican Constitution in order to allow President Chiluba to run for a third presidential term of office. The resulting conflict within MMD led to the formation of the following political parties which split from MMD: the Forum for Democracy and Development (FDD), led by Lt. Gen. Christon Tembo; Heritage Party (HP), led by Brig. Gen. Godfrey Miyanda; and the Patriotic Front (PF), led by Michael Chilufya Sata.

Further, 42 of the parliamentary election results were petitioned in the High Court, out of which four petitions resulted in the nullification of the elections. The presidential election result was also petitioned by the United Party for National Development (UPND), FDD and HP. The petitions were consolidated into one, and hearing of the presidential election petition commenced in January 2002. It was determined and concluded by the Supreme Court, on 16th February, 2005 and the MMD presidential candidate was declared duly elected.

9.5 Electoral system reform debate

For Zambia, the 2001 elections were perhaps the turning point in terms of arousing many stakeholders towards the need to reassess a number of issues in the electoral process. The 2001 election heightened the debate around the legitimacy and quality of electoral outcomes in the electoral process and many stakeholders questioned the efficacy of preserving an electoral regime that they argued was no longer relevant in the current environment in the country.

Among others, the main contentious issues that prompted the debate on electoral reforms were the following:

- The issue of setting of the date for the general elections by the President who is an interested party;

- The non-comprehensive nature of the Electoral Act as the principle law governing the electoral process;

- The continued violation of the Electoral Code of Conduct posed by limitation in enforcement. There were no clear provisions as to the enforcing authority (whether ECZ or police);

- The apparent selective ("unfair") application of the Public Order Act among stakeholders by the police;

- The unrepresentative nature of the FPTP electoral system which, under the Third Republic, seemed to give rise to other common problems such as:

1 Wastage of the votes;

2 Institutionalised "minority electoral victories" (defeating the principle of majority rule);

3 High prevalence of electoral malpractices, electoral disputes/conflicts;

4 High prevalence of "instigations," unnecessary and costly by-elections;

5 Lack of guarantee for equitable representation (e.g. women, youth, PLWHAs, etc.);

- The perception by some stakeholders of the ECZ not being sufficiently independent to inspire total confidence of all electoral stakeholders;

- Registration of voters and administration/security of voters' cards;

- The occurrence of disorderly conduct and even violence during campaigns, especially for by-elections;

- Abuse of public resources (human, financial and material) with culprits unpunished;

- Un-equitable coverage of electoral campaigns and political parties by public media;

- Violation of electoral rules with impunity; and

- The system of not punishing offenders on the spot.

As a response to the above concerns, many stakeholders and civil society joined hands in calling for comprehensive electoral reforms in the country. FODEP commissioned a nationwide campaign in 2002 to agitate for a serious review of the entire electoral process in the country arising from the main problems noted during the successive elections held after the historic first round multi-party elections in 1991.

In an apparent show of responsiveness, the government acted by undertaking to review the legal framework governing the process. Early in 2003, the government constituted the Constitutional Review Commission (CRC) and the Electoral Reforms Technical Committee (ERTC) was constituted later in the same year to deal specifically with electoral legislative reforms.

9.6 Constitution Review Process

In its quest to strengthen the Republican Constitution, the government appointed the CRC to spearhead the process of consultations with members of the public and other stakeholders on the kind of Constitution they needed.

From the start, the work of the CRC was characterised by controversy and stand-offs between government and other stakeholders, particularly on the criteria used in selecting CRC members and on the question of the mode of adoption of the new Constitution, with many civil society and interest groups pressing for a Constituent Assembly (CA) while the government maintained a determined and sustained position against the CA in preference for the adoption of the new Constitution exclusively through the National Assembly (FODEP, 2006).

The CRC conducted its work and released its Interim Report and Draft Constitution in June 2005. Many stakeholders acknowledged that the documents were very good drafts. The Final Report and Draft Constitution were released in December 2005. Both the Interim and Final documents of the CRC recommended a CA to adopt the Constitution.

Early in 2006, the government announced its decision to embrace the need to adopt the constitution through the CA, but only on condition that this would be after the 2006 tripartite elections. The government claimed there was not enough time to carry through the processes before the 2006 elections. However, many observers and critics charged that

government was just trying to have its own way in the constitution-making process and that the delays had been well calculated and deliberately designed to restrict the recommendations of the CRC and stagger the process beyond the 2006 elections so that they should be held under the old constitution. Many stakeholders alleged that this was deliberately designed to enhance the chances of the incumbent President winning the second term of office (FODEP, 2006).

It is worth noting that while the CRC did address the need to secure basic human rights, and considered gender, youth, persons with disability and majoritarian electoral system in the draft constitution, there is no specific provision devoted to issues around HIV/AIDS, its implications for the electoral system and the participation of HIV-positive persons in governance. In the context of this report, this is one aspect that the reform process will need to address as the processes continue after the elections. There is need to reform the reform process itself so that all the pertinent issues are incorporated because continuing without doing this will mean a very timely opportunity to address this oversight being missed.

9.7 Electoral Reform Process

In responding to the shortcomings in the electoral process as highlighted earlier in this chapter, government constituted a broadly representative ERTC late in 2003 and mandated it with the responsibility of consulting and recommending necessary review in the electoral process.

The ERTC conducted its work for almost one year and released its Interim Report in August 2004 with a number of what most stakeholders described as "progressive recommendations". The interim recommendations were subjected to countrywide public discussions over a 90-day period and this elicited a lot of reactions on the key issues, with the majority endorsing most of the interim recommendations. However, government also issued its reactions and opposed many of the ERTC recommendations. This affected the quality of the final report, which many stakeholders have said had been watered down to suit government preferences (FODEP, 2006).

The ERTC final report, released late in 2005, has therefore been criticised by many stakeholders, as projecting a compromised position favourable to government's position on many of the major recommendations compared to its interim report. Some of such key issues include the need for 50%+1 majority electoral system for presidential elections, MMP electoral system for parliamentary elections, and independence of the legislature. Regardless of the many complaints from various stakeholders, government proceeded to enact a new Electoral Act No. 12 of 2006 based on the diluted ERTC report (FODEP, 2006).

Although many of the new issues in the Electoral Act hinge on administrative matters, one of the key provisions introduced allows for special votes for the sick, disabled or those who for one reason or the other are not able to vote on election day. It is regrettable however that despite the new Electoral Act providing for the special vote, the ECZ failed to put in place measures to implement this provision during the 2006 elections.

Stakeholders and CSOs are thus still set to continue exerting pressure on the continued need for electoral reform beyond the 2006 elections. There is an opportunity, therefore, for the findings from this study to influence the course of the reforms, especially in the context of the pressure exerted by replacement costs for political representatives, both in parliament and at other levels of representation under the FPTP system (FODEP, 2006).

For example, many stakeholders who submitted to the ERTC were unanimously of the view that most by-elections held recently were a drain on national resources and made various proposals, which included:

- Change the electoral system to do away with by-elections;

- Introduce a mandatory requirement that aspiring candidates present HIV test results;

- Restrict the holding of by-elections only to specific times of the year (ERTC, 2006b).

It is important to note here that implementing this highly consultative exercise is quite expensive. As Mutasa (2005) observes in his paper on sustainable electoral system design, there is no doubt that engaging in consultations for electoral and constitutional reform processes and managing elections themselves are costly exercises potentially competing with the need to meet social service expenditures. The irony however is that, done properly and in a responsive manner, electoral reforms can provide a country with a sound basis of governance, within which it is better able to realise its social and human development targets. A state seen as having accessed power legitimately, operating within an acceptable constitutional and electoral framework that fosters accountability is a better custodian of a

national development agenda than any other because resources would be less prone to be lost through corruption, patronage or depletion (Moonga, 2003).

Thus, the imperative is self-evident. There is a need to establish sustainable forms of democratic participation, particularly in the face of the epidemic. An electoral system that seeks to control the replacement costs that come with the increasing incidence of by-elections would be most suited, and ought to be on the electoral reform agenda for the country.

9.8 Impact of HIV/AIDS on governance

Broadly, governance is a term applied to the exercise of power and the process of decision-making and implementation in a variety of institutional contexts. It involves building consensus, or obtaining consent or acquiescence necessary to carry out a programme in an arena where many different interests are at play (Alcantara, 1998: 104). Good governance needs to fulfil two important purposes. Firstly, its role is pushing rulers to become more accountable to the populations over which they claim authority. Secondly, it facilitates a relationship of bargaining through which the interests of the state and those of society can be adjusted to each other so that the exercise of state power becomes more legitimate in the eyes of those subjected to it (Apter and Roseberg, 1994: 91).

In Zambia and in the context of this report, good governance entails genuine participation of citizens in the choice of their leadership, programmes, and the pattern of resource utilisation. It also means judicious application of scarce resources towards the reduction of HIV/AIDS. Similarly, the fight against HIV/AIDS in the area of governance must be guided by a vision of a Zambian society in which all citizens have equal opportunity to fulfil their potential and co-exist in dignity and harmony (Moonga, 2003). The goal should be to transform all the private sector and public institutions into instruments for good governance. Without good norms and practices at all levels and in all institutions, HIV/AIDS would remain a problem even with the ideal endowment of resources. Good governance therefore comprises the mechanisms, processes and institutions through which citizens and groups articulate their interests, exercise their legal rights and mediate differences in the country, including those relating to the HIV/AIDS epidemic.

However, evidence from this study and others indicates that the HIV/AIDS epidemic could be affecting all these processes as formal state institutions, civil society, and the general citizenry are incapacitated due to illness, death, and extra costs in form of medical fees and loss of income. Such developments are likely to compromise the long-term sustainability of democratic political processes and people's confidence in democratic principles. It also becomes very difficult to promote development and does not provide an encouraging environment for economic and social investment. The result is a vicious cycle that recreates a nexus of destructive forces - ineffective governance, leading to more poverty, which worsens the HIV/AIDS situation, which in turn worsens the governance situation even further. It is this self-reinforcing nexus that is threatening the viability and sustainability of democratic governance in many South African countries, Zambia among them.

It can be seen from this discussion that Zambia's governance and democratic development bears a lot of the signs of its historical relationship with colonial Britain. The political and electoral systems that Zambia uses today were mainly inherited from Britain. The FPTP electoral system is one of the many systemic structures that have been inherited, almost without any adaptation. It has also been noted that the adoption of these systems lacked significant consultations with the various stakeholders involved in governance and electoral processes.

It is also clear that since independence, Zambia has gone through rounds of trying to review both the constitution and electoral laws. Unfortunately, it is sad to note that most of the substantive or contentious issues are rarely touched on and many stakeholders assert that at any given time, the government in power has only tended to touch on those aspects that gives it more control in maintaining the status quo. For example, a number of issues have been raised with regard to reforming the current electoral system but government has been resistant. It was the wish of many stakeholders that the 2006 general elections could be held under a new constitution and new electoral laws in areas highlighted in this and other chapters. However, government resisted most of the contentious issues and delayed the reform process until the elections were held under the old legal regime. In the next section, we discuss the implications of HIV/AIDS for the sustenance of Zambia's electoral model.

10. Impact of HIV/AIDS on electoral system

This section examines the relationship between the HIV/AIDS epidemic and the electoral process in general and more particularly the impacts the epidemic could be having on the electoral system in Zambia. The discussion focuses on issues surrounding the debate on the suitability and sustainability of current electoral models and systems design in the context of the HIV/AIDS epidemic.

The argument is premised on the proposition that a sustainable electoral system should be one whose ongoing existence and viability can be carried through within the limits of available resources (financial, human and technical). To what extent is an electoral system in an environment of the type generated by HIV/AIDS responsive to the need to adapt to ensure sustainability and cost effectiveness on the one hand, and continued relevance and effectiveness as a critical elections tool on the other?

We discuss this matter within the context of Zambia's electoral reform process. In particular, the costs associated with replacement of representatives through by-elections as in the case of the FPTP model, which Zambia uses, are discussed and their implications analysed.

10.1 Zambian Electoral System

The Zambian electoral system is stipulated in the 1991 Constitution as amended in 1996, and also the new Electoral Act of 2006. Prior to the 1996 elections, the electoral system for electing the Republican presidential was the absolute majority (50%+1) system, while at parliamentary level the system was the simple majority FPTP.

In 1996, the government of President Chiluba amended the presidential electoral system to bring it in line with the parliamentary system's FPTP. The electoral system is based on Majority Single Member Constituencies with one round of elections. The FPTP principle is used in determining the winner, and the candidate who obtains the highest number of votes is elected.

Attempts were made through both the ERTC and the CRC to revert the presidential electoral system to 50%+1 majority system but this did not succeed due to the fact that the constitution review process was deferred to after the 2006 elections. Consequently,

Zambia went to the 2006 tripartite polls under the same FPTP system in all the three elections: local government, parliamentary and presidential.

10.1.1 Impact of HIV/AIDS on FPTP system

Electoral democracy, premised on the mass participation of people in governance has not been spared the ravaging effects of HIV/AIDS, though the effects in this sphere may be unique and mostly centred around the participation variables in the process and the costs associated with participation and representation.

10.2 Economic, political costs

10.2.1 Costs associated with by-elections

From its recent research, Idasa has postulated that the FPTP system practised in Zambia and other countries in the region may no longer be sustainable in the light of AIDS-related mortality and morbidity, which could increase the incidence of by-elections as local government and national parliament's representatives are affected like any other cohort of the population. The costs to the state of the loss of elected representatives can be understood in both political and economic terms.

10.2.2 Political costs

The constituencies affected by by-elections suffer political costs. The political costs relate to the loss of political representation in the legislature usually for the duration of up to 90 days, and in some cases, replacements have taken even longer.

An example is the Lusaka Central and Mandevu Constituencies whereby the incumbent MPs who at the time of the general elections in 2001 belonged to and won their seats on the FDD ticket, were later expelled. Following their expulsions from the political party, they however held on to their seats in parliament on the basis of a legal technicality, and the failure by the Speaker of the National Assembly to declare the seats vacant as per the electoral laws. Critics charged that the only reason the seats were not declared vacant was that the ruling party was not so confident of retaining the seats in the city given the political consciousness of the electorate.

Other seats that were later lost in similar circumstances, such as Milanzi in Katete district, were quickly declared vacant and the ruling party won the by-election that resulted. The people of Mandevu and Lusaka Central could not be considered to have had effective political representation at that time because the MPs who had accepted ministerial positions were now considered to have shifted their loyalty to the ruling MMD as opposed to the aspirations of the people who voted then into power by virtue of being opposition party candidates.

In addition, where replacements are occasioned by by-elections, the representation may not always be based on the same policy agenda, causing disruptions with obvious disillusionment and frustrations among the electorate. The disruptions in some cases result in changes in development priorities and even in the reversal of popular priorities, especially where a different political party takes office, leading to stagnation in development in the area concerned. The consequence is that the masses end up being disadvantaged and demoralised.

This fact can further be illustrated by the fact that by-elections in Zambia have often been characterised by higher voter apathy than general elections. The disillusionment posed by the loss of a favoured MP and voter fatigue could be the contributing factors to this kind of scenario.

10.2.3 Economic costs

Another dimension of the costs is economic in character, imposed by the increased incidence of by-elections. These mainly relate to the financial and material costs incurred by the ECZ and other stakeholders in conducting and participating in the by-elections.

The ECZ has estimated that an average parliamentary by-election in Zambia costs them K1 billion or US$235 850. A ward by-election at local government level costs K450 000 or US$106 000[1]. These are, by any standard, very significant costs and in the era of HIV/AIDS where the incidence of mandatory by-elections as the only mechanism for replacing political representatives, this could pose a potential unsustainable drain on scarce national resources. It has to be said that the ECZ figures represent costs to the state. They do not account for what political parties, civil society organisations and election monitors invest in the process.

Figure 10.1: Cause of by-elections

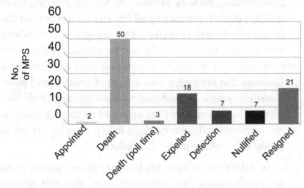

Source: Zambia Electoral Commission, 2007

10.2.4 An analysis of by-election cost components in Zambia

In trying to ascertain the actual costs of what goes into a by-election, the following analysis is ideal. The estimates of costs of a typical by-election in Zambia are made based on the criteria below:

- Constituency location (rural);
- Average size/expanse (130km x 160km);
- Polling centres (approx. 60 polling stations, and 84 voting streams).

10.2.5 Costs according to the ECZ

Announcements and publicity

For each by-election that falls due, the ECZ is obliged to publicly announce the by-election in both the print and electronic media. The ECZ employs mostly the public media institutions to carry out most of its publicity campaigns. A number of announcements are made and repeated for maximum impact, and mostly, these are targeted for prime time in the case of electronic media (radio and TV) and at least half-page in the print media.

Our barest estimations on the number of advertisements in such publicity activities would be as follows:

- Television (a minimum of three times per day, for three days);
- Radio & TV (a minimum of five times per day, for five days);
- Print media (a minimum of two quarter-page

insert-advertisements, in all the three daily papers);

- Posters and flyers (a minimum of five reams of posters and ten reams of flyers).

Taking the current average estimates based on recent similar activities undertaken by FODEP, it is possible to estimate the costs for the above activities, which should be not far from the following inference (expressed in US$s):

- Radio advert (average cost is US$190 per 45 seconds) for peak time: x 3 x 3 = US$1 710;
- TV advert (an average cost is US$680 per 45 seconds) for peak time x 3 x 5 days = US$10 200;
- Print media (three widely read newspapers) at US$1 340 per 25% of the page = US$12 060;
- Posters and flyers (average cost would be US$1 570 per ream) 5 x reams = US7 850;
- Flyers (average cost would be US$1 090 per ream) 10 x reams = US$10 900.

The total average cost estimates for announcements and publicity activities, within reasonable limits, and excluding other elements not mentioned above, would ideally be not less than K146 305 000 or US$42 407.25 at the current exchange rate (K3,450 per US$1).

Nominations

For each by-election, the ECZ normally sends a team of officers and at least one commissioner from Lusaka, and these join the district electoral and returning officers who conduct the nominations at a central constituency location. The costs in this task include the cost of transport (if hired) or costs for fuels and lubricants for the Lusaka team. (Transport costs are usually overlooked when talking about the cost of a by-election).

Nominations normally last one day, and officers from Lusaka require a minimum of two nights away from their station. The estimates of costs in payments to the individuals involved include:

- Daily subsistence allowances to the team (about four people) at the rate of about US$95 per day for three nights costs US$1 140;
- Daily subsistence allowance and accommodation cost for a commissioner at the average of US$190 per day for three days is US$560;
- Fuel costs to and from the designated district (not less than 320 litres on average) is US$700;
- Payment of allowances for about five electoral

personnel in the district and four ECZ personnel conducting the nominations (US$95 each) costs US$835.

The total average cost estimates for announcements and publicity, within reasonable limits, without considering the cost of hire of vehicle and other elements not mentioned, would be not less than US$3,200 at the minimum.

Recruitment, orientation/briefing of electoral personnel

The ECZ needs to mobilise the following personnel for the by-elections, and these are briefed or oriented ahead of any by-election.

- Electoral Officer;
- Returning Officer;
- Presiding Officers;
- Polling Assistants;
- Security Personnel.

During the briefings, all electoral personnel listed above are usually entitled to one day's subsistence allowance at the minimum rate of K160 000 (about US$50). Each polling station requires about five polling personnel and one security officer (six persons in total). With the introduction of voting streams for large polling stations, most of the polling stations would have double streams, with each stream requiring five persons and a security officer, which implies twice as many personnel.

On average therefore, a constituency with about 60 polling stations would have at least 40% of the polling stations with double streams, which gives a total of 84 voting streams in an average constituency. Multiplying this by five electoral personnel and one police officer, the total number of electoral personnel comes to 420. This is besides the electoral officer, returning officer and an average of five ECZ staff from Lusaka.

The cost estimate for this stage would therefore be about the cost for the nominations (US$3 200) added

to the daily allowances for about 420 assistants, i.e. US$19 540. This brings the total average cost to about US$22 620 for the recruitment and briefing of electoral personnel. This does not take into account the costs associated with the identification, publicity and recruitment process done at district level by electoral officers. It also excludes the transport costs at district level.

Briefing of electoral stakeholders

The ECZ sends its officers to the district designated for a by-election to hold briefings with the stakeholders in the by-elections, which include political parties, security personnel, election monitoring NGOs and other interested groups.

The costs associated with this part of the exercise relate closely to the costs under nomination: i.e. about US$3,200.

Printing of electoral materials:

Ballot Papers

Following the nominations and briefings, the ECZ then prints ballot papers and other materials necessary for conducting the by-elections, such as forms, booklets and other election guides.

Ordinary ballot papers (with no portrait – black & white): for a constituency with an average of 27 000 voters, according to the government printers' rate would cost K3 325 000 (US$1 090 at the exchange rate at the time of writing).

The cost for printing ordinary ballot papers for a ward by-election with an average of 8 000 voters would be K1 000 000 (or US$330 at the exchange rate at the time of writing).

This is based on actual quantity of the estimated 27 000 voters. In reality, the printed quantities would be higher to allow for an excess number of ballots in case of spoilt ballot papers.

Table 10.1: Costs as estimated by private printer (Golden Touch Printing Co Ltd)					
By-election type	Average voters	Black & white		Colour	
		ZMK	US$	ZMK	US$
Parliamentary	27,000	3,950,140	$985.07	6,138,570	$1,530.82
At reporting time's Rate (US$)			$1,295.13		$2,012.65
Local government	8,000	1,700,150.00	423.98	2,445,896.00	$609.95
At reporting time's Rate (US$)			$557.43		$801.93
NB: For the last elections in 2006, colour ballot papers were used for the first time. The printing was outsourced in South Africa.					

The above does not include costs for other relevant election forms such as:

- Ballot paper account forms;
- Results forms;
- Oath forms, other stationery, etc.

Voter registers

Each voting station is supplied with the current fresh copy of the voters' register. For an average constituency with 84 voting streams, 84 copies of the registers would be required. Going by the ECZ rates of the cost of one register during the 2006 elections being K25 000 per copy, the 84 registers would cost US$640.

10.2.6 Deployment of personnel

Deployment involves the dispatch of materials and personnel from Lusaka and from the district centres to the respective polling stations to be in time for the opening of polls at 06:00hrs. This entails an intensive demand for transport at both the national and district level.

Transport for materials (Lusaka to field)

Election materials such as ballot papers, ballot boxes, and ballot booths, as well as other electoral stationery (ink, marked envelopes, seals, official stamps, etc) have to be transported from Lusaka to the respective districts. This usually involves hiring additional vehicles, as other ECZ vehicles in Lusaka have to remain there to fulfil logistical requirements during the election time.

The costs involved in this category are quite difficult to quantify in precise terms, but the barest estimates would include the fuel costs of not less than 640 litres per vehicle for a minimum of three vehicles over a period of five days prior to election day. Going by the current rate, a reasonable estimate of US$2 900 just for fuels and lubricants for the three vehicles prior to the election is close. This excludes the costs related to the actual hire of the vehicles that we have assumed the ECZ provides from among its fleet (though in the strict consideration, such costs are necessary to quantify and consider).

The applicable personnel costs at this stage relate to the daily subsistence allowances or per-diems for the personnel from headquarters and electoral

officers, estimated for about six officers and one commissioner over a five day period at the rate of about K400 000 each: US$3 480. This is exclusive of the applicable allowances that are due to personnel when conducting elections.

Transport for personnel and materials to polling stations

During the election period, starting a day prior to the polling day through the polling day itself up to the day after the polls (a period of three days) the electoral personnel at the district level require a relatively higher level of logistical support than on any other day. The actual requirements vary from district to district. However, taking an average rural district, there would be need for about six vehicles: (at least three vehicles devoted to the deployment of electoral materials and personnel [electoral & security] to the polling stations; one vehicle for use by the returning officer, one vehicle for the district electoral officer, and another for the ECZ mobile team). This part of the operation may cost up to US$2 320 in fuels and lubricants. We have not factored the costs incurred in hiring helicopters for some remote areas that are difficult to access, such as parts of Muchinga constituency in Serenje, and Kanchibiya and Mfuwe constituencies in Mpika, and some parts of Shangombo, Chama and Kalabo districts where the ECZ has always had to rely on chartered air-transport (helicopter) to ferry materials and personnel. Where these are required, the costs could be in excess of US$69 600 on air-transport alone.

10.2.7 Allowances for electoral personnel

In addition to logistical costs, the ECZ pays allowances to electoral personnel, (and also, perhaps facilitates the payment of allowances to security personnel).

Subsistence Allowances for Lusaka-based officials

As noted above, the ECZ normally sends its personnel from Lusaka to the field to oversee the conduct of by-elections. The number ranges between three and five personnel inclusive of drivers, and usually one commissioner.

Allowances for field-based electoral personnel

A large number of the electoral personnel are deployed in the evening prior to the elections, and these would be entitled to night allowances for two days (i.e. the evenings before and after the elections). According to the rates applied by ECZ, various categories of electoral personnel are entitled to the following on a daily basis when on electoral duties.

- Electoral officers: US$60 per night;
- Returning officers: US$55 per night;
- Electoral assistants: US$50 per night;
- Security personnel: US$50 per night.

A typical by-election would entail that each of these personnel are paid for two nights and one full day, with an additional number of days for electoral and returning officers as a result of their longer term (about seven days) involvement covering the preparatory period.

A good estimate would therefore be:

- For one district electoral officer: US$60 x 7 x 1 = US$420
- For one constituency returning officer: US$55 x 7 x 1 = US$385
- For about 84 electoral assistants US$50 x 3 x 84 = US$12 600
- For about 84 security personnel US$50 x 3 x 84 = US$12 600
- For about 6 drivers US$50 x 3 x 6 = US$900
- Sub-total (allowances) =US$26 915

10.2.8 Communication expenses

In addition to telephone and fax communication between field personnel and ECZ headquarters, there is usually a high level of communications necessitated by a by-election, particularly between the ECZ Secretariat and the district personnel. This would be in terms of fax, telephone and mobile phone communication, which by Zambian standards are quite high. These costs are not easy to quantify and estimate, but they amount to a significant amount. There is also mobile communication, where network coverage is available, among the district electoral officers, returning officers and the presiding officers during election time, adding to the costs. We would believe that a round estimate of not less than US $1,450 on communication would not be an underestimate.

10.2.9 Costs by political parties/contestants

Apart from the costs incurred by the ECZ, other key electoral stakeholders do incur costs in relation to their participation in a by-election. Among such key stakeholders in every election are political parties and candidates.

The political parties do incur costs in varying degrees on the following processes as part of their involvement in by-elections.

Adoption process

The various party structures have to meet and engage in processes of evaluating and adopting sellable candidates for the by-election.

Nomination fees

Political parties also have to pay nomination fees. The current nomination fees as revised by the ECZ are as high as K500 000 per candidate, and these are non-refundable. This is a significant amount for most political parties.

Briefing and accreditation of polling agents

Political parties have to mobilise, orient and train their party polling agents. They also have to mobilise funds to pay their polling agents as allowances, transport and food.

Deployment and fees for polling agents

The deployment of polling agents for political parties brings in transport and upkeep costs on the political party. Given that these have to maintain a continuous presence in every polling station from the start of the poll to the end of the count means that the parties need to mobilise for each polling station about two polling agents.

Transport and logistics for campaigns and mobilisation costs

Political parties also have to mobilise and deploy teams in the field for campaigns over periods ranging from four to six weeks or more. These teams require logistics, materials and upkeep, which imply a lot of costs to the political parties.

Buying voters' register and printing campaign materials

Political parties also spend resources on buying voters' registers for the party agents, printing their campaign materials, and a range of other costs associated with campaigns.

Estimates

It is very difficult, even to a very rough extent, to arrive at a fair estimation of how much on average, a political party spends on a by-election. This is due to the fact that political parties do not keep records of their spending and that some of their income used for campaigns is not well accounted for.

However, what is certain and acknowledged by all political parties is the fact that there is a discrepancy in the extent to which they spend for by-elections, especially in terms of how much the opposition spends in relation to the ruling party. The ruling party is alleged to spend much more in a by-election than the opposition parties.

The ruling party, by virtue of it being in a privileged position to access or influence the spending of public funds, has been known to always maximise its advantage to the extent of deriving the benefits from projects and activities undertaken from public funds.

Comment

While these costs are not necessarily incurred from public funds by a public body such as ECZ, their costs cannot be ignored, as they are critical to ensuring that a by-election happens. Without the participation of political parties, there cannot be a by-election, and where there are no by-elections, candidates from the ruling party are likely to win the seats unopposed, rendering the quality of representation and democracy poor, and the level of interest and participation by citizens would die away.

Yet, whereas all political parties invest money in contesting by-elections, only one political party emerges victorious and in that sense, all the money invested by other contesting parties in campaigns is "wasted", especially in the context of the FPTP electoral system in place in Zambia. Usually, such wastage mainly affects opposition political parties, given the high frequency of by-election victories by the relatively well-resourced ruling party.

10.2.10 Costs by other organisations (monitors)

Apart from the political parties, each by-election that occurs entails some costs for election monitoring civic organisations like FODEP. Civic organisations mobilise, train and deploy election monitors for by-elections to ascertain the extent to which the stipulated electoral laws are observed in the electoral process.

Among the key cost areas for a monitoring operation include the following:

- Monitoring the nomination process;
- Orientation of monitors;
- Voter education materials;
- Voter education campaigns;
- Deployment costs for monitors;
- Transport and logistics for campaigns and mobilisation costs;
- Voters' register costs.

A civic election monitoring organisation such as FODEP spends up to US$9 500 on an average by-election.

As noted under the section on political parties, these costs, while not necessarily incurred from public coffers or government, are necessary to consider as their contribution to the quality of the election and the outputs thereof do add value to the electoral process and part and parcel of the investments devoted to the by-election by stakeholders.

10.2.11 Costs associated with electoral system

Various electoral systems impose different kinds of requirements on the electoral regime. Electoral systems vary in terms of the costs they impose on a nation. The FPTP system has been identified as being more prone to extra costs of replacement than any other system. This section examines this factor in relation to the experience of the tripartite elections held on September 28, 2006, with the focus on the candidates and the experiences noted prior and after the elections.

During the Zambian tripartite elections of September 28 2006, a number of incidents hinging on the loss and stigmatisation of electoral candidates were noted in various instances, denoted by the dropping of some aspirants considered unhealthy. While no evidence exists that such cases had anything to do with HIV/AIDS, the manner in which they aspirants were discarded exposed them to unsavoury scrutiny. In some cases the nominated representative died prematurely of unexplained causes.

Prospective candidates

Ahead of the 2006 elections, at least one known case of a prospective parliamentary candidate being withdrawn on the basis of ill health was noted. The United Democratic Alliance (UDA) candidate for Bweengwa constituency in Southern province was withdrawn by the alliance on grounds of ill health. The replacement candidate managed to win the election for the alliance, but the discarded representative died a week after being dropped.

This incident goes to demonstrate both a classical example of how those who may be ill could be discriminated against in terms of standing as candidates, and the potential strain the vacancy causes in terms of replacement costs to the party and the state.

The observation that the health of a potential candidate is a factor in considering adoption of prospective candidates, as noted in the focus group discussions held in Mansa, Petauke and Ndola districts, seems to have lent credence to this incident.

Nominated candidates

The second example is the case of death of candidates after nomination, just before an election. During the run-up to the 2006 elections, the nominated candidate for the Reform Party (RP) for Lupososhi, Elpidius Mweni, died on Tuesday, September 5th 2006, at Luwingu General Hospital after an undisclosed illness. Announcing the death of the candidate, the RP spokesperson described him as one of the strongest candidates the party had fielded for the general elections.

Following his death, the party wrote to the ECZ requesting a postponement of the election to allow for time to find a replacement candidate. The party acknowledged that Mr Mweni had sacrificed a lot for the party and would be a great loss.

The death of Mr Mweni was the second experience of a nominated MP dying before the elections. The first case ahead of the 2006 tripartite elections was the death of the ruling MMD's aspiring candidate for the Kabompo East constituency seat, Mr Jonathan Munengu, about one week earlier.

As there is no obvious provision in the electoral laws of Zambia on how to handle such occurrences, the ECZ relied on a provision in section 28 of the Electoral Act and requested the two political parties whose candidates had died to find replacements in the spirit of levelling the playing field. Section 28 of the new Electoral Act No. 12 of 2006, provides that "... the Commission may postpone the polling day for an election provided it is satisfied that the postponement is necessary for free and fair elections and the new polling date shall still fall within the period as required by the constitution..."

The electoral regulations drawn up by the ECZ provide for the postponement of the election in the event of death of a nominated candidate.

A similar incident was recorded at the level of ward councillor in Chipata where an MMD nominated candidate for a local government ward died about one week before the elections, prompting the ECZ to defer the elections to 26 October 2006.

10.2.12 Parliamentarians and councillors

The case of a by-election being required immediately following a general election was also noted during the 2006 elections. This followed one case of the death of MMD MP-elect for Liuwa Constituency, who died of a short illness five days after being declared winner of the parliamentary seat. This happened even before the new MP could assume his position in parliament. At local level, data from the ECZ shows that by-elections occur with startling regularity. This further accentuates the "fatigue" and cost factors.

Figure 10.2: Number of elections

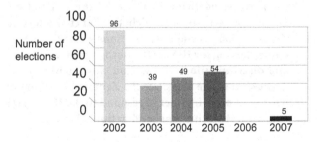

Source: Zambia Electoral Commission, 2007

For all the above cases, the various electoral models have different ways of addressing the situations. For instance, while under the FPTP the only practical option available is that of seeking to replace the candidates through a by-election, the Proportional Representation (PR) system would simply require the affected political party to replace the candidate or MP-elect with the next person on their approved party lists without the cost of holding by-elections. By-elections at local level in Zambia happen almost monthly.

It has been sufficiently established that the FPTP electoral system appears to be the most vulnerable system in the context of the HIV/AIDS epidemic. This system is likely to be even more expensive to sustain as the epidemic spreads and for poor countries, as are the majority in Sub-Saharan Africa, this could be a major strain on national development. The increasing by-elections also have an added effect: decreasing the policy influence of political parties that are unable to retain seats that fall vacant. These "power shifts" have a tendency of reconfiguring parliamentary power distribution and as already alluded to in the first chapter, may affect how governance decisions are reached.

11. Impact on parliamentary configuration

This section examines how HIV/AIDS is impacting on parliament vis-à-vis power shifts due to ever-increasing incidence of by-elections resulting from high mortality among political representatives. We assess the extent of power shifts as a result of the failure to retain parliamentary seats in by-elections by the party concerned and whether the process of holding new elections to replace deceased representatives do systematically disadvantage some political players, particularly those in the opposition. Further, we scrutinise the debates that characterised the pre-2006 presidential elections regarding mandatory testing for HIV/AIDS, notification, treatment and discrimination. The section closes with a brief discussion of the measures the Zambian Parliament has put in place in order to respond to the HIV/AIDS epidemic at institutional and national levels.

11.1 Parliament and HIV/AIDS

It is now widely acknowledged that HIV/AIDS are negatively impacting on the legislature in Zambia. HIV/AIDS are causing MPs, key legislative personnel and administrators, and other support staff to fall ill and/or die, leaving gaps in different positions, skills, experience and talent. Government has now acknowledged that the inefficiencies that the country was facing in implementing development and other interventions could be a result of the large numbers of people who are dying or suffering from HIV/AIDS.

As discussed in the previous section, the loss of elected representatives imposes strains on the electoral system. The added effect is that parties that fail to recapture seats through by-elections may also lose influence as a result of declining numbers in Parliament.

11.2 National Assembly

At the end of the 2006 presidential and parliamentary elections, the distribution of seats in the Zambian National Assembly showed a significant gain in the number of parliamentary seats held by opposition political parties, particularly the Patriotic Front (PF), which won 43 seats and the United Democratic Alliance (UDA), which won 23 seats. This left the ruling MMD with 72 seats of the 150 member parliament. Three seats remained vacant as they were awaiting the holding of by-elections as a result of the death of parliamentary candidates and the death of a newly elected MP, who passed away only five days after being elected.

The ruling MMD scooped all the three seats left vacant before the general elections. The opposition PF even lost the Lupososhi parliamentary seat to the ruling MMD, a seat in a province where PF won almost 100% of seats during the general elections. Only a month after the general elections, the power of the ruling party to win seats through by-elections was beginning to affect the configuration of parliamentary representation.

11.3 Death rates

The frequent deaths of MPs and other political representatives as a result of illness have only become common in the last ten to fifteen years in Zambia. As a result, the number of by-elections as a result of death of incumbent MPs and councillors has also increased during the last 15 years. According to official records made available to us by parliament and the Electoral Commission of Zambia, there were 46 by-elections between 1964 and 1984, (of which 6.4%

resulted from the death of the incumbent MPs). A total of 146 by-elections were held between 1985 and 2006, (of which at least 60% of them are attributed to natural deaths (disease-related) amongst incumbent MPs).

In the more recent by-election statistics for which disaggregated data are available by cause of death, it is very clear that the death of the incumbent MP is becoming a more significant contributor to frequency in by-elections in Zambia. For example, there were 106 parliamentary by-elections between 1992 and 2006 and 53 out of these were a result of the death of the incumbent MP. Three deaths occurred during the general elections of 2006. In addition, there have been 243 local government by-elections between 9th July 2002 and February 2007. In Zambia therefore, the frequency of by-elections increased with a correlated increase in the number of deaths among MPs and this occurred during the 1985-2006 period, a period within which HIV/AIDS had its most significant toll on the Zambian population as opposed to the 1964-1984 pre-HIV period.

One could argue that it is no coincidence that mortality rates among MPs, and consequently the number of by-elections, have become significant in the period 1985-2006. Relating these development to the general trends in mortality rates in the country and the significant role that HIV/AIDS are playing, it could safely be inferred from this that HIV/AIDS may have been a significant factor in some of the deaths of MPs. This is exemplified in the graph below:

Figure 11.1: Parliamentary by-elections by cause

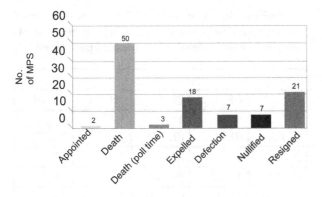

Source: Foundation for Democratic Process

Although it is usually difficult to establish the actual cause of such deaths, mainly due to confidentiality that goes with the HIV/AIDS status, the fact

that these trends correlate with the progression of the spread of HIV/AIDS in Zambia, it is not unfounded to make inferences that most of the deaths may be due to AIDS-related conditions. HIV/AIDS seemed to peak during the period 1993 and 2003, the period within which the death and mortality rates have shown an exponential increase. Moreover, the high death rates have usually occurred in the 40-60 age band, which is most vulnerable to HIV/AIDS.

The frequency by which MPs are dying is even a more worrying phenomenon today and may underline the seriousness of the potential impacts of HIV/AIDS. In one notable case, an MP died within months of winning a by-election, which means two by-elections had to be held in the same constituency within a short space of time, exerting undue financial burden not only on the treasury but also on the political parties that contested the by-elections.

The happenings of the pre-2006 presidential elections are also indicative of the fact that mortality and morbidity rates are worsening and that HIV/AIDS is starting to tilt the playing surface to the extent that the final electoral outcomes will be significantly affected. To start with, one of the leading opposition leaders, Anderson Mazoka, died only a few months before the 2006 tripartite election could be held.

We are not insinuating that his death had anything to do with the pandemic as no such evidence is in our posssesion. What we seek to illustrate is the consequences that come with the death of a prominent leader, regardless of the cause of death.

The death of political leaders can have a telling effect on the electoral viability of a political party, regardless of the cause. Given that most parties in Africa, Zambia included, are not institutionalised, and therefore depend on prolific figures to finance and manage them, the premature deaths of such individuals could derail an entire campaign. The death of Anderson Mazoka, president of the UNDP, just months before Zambia's 2006 general elections, had far-reaching consequences for his party. It is widely thought that the party may have been compromised in its performance in the elections as it did not have enough time to sell the newly elected candidate to the electorate. Mazoka, who succumbed to an undisclosed illness, had lost his earlier presidential bid in 2001 to the MMD's Levy Mwanawasa by a slender margin.

There are other more compelling ways in which the strong possibility of HIV/AIDS causing disruptions to the electoral process may arise. For instance, three weeks before polling day, two political parties applied for permission to replace their parliamentary candidates, and one local government candidate, because they had died within two months of being nominated. The ruling party, MMD, lost one nominated candidate for Kabompo East Constituency and one candidate nominated for local government elections in Chipata.

At the same time, the opposition National Democratic Focus (NDF) lost its nominated candidate for Lupososhi constituency during the campaign period due to an undisclosed illness. In addition, a few weeks before the 2006 presidential elections, the opposition United Democratic Alliance (UDA) dropped its nominated MP for Bwengwa constituency in Monze district, allegedly on consideration of ill-health. The candidate died only five days after being dropped. All these deaths occurred within the period between nomination of parliamentary and local government candidates and election day, a maximum of three months.

In addition to all this, while the ECZ was making preparations for by-elections in the three constituencies, as polling was postponed to give parties and their new nominees time to prepare adequately, the ruling MMD lost its newly elected MP for Liuwa constituency within four days of being elected, due to a short illness. Inevitably, this means that by-elections will need to be held in the three affected constituencies and one ward.

11.4 Power shifts in Parliament

As has been observed already in earlier chapters, Zambia's FPTP electoral system requires that a by-election be held every time an incumbent elected political representative dies, either at parliamentary or local government level. According to findings from this study, political players, especially those backed

by opposition political parties, are suffering from what was termed double impact of the epidemic. To start with, HIV/AIDS has made political parties very weak in many aspects.

As the epidemic continues to deplete dependable personnel both in terms of organisation, mobilisation and financial support, most political parties have become relegated to what was termed "ad hoc assemblies that only become alive for election purposes." As a result, when there are no elections in sight, most opposition political parties are dormant for most of the time while the ruling party remains relatively more active and visible throughout even when there are no elections as they are usually called upon to perform national and local government functions from time-to-time by virtue of being in power. Secondly, given the fact that the ruling party often has financial, organisational and political advantage over the opposition, by-elections or sudden disruptions in plans have tended to skew the playing field in favour of the party in power.

Thus, when a by-election is to be held suddenly due to the death of the incumbent MP, most opposition parties are somewhat caught off-guard. It was observed that by the time opposition parties begin to re-organise, the ruling party would have gained a lot of advantage as they even have the capacity to transport organisers, campaigners and resources from other parts of the country just to make sure they win the seat, a privilege which most opposition parties may not have due to limited funds and logistical capacities.

The case of the 2006 presidential and parliamentary general elections in Zambia could be reinforcing fears that by-elections could be tilting the political playing field in favour of the ruling party.

Polling in by-elections for Lupososhi and Kapompo East constituencies which were postponed due to the death of nominated parliamentary

Table 11.1: Power shifts in Parliament, 2001-2006									
	MMD	UPND	FDD	UNIP	HP	PF	ZRP	INDPT	Totals
2001 election seats	69 (46%)	49 (32.7%)	12 (8%)	13 (8.7%)	4 (2.7%)	1 (0.7%)	1 (0.7%)	1 (0.7%)	150 (100%)
Seats lost	2	7	1	4	2	1	0	0	15
Seats retained	11	1	0	0	0	1	0	0	13
Seats gained	14	0	1	0	0	1	0	0	16
Net gain	12	-6	0	-4	-2	0	0	0	
Pre-2006 election seats	81 (54%)	43 (28.7%)	12 (8%)	9 (6%)	2 (1.3%)	1 (0.7%)	1 (0.7%)	1 (0.7%)	150 (100%)
Source: Foundation for Democratic Process									

candidates were held on 26th October 2006 and the ruling MMD won both seats, including Lupososhi, a constituency in Northern province in which the opposition PF won almost 100% of the seats less than a month earlier during the general election. Just one month after the 2006 presidential and parliamentary general election, the configuration of Zambia's National Assembly was already being influenced by results from by-elections. This may be confirmation of the argument about the power of a ruling party to wrestle parliamentary seats from opposition parties during by-elections.

The net outcome of this two-thronged impact of the epidemic has been that opposition parties have generally been losing the majority of the by-elections, most especially in rural constituencies, partly because they have not been able to compete with the well-resourced ruling party. For example, the table above reveals that out of the 29 by-elections held between 26th June 2001 and 12 April 2006, the ruling MMD retained 11 of the 13 seats they held before the by-election and wrestled 14 seats from the opposition out of a total of 16 seats held by the opposition before the by-elections while they

Table 11.2: Power shifts in Zambia's National Assembly between 26 June 2001 and 12 April 2006			
Constituency	Cause of MP replacement	Affected Party	Winning Party
Mkushi North	Death	MMD	MMD
Chawama	Expulsion	MMD	MMD
Kabwata	Expulsion	MMD	FDD
Isoka East	Expulsion	MMD	MMD
Lufwanyama	Death	MMD	MMD
Bwacha	Defection	HP	MMD
Kabwe Central	Defection	HP	MMD
Mwandi	Expulsion	UPND	MMD
Keembe	Death	MMD	MMD
Mwansabombwe	Death	MMD	MMD
Nangoma	Resignation	UPND	MMD
Kantanshi	Death	MMD	PF
Solwezi Central	Resignation	UPND	MMD
Kaoma Central	Resignation	UPND	MMD
Lukulu East	Nullified	UPND	MMD
Msanzala	Nullified	UNIP	MMD
Mulobezi	Nullified	MMD	MMD
Mpika Central	Nullified	MMD	MMD
Mwinilunga East	Defection	UPND	MMD
Kantanshi	Death	PF	PF
Kantanshi	Death	PF	MMD
Kasempa	Death	MMD	MMD
Sinjembela	Death	UPND	MMD
Kalulushi	Resignation	MMD	MMD
Mapatizya	Death	UPND	UPND
Roan	Death	UNIP	MMD
Chama South	Death	UNIP	MMD
Milanzi	Resignation	UNIP	MMD
Mporokoso	Death	MMD	MMD
Source: Foundation for Democratic Process			

lost only 2 seats, leaving them with a net gain of 12 seats. This represents significant power shifts in the National Assembly, with the MMD shifting from 46% to 54% representation in Parliament between the 2001 and the 2006 presidential and parliamentary general elections. As for the opposition, the UPND and UNIP dropped from 49 to 43% and 8.7 to 6% parliamentary representation respectively while the others remained the same. This could mean that the more by-elections become frequent, the more the larger parties, which often tend to be the parties in power, are likely to gain influence in the National Assembly.

11.5 Parliamentary debates

11.5.1 Testing

In 2005, there was a heated public debate on the need (especially for presidential candidates) to undergo mandatory VCT. Provoked by the influential Medical Association of Zambia, the debate arose as a result of the prolonged illness of the leader of one of the main opposition parties, the UPND. Many politicians outside the UPND made insinuations that the leader in question would be constrained by illness to campaign in the 2006 elections, let alone rule the country effectively.

However, the general reaction from many political party leaders and some independent stakeholders was that mandatory testing for presidential candidates or any other category would be a violation of their human rights and that this would unnecessarily disadvantage those who test positive in the electoral process.

11.5.2 Notification or disclosure

There have also been debates on the extent to which disclosure of the status of a political leader could help reduce stigma and discrimination, and how this could encourage ordinary Zambians to go for VCT. Views on this issue have been mixed and the debate, to a large extent, remains unresolved. Both members of the public and MPs were asked to comment on whether disclosure of a political leader's status could help reduce stigma and discrimination and if this could encourage the general population to want to know their status too.

While a few members of the public felt this could be a good idea, the majority argued that disclosure would be suicidal on the part of the political leader because HIV/AIDS, unlike other debilitating illnesses, still generates significantly higher levels of stigma ands discrimination due to its incurability. The general view was that once the electorate learnt about a candidate's status, especially where it is positive, that would be the end of the political career of the individual concerned. There were strong views indicating that HIV/AIDS is still viewed as a death sentence.

Where such an individual is aspiring for political office, it would be almost impossible for them to win an election. The majority of people interviewed (selected members of the public) said that they would not vote for an HIV-positive person because "it is a waste of time and resources as that would mean voting in a by-election sooner rather than later." Members of the public noted that this is why only leaders who have tested and have found themselves to be negative announce their status. There is no political leader in Zambia who has announced that they are living with HIV and many members of the public wondered if, of all those who have opted to test, not a single person has been found to be positive.

It was not possible to capture the number of MPs who have gone for VCT. It was difficult mainly because these figures were not readily available. There are no official records of people who have tested or who are HIV-positive. Moreover, it was observed that VCT was a personal matter and that the institution does not have the power to test or collect information to that effect. Only a few examples were cited of MPs who had voluntarily tested and made their results public. These were only captured through public media and as comments from members of the public indicate, all of them have been negative.

The general conclusion among members of the public was that there was a possibility that there are some political leaders who have been found to be HIV-positive but that they opt for the safer way, to hide their status in order to keep their chances of continuing with their political lives. Many participants observed that many of these fear to be stigmatised and discriminated against. Thus, the safest thing to do is to keep the electorate ignorant about one's HIV-status. As one participant put it, "if they don't know, they would give you the benefit of the doubt even if they may suspect that you are sick."

These sentiments were also echoed by responses from MPs who observed that announcing one's status would be disastrous, especially when someone is HIV-positive. Many MPs stated that stigma was a very serious problem that could affect both the effectiveness of an MP and their participation in national affairs. The opinion of most MPs was that disclosure of a leader's positive status would neither help reduce stigma nor encourage citizens to go for VCT. Most MPs observed that one's status is a very personal matter and that whether somebody goes to test has nothing to do with what other people have done. It was emphasised again that disclosure, particularly for a positive HIV status, would come at a very high cost for the leader concerned. The issue of stigma and discrimination, both by fellow MPs and members of the electorate was again highlighted. As one MP put it, once you declare your positive HIV status, people would look at you like you are dead already. In fact, most MPs believed that it would be their fellow parliamentarians who would aim to finish them off rather than the electorate.

Thus, disclosure or notification of one's status depends, to some extent, on the perceived stigma and discrimination by the people concerned.

11.5.3 Stigma and discrimination

Findings from this study reveal that disclosure will remain problematic as long as levels of stigma and discrimination remain high. Therefore, measures aimed at increasing disclosure should also aim at reducing stigma and discrimination at all levels of society.

One aspect that should be emphasised here is that stigma and discrimination are very sensitive topics to discuss in public, especially with the increased information against these attitudes towards PLWHAs. The other problem is that stigma and discrimination often manifest themselves in very subtle ways that may not be obvious even to the people manifesting them or those being stigmatised or discriminated against. As a result, capturing the magnitude of the problem in certain and specific terms is difficult.

Findings from the study reveal contradictions within and between certain categories of respondents. For example, almost 100% of the people interviewed (both in the workplace and in communities) said they would not stigmatise or discriminate against PLWHAs in any way. There seemed to be a general consensus that doing so would be wrong and immoral. Interestingly, for many, their argument was that there was no stigma or discrimination. This should not give the impression that attitudes towards PLWHAs have changed substantially from negative to positive.

Although the extent of stigmatisation is difficult to capture, it was also obvious that stigma and discrimination are real life experiences for PLWHAs and that these may already be affecting the participation of these people in the social and political arenas of life. When views that there was no stigma and discrimination were shared with PLWHAs who participated in FGDs, these claims were strongly challenged. The majority of PLWHAs noted that stigma and discrimination was rife, though manifesting in less conspicuous and subtle ways. They argued that most people could not openly agree that they do stigmatise or discriminate because they know the moral implications of doing so.

In addition, interviews with selected members of the communities revealed that stigma and discrimination towards PLWHAs and HIV/AIDS as a disease were still high. Respondents revealed that discriminatory attitudes and practices are evident towards whoever is suspected to be suffering from the disease. It was noted that even where people have not come out to disclose their status, the experience people have had with the epidemic makes them carry out what they call "social diagnosis" and that they are able to speculate about which people may be suffering from AIDS. Unscientific as this could be, it just points to how negative attitudes could easily translate into negative "labelling" and stigmatisation, which may result in different aspects of discrimination. Even where the so-called "social diagnosis" is right, these attitudes and practices amount to stigmatisation and discrimination of the people so diagnosed.

Evidence of stigma could also be seen in such responses as: "Even where somebody is stigmatised or discriminated against, it was unlikely that the individual would do anything to seek redress. An HIV-positive person cannot speak out because they do not want to be known and labelled as being positive." Further, the use of such phrases as there is no stigmatisation against "these people" constitutes some stereotyping or labelling of some sort and this, though not obvious, constitutes stigmatisation. Thus, there are still a number of ways in which the rights of PLWHAs are infringed upon, both at the workplace and community levels. Thus, there is a need to improve human rights observation with regard to stigma and discrimination. This should be as practical as possible so that the affected individuals feel and/or experience this.

Thus, while in theory people appear to be more aware and informed about the need to stop stigma and discrimination, in practice, stigma and discrimination remains high and an important factor in determining the level of and willingness to participate, both in workplaces such as Parliament and in communities at large. It was further observed that HIV/AIDS remains a difficult issue for people to discuss openly. It was observed by the majority of people interviewed that although stigma and discrimination happen, "people do not want to openly discuss them, including the majority of those who are personally affected."

11.5.4 Treatment

As has been noted elsewhere in this book, perhaps the most important factor in changing the epidemic's course is the willingness of political leaders to acknowledge the crisis and urgently implement needed interventions as swiftly as possible. One country that prides itself on such a response from the highest level is Uganda. On the other hand, empirical evidence also shows that where political leaders have been slow to act effectively, the virus has continued to spread unchecked, usually with very devastating effects.

In Zambia, at least in theory, there have been efforts towards improving support, care and treatment of HIV and AIDS in Parliament. Programmes have been put in place to ensure adequate and effective support, care and treatment programmes in Parliament. The provision of ARVs has been the main thrust as far as treatment of HIV/AIDS is concerned. However, although by virtue of their status in the country, most MPs are likely to have relatively easy and adequate access to ARV and other life-prolonging treatments, the adequacy and effectiveness of current support, care and treatment programmes for ordinary employees in Parliament remain questionable.

Additionally, training programmes have been conducted for MPs in order to increase their awareness and knowledge of HIV/AIDS initiatives going on especially in their constituencies. Programmes have been put in place also to improve MP involvement in initiating HIV/AIDS activities in their constituencies. Further, VCT is another key intervention being implemented at Parliament. Individuals need to volunteer for testing; no one can be coerced. All results remain confidential. Parliament has implemented a VCT training programme and educated personnel within Parliament in VCT issues in order to enhance the provision of support, care and treatment within the workplace. Counselling is provided to all members of staff, including MPs, on the advantages and disadvantages of testing and knowing one's status. In Zambia, it is now possible to use the rapid test methodology which enables the individual to receive the results in a single visit to the counselling and testing centre. This is important because, before people can start receiving treatment, they have to know their status and that could only be achieved through testing.

Despite the importance of VCT in controlling the HIV/AIDS epidemic, the interviews revealed that most employees at Parliament have not been tested for HIV. Most MPs interviewed could not even comment on whether they have tested or not. This low level in testing is similar to what is prevailing in the country as a whole. According to the Demographic and Health Survey, 2002 - 2004, only 9% of men and 14% of women (12% of adults) had ever been tested. Another 69% of women and 64% of men want to be tested but have not done so yet. Testing is more common in urban areas (14% of women and 17% of men) than rural areas (6% of women and 12% of men). VCT is also more common among the better educated. Therefore, it could be that the perceived low level of testing at Parliament could be a result of non-disclosure rather than not having tested at all. This could be helped by the introduction and expanded delivery of ART within Parliament.

The introduction and expanded use of ART in the country was one of the most momentous single step in the fight against HIV/AIDS. Parliament is in the process of expanding the use of ART among all infected personnel. ART could decrease illness and improve survival time for individuals infected with the virus. The therapy is designed to reduce the viral load (level of virus in the blood) to the lowest level (often undetectable) for as long as possible. For almost all users, this slows down the progression of HIV/AIDS and infected people are able to live healthier and longer lives. Because of confidentiality concerns, information on how many people are using ART among MPs and ordinary Parliamentary employees was not available. However, in any case, ART is bound to improve the lives of those benefiting from the treatment and this is likely to slow down the adverse impacts of the virus on Parliament as an institution.

The effectiveness of these programmes remains questionable. The study revealed that most of these activities have been in their formative stages for many years. For instance, the HIV/AIDS draft policy has remained on the shelves of the Parliament building for more than five years.

11.6 Institutional response

As has been noted already in the early sections of this chapter, the availability of strong and committed political leadership is a major factor in any institutional or national response to HIV/AIDS. The call for stronger political leadership to confront HIV/AIDS has been sounding since 1987 when the World Health Organisation's Global Programme on AIDS (WHO/GPA) urged all national governments to make AIDS an official priority, emphasising the importance of vocal political commitment from the highest levels of government.

11.6.1 How MPs influence HIV/AIDS policy

The table below summarises what political leaders, particularly MPs, can do in order to influence the HIV/AIDS policy at its various stages. It also includes information on how networks can help in influencing policy.

With regard to what is actually happening at Parliament vis-à-vis an institutional response, the study reveals that Parliament has been in the process of setting up the HIV/AIDS response for a number of years, although little progress has been made so far. Although Parliament has not done very well in terms of eliciting policy, there have been efforts to build strategic coalitions of key players such as legislators, bureaucrats, public health experts and caregivers through the establishment of a Parliamentary Health Committee and the review and enactment of pieces of legislation, such as the HIV/AIDS/STI/TB Council Act of 2002 that established the National AIDS Council (NAC) and mandated it to co-ordinate a multi-sectoral response against HIV/AIDS in the country. In general, therefore, participants observed that Parliament was trying to be responsive to the HIV/AIDS epidemic, although many respondents were of the view that more needed to be done.

In addition, Pact Zambia implemented a five-year Democratic Governance Programme called A-Watch Project. The A-Watch Project is being implemented from September 10, 2004 until September 30, 2009. The development objective of this project is a sub-set of the USAID/Zambia 2004-10 Strategic Plan addressing Strategic Objectives that include

Table 11.3: How Parliament (MPs) can influence HIV/AIDS policy		
Stage of the policy process	Key objectives for actors aiming to influence policy	How networks can help
Agenda setting	Convince policymakers that the issue does indeed require attention	• Marshall evidence to enhance the credibility of the argument • Extend an advocacy campaign • Foster links among researchers, NGOs and policy makers
Formulation	Inform policymakers of the options and build a consensus	• Collect good-quality representative evidence and act as a 'resource bank' • Channel international resources and expertise into the policy process • Build long-term collaborative relationships with policymakers • Bypass formal barriers to consensus
Implementation	Complement government capacity	• Enhance the sustainability and reach of the policy • Act as dynamic 'platforms for action'
Evaluation	Collect quality evidence and channel it into the policy process	• Provide good quality representative evidence and feedback • Link policymakers to policy end-users
Source: WLSA 2006		

enhancing the capacity of citizens to demand accountability from their elected leaders, particularly MPs in the National Assembly. The project also aimed at enhancing the overseeing ability of oversight institutions in Zambia in order to provide checks and balances in the governance of the country.

Further, in line with the Mission's requirement to mainstream HIV/AIDS, the project sought to "reduce HIV/AIDS impact through an integrated response". This component specifically focuses on "improving care and support for PLWHA" and "improving the policy and regulatory environment". This project is being implemented at Parliament and in the judiciary.

The project's main objective is to enhance MPs' leadership role in the national response to HIV/AIDS by increasing their involvement in HIV/AIDS activities in their constituencies. The effectiveness and specific impacts of these interventions are yet to be evaluated.

Document reviews however suggest that not much has been done at Parliamentary Committee level. The chairperson of the Parliamentary Health Committee disclosed that the HIV/AIDS draft policy was left in its draft form for more than five years. It was observed further that the legal and institutional environment remains unfavourable, making it difficult to ensure effective responses on the part of MPs. Many stakeholders interviewed were of the view that there was need for new laws that should specifically respond to the new challenges brought about by the worsening epidemic. These new laws should include those that will protect citizens who may be living with the virus, that will provide for a holistic and multi-sectoral response, and that will deal with unfair stigmatisation and discrimination, both in the workplace and in society.

However, while the majority of respondents gauged Parliament as an institution favourably, they were of the view that MPs as individuals appeared to have a negative attitude towards HIV/AIDS going by the relative silence on the matter. Many respondents observed that genuine commitment on the part of MPs should be seen in the way they are ready to discuss the problem in different fora, including Parliamentary debates. It was noted that discussion of HIV/AIDS was largely limited to official roles performed by Ministers designated to the Health portfolio or when there was commemoration of such days as the World AIDS Day. The general view therefore was that MPs were not very committed to issues of HIV/AIDS.

The study reveals that MPs were not doing much in providing leadership in the multi-sectoral response to HIV/AIDS and service delivery in the country. In an interview with the Parliamentary Committee for Health, it was confirmed that although there were some activities going on, Parliament could do much better to respond to the HIV/AIDS problem in Zambia. It was observed that at the moment, Parliament does not have funds to even carry out outreach visits to constituencies to implement programmes on HIV/AIDS. Further, MPs' awareness of constituency HIV/AIDS issues remains very low and very few have initiated any sustainable activities in their constituencies. For many respondents, MPs were just not accountable to their electorate. They observed that going by the extent to which the epidemic was affecting society, any accountable MP would inevitably be sensitive to issues of HIV/AIDS.

It was therefore argued that, although Parliament could be an effective instrument in a national HIV/AIDS response that could affect the course of the disease in the country, this is yet to be achieved in practice. Commitment on the part of MPs is erratic and the institutional and legal requirements for ensuring that Parliament takes the lead in responding to the epidemic remain undeveloped. Many respondents observed that the greatest challenge to an effective HIV/AIDS response in Parliament, and in the country in general, rests upon individual MPs. It was noted that without genuine commitment at individual level, it would be unfounded to expect anything tangible in terms of an institutional response.

The majority of respondents also noted that the calibre of MPs could be affecting how Parliament responds to different issues of national interest, including HIV/AIDS. It was observed that there were a significant number of MPs who find their way into Parliament by virtue of belonging to a popular political party rather than their ability to represent the electorate effectively. Many respondents noted that this has led to people who cannot articulate complex issues such as HIV/AIDS being in Parliament. Thus, it was recommended that interventions to ensure that Parliament responds effectively to the HIV/AIDS epidemic should be targeted at individual MPs first before Parliament could develop the required culture of responsibility and commitment that is required in the multi-sectoral response to HIV/AIDS in the country.

The majority of respondents, including MPs, were of the view that there is a need to increase MPs' awareness and involvement in HIV/AIDS initiatives in their constituencies and at the national level. An assessment of the number of HIV/AIDS policy and strategic proposals initiated by MPs and submitted to/and adopted by Parliament shows clearly that not much was happening in the Zambian Parliament. It was further observed that for any political commitment to be effective it should be translated into broader societal mobilisation efforts. It was therefore felt that MPs should take up their strategic position and strengthen their role in generating policy and legislative responses through informed and open discussions. They need to take the lead in educating the public in order to alleviate stigma, and to generate an environment conducive for NGOs and communities to respond to the epidemic. Respondents also emphasised the need to decentralise government operations vis-à-vis the multi-sectoral response to HIV/AIDS. Effective participation of the civil society and other private sector stakeholders was another imperative noted.

Respondents further highlighted the imperative of ensuring improved care and support for PLWHAs. Many were of the view that without improved access to appropriate treatment, care and support, the multisectoral response to HIV/AIDS would fail to achieve the desired results. To attain this, an improved policy and regulatory environment is also essential. Again, MPs are very strategic in this regard.

The importance of institutions such as parliament in a democratic dispensation cannot be overemphasised. It provides a forum for discussing and negotiating important national issues and deciding upon resource distribution, policy direction and shaping appropriate legislation. However, it is important to note that this role and strategic position of parliament is being compromised by the adverse impacts of HIV/AIDS.

The preceding section has endeavoured to analyse the potential and actual impacts of HIV/AIDS on the configuration of Zambia's National Assembly and how this relates to power shifts between competing political parties, with specific focus on how power and/or influence in parliament is affected due to the failure by opposition parties to retain parliamentary seats in by-elections. It is now sufficiently established that the increasing death rates among MPs and other elected political representatives is not a coincidence, but could be a result of the general toll that HIV/AIDS is having on the general population in the country. This argument is strengthened further by the fact that these increases in death rates fit logically in the general trends in HIV/AIDS prevalence in the country.

This section has indicated that the impact of

HIV/AIDS on the National Assembly in Zambia is now evident. The loss of qualified and talented staff, MPs, experience and institutional memory have been highlighted as some of the obvious institutional losses. Beyond these obvious losses, there are also more subtle impacts that are only evident in the loss of operative capacity at institutional level. HIV/AIDS is causing MPs, key legislative and administrative personnel and other support staff to fall ill and die at a significantly accelerated rate, leaving gaps in different positions and depleting the resources for skills, experience and talent.

12. Electoral administration and management

This segment highlights the legal and institutional framework governing elections, explains the structure and staffing portfolios of the ECZ and proceeds to elucidate how these institutions inter-face with the HIV/AIDS pandemic.

12.1 Zambia's electoral system

As alluded to earlier, Zambia's FPTP system is stipulated in the current 1991 Constitution of the Republic of Zambia, as amended in 1996. The Constitution, the new Electoral Act of 2006, along with the Electoral Code of Conduct 2006 and the Electoral Commission Act of 1996 constitute the electoral legal framework governing the whole electoral process in Zambia. The Electoral Act (2006) further provides for the institutional framework, the electoral system procedures for delimiting constituencies, qualifications and requirements for candidates and guidelines on all matters relating to the electoral process. Zambia's electoral process therefore involves the following basic stages:

- Legislation (legal framework);
- Delimitation of constituencies, wards and polling districts;
- Voters registration (and education);
- Adoption of candidates, nomination and registration of parties and candidates (including designing of ballot papers);
- Elections campaigns regulation;

- Polling (voting process);
- Counting and tabulation of votes;
- Results and declaration of the results; and
- Verifying results and resolving election-related disputes/complaints (including petitions).

12.2 Legal framework

The Constitution of Zambia, Article 76 and 77, provides for the promulgation of various Acts for the management and administration of elections in Zambia. These Acts include the Electoral Act, Cap 139, the Electoral Commission Act No. 22 of 1996, The Local Government Act and the Referendum Act Cap 14 of the Laws of Zambia (Constitution of Zambia, 1991).

The Electoral Commission Act establishes the Electoral Commission, which is charged with the responsibility of conducting elections; supervising registration of voters; conducting all public elections; and reviewing boundaries of constituencies, wards and polling districts for purposes of elections.

The ECZ comprises five Commissioners who are appointed by the President of the Republic of Zambia, subject to ratification by Parliament. Section 17 of the Electoral Act confers upon the Electoral Commission administrative and regulatory powers to initiate legislation pertaining to the conduct of elections. Upon enactment by parliament, these become part of the electoral laws of Zambia. The other related legislation that has a significant bearing on Zambia's electoral process includes the Electoral Code of Conduct (2006) and the Public Order Act.

12.3 Electoral Code of Conduct

The Electoral Code of Conduct, first enacted in 1996, has since been revised and replaced by the Electoral Code of Conduct 2006, enacted in August 2006 subject to the Commission's exercise of its regulatory powers in consultation with civil society and political parties. Statutory Instrument No. 179 of 2006 is a legal document that provides the Zambian Electoral Code of Conduct. Deriving its authority from sections 17 and 18 of the Electoral Act No 12 of 2006, the Code of Conduct outlines a set of principles that all stakeholders must abide by when taking part in the electoral process. All persons wishing to be elected, all political parties, media institutions, election monitors and any other interest groups wishing to participate in the electoral process have to abide by this set of guiding principles (ECZ, 2006).

The Code of Conduct provides that every person shall during campaigns and elections promote conditions conducive to the conduct of free and fair elections, and guarantees rights and freedoms of both the electorate and contestants. It also forbids intimidation and violence, bribery, corruption, and office inducement as means of wooing voters during elections. The Code also forbids the use of government facilities for campaign purposes (ibid).

However, in its current form, the Code of Conduct has proved problematic in terms of enforcement. The main weakness lies in the lack of a clear complaints mechanism and the absence of an enforcement authority. Additionally, in the context of the current subject in this report - HIV/AIDS and PLWHAs and those affected by the disease are not provided for in the Code. As a result, incidences of corruption, vote-buying, bribery, abuse of office, and stigmatisation of PLWHAs continue unabated in the Zambian electoral process.

12.4 Management of electoral process

This section discusses the management of the electoral process in Zambia. It presents the legal and institutional framework that created the ECZ and analyses the impact of HIV/AIDS on the ECZ as an institution and on the general management of elections at both the national and local levels. The section also discusses, generally, the implications of the HIV/AIDS epidemic for democracy in the country.

12.4.1 Legal and institutional framework

The management of the electoral process in Zambia is the responsibility of the ECZ. The ECZ was established under Article 76(1) of the Zambian Constitution, while Article 76(2) provided legislation regarding its composition and operations. In fact, pursuant to Article 76(2) of the Constitution, the Electoral Commission Act No. 24 was enacted on 14 October 1996 to provide for the composition of the Commission (ECZ, 2006).

Prior to the 1996 Constitution, the conduct and

supervision of presidential, parliamentary and local government elections was the responsibility of the Electoral and Local Government Commissions, which were constituted on a part-time basis. These two commissions operated in liaison with the Elections Office in the Office of the Vice-President.

When the Electoral Commission Act was enacted in 1996, the Elections Office was de-linked from the Office of the Vice-President to form the Electoral Commission and their staff was transferred to the Electoral Commission. The Electoral Act empowers the ECZ to make regulations providing for the registration of voters, conduct of presidential and parliamentary elections, electoral malpractices, penalties and petitions. Furthermore, section 13 of the Electoral Act states that the Commission shall not be subject to the direction or control of any other person or authority (ECZ, 2006).

12.5 Functions of Electoral Commission of Zambia

The Electoral Commission's statutory functions are to:

- Supervise referenda pursuant to the Referendum Act, Chapter 14;
- Supervise the registration of voters;
- Conduct presidential and parliamentary elections;
- Conduct and supervise local government elections as provided under the Local Government Act;
- Formulate and review the Electoral (General) Regulations;
- Review the boundaries of the constituencies into which Zambia is divided for the purposes of elections to the National Assembly; and
- Perform any other statutory functions that the National Assembly may call upon it to undertake.

12.6 Organisational structure of Electoral Commission

As earlier mentioned, prior to 1996, the Elections Office operated under the direction of the Office of the Vice-President and that staff of the secretariat

were appointed by the Public Service Commission and were subject to civil service conditions. Such a structure caused the Elections Office to be perceived as a central government department with the sole responsibility of representing government interests in the electoral process. Hence, the ECZ was established in 1996 and mandated to employ its own staff by the Electoral Commission Act. This was intended to make the ECZ operate autonomously within the principles of an independent management body (ECZ, 2006).

Therefore, since 1997, the organisational structure of the ECZ took into consideration the functions stipulated in Article 76(1) of the Constitution which are: "to supervise the registration of voters, conduct Presidential and Parliamentary Elections and to review the boundaries of the constituencies into which Zambia is subdivided for the purposes of elections to the National Assembly."

Initially, seven departments were recommended, though by the end of 2005, nine departments were in place. These include:

12.6.1 Office of the Director

The appointment of the Director by the Commission is provided for by the Electoral Commission Act, No. 24, Section 12(1) of 1996. In addition, section 12(2) of the same Act states that the Director shall be the Chief Executive Officer of the Commission and shall be responsible for the management and administration of the Commission, and implementation of the decisions of the Commission.

12.6.2 Elections and voter education

The 1997 ECZ organisational structure proposed that the Elections and Civic (Voter) Education Department be established to undertake training, civic education, registration of voters, management of elections and delimitation functions. Specifically, these functions were performed under the following special sections:

Training and voter education

This section is responsible for conducting training programmes for Electoral Officers in all the provinces as well as conducting and monitoring voter education programmes for Members of Parliament.

Elections

This section is to supervise and administer elections and all related matters such as delimitation and voter registration.

Staffing for the Elections and Civic Education Department is to comprise a Deputy Director, two Principal Electoral Officers, two Senior Electoral Officers and an Assistant Electoral Officer. Currently, the Deputy Director - Elections and Voter Education, heads the Department of Elections and Voter Education, and is assisted by two Principal Electoral Officers, one Senior Electoral Officer and three Assistant Electoral Officers.

Apart from these, the ECZ usually hires a temporary workforce from local authorities, the Ministry of Education and other government ministries and departments countrywide to carry out electoral functions as and when need arises.

12.6.3 Department of Human Resources and Administration

The Department of Human Resources and Administration is mandated to manage and develop human resources, provide adequate and suitable transport, and provide other administrative services for the efficient operation of ECZ. This is to be done through the Human Resources, Administration sections.

The Department is to be headed by the Human Resources and Administration Manager who is to be in charge of human resources management and development, and administration. Supporting the Manager would be a Human Resource Officer, Administrative Officer, Transport Officer, Registry Officer and a Registry Clerk.

The Human Resources and Administration Manager is currently in charge of the Department and is assisted by one Administrative Officer and an Administration Assistant. The Department incorporates the Central Registry and Transport Unit. All the secretarial personnel fall under this Department.

12.6.4 Procurement and Supplies Department

This department is mandated to procure and disburse requisites for the efficient operation of the Commission. The Head - Procurement and Supplies - is in charge of the Department and is assisted by two Procurement and Supplies Officers. In addi-tion, the Department has one Stores Officer and an Assistant Stores Officer.

12.6.5 Finance Department

The role of this Department is to ensure the timely production of annual financial management reports, and enhance accountability and transparency and the development of a financial base for the operations of the Commission. The Department is to comprise a Finance Manager as the head, supported by an Accountant, Assistant Accountant, a Cashier and two Account Assistants.

However, the Department consists of the Finance Manager as head of the department, who is assisted by a Management Accountant and a Financial Accountant. Each of these has an Assistant and below them are two Accounts Clerks.

12.6.6 Internal Audit Department

The Internal Audit functions of the Commission are superintended by an Internal Auditor who reports directly to the Director. The Internal Auditor is deputised by an Assistant Internal Auditor. Although the two positions are filled by appropriately qualified officers, there is need for additional staff in order to ensure prudent accounting of the financial and material resources of the ECZ.

12.6.7 Information Technology Department

This Department was created to ensure timely, accurate and concise collection of data and the processing, storage and utilisation of information for the effective operation of the Commission. Specific functions of the department included data processing, systems development, computer operations and maintenance, information dissemination and project planning and coordination. The department has the following sections: Systems Development; Computer Operations; and Planning and Donor Co-ordination. The Department is to be headed by a Deputy Director, supported by a Principal Systems Development Officer responsible for analysis, design and implementation of electoral system applications, a Computer Operations Officer, who is in charge of computer hardware and system software maintenance, a Planning Officer or Donor Coordinator in charge of coordinating the ECZ planning activities and donor support, two Programme Analysts, and two Computer Technicians.

The current structure has the Deputy Director of Information Technology as head of Department, assisted by one Senior System Analyst or Programmer, two Geographical Information Systems Officers, two Data Entry Supervisors and three Data Entry Operators. During peak periods, such as voter registration, temporary employees are engaged to supplement the work of permanent staff

12.6.8 Public Relations Unit

The Public Relations Unit was established to promote and maintain a good image of the ECZ and its functions by ensuring that the electorate and stakeholders were provided with the necessary information concerning the operations of the Commission. The Public Relations Unit is to be managed by a Public Relations Officer.

Presently, the Department is currently headed by a Public Relations Manager who is assisted by a Senior Public Relations Officer and a Public Relations Officer.

12.6.9 Legal Department

The Commission Secretary and Legal Counsel heads this department and is assisted by a Legal Counsel and a Research Officer. Although the department is managed by appropriately qualified professionals, the Attorney General's Chambers attend to most of the legal matters of the Commission.

In order to enhance efficiency of the operations of the Commission, the 1997 institutional and managerial structure envisaged a decentralisation of the operations of the ECZ to the provinces, and to that effect, it was proposed that Provincial Electoral Offices be established at all provincial headquarters. These offices were to perform the following functions: training, civic/voter education, registration of voters, administration, elections management and data processing.

Staff for the Provincial Office was to comprise: a Senior Electoral Officer as the overall supervisor for the office, who was to be assisted by an Electoral Officer responsible for administrative affairs of the office; and a Data Processing Officer responsible for the collection, processing and transmission of electoral data to the Commission's headquarters for consolidation. These positions were to be supported by

Data Entry Clerks, Registry Clerks, Typists, Drivers and Office Orderlies. These structures and positions were by end of 2005 not yet functional.

The implementation of the structure of the independent ECZ had implications in terms of staffing and finances. The structure comprising specialised departments, such as Elections and Voter Education, Finance and Information Technology, demanded that the Commission employ highly qualified personnel in these specialised fields. With the coming of the HIV/AIDS pandemic the pressure of employing specialised personnel can only be assumed.

It was recommended that the Commission's establishment be increased from 17 members of staff, under the old civil service complement, to 125 under the new structure. This had financial implications in terms of costs to cover personal emoluments, office accommodation and procurement of plant and equipment to support the new structure.

Due to these and many other factors, the target of employing 125 members of staff was not completely achieved. In addition, the envisaged decentralisation of the Commission to the provinces through the establishment of Provincial Electoral Offices has not taken effect. This means that ECZ continues to rely on other institutions (such as the Ministry of Education [MoE]) to perform electoral duties at provincial and district levels, as and when required.

Therefore, by the first quarter of 2006, there was a total of 109 personnel employed by the ECZ. Among these, nine were part-time officers at each of the nine provincial headquarters. In terms of gender, only 35 of the 109 were female.

12.7 Impacts of HIV/AIDS on electoral management and administration

A credible electoral administration framework is necessary for effective management and implementation of electoral processes in any democracy. Electoral management should be trusted and deemed worthy of its authority by the public.

However, as has been discussed in other sections of this report, HIV/AIDS may have had adverse impacts on the political institutions such as political parties, civil society organisations and such strategic institutions as media. The ECZ might not be spared either. The HIV/AIDS epidemic may have adversely impacted on the ECZ in many respects, although the exact extent is difficult to establish due to unavailability of the relevant information. There is evidence however that the organisation has been experiencing a relatively high rate of deaths; absenteeism due to persistent illnesses; caring for those who are ill; and attending to funerals; all of which may be resulting from the worsening situation of the HIV/AIDS epidemic in the country. The loss of well-trained personnel, experience, institutional capacity and the financial costs of replacing staff and conducting ever-increasing numbers of by-elections to replace elected leaders who are dying, could all conspire to deplete the institution's capacity to function effectively.

The problem of attrition is more disruptive at provincial and district level where the ECZ depends on other government ministries and departments to administer elections. At this level, the ECZ relies heavily on part-time staff from the Ministry of Education (MoE) in order to carry out its activities. The MoE has particularly been singled out as one ministry in Zambia that has been adversely affected by the HIV/AIDS pandemic and statistics are easily available.

For instance, according to the Anti-AIDS Teachers Association of Zambia (AATAZ), an organisation established in 2001 to help prevent and mitigate the impact of HIV/AIDS on the teaching profession, the number of teachers who have died as a result of HIV/AIDS has been increasing over the years. In 1996 alone, there were 624 recorded HIV/AIDS-related deaths in the MoE. The number rose to 680 deaths in 1997 and by October 1998, the number of teachers who had died as a result of HIV/AIDS-related illnesses totalled 1 300 in a year. According to AATAZ, every school records at least one or two deaths each as a result of HIV/AIDS every year. And of the 37 117 primary teachers in Zambia in 1999, 8 100 (22 per cent) were HIV positive and 840 died from AIDS that year (Grassly et al, 2003). Furthermore, the figure on record by the end of 2003 was 1,400 deaths that year. It is projected that the HIV/AIDS epidemic is likely to reduce the number of teachers in Zambia from an expected 59 500 to only 50 000 by 2010, while teacher absenteeism due to HIV-related illnesses will cost 12 450 teacher-years over the next decade.

The Electoral Act (1991) provides for the institutional framework, the electoral procedures and guidelines on all matters of the electoral process, while the Electoral Commission Act No. 22 of 1996 establishes the ECZ, which is charged with the responsibility of, among other things, conducting elections, supervising voter registration, and delimi-

tation of boundaries of constituencies, wards and polling districts for purposes of elections.

However, to a large extent, an assessment of the legal and legislative frameworks for the administration and management of the electoral system shows that these frameworks are quite inadequate in a number of ways. For example, there is need to enhance the independence of the ECZ and to provide it with adequate capacity to deliver free and fair elections, an important ingredient in any democratic process. These handicaps have been exacerbated by the fact that the advent of the HIV/AIDS epidemic has brought into play new challenges which have so far been omitted in all efforts to improve the electoral system in Zambia.

13. Impact on parties, policy proposals

We focus on the impacts of HIV/AIDS on political parties as significant players in the electoral process. The section looks at how far political parties have been affected by the epidemic and the likely consequences of such impacts.

We then explore what the political parties are involved in in relation to HIV/AIDS policy both at national and party levels. Issues of stigma and discrimination and how they affect the participation of citizens in political spheres are analysed in the context of what is happening on the ground in Zambia.

13.1 Political parties, HIV/AIDS

Since the re-introduction of multi-party politics in 1991, Zambia has seen a mushrooming of political parties. As of September 2006, more than 40 registered parties were in existence. Political party stability encourages citizens' political participation and promotes faith in the political system. The specific administrative structures that can advance institutional stability will vary, but consistent elements will include the existence of and reliance upon by-laws (rather than personalised control) and effective communication systems.

In the Zambian context however, the party system is relatively undeveloped. The current scenario exhibits a situation where party politics are heavily influenced by the dominance of strong personalities and patrons, who provide both leadership and party finance (Van de Walle and Butler, 2003). As a result, most political parties have been grappling with the challenges of institutionalisation. This reliance on strong personalities and lack of institutionalisation has implications when these individuals are either chronically ill or they die. In most cases, parties whose leaders have died have also disappeared. In this context therefore, the impact of the HIV/AIDS epidemic on political parties cannot be underestimated.

Zambian parties also lack the resources to sustain themselves as institutions and are thus most visible during elections. This lack of visibility is partly due to the fact that party members view other activities as being of higher priority than party organisation. One contributing factor is that the time and money that an average Zambian can spare after they have spent on funerals, treatment for the sick and looking after orphans of HIV victims is not enough to sustain the individual, let alone contribute meaningfully to the party.

Closely related to the above, whatever pronouncements parties make about their policies on HIV can only hope to be implemented if the party wins elections and assumes government office (where they will have access to government funds and civil servants to implement their pronouncements). For those that remain in opposition, the pronouncements have to wait to be repeated at the next campaign rally or in the next manifesto.

Political parties play a key role as intermediaries between the electorate and the elected. However, in order to be viable, parties need well-vested, skilled, talented and experienced personnel who can volunteer their time and expertise. As has been discussed in the previous section however, the HIV/AIDS epidemic has not spared political parties. All the major political parties in Zambia do acknowledge that the HIV/AIDS epidemic has had a serious impact on their organisations. Unfortunately, the majority of these potential "pillars of strength" are within the age group most affected by HIV. The rise in the mortality rate among MPs is a worrying phenomenon for political parties to which they belong. The death of an MP has cost and political implications for political parties too. This is mainly because they usually would need to return to the drawing board, start looking for possible replacements, funds to re-campaign for the chosen replacement and just the disruption that comes with an election, especially where these by-election are frequent.

The HIV/AIDS epidemic also affects the electoral process from this different angle. The loss of party representatives (at various levels such as counsellors, MPs, and even presidents) through illnesses and death is quite disruptive. By threatening to wipe out this kind of personnel, the HIV/AIDS epidemic indirectly threatens the sustainability of these critical institutions of the democratic environment.

Beyond these personalised impacts, there are other institutional effects as well. As more and more of the vested personalities in any political party die away, it affects the institutional capacity of the party. In order to fulfil its role as intermediary between the electorate and the elected, a political party must have the ability to reach out to its constituency. Usually, this is achieved through a few gifted and well-vested individuals who sacrifice themselves for the further development of their party. Losing such skilled and experienced party organisers, in most cases, invariably translates into loss of 'institutional memory' and decreased institutional capacity to organise and mobilise membership.

There is also the question of stigma when a party leader or member is chronically ill. As indicated earlier, there has been a nation-wide debate in Zambia on whether chronically ill party leaders should be subjected to HIV tests or be permitted to continue leading their parties and even contesting elections. There has also been a demand that government ministers, including the President, should undergo HIV tests to determine their status. The question is, when one is found positive, what next? Is the political landscape mature enough to accept HIV/AIDS as just another illness? Is knowing the HIV status of political leaders beneficial to the fight against stigma and discrimination?

Findings from other studies reveal that this may not be so. In fact, there are arguments that the announcement may work against the leader concerned, especially when the result is positive (Pact Zambia, 2005). As the report notes, "this is why only those leaders who test negative announce their statuses". This may be the reason why while a few political leaders and ministers have voluntarily undergone VCT, the majority of them have not, for fear of stigma and the political implications of a positive outcome being made public. Thus, although no official connection has been established in this regard, analysis of public opinion as expressed in different fora, including the public media, may provide insights on the status of political party leaders at different levels and how this may be impacting on this important institution of democracy.

Such uncertainties have heightened speculations

that some key political party leaders may actually be HIV-positive and may be even suffering from AIDS. The complication, many stakeholders calling for mandatory testing have said, is that should such leaders be elected into office, they may not live long, prompting unnecessary by-elections. There have therefore been intense debates about mandatory HIV-testing among aspiring political candidates. The general view of most stakeholders however has been that mandatory HIV-testing would be unfair to PLWHAs and that this would constitute an infringement of their human rights. Mandatory HIV-testing of political candidates has therefore been dropped on human rights grounds.

Party officials in Zambia also noted that the HIV/AIDS pandemic has placed considerable pressure on parties and party leaders and elected representatives, such as MPs and councillors who are forced to devote a good amount of their time and resources to funerals. Party officials and elected representatives have had to attend to multiple funerals and parties have had to contribute towards funeral expenses. The constant demands of funerals have negatively affected party resources, organisation and officials' ability to attend meetings and respond to the needs of their constituents.

Contributing to a focus group discussion in Mumbwa, one party official noted that, "the rate at which people are dying was like flies. We bury at least one party official (potential parliamentary candidates) or party supporter every week…. In Mumbwa alone, there are at least 4-5 burials per day, which is quite high for such a small town". From this statement it is clear that the impact of HIV/AIDS on political parties is clearly acknowledged by party officials. As to what extent the epidemic was affecting the practical functionality and performance of political parties in elections, this could be left to conjecture. What is unquestionable is that the epidemic is affecting the human resources that are necessary for the effective performance of vital functions of political and electoral processes either as voters or as candidates.

13.2 Responses to HIV/AIDS within political parties

All political party officials and other stakeholders agreed that HIV/AIDS is a national issue and therefore was a potential campaign issue on which parties could mobilise support during the 2006

elections. This, however, is in contrast with the fact that most senior party leaders are not known to make public pronouncements on the HIV/AIDS epidemic and what their parties plan to do about it. In theory, political parties have made general expressions of their readiness to adopt supportive measures towards the participation of women and other disadvantaged groups (including people living with HIV/AIDS) in political processes. This refers to the inclusion of women and disadvantaged groups in the decision-making structure of political parties and their willingness to back members of these groups as political candidates. At a minimum, parties should exclude no member based on HIV-status in the equal participation of party activities, both in terms of the written regulations and the behaviour of the membership.

However, information from interviews indicate that no political party had a clear policy on HIV/AIDS with regard to prevention, treatment, care and support for those infected and affected by the epidemic so far. Further, the study revealed that political parties do not have any internal policies or programmes on HIV/AIDS at party level. This is not only a problem of lack of interest in the subject, but mostly, lack of capacity.

A quick look at party policy positions clearly indicates their recognition of the HIV epidemic and a clear lack of practical strategy to mitigate the scourge. For example, in relation to HIV, the PF has as part of its vision:

> "….. a nation free of HIV/AIDS and corruption; enhanced democratic governance and economic growth."

The UPND Manifesto states: "Providing accessible, affordable, and quality health and social care services to reduce mortality and morbidity from preventable and communicable diseases such as malaria, cholera, T.B, small pox and measles. AIDS will be declared a national disaster in order to reawaken citizens to the danger that the disease poses whilst putting in place a rigorous and sustainable behavioural and medical intervention to mitigate and reduce the impact of the HIV/AIDS pandemic."

The FDD notes that, "The HIV/AIDS pandemic is a crosscutting issue affecting the Zambian society in many ways".

As has been indicated earlier in this chapter, around 16% of the Zambian population is infected with HIV while everybody is affected. The 16% infection rate has been contained for a few years now in Zambia due to the work of the NGOs that have been involved in sensitisation campaigns and prevention of HIV/AIDS. The challenge for political parties on the HIV/AIDS is not so much of sensitisation to the epidemic as almost all Zambians are already aware about it. The challenge now is to educate the communities on HIV/AIDS and encourage them to take up VCT so that they could access ART. The other challenge of this epidemic is also to reduce the infection rate from the present 16% to a single digit through continuous HIV/AIDS education.

Although all political parties profess to be concerned about HIV, there are almost no tangible efforts being made to curb the scourge. The pronouncements about commitment only go as far as the party manifestos, which only become visible during election campaigns. In between elections, there is a deafening silence on activities within parties aimed at mitigating the epidemic. Perhaps the only audible effort is from the party in government (the MMD), which, through its Minister of Health, uses every opportunity to remind the public about its commitment to fighting HIV.

The MMD manifesto (2006) states on the health sector, "...the aim is to ensure visible but affordable improvements in health care utilisation as an overriding goal of Zambia's health reform process." The party goes on to outline their achievements in the health sector. More relevant to this discussion are the following:

The review and enactment of pieces of legislation (such as the HIV/AIDS/STI/TB Council Act of 2002) that mandated the NAC to co-ordinate a multi-sectoral response against HIV/AIDS in the country.

The implementation of the WHO 3x 5 HIV/AIDS initiative that targeted three million people globally to be put on ARVs by 2005. The MMD states that they increased the number of people receiving ART from as low as 10 000 patients in 2003 to 45 000 patients by the end of 2005 (MMD Summary Manifesto 2007-2011). This figure had increased to 60 000 in 2006.

Sadly, apart from mentioning the continuation of the WHO 3x5 HIV/AIDS initiative, the party's manifesto does not outline any other strategies or internal improvements in combating HIV/AIDS.

In the same vein, the All People's Congress Party (APC) recognises the need to get involved in the fight against AIDS. The party promises to prioritise HIV/AIDS treatment, care and prevention. It also promises to introduce free, voluntary and comprehensive HIV/AIDS testing and counselling as well as provide free ARVs to those in need.

Thus, in terms of contribution to public policy on HIV/AIDS, parties in Zambia are not engaged in a sustained policy debate on the epidemic. Almost all opposition political parties endorsed the way government was handling the HIV/AIDS problem and argued that they would continue on the same lines if they were to be in power. However, there are some complaints with regard to the non-availability of antiretroviral drugs (ARVs) and insufficient supplies of testing facilities for CD-4 counts, especially in rural outposts.

It should be noted also that there is a great deal of political denial on the part of political party leaders on the necessity of VCT and encouraging positive living among those who are HIV-positive. Following the example set by former South African president Nelson Mandela, who avoided the subject to appease the voters in order to win the 1994 elections, in Zambia HIV/AIDS is considered a sensitive subject by politicians.

Stigma and the risk of losing elections were noted as the main factors affecting political leaders' attitude towards the epidemic. Many felt that the knowledge that a certain party leader was HIV-positive would be exploited by rival political parties to maximise political mileage. This can also explain why the few political leaders who have volunteered to go for VCT and publicise the results are only those whose results came out negative. Zambia has yet to experience a political leader declaring themselves HIV-positive and still wishing to compete in the political realm.

Within political parties, there has not been an attempt by members living with HIV coming out publicly to demand equal rights and treatment, as have some disadvantaged groups such as the youth and people with disabilities. The social distance that political leaders maintain from those infected is far greater than that with other marginalised groups. A party leader would be comfortable being seen making a donation to a school for the blind but will avoid taking a photo opportunity with party members that are infected. This uncertain situation does not encourage those HIV-positive members to lobby for internal policies and programmes that would improve their wellbeing.

Parties have sadly not appreciated the direct benefits of investing in internal prevention and counselling programmes within the institution. The cost of helping their members live longer and more productive lives would eventually be recovered by reducing the costs of funerals and by-elections and would eventually guarantee the party a strong and sustained support base. One argument raised by one political leader was that with the trend of rampant defections from one party to the other, the party would not be guaranteed that the investment reaps the desired benefits.

Perhaps the greatest challenge facing the Zambian political parties is their inability to translate their manifestos into tangible actions in between elections whether they are in government or opposition. The lip service they pay to fighting HIV as they are campaigning suddenly disappears once they are elected into office. Worse still, once they lose an election, the opposition parties do not continue to interact with the public by implementing practical activities that would show that they have a better approach to dealing with the pandemic than the party in government.

In addition, the internal functioning of the parties does not reflect any mechanism for care and support of infected members. Talking to Zambian politicians, one hears a long tirade of how many funerals they have had to attend which, (in some cases) is a result of HIV. They openly admit that the parties have no internal mechanisms for sensitisation, care and treatment. Parties blame this situation on lack of resources and the fear that their rivals would make political mileage out of the public portrayal of their members as being infected. Party leaders, therefore, prefer to present an image that says all their members are not infected.

Parties also are concerned that the demand for resources that comes with caring for their HIV-positive members may be too enormous for them to afford. They worry that once they advertise themselves as care-givers for AIDS victims, their membership structure will be dominated by people looking up to the party leadership for good nutrition, ARVs and other support. Considering the limited resources already prevalent in the parties (especially the opposition), the common response has been diplomatic silence on internal party strategies on HIV.

Parties, in spite of their denial, still take advantage of the opportunity offered by funerals to propagate their ideologies and to campaign for more members. At most funerals in Zambia, time is allocated for speeches to be made at the graveside. A senior leader of the party of the deceased is usually allowed a few minutes to say a few words. These few words are usually to praise the deceased for their tireless efforts in organising the party and to inform the mourners of the plans that the party had for the deceased (usually a promotion) had God not taken them away from the party.

14. Political opinion, civic participation

The behaviour and effective operation of formal state institutions is an essential determinant of the degree of success or failure of developmental and democratic processes. Transparency requires that governments consult broadly to ascertain citizen interests, publicise plans and decisions, share information widely and in good time, and consistently act in an open manner. Accountability, on the other hand, depends on governments taking full cognisance of, responding to, and being monitored by, organised public opinion, including civil society.

This section analyses the political opinion surrounding HIV/AIDS in Zambia and civic participation in the context of the epidemic. The first part uses Afrobarometer public opinion data from Zambia to capture the prevailing scene regarding HIV/AIDS and governance in the country.

The second part focuses on civic participation and the impact these civic players are having in elevating HIV/AIDS issues on the list of priorities in the nation.

14.1 Public opinion

A detailed analysis of Afrobarometer public opinion data collected in 2003 in Zambia was undertaken to develop an understanding of public opinion regarding HIV/AIDS in the country. The results of this analysis revealed that there has been a marked increase in awareness and prioritisation of HIV/AIDS as a major socio-political problem that calls for urgent measures to reverse the worsening trends in HIV/AIDS progression. In general therefore, the Zambian society and leadership has become more sensitised about HIV/AIDS, how the epidemic is impacting on different spheres of the nation, and the urgency with which to respond to it.

However, one finding that is of significance to the study is that there is no definite body of public opinion leading Zambian politics at the time of the study. The diversity of issues noted as being the most important problems for many people is indicative of the complicated and diverse nature of public opinion in Zambia. It should also be observed that this study was undertaken at the time the country was preparing for a major national presidential and parliamentary election, which could have shifted the emphasis and focus of most people's views in the interviews.

14.1.1 Zambia's Public Agenda - 2006

Members of the public were asked to name the most important problem in Zambia. Analyses of Afrobarometer opinion data indicate that although the most highly rated problem was health, AIDS did not feature in the top 15 priority problems listed by participants in the study. Out of a total of 1 200 respondents interviewed to capture the Afrobarometer data in 2003, only 18 (that is, 1.5%) listed AIDS as the most important problem in the country. This does not necessarily mean that AIDS is not important in reality. There may be other factors that may explain the low rating that AIDS got in the research. This should be contrasted with the high rating for health. The table below shows the top 15 rated problems and their corresponding percentages.

Because of the stigma that goes with AIDS, many people are not ready to relate themselves to it directly and would rather mention health in general. A cross-reference analysis of other sets of Afrobarometer data, such as time spent caring for own illness, time spent caring for sick member of household and AIDS-related deaths in their households indicate that there was a very high rate of morbidity among participants who answered the questions. For instance, in spite of the fact that many respondents did not rate AIDS highly among the most important problems in the country, the majority (520 of the 1 200 or 43.3%) said they spend more than five hours tending to their own illnesses. It could be seen therefore that in spite of the lower rating of AIDS, the epidemic could even be affecting a large number of the respondents.

This reality appears to be common in all African countries included in the first of its kind pan-African poll started in 1991. Based on the results from this survey, De Waal noted that AIDS is rarely a top ranking concern in almost all the countries covered by the survey. He observes that the time delay between infection and becoming sick, the abstract quality of population based numbers, and the many religious condemnations of AIDS and its sufferers have all

Table 14.1: Most important problems in Zambia

Priority problem	Frequency	Percentage	Valid %	Cumulative %
Health	240	20	20	20
Education	138	11.5	11.5	31.5
Farming/agriculture	89	7.4	7.4	38.9
Water supply	70	5.8	5.8	44.7
Children/homeless children	59	4.9	4.9	49.6
Poverty/destitution	55	4.6	4.6	54.2
Infrastructure/roads	51	4.3	4.3	58.5
Food shortage/famine	47	3.9	3.9	62.4
Unemployment	46	3.8	3.8	66.2
Wages, income/salaries	40	3.3	3.3	69.5
Transport	38	3.2	3.2	72.7
Corruption	29	2.4	2.4	75.1
Management of economy	25	2.1	2.1	77.2
Housing	21	1.8	1.8	79
Loans/credits	20	1.7	1.7	80.7
Crime and security	19	1.6	1.6	82.3
Communication	19	1.6	1.6	83.9
AIDS	18	1.5	1.5	85.4
Others	176	14.6	14.6	100
Total	1200	100	100	

Source: Afrobarometer data - 2003

had a role to play in the denial of the epidemic (De Waal, 2006).

Therefore, although there is no certain connection between these levels of morbidity and HIV/AIDS, by inference, it is possible that a large number of people who listed health as the most important problem in Zambia could invariably be basing their decision on the impact of HIV/AIDS on the general population in the country, and even their own experiences.

When respondents were asked to state how much time they spend caring for sick members of their household, 357 of the 1 200 or 29.8% said they spend more than five hours. When we factor in the time spent caring for sick household members, the morbidity percentage goes beyond 70%. It is therefore surprising that AIDS could receive such a low rate while its impacts could be contributing to such high morbidity rates among respondents and their households.

The other factor that could have led to the low rating of AIDS among the most important problems in the country could be that poverty and other immediate problems of unemployment, education, roads and other infrastructure, water, transport, and agriculture for rural areas, are looked at as survival capacity builders, whether one has AIDS or not. Therefore, most Zambians are pre-occupied

with these immediate requirements such that anything whose effects could only come in the longer term is put on hold, not necessarily because they are unimportant but because they could wait one more day without catastrophic effects on the individuals concerned. The question then arises as to whether individuals who spend so much time daily tending to the fallout of the AIDS pandemic, would necessarily dedicate much effort to participating in political rallies, forums and elections. Analysis of Afrobarometer data indicates that the majority of participants in the survey that produced these data (88.6%) earn K1 000 000 (approximately USD$240) or less and 39.8% said they did not have income at all. For such individuals, issues of poverty, unemployment, and other immediate problems are likely to be placed high on the list of problems needing urgent attention. The following table presents the distribution of income levels among participants.

However, in spite of the under-reporting, generally speaking, AIDS has become a relatively important issue in the lives of many Zambians than was captured in the Afrobarometer opinion data of 2003. The ratings in the Afrobarometer opinion data set could therefore be misleading in many respects.

The case to put HIV/AIDS on the national agenda has been assisted by the announcement by first

Table 14.3: Time spent tending to own illnesses

Time spent	Frequency	Percentage	Valid %	Cumulative %
Spend no time	290	24.2	24.2	24.2
Less than 1 hour	167	13.9	13.9	38.1
1-2 hours	118	9.8	9.8	47.9
3-5 hours	75	6.3	6.3	54.2
More than 5 hours	520	43.3	43.3	97.5
Don't know	30	2.5	2.5	100
Total	1200	100	100	

Source: Afrobarometer data - 2003

Table 14.4: Time spent caring for sick member of household

Time spent	Frequency	Percentage	Valid %	Cumulative %
Spend no time	303	25.3	25.3	25.3
Less than 1 hour	190	15.8	15.8	41.1
1-2 hours	203	16.9	16.9	58
3-5 hours	131	10.9	10.9	68.9
More than 5 hours	357	19.8	19.8	98.7
Don't know	16	1.3	1.3	100
Total	1200	100	100	

Source: Afrobarometer data - 2003

Table 14.5: Household income of participants

Income	Frequency	Percentage	Valid %	Cumulative %
None	477	39.8	39.8	39.8
Less than K100,000	202	16.8	16.8	56.6
K100,000 - 200,000	131	10.9	10.9	67.5
K200,001 - 300,000	57	4.8	4.8	72.3
K300,001 - 500,000	72	6	6	78.3
K500,001 - 700,000	64	5.3	5.3	83.6
K700,001 - 1,000,000	60	5	5	88.6
K1,000,001 - 2,000,000	43	3.6	3.6	92.2
K2,000,001 - 3,000,000	4	0.3	0.3	92.5
K3,000,001 - 5,000,000	3	0.3	0.3	92.7
Refused to say	21	1.8	1.8	94.5
Don't know	66	5.5	5.5	100
Total	1200	100	100	

Source: Afrobarometer data - 2003

Zambian Republican President Dr Kenneth Kaunda that one of his sons, Masuzyo Kaunda, died from an AIDS-related illness as early as the mid-1980s. This pronouncement ignited a very emotionally loaded debate in the country on the efficacy of announcing AIDS as a cause of death for people. At that time, AIDS was hardly discussed and it was something of a surprise that such an announcement could come from the then President of the country. The debate in a way helped elevate issues of HIV/AIDS higher on the agenda of national priorities. Since then, Dr Kaunda has personally and publicly committed himself and has been involved in HIV/AIDS efforts in the country.

Prior to the 2006 general elections, HIV/AIDS were raised as a serious election issues. A number of NGOs and other stakeholders formed an advocacy group that set out to "force HIV/AIDS issues onto the agenda in the run-up to the general elections". They were advocating that all aspiring candidates should make clear their personal commitment to tackling HIV/AIDS. Their main objective was to compel "Zambian politicians to take a leading role in fighting the HIV/AIDS" epidemic. So, all aspiring candidates were required to say what they would do about the epidemic if they were elected into office "because they should recognise that HIV/AIDS are as much election issues as is a better economy or improved education" (Mwanza, 2006).

Zambians living with the virus distributed over 10 000 questionnaires among electorates and to all the aspiring candidates for presidential, parliamen-tary, and local government elections (approximately 1 200 of them). The intention was to make sure that all candidates, from presidential to ward counsellors, filled in these questionnaires and then PLWHAs used the responses in the questionnaires to make the electorate decide whom to vote for. This effort was very similar to what the Citizens Forum was doing. It had also requested all candidates to sign social contracts with their communities, outlining priority areas for development. It was strongly emphasised that candidates who do not show serious commitment to HIV/AIDS would not stand any chance of being elected as HIV/AIDS is a national issue since every voter either had someone with HIV or had been affected by it in some way.

How far this affected election results could not be established. However, the political significance of such efforts are that every politician was forced to think, and most significantly, to talk about HIV/AIDS in their campaign messages throughout the election period.

Further, as the figures in the tables below show, people are now more interested in discussing HIV/AIDS than they were a decade or so ago. Out of all the participants interviewed in the Afrobarometer opinion survey, 69.7% were interested in the topic while 27.2% were in between interest and boredom. Only a meagre 3.2% exhibited signs of disinterest. Further, opinion data indicate that 79.2% of the participants were extremely cooperative to the interviewers while only 1.4% were not cooperative. The majority also discussed the subject with ease rather

Table 14.6: Level of interest in discussing HIV/AIDS issues

	Frequency	Percentage	Valid %	Cumulative %
Interested	836	69.7	69.7	69.7
In between	326	27.2	27.2	96.8
Bored	38	3.2	3.2	100
Total	1, 200	100	100	

Source: Afrobarometer data - 2003

than with suspicion. Sixty-nine point two per cent (69.2 %) of the respondents were at ease to discuss HIV/AIDS while only 3.9% exhibited suspicion during the interviews.

This shows that issues of HIV/AIDS are becoming common discussion topics for most Zambians and that many are now accepting it as something that can be discussed publicly, even with people not very well known to them. Although a lot needs to be done to achieve the desired public position, there are encouraging signs indicating that the country could be headed in the right direction as far as influencing public opinion is concerned.

14.2 Government performance on HIV/AIDS

Respondents were also asked to gauge the performance of government in handling the HIV/AIDS epidemic in the country. The majority rated government's performance in combating HIV/AIDS as fairly well (44.3%) and very well (21.9%). Thus, most citizens who participated in the opinion survey in 2003 are fairly satisfied with the way the government was responding to the epidemic. It is also encouraging to note that overall, the majority of participants were able to categorically rate government's performance as opposed to only a few (2.4%) who said they did not know. This could be a sign that most Zambians

are becoming more aware about HIV/AIDS and what government was doing about it.

14.3 Civic participation

Civic participation includes NGOs, community based organisations (CBOs), faith-based organisations (FBOs) and individuals, each of which has a different comparative advantage based on its role, function, and position in society. Civil society helps ensure widespread representation of views, interests, and expertise in the fight against AIDS. Civil society groups also coordinate and implement activities of their members.

The Zambia National AIDS Network (ZNAN) for example promotes liaison, collaboration, and coordination among AIDS service organisations. To strengthen its coordination of the response by religious groups, the Zambia Interfaith Network Group on HIV/AIDS (ZINGO) gained registered NGO status.

14.4 Public and private sector participation

Great efforts have been made in the establishment of workplace-based HIV/AIDS programmes in both public and private sectors. For the public sector, all

Table 14.7: Government's handling of HIV/AIDS

	Frequency	Percentage	Valid %	Cumulative %
Very badly	181	15.1	15.1	15.1
Fairly badly	195	16.3	16.3	31.3
Fairly well	532	44.3	44.3	75.7
Very well	263	21.9	21.9	97.6
Don't know	29	2.4	2.4	100
Total	1, 200	100	100	

Source: Afrobarometer data – 2003

line ministries have accessed funding for their HIV/AIDS programmes. All government ministries now have HIV/AIDS focal point persons who are tasked with implementing HIV/AIDS activities according to the annual action plans that they develop. The performance of the focal persons varies and systems would have to be developed to systematically capture what the focal point persons specifically and what the different ministries are actually doing.

For the private sector, organisations such as Zambia Health Education and Communication Trust (ZHECT), CHAMP and ZBCA have been able to support over 100 companies to establish HIV/AIDS workplace policies and programmes. Some of the companies that have policies and HIV/AIDS workplace activities include: Barclays Bank, Standard Chartered Bank, Bank of Zambia, Dunavant and Cotton, Konkola Copper Mines, Zambia Chloride Batteries, Phoenix Constructors, and Zambia Sugar Company.

In January 2001, the Zambia HIV/AIDS Partnership in the Workplace was formed. Members include the Zambia Business Coalition on HIV/AIDS, the ZHECT, the Zambia HIV/AIDS Business Sector, Comprehensive HIV/AIDS Management Programme, capacity-building organisation INWENT, Zambia Integrated Health Programme, government ministries, small-scale enterprises, and host communities. The Zambia Business Coalition on HIV/AIDS acts as the coordinating umbrella body for the private sector response.

For example, the case of Zambia Chloride Batteries gives an indication of how private sector players could contribute to the fight against HIV/AIDS. Chloride Batteries, with an establishment of 42 employees, started their HIV/AIDS workplace programme and policy formulation in 2003.

The programme started with sensitisation workshops and was followed by an HIV prevention survey among all its employees, including senior management. Peer educators were trained and they started their activities within the company. Staff started bringing their spouses for couple VCT. The company encourages good nutrition as opposed to medical treatment unless the situation requires ART. HIV-positive employees are encouraged and supported to go for monthly CD-4 counts, paid for by the company.

The media fraternity has also realised how susceptible it is to the epidemic given the high mobility involving their work. This has resulted in Zambia institute of Mass Communication (ZAMCOM) spearheading the formation of the HIV/AIDS Policy Framework under the auspices of the Danish International Development Agency (DANIDA).

The key challenges for workplace HIV/AIDS activities are the lack of partnerships for small organisations, scarcity of ARVs in public institutions, lack of multi-sectoral and interdisciplinary forum for strengthening public and private partnerships. In addition, lack of funds to support partnerships and gaps in the draft national policy have been slowing down progress.

The recommendations are that more awareness about the Business Council should be created, that information on how to access ARVs in the public sector should be widely disseminated and that organisations that can assist institutions with implementation of workplace programmes should be identified.

15. Exploring impact on voter turnout

This section explores the impacts of HIV/AIDS on voter participation and turnout levels in Zambia. It begins by tracing trends in voter participation and turnout from the pre-HIV period to date. It then highlights the implications of the epidemic for voter participation and turnout levels during elections.

The section indicates that the worsening HIV/AIDS epidemic in Zambia is likely to adversely affect citizens' participation in electoral processes. The impact would result from a number of direct and indirect impacts that the HIV/AIDS epidemic is having on society. To start with, as more people fall ill and become physically incapacitated as the illness progresses, they are bound to be constrained from participation in many different processes and activities in the electoral process.

Further, the high death toll would continue to deplete the voters' roll. In addition, commitments of caring for sick relatives would mean that more people than are directly affected by infection would be hindered from active political participation. Beyond nursing commitments, the high levels of stigma would also negatively influence infected persons and some could stay away from public participation in electoral processes.

Figure 15.1: National Population, Voter Participation/Turnout Trends – 1964-2006

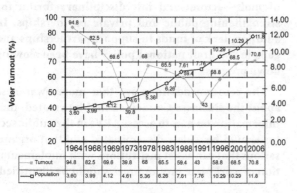

Voter Turnout & National Population 1962 - 2006

Election Year	1964	1968	1969	1973	1978	1983	1988	1991	1996	2001	2006
Turnout	94.8	82.5	69.6	39.8	68	65.5	59.4	43	58.8	68.5	70.8
Population	3.60	3.99	4.12	4.61	5.36	6.26	7.61	7.76	10.29	10.29	11.8

Sources: Computed from ECZ Parliamentary Provisional Results (1991, 1996, 2001 & 2006), and CSO Population Census Data (1964-2006)

15.1 Voter practices

15.1.1 First Republic

During the First Republic from 1964 to 1973, Zambia was a multi-party state. Parliamentary elections were contested amongst the political parties under the FPTP electoral system. Election competition both among and within political parties was characterised by factional conflicts and division mainly along ethnic lines (Chikulo, 1996: 25-27). In fact, ethnic factionalism was the main reason used by the UNIP government to justify the introduction of the one-party state.

In the First Republic, voter turnout was generally very high. In the 1964 general elections, an all-time high turnout of 94.8% was recorded while the 1968 elections had 82% turnout. At this stage, Zambians were still enthusiastic about their newly-acquired independence and self-rule. They were still expectant of the new government. Hence, voter turnout was still very high. However, as people became disillusioned with their failed hopes and aspirations, voter participation begun to decline until it reached its lowest (at 39.8%) around 1973.

15.1.2 Second Republic

The Second Republic, between 1973 and 1991, entailed the entrenchment of a political monopoly for one party, UNIP. The main stages for the electoral process for parliamentary elections involved the nomination process, primary elections and the general elections. Since there were no opposition political parties, only up to three UNIP candidates contested the general elections. Primary elections produced three candidates per constituency out of those who presented themselves. No primary elections occurred if only three or less candidates stood. Voters in the primary elections were electoral colleges comprising UNIP officials from all local executive committees in the constituency.

Candidates emerging from primaries were approved by the party's Central Committee, which, under the electoral laws, had discretionary powers to disqualify any candidate considered to be inimical to "the interests of the party". In general elections, every registered voter was qualified to vote. The FPTP was the electoral system used. Voter participation saw a marked increase from 1973 onwards.

Kaunda's policy of "One Zambia, One Nation" became a huge unifying factor and participation (or voting) was almost mandatory at that time. This could explain the sudden increase in voter participation from 39.8% in 1973 to 68.0% in the next election. However, beyond that, voter participation went through a downward trend, first slowly to 65.5%, 59.4% and then rapidly (43.4%) towards 1991. Around this period, Zambians had become highly agitated and were calling for a referendum to change both the system of government (the one-party state to multi-party state) and the government itself. Due to continued and worsening public pressure, Kaunda gave in and repealed the Zambian constitution to allow for the formation of political parties and a general election was announced for 1991.

15.1.3 Third Republic

A trend analysis of the voter turnout over the three general elections during the Third Republic (1991-2001) reveals that there has been an upward trend over the years. In 1991, the national average turnout was 43.6% of the registered voters. The turnout for the 1996 general elections was 58.8% while in 2001, the turnout rose to 68.5% of the registered voters in the respective years.

The findings appear very favourable at face value. This may even tempt some to dispel the argument that the FPTP in Zambia has led to low voter participation in elections. However, two very important points are worth noting before one makes any conclusions: (i) that the turnout is a percentage of registered voters in respective election years; and (ii) that voter registers in the successive years underrepresented the actual number of eligible voters.

Thus, a critical examination of the trend against the overall national population growth and the corresponding rates of registered voters reveal that whereas the national population was increasing, the numbers of registered voters in the successive years kept decreasing. In other words, whereas in 1991 voter turnout was 43.6%, the proportion of the population that was registered as voters was significantly higher than in both 1996 and 2001. In 1991, 37.6% of Zambians had registered as voters compared to 24.6% in 1996 and 25.3% in 2001. The table that follows below illustrates this clearly.

Figure 15.2: National Population and Levels of Registered Voters

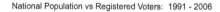
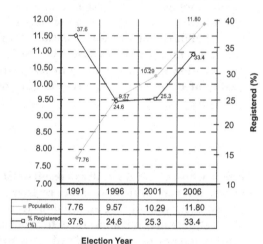

Source: Computed from ECZ Election Results – 1991, 1996, 2001 & 2006; and CSO National Population Data

Therefore, since voter turnout is based on the numbers registered, the number of registered voters becomes a more appropriate indicator of voter participation because it gauges the proportions of those registered against the total number of eligible voters. Overall, analyses of the voter registration and turnouts, especially over the three general elections since the beginning of the Third Republic in 1991, indicate that in spite of a seemingly positive upward trend in voter turnout over the years, there has been a consistent decline in voter participation in Zambia. A closer re-examination of the trend against the rate of overall population growth and the corresponding proportion of registered voters reveals a sustained downward spiral in overall citizen participation in elections. There is evidence showing that fewer Zambians are interested in registering as voters. While this could be a result of many other factors, the impact of the HIV/AIDS epidemic is likely to be high on the list of factors contributing to declining voter participation in elections. It is now more probable that most of the voters ticked absent on election-day may actually have died between registration period and polling day. The experience we are having with MPs dying within the three-month period between nominations and polling is not uniquely limited to that category of Zambian citizens.

One other issue that needs outright acknowledgement is that it was not possible to establish the real impacts of the HIV/AIDS epidemic on voter participation on a longitudinal basis. A number of factors conspired against this, but most important is the fact that the ECZ has not been able to consistently maintain their voters roll over time. The trend has been that voters' rolls have been compiled and discarded a number of times and completely new ones compiled. For instance, during the UNIP era (1964-1995), a different voters' roll was used for elections purposes. This was discarded in 1996 when a completely different voters' roll (popularly known as the NIKUV voters' register, (named after the Israeli Company

Year	Eligible voters	Registered voters	Votes cast	Voter turnout as % of registered voters	Voter turnout as % of eligible voters
1973	3,200,800	1,746,107	688,501	39.4%	21.5%
1991	3,863,769	2,931,909	1,323,790	45.1%	34.2%
1996	4,773,000	2,267,382	1,325,053	58.4%	27.7%
2001	5,267,483	2,604,761	1,737,948	66.7%	38.0%
2006	5,740,120	3,904,053	2,740,178	71.2%	47.7%

Table 14.8: Eligible voters, registered voters, voter turnout in Zambia, 1973-2006

Source: Electoral Commission of Zambia, Facts and Figures, 2006; CSO, 1990; and 2000 Census.

that was contracted by government to establish it) was compiled.

The NIKUV voters' register had great potential for timely and accurate purging of voters that die and the inclusion of those that register - even effecting changes for those who change residence, as it was completely computer-based. However, this same potential for easy review was seen as a disadvantage, especially by opposition political parties who claimed that the system was vulnerable to manipulation, making rigging very easy on the part of those with the power. Moreover, it was alleged that the system was designed with mechanisms that gave an in-built advantage to the ruling party. Thus, although the system was used in the 1996 general elections, it was very unpopular in the eyes of opposition parties and many stakeholders in the country. In spite of all these opposing views, government continued to use the NIKUV voters' register. It was updated in 2001 and used in subsequent elections until just before the 2006 general elections when another, completely new voters' register - the Optical Mark Recognition (OMR) system was introduced for the 2006 general elections.

Because of this lack of consistency in the voters' roll, it was difficult to track the actual impacts of the HIV/AIDS epidemic in terms of voters who are dying away from the register as a result of the epidemic. This shortcoming should however be balanced with the realities facing the Zambian population, as is shown in the following sections, that even in the absence of actual figures of the number of registered voters who may have died or are sick, it is clear that the epidemic has wrought havoc on the voting population in the country.

15.2 Voter participation

Democratic governance implies popular participation, including by disadvantaged social groups, in both public policy-making and its implementation. In this process, civil society (driven by the citizenry) performs its classic role of complementing, and sometimes countervailing, the state. By promoting and protecting civil rights, CSOs ensure that citizens have the means to express their preferences, engage in dialogue with policy-makers, and affect decisions in the public realm. Therefore, participation here is understood in its comprehensive form. This refers to citizens' engagement and participation in the political process, including party membership, volunteer service, voting, talking about politics and member-

ship in NGOs that advocate for various policies. It represents the notion that political involvement goes far beyond the act of voting.

It has been already noted that it was very difficult to capture the longitudinal impacts of HIV/AIDS on the voters' roll. This is mainly because Zambia has not maintained a single voters' roll over the period 1964 to 2006. Voters' rolls have been developed and discarded more than three times and completely new ones developed. This lack of continuity hindered a meaningful longitudinal evaluation of the impact of HIV/AIDS on the death rates among registered voters.

However, views from participants indicate that by its very nature, in that it affects large numbers, the HIV/AIDS epidemic is likely to have direct impacts on voter participation and electoral processes in the country. What we are saying is that exposure to HIV/AIDS is more often than not likely to lead to reduced participation in governance and electoral processes by those affected, either because they are too ill and bedridden, they are caring for the sick, attending to funeral commitments or because stigma makes them unwilling to go out and get involved. As participation of all eligible citizens is the foundation of legitimacy in a democratic system, exclusion due to HIV/AIDS complication is therefore likely to compromise the quality of democratic and electoral governance in the country.

15.2.1 Voter morbidity

People who are terminally ill as a result of HIV/AIDS may find it very difficult to either register as voters or cast their vote during an election because their physical state may not allow them to stand and wait in long queues usually associated with voter registration and/or voting on election day. The rules governing voter registration and voting can be very demanding in terms of the direct and indirect costs they involve for the prospective voter. The physical demands that lining up to register and/or votes puts on individuals are likely to be too much for those already weakened by illness. As a result, many PLWHAs whose health is severely compromised are bound to stay away from participation in electoral processes, be it registration as voters, campaigning for political parties of their choice, voting on election day, and even as election monitors, observers, and retaining officers. The hindrance here is more physical than attitudinal or psychological.

This is even exacerbated by other physical factors such as long distances to and from registration offices and polling stations, lack of transport, lack of funds for bus or taxi fares, and lack of relevant facilities at registration and polling stations such as toilets, clean water, and resting requirements like seats. For instance, the costs of travelling and acquiring the necessary documentation even before election-day could prove to be too high for those already burdened by HIV/AIDS. In any case, costs should include not only financial but also time, energy, and other less tangible outlays.

15.2.2 Caring for the sick

Related to the above issue of high morbidity is another problem of commitments of caring for sick relatives. It was highlighted in the study that to the extent that HIV/AIDS could be hindering infected persons from participating in electoral processes, they could be affecting one or more other persons who are nursing the sick, who are usually bed-ridden in the homes. The impact of caring commitments on participation is therefore likely to be more adverse than even the direct impacts of HIV morbidity.

It was indicated that for every single individual bed-ridden due to sickness with HIV/AIDS, more people are likely to be hindered in their capacity as caregivers. The majority of caregivers interviewed in this study observed that, "it would be unwise to leave a critically ill patient even for a minute because our patients need a lot of attention which they cannot do away with. For example, they need to take their medication at specific times." So, it was said that caring commitments for sick relatives, whether in hospital or in the homes, is more likely to hinder many more people from participating in politics, specifically the electoral processes of registering as voters, campaigning and voting.

It was observed that this is made even more significant because the ECZ does not have facilities or mechanisms to enable those who are physically incapacitated, due to illness or other reasons such as caring for the sick, to attend the voter registration process or to vote. This is despite many people approaching ECZ and district local government officials for assistance with registration because they are unable to physically vote or attend a voter registration exercise.

15.2.3 Voter mortality

Additionally, although this research was not able to establish the exact impact of HIV/AIDS on the vot-

ers' roll, analysis of HIV/AIDS trends in the general population in the country indicate that the epidemic could have significantly increased morbidity among registered voters as the majority of voters in Zambia fall within the 15 to 49 year old band. Certainly, as more and more people die, this robs electoral democracies of potential participants, both as candidates and as voters, in the elections. There are examples from other countries like Uganda where entire communities were wiped out by the epidemic, leaving only children and the very old. Such an occurrence has huge and direct implications for electoral democracies. Already, there are indications of declining voter participation and overall citizens' participation in the electoral process.

Although there is no proven direct connection between this decline in voter participation and the incidence of HIV/AIDS, stakeholders interviewed observed that it will not be long before the epidemic starts contributing to declining voter numbers and ultimately voter participation levels in Zambia. It was observed that the death toll from AIDS has been high and that it continues to rise. In 1990 for example, about 10 600 persons died from AIDS. The annual number of AIDS deaths then soared to 76 700 in 2000, and then 95 400 in 2005. It is projected that the death toll could be 94 100 in 2010. The devastating impacts of AIDS on citizens participation is likely to be even more adverse in the future. This can be seen by considering cumulative AIDS deaths in the country over time. From the beginning of the epidemic until 2000, the CSO reports that an estimated 482 000 Zambians have died from the disease. In the ensuing 10 years, 2000 - 2010, another 928 000 are projected to die from the disease in the absence of widespread use of ART. This would result in a cumulative total of 1.4 million deaths by 2010.

With such figures, it was noted that death as a result of HIV/AIDS could be depleting the voters' roll of voters almost at a similar proportion since the majority of voters in Zambia fall within the most affected age-band, the 15 to 49 years category.

It was also highlighted that apart from affecting overall participation, these high death rates may complicate the management of the voters' roll, which would compromise its integrity. It was observed that the ECZ does not have swift mechanisms in place for purging dead voters from the voters' register. Going by the rate at which Zambians are dying and considering that the voters' roll is not continually updated, the numbers of "ghost" voters on the register is bound to be significant. This makes the electoral process vulnerable to malpractice and vote rigging as this makes it easy for relatives, friends and/or other individuals to manipulate and use voters' cards of those who are dead in an election. Participants observed that the loss of integrity in the voters' roll could indirectly lead to further reductions in participation.

15.3 Stigma

Stigma was also highlighted as a major hindrance to participation that was affecting a significant number of PLWHAs and those close to them, especially when participation involved candidature in elections. Participants acknowledged that the worst forms of stigmatisation and discrimination that characterised the HIV/AIDS epidemic in the mid-1980s are no longer evident. It was observed that at that time, PLWHAs were "chased out of homes - that relatives abandoned them with no one to support them". People would not share house utensils with PLWHAs and stigma and discrimination was at its worst level. It was noted that these forms of stigmatisation and discrimination are no longer evident in most societies in Zambia. However, in spite of these improvements, stigma remains high and as long as it remains high, those who are infected would stay away from public participation. This is in spite of their desire, potential and capacity to perform just as well, and in some cases even better, than those who are not infected, or at least whose status is not known. Considering the high rates of HIV/AIDS infections and the correspondingly high levels of stigma, stigmatisation is therefore likely to have significant impacts on participation in the electoral process.

Although some respondents did not see any reason why an HIV-positive person could be discriminated against as a candidate in an election, most political actors and citizens alike felt that "it would be a political (or tactical) blunder to adopt an HIV-positive person to stand in an election in such an environment of high stigma among both the opponents and the electorate." They argued that adopting an HIV-positive person would only serve as political ammunition for the competitors as it would fuel negative campaigns that there would soon be a by-election. The fear of losing a parliamentary seat due to the positive status of a candidate is considered to be a very high price for political parties to pay. HIV-positive people are therefore more likely to be constrained from participating by virtue of their HIV status, especially where they want to stand as candidates. Participants noted that, "society still has a negative attitude towards HIV infection. Many people in society usually associate fielding an HIV-positive as a candidate with the cost of by-elections. For political parties, the cost may even include the loss of a seat when they fail to win the by-election." The general argument in this study is therefore that, although there are no laws or policies that discriminate against HIV-positive persons as political candidates, society still has imbedded attitudes and practices that give PLWHA whose status is public no chance of winning an election.

With regard to HIV-positive persons participating in voter registration, voting, campaigning, etc, it was observed by respondents that there was nothing that could hinder them from doing so. It was noted that HIV-positive persons were normal human beings who were free to exercise their political rights. However, it was also acknowledged that there was a perceived tendency, though not in every case, for some people who know they are HIV-positive or have AIDS to withdraw from any commitments for the longer-term future. As such, respondents observed that such people would not consider participating in an election as important or a priority. This is mainly because of the stigma and wrong beliefs associated with being HIV-positive. For many people in Zambia, in spite of the sensitisation that has taken place, being HIV-positive, to a large extent, is still considered a death sentence. As such, being pronounced positive is synonymous with being asked to start preparing to die. This makes many affected individuals lose hope and stop investing in the future and voting is one thing they are bound to cut out of their lives, especially as the illness progresses. This was however said to be limited to a few individuals. Therefore, giving up on life was not given significance in affecting participation compared to the fear of being known to be HIV-positive.

Here, it is important to acknowledge some other factors that may be affecting participation levels in Zambia. As has been noted elsewhere in this chapter, HIV/AIDS has a backdrop of many other problems. Specifically, poverty is one such factor which is worsening the impact of HIV/AIDS on the Zambian population. This has created an environment that has made politics become what Fortman describes as "a dominant social good." This could either be good for participation or bad, depending on how this "dominant social good" is applied. To start with, it means those with political power have great influence and capacity to command a wide range of other goods and processes.

Thus, these people who hold power could play a very critical role in realigning policy and institutions and functions of governance and the electoral process to adequately and timeously respond to the challenges brought about by the HIV/AIDS epidemic. These powerful people could also influence resource and community mobilisation for responding to the epidemic and sustaining (and even increasing) participation in the electoral process. At the mass level, there has to be a broad normative and behavioural consensus - one that cuts across class, political inclination, and other cleavages - on the importance of incorporating efforts of tackling the HIV/AIDS epidemic in the electoral systems and processes.

On the other hand, and as is mostly the case in Zambia, the "dominant social good" is being abused by those in power. Today, politics is looked upon largely as a means to wealth, influence and position rather than a service, reinforcing the tendency of politicians to put personal gain ahead of national development goals. In this regard, the "dominant social good" has become the "dominant social bad".

It is no wonder most politicians and candidates stop at nothing in trying to enhance their chances of election victory. Many go as far as engaging in illegal practices such as bribing voters, vote-buying, corruption, etc. They must secure victory at all costs. Once elected, most representatives have acquired immense personal benefits and improvements in their livelihoods, which in many cases is out of proportion to their legitimate earnings. Contrasted with the deteriorating socio-economic realities in the lives of many Zambians, mainly due to increasing poverty and the worsening HIV/AIDS epidemic, many citizens now look at voting only as a way of enriching others while they remain poor. As such, for many Zambians, if they cannot stand so that they can benefit from the privileged position that comes with political office, they would rather stay away from participation than enrich others. This is therefore another factor that may be contributing to declining participation in elections by the citizenry.

16. Role of stigma, discrimination

This section presents findings from Focus Group Discussions (FGDs) held with PLWHAs, caregivers and registered voters from the communities visited, both in urban and rural areas of Zambia. The first part provides a brief description of the methodological issues on how FGDs were constituted and the main issues discussed. Thereafter, stigma and discrimination are discussed in a theoretical perspective and in relation to HIV/AIDS. It is argued here that stigma and discrimination associated with HIV/AIDS leads to social and political ostracism and alienation and to the deterioration of civil, economic and political rights of the individuals concerned.

The last section presents a detailed discussion of the main findings from FGDs. The section reveals no evidence that people infected by HIV/AIDS tend to be demotivated by their HIV status to the extent that they give up on social and political involvement. PLWHAs are more likely to stay away from active involvement in politics largely because they are physically challenged as their physical state gives in as the disease progresses rather than deliberately deciding to stay away. It is also noted that whether one becomes apathetic depends on the individual. There was no systematic apathy among PLWHAs to justify the argument that PLWHAs are likely to be more apathetic than people without the disease.

16.1 Designing Focus Group Discussions

The main objective of undertaking FGDs was two-fold:

- To determine whether or not there are structural factors that prevent PLWHAs and their caregivers from participating in elections (long processing time, long distances to polling stations, lack of ablution facilities, long queues, time constraints due to care-giving responsibilities, lack of special voting provisions, etc).

- To determine whether there are attitudinal factors that prevent people from freely participating in elections (stigma, discrimination; marginalisation, general apathy).

To capture these issues, a number of topics were included in the FGD guideline that was used during the discussions. The main topics included the following:

- Knowledge of whether the ECZ had any facility to help those who were pregnant, infirm or disabled to vote in the 2001 elections.

- Whether the ECZ was doing enough to assist people infected and/or affected by HIV/AIDS to participate in elections.

- What should be done to increase the participation of those infected and affected by HIV/AIDS in elections.

- Whether people infected or affected by HIV/AIDS are more or less likely to participate in politics.

- Whether people infected or affected by HIV/AIDS are more or less likely to participate in elections.

- How the involvement of PLWHAs in the leadership and the election process affect their decision to vote.

- Whether HIV/AIDS are political problems that people must try and resolve together through elected politicians or personal and private problems that everyone must try and resolve in his/her own family.

- The strongest change agent on issues of HIV/AIDS and why?

- Involvement in community-based organisations that campaign around HIV/AIDS issues.

- In general, how important elections are to improving the quality of their life.

Every FGD was closed with a request for a general comment on the involvement of people infected by HIV/AIDS and other illness in elections.

It was a deliberate requirement of all FGDs that:

- All participants should be either eligible or registered voters;

- The majority of participants are living with HIV/AIDS and a lesser proportion of caregivers (ratio of 6:4);

- At least one-third to half of all participants must have voted in the 2001 general elections.

A total of eight FGDs were held with PLWHAs, caregivers and registered voters from the communities visited, four in rural areas and four in the urban areas. Each FGD constituted eight to ten participants, though in most rural FGDs participation per FGD was lower, between six and eight, as it was not easy to assemble PLWHAs due to limited numbers in some areas.

Overall, a total of 72 participants took part in the FGDs, with a comparatively larger proportion (40) coming from the urban areas.

16.2   Context of stigma and discrimination

Stigmatisation has been defined as "a process of

devaluation within a particular culture or setting where attitudes are seized upon and defined as discredible or not worthy" (PANOS/UNICEF, 2004). In many regards, this would imply that specific categories of people are systematically and consistently cast aside based on the assumption that they are different (usually in the negative) and therefore a departure from the "normal social order" of things as is generally acceptable in the society concerned. Stigmatisation is to a larger extent attitudinal, very subtle and usually becomes part of the socialisation process. Through the socialisation process, stigmatisation is internalised among the people concerned, making it appear natural and correct. This process not only affects those who stigmatise but also affects the stigmatised, making them feel unworthy and, in most cases, unable to challenge the violation of their rights. Stigmatisation therefore connotes a sense of shame and unworthiness.

On the other hand, discrimination is the process of exclusion that grows out of stigmatisation. At individual level, this could be internalised, just like stigmatisation, making it appear part of the normal functioning of society. Discrimination can also be institutionalised, a situation where it is built into the day-to-day functioning and operation of institutions. It is this internalisation and institutionalisation of stigma and discrimination that make it difficult to change individuals and institutions. It is with this understanding that any effort to overcome stigma and discrimination should take a long-term approach towards de-socialising and de-institutionalising these normally deep-rooted attitudinal biases against specific individuals or groups of people.

16.3 Effects of HIV-related stigma

Whether affected or infected, many people in Zambia still avoid any mention of HIV/AIDS because of the stigma attached to the disease, and the fear of the resultant discrimination. One of the fundamental principles underlying the National HIV/AIDS/STI/TB Policy is that the human rights and dignity of HIV-infected people should be respected and that all stigma and discrimination against PLWHAs should be eliminated (NAC, 2004). This is not only compassionate and humane but also good public policy. It is now generally recognised that when human rights are upheld and protected, and when stigma and discrimination are reduced, PLWHAs and their families are able to cope better with the disease and they are more likely to remain active participants in public life than otherwise.

HIV/AIDS-related stigma is both widespread and is a significant obstacle to effective care and support measures (NAC, 2005). Stigma could occur at the political, institutional, social and psychological level. All FGDs discussed a series of questions to determine the degree of HIV/AIDS-related stigma. Although stigma was not listed as the main challenge faced by PLWHAs in the electoral process, it was described as "a scar that you cannot get away from", being labelled as "a person who has been doing 'that thing'" - "it is a stain in the mind."

During FGDs, some participants living with the virus reported disclosing their HIV status to their relatives or their pastors (counsellors). However, generally, disclosure of HIV status was found to be very uncommon. Very few participants indicated that they had disclosed their HIV status - some said they took very long before they even disclosed their statuses to their spouses. Many participants living with HIV believe disclosure of results should be left to the individuals concerned. Health and community caregivers who participated in FGDs expressed the same view.

The study revealed that testing and receiving test results is a sensitive process and could signal the beginning of HIV-related stigma, especially where the individual tests positive. Stigma associated with HIV/AIDS and discrimination against PLWHAs usually leads to social ostracism and alienation and to the deterioration of civil, economic, and political rights of the individual(s) concerned. A major problem in attempting to address this epidemic is that people often avoid learning about or admitting to being infected with HIV because of the stigma attached to the disease and the fear of discrimination (NAC, 2005).

Such avoidance limits diffusion of knowledge about HIV/AIDS in the general population and increases the risk of transmission to loved ones and others. In addition, in the area of prevention, stigma and discrimination makes people shy away from knowing their status, thereby delaying treatment for those who may need it. Even those who may know their positive status may shy away from accessing treatment for fear of being identified as being HIV-positive.

HIV/AIDS-related stigma and discrimination also affect the workplaces. HIV/AIDS-related stigma and discrimination in the workplace in Zambia manifests in the following consequences (1) not having an opportunity to be picked for a job; (2) manda-

tory testing at recruitment; (3) questions on recruitment forms or interviews related to HIV status; (4) unjustified restrictions relating to promotion, job location, or employment benefits; or (5) summary dismissal from the job (NAC, 2005). As a result, many people avoid learning about or admitting their status because they fear the economic consequences of losing a job.

AIDS-related stigma and discrimination also affect the number of people accessing VCT services. Research has revealed that many people do not feel comfortable going for VCT because they are concerned that their results will not be kept confidential and that stigma and discrimination would follow the disclosure of the status. Clearly therefore, the more openness that exists about the disease and the less people fear stigma and discrimination, the more likely they would utilise VCT services and ultimately, disclosure would become a normal part of life.

Stigma and discrimination also affects those who give care and support to the infected. Because of the stigma associated with the disease, some people may not wish to be seen to be caring for those who are infected with the HIV, even when the infected persons are family members. This may make them discriminate against those infected and this has led to some PLWHAs losing hope in life, withdrawing from society and in the worst case scenario, even committing suicide.

As a cross-cutting issue therefore, stigma and discrimination has to be addressed as a barrier to successful intervention in HIV/AIDS programming. HIV/AIDS-infected persons also have the right to non-discrimination and equality before the law; they have the right to health, so as not to be denied health care and treatment; and they have the right to educational opportunities. There are indications, as will be seen in discussions of FGD findings, that in some cases these rights are being compromised due to HIV-related stigma and discrimination. Without respect for these rights, people have less motivation to find or divulge their HIV status. In this context, recognising and respecting the human rights of PLWHAs and those affected by the epidemic, and opposing stigma and discrimination in all its manifestations, makes good political and governance strategies towards increased participation of PLWHAs in politics and electoral processes.

In Zambia, this would only be possible when HIV/AIDS are mainstreamed in the broader human rights efforts of the Permanent Human Rights Commission of Zambia. Many efforts to reduce stigma and discrimination are not a mutter of courts and laws.

Therefore, many efforts could be put in place without waiting for the policy and legal environment to shift. For instance, employers are already practicing "affirmative action," where HIV-positive employees receive psychological and medical support and are not discriminated against. The Bank of Zambia, Finance Bank and Barclays Bank are examples of employers with affirmative workplace policies.

Further, faith-based organisations (FBOs) and other NGOs are promoting openness about the epidemic and tolerance and support for the infected and affected among their own membership and communities. PLWHA organisations such as NZP+ do promote "speak out" campaigns and advocate for fair treatment of PLWHAs. It is clear from Uganda and other experiences that openness and tolerance can be significant factors in lowering HIV prevalence over time.

16.4 Findings

All participants were asked to express their opinion on whether HIV/AIDS resulted in political problems that needed a concerted national effort together with elected politicians, or whether it was a personal and private problem that everyone must try and resolve in his/her own family. The outcome from discussions was unanimous. All participants observed that, going by the way the epidemic was progressing, HIV/AIDS is no longer a personal issue. Participants indicated that although HIV/AIDS is contracted and experienced more at the personal and private level, its impacts are more national, if not global, in their implications.

It was therefore strongly noted that HIV/AIDS should be considered as a critical national development-governance issue. It was against this background that the majority of participants felt that it was equally the duty of government and all elected political leaders to be seriously involved in all efforts to fight the epidemic in the country. Participants wondered why government seems to show minimum concern "when the epidemic is spreading like wild fire in the country".

When asked to comment on whether being HIV-positive would affect one's capacity to belong to a political party, participate in such activities as political rallies, campaigning, registering of voters, observation and monitoring, and voter education, participants observed that there was no evidence that positive status would be a major determinant of whether somebody participates or not. The general argument was that people infected or affected by HIV/AIDS could freely participate in politics and elections. It was highlighted that as long as the individual was physically able to participate, there was no reason why they should not. So, what determines one's participation in these activities is not the HIV status per se, but their physical state.

It was noted that where someone was unwell, regardless of whether they are HIV-positive or not, they are likely to be more physically challenged and may therefore be more likely not to participate in those activities that require physical well-being for someone to make a meaningful contribution. Thus, as long as someone is physically able, one's HIV status was almost inconsequential. It was observed that, "there were so many people today who were actively participating in politics and yet they are sick - they don't just know." It was therefore not logical how someone who knows would be unable to participate even when the disease has not yet taken its toll.

Participants were also asked to comment on the factors that could play a key role, if at all, in impeding participation by people who are affected by or are sick from AIDS. This was meant to capture how political apathy is related to HIV/AIDS. In this regard, both attitudinal and structural factors were highlighted.

16.5 Structural challenges for PLWHAs

16.5.1 Inaccessibility of the polling station

Inaccessibility to polling stations was mainly attributed to a combination of long distances and lack of transport or transport money. Many participants observed that, as PLWHAs, they are challenged on many fronts. They argued that HIV/AIDS usually led to loss of income and physical strength, especially where the disease is advanced. As a result, because of the long distances usually involved, many PLWHAs could not walk to polling stations even where those who are well are able to walk. Further, financial challenges also entail that they cannot afford to pay the fares to go to the polling station.

One salient argument that was emphasised, even in urban areas, is that even where there is transport such as public transport mini-buses, it is not ideal when somebody is very sick. Many participants noted that when one is very sick, even the mini-buses become unusable. So, one would need to get a taxi, which is even more expensive. Thus, inaccessibility to polling stations remains a huge challenge for the PLWHAs and this may be contributing significantly to their failure to participate in elections.

16.5.2 Too much time spent in voting queue

Time is another factor that was highlighted as contributing to the failure to participate in elections by PLWHAs. They observed that when they are unwell, they need a lot of things which could not be found at the polling station. So, if they are to go out to vote, they need to vote quickly and get back home where they have those facilities. While people who are well could wait for hours before casting their vote, this was not practical for PLWHAs. They need such things as ablution facilities, clean drinking water, food or snacks, a place to rest, etc. It was observed by many participants that sometimes when they are unwell, their physical state could allow them to stand in a queue for hours. This problem brings us back to the earlier suggestions of making the voting process swift and efficient so that people do not spend long periods waiting to vote.

The other time aspect that was noted related to caregivers. When you have someone who is critically ill, it is very unlikely that you could leave them for hours unattended to. Thus, the impact of HIV/AIDS is always wider than just affecting the infected individual. It was noted that caregivers are also affected by almost the same problems that affected PLWHA. Long distances, lack of funds for fares, time factor, etc. It therefore argued that HIV/AIDS could be hindering the participation of more than just the infected.

16.6 Attitudinal challenges for PLWHA

16.6.1 Stigma and discrimination

Although the majority said stigma and discrimination were not a major impediment, they were noted among the factors that could affect the participation of PLWHAs in elections, both as a voter and as a candidate. Participants argued that stigma was still high in the country. A number of participants personally shared experiences when they were made to feel "shame", "out-of-place", "unwelcome", etc, because they were sick (not necessarily HIV-positive).

One participant noted that, "when you are not feeling well and you go out, even the way you walk would show that you are not okay because we do not have strength. So, people would stare at you like they are asking 'What is this one doing here?'"

Some participants blamed the negative television adverts on HIV/AIDS as providing negative messages, which they said only worsen stigma among citizens.

Another aspect highlighted with regard to stigma was that women were most adversely affected. It was revealed that whenever a woman declared her HIV status, the consequences are far more adverse than for men. Most women who have announced their status have ended up losing their marriages. Many are in fact accused of infidelity as their spouses refuse to go for VCT, claiming they are negative.

So, it was generally agreed that, although usually unspoken, stigma and discrimination could be discouraging PLWHAs, especially those at an advanced stage of the illness, from going out to be involved in public arenas.

The study therefore revealed no evidence that people infected by HIV/AIDS tend to be demotivated by their personal circumstances to the extent that they give up on social and political involvement. PLWHAs are more likely to stay away from political rallies, campaigns, voting, etc, mainly because they are physically challenged because of their physical state as the disease progresses rather than deliberately deciding to stay away. The study also indicated that whether one becomes apathetic depends on the individual - there was no systematic apathy among PLWHAs to justify the argument that PLWHAs are likely to be more apathetic than people without the disease.

Participants were also asked to discuss whether the involvement of PLWHAs in the leadership and the election process would encourage or discourage them to participate in politics as well. Participants revealed that it was more likely than not that there were many PLWHAs who are actively participating in politics at all levels. So participants observed that it was not the question of whether the involvement of PLWHAs would encourage them but rather whether the announcement or disclosure of one's positive status by those already involved would encourage those that are not yet involved.

Participants noted that the outcome of disclosure would depend on the circumstances, though there was a strong argument that disclosure would more likely discourage than encourage. It was stated that stigma towards HIV and AIDS and those infected is still high in the country. It was argued that it would be very unlikely that an HIV-positive person would be well received by both fellow politicians and the electorate. There was an expressed fear that once people know one's positive status, you are likely to be maligned and discredited. Examples were given of how senior political leaders in the country have been making jokes about each other's sickness and how a positive status could be taken advantage of as ammunition by opposition candidates. It was therefore concluded in many FGDs that the environment is still very unfavourable to encourage the participation of PLWHAs in leadership, especially at a higher level. It was highlighted that one could only be involved on the pretext that everyone thinks they are negative.

Participation in politics was however divided into two spheres - participation as a voter, which almost all participants said was easily attainable; and participation as a candidate, which the majority of participants said was very difficult to attain, especially when follow candidates and the electorate are aware of one's positive status. This somehow corroborates responses from other categories targeted by this study, such as political parties and members of the public. Political parties made it clear that although they do not encourage discrimination by HIV status, it would be suicidal to field somebody everyone knows to be HIV-positive. The majority of members of the public also indicated that they would not elect an HIV-positive candidate. The main explanation for this negative attitude towards electing HIV-positive people had nothing to do with their capacity to function but that many people would want to avoid by-elections, which they view as inevitable when you elect a HIV-positive candidate. So, the general understanding was that this sense of stigma, discrimination and despair is more likely to discourage PLWHAs from participating, especially where they see or hear how those already involved are maligned and taunted in public.

Participants were also asked about whether the ECZ had a facility to help those who were sick, pregnant, infirm or disabled to vote, with specific reference to the 2001 elections. Almost all participants expressed ignorance of the availability of such a facility. They noted that the ECZ was not doing much in facilitating the participation of those who are challenged, physically, logistically and even by illness.

Examples were given of pregnant women queuing for hours without any consideration from anyone on how burdened such people were just to make sure they vote. Other examples of people who are disenfranchised due to the lack of mechanisms for assisting them to participate are the sick (those admitted in hospitals, clinics and other health facilities, and even in homes); those in prison; the blind; pregnant women; and even those who are tending to them.

The majority of participants were of the view that many people are hindered from registering as voters and voting mainly because of the complicated and inefficient processes involved. It was highlighted that starting from the National Registration office, which gives National Registration Cards (NRCs), the processes are very time consuming, demanding and discouraging. This is even worse when somebody is physically challenged, sick or pregnant.

So, the general perception in all the FGDs was that there was need for those responsible, the ECZ in this case, to ensure that they improve the efficiency of all processes that are related to elections, from obtaining NRCs, registering as voters, and voting on polling day. If these processes could be improved so that they run swiftly, it will reduce the burden on individuals willing to participate and this will make the whole electoral process acceptable to these challenged categories of voters.

In addition, there was a general complaint about how government hospitals treated PLWHAs. Many participants were of the view that there was a lot of neglect in Zambian hospitals once health personnel know that one has the virus, especially where the disease has developed into AIDS. It was noted that there was a tendency to send sick people home when they should be tended in the hospitals. It was observed that if the sick were to be tended in hospitals, it would free those who are made to tend to them in the homes to go and register and vote because they would know that there are professional people taking care of their sick relative. There was therefore a strong feeling that government should do something about this tendency, especially in government health facilities.

When they were asked to comment on the need to come up with mechanisms to ensure that these categories of voters are specifically catered for in the electoral process, many participants suggested that this may lead to further disenfranchisement, especially if such mechanisms were to be targeted at those living with HIV. Many felt that PLWHAs were already facing challenges such as stigma and discrimination and they argued that creating a parallel system for them to vote would only enhance their exclusion from the mainstream electoral process.

What many participants observed was that in fact there is a need to incorporate PLWHAs and any other excluded categories such as the blind in the system by making it responsive to their special needs rather than establishing parallel structures such as the "special vote" to specifically cater for them.

Suggestions for improving the efficiency of the processes ranged from establishing many national registration offices (or mobile registration offices) making voter registration continuous so that distances and queues are significantly reduced; increasing the number of polling stations and putting them as close to the people as possible. The other suggestion was that, even within a polling station, there was need for many polling booths rather than people queuing up for two or so booths for hours.

As far as stigma and discrimination are concerned, there is a need to do more to fight their negative manifestations, especially where malignant statements are included in election campaign messages. There was a need for serious campaigns among and within political parties to sensitise them and their candidates against derogatory statements, which had been rife in the presidential and parliamentary elections. The implementation of the "Code of Conduct" clause of the Electoral Act should include things that border on stigmatisation and discrimination, be it by tribe, race, HIV status, and gender.

At another level, there is a need for more vigorous voter education, not only focusing on electoral processes and responsibilities but also ensuring that issues of stigma and discrimination are adequately covered. As was indicated earlier in this chapter, stigma and discrimination are deeply entrenched through our socialisation and usually institutionalised in various social-political institutions. To uproot such internalised attitudes and practices requires a very sustained and rigorous effort targeted at all relevant fronts.

When asked to comment on the need to institute mandatory testing for aspiring candidates, many respondents were against the idea. However, others argued that if a medical report is to be presented by all aspiring candidates then medical testing should not be confined to one's HIV/AIDS status only. Medical testing in this case should cover other health ailments, of which HIV/AIDS should only be a part.

Participants also discussed who they felt would be the strongest change agent on issues of HIV/AIDS in the country. Among those ranked high were religious leaders, traditional leaders and politicians, in that order. The majority of participants were of the view that in spite of their privileged position in their societies and the nation in general, most politicians were not playing their role as change agents vis-à-vis the fight against HIV/AIDS. Many even alleged that most politicians were in fact culprits in worsening infection rates due to their dubious sexual behaviour. Participants noted that elected political leaders were a disappointment in many respects. It was highlighted that many politicians were not accountable to their electorate and that they go into politics just for their personal agendas. It was revealed that it was much harder to access political leaders and many wondered how they would effectively represent them whether in Parliament or at national level when there was no contact whatsoever.

However, in spite of all these shortcomings, participants indicated that elected political leaders were strategically positioned to change the course of the epidemic and that they needed to take it upon themselves to do that. The role of MPs was singled out. It was revealed that MPs have the power to determine many factors that are relevant to the desired national response to HIV/AIDS. For instance, MPs make legislation, they debate and decide resource allocation, they approve national policies - in other words, they determine the overall national environment within which the HIV/AIDS epidemic is impacting on the nation, while at the same time they could create the kind of environment and direction with which the nation responds to the epidemic.

Participants therefore argued that MPs needed to be proactive in creating the right environment within which the nation should respond to the epidemic. It was observed that there was a need for appropriate policies and legislation to guide the nation in its response to HIV/AIDS. The majority of participants noted that most of the challenges discussed earlier in this section could be handled by that kind of high-level leadership. Beyond creating a conducive legislative and policy environment, it was also noted that political leaders such as MPs needed to be above board morally because that is the only way they could be an effective agent of positive change.

Therefore, the majority of participants were more confident about the role religious and traditional leaders could play in the fight against HIV/AIDS. It was noted that religious and traditional leaders have the moral advantage of guiding the nation. Moreover, the majority of participants indicated that these categories of leaders were more accessible at all times, and that their operations are usually at the grassroots level where the majority of people are.

Thus, the majority of participants felt that religious and traditional leaders needed to get more involved in efforts towards fighting HIV/AIDS both at local and national levels.

The main conclusions from this chapter are that, although people in Zambia have become more sensitised and aware of HIV/AIDS issues, stigma and discrimination have remained a significant factor in the lives of PLWHAs. It has been argued that in fact, instead of reducing stigma, more awareness has only made it more subtle and invisible, making it even more difficult to investigate. Stigma continues to significantly affect the lives of PLWHAs at an individual and institutional level, and in social, economic and political spheres.

The discussion has also highlighted a number of structural and attitudinal factors that do impact negatively on the participation of PLWHAs and caregivers in governance and electoral processes. Among the structural factors mentioned are inaccessibility to polling stations due to long distances, lack of (appropriate) transport, lack of transport money, lack of ablution blocks at polling stations, lack of seating or resting facilities for people waiting to vote and many other factors related to a lack of other facilities. In terms of attitudinal factors, stigma and discrimination were the major factors highlighted. These factors would continue to affect PLWHAs' ability to effectively participate in governance and electoral processes as long as they remain unresolved.

The study has also revealed that it was the view of many participants that the ECZ was not doing much to facilitate the effective participation of PLWHAs in the electoral process. There is therefore a need for more work on the part of government and the ECZ to ensure that facilities and other logistics are improved to ensure enhanced participation of PLWHAs in the electoral process.

17. Conclusions and recommendations

17.1 Conclusions

The fact that the HIV/AIDS epidemic is having a devastating effect on Zambia's population has been clear for over a decade now. However, what this study has achieved is to use empirical data and life experiences of those infected and/or affected by the disease to show that there is clearly a significant connection between HIV/AIDS and the realms of governance and electoral management and processes, and that if Zambia continues with a lukewarm response to HIV/AIDS, more disastrous consequences are likely. Understanding these challenges and the opportunities open to us is crucial in determining whether we win the fight against the epidemic.

The study has illustrated that the HIV/AIDS epidemic is affecting governance institutions and the electoral processes in Zambia in ways that have not been considered either in HIV/AIDS policy or in governance and electoral legislation and practices. As a result, this study concludes that there is an imperative to urgently reconcile both the HIV/AIDS policy and governance and electoral legislation and practices in order to incorporate the insights emanating from the findings presented in this report. The study acknowledges the difficulty of reconciling the dual necessity of a comprehensive HIV/AIDS response that is technically effective for public health yet also supportive of electoral management and democratic governance.

Although we acknowledge that there is a need for even further in-depth research in the specifics of certain relationships between the various factors and/or components of the HIV/AIDS epidemic and electoral and governance institutions and processes, this study concludes the following:

- Although relatively lower than some of the neighbouring countries in the region, HIV/AIDS prevalence in Zambia has remained high for a long time. This, it has been noted, has many disruptive implications for governance and electoral institutions and processes in the country. Further, although Zambia prides itself on its extensive national response to HIV/AIDS, there is a huge omission as far as the many concerns raised in this report are concerned. As a result, the current national response to HIV/AIDS falls short of the required breadth and depth of responses.

- The study also reaffirms that the FPTP electoral system being used in Zambia appears to be the most vulnerable to the adverse effects of the HIV/AIDS epidemic. This is mainly because of the replacement costs that go with by-elections. It has been noted that these costs are likely to spiral out of control as the death rates among elected political leaders due to HIV/AIDS and related illnesses continue to worsen. The heavy burden this is likely to place on national resources and the decreasing effectiveness in institutions and processes resulting thereof are likely to render participatory democratic governance unsustainable in the long run.

- The impacts of the HIV/AIDS epidemic on governance and electoral processes are wide and deep. What this means is that the HIV/AIDS epidemic is not only affecting a single institution, such as the ECZ, but that it is affecting all critical institutions and individuals alike. Parliament, political parties, and all other stakeholders involved in governance and electoral processes have all been hard hit, thereby compromising their effectiveness and functioning. As a result, all these institutions and individuals cannot act to respond to the epidemic in isolation. There is need for a concerted effort within and across institutions. This however will need leadership – a role political leadership, electoral institutions such as the ECZ, political parties, and the CSOs can take up to spearhead a national response to the epidemic.

- Although this study does not claim to have provided empirical statistics to prove the actual impacts of HIV/AIDS on voters' roll and voter participation, we have enough qualitative evidence showing that the epidemic is having significant impacts on the voters' roll and voter participation in governance and electoral processes. The high morbidity and mortality rates resulting from HIV/AIDS-related complications are incapacitating many citizens, thereby reducing the number of people available to participate in electoral processes in various capacities.

- The other major conclusion is that, although stigma has been cited as one of the factors hindering the participation of PLWHAs and affected individuals, structural impediments are more effective barriers to participation. Such structural factors as long distances, lack of appropriate facilities at polling stations, inefficiency in registration and voting processes, lack of trans-

port, etc., are more likely to hinder physically drained individuals than stigma per se. However, the study has also shown that the impact of HIV/AIDS-related stigma on participation is more and clearly intense regarding participation as candidates compared to participation in other activities. This distinction was very clearly evident and it is important in guiding future programmes and interventions in the country.

- Overall, the report concludes that, in spite of this pessimistic picture of the interaction between HIV/AIDS and electoral processes in Zambia, there is a great opportunity for responding to the epidemic with seriously considered institutional and national programmes to avert the many consequences perceived by this study.

17.2 Recommendations

- It must be re-emphasised here that this realm of knowledge i.e. the relationship between HIV/AIDS and electoral process is still new and under-researched. As a result, our understanding of most critical issues on this topic remains, to the large extent, incomplete. As a result, the first major recommendation is that there is an imperative to delve more into the different issues and factors unveiled in this study, through both quantitative and qualitative research.

- Secondly, it is not necessary to wait until we have a clearer understanding of the problem at hand before instituting corrective measures. It is clear that the current institutional and legal framework does not respond to the special needs of PLWHAs. Given the extraordinary constraints on the functioning of national and local institutions, we may need to re-look at electoral institutions and processes themselves – to re-invent or reconstitute them in order to respond to the new challenges in the age of HIV/AIDS. As a result, based on the current information, there is an urgent and serious review of both the HIV/AIDS policy and governance, electoral and related legislation and practices in the country needed to fill in the gaps and reconcile the two realms which have until now been considered as completely unrelated. It would be an enriching experience to undertake these reviews while simultaneously carrying out further studies so that the two processes can feed into and from each other. The end result should be a reconstituted institutional (ECZ, Parliament, political parties, etc) and legal (legislation, laws, practices, etc) framework in order to recreate a conducive environment for PLWHAs to participate effectively. In other words, there is a need for a strong watchdog system (legal and institutional) to watch over and protect the rights of PLWHAs in all spheres of life.

- At an institutional level, there is an urgent need for comprehensive treatment and care programmes for employees already infected by the disease so as to slow down its progression and ultimately minimise the adverse impacts of the epidemic in the interim. If we can make those already infected lead better and longer lives, then we would be succeeding in helping to mitigate many of the more dangerous secondary impacts of widespread adult mortality. For example, by keeping skilled people alive longer, it will make it easier to sustain complex institutions by reducing attrition rates among workers. However, in the longer term, all relevant institutions should put in place programmes to prepare for the likely higher rates of staff attrition in the future. Some government departments such as the judiciary are already working on similar programmes.

- These should be expanded and re-aligned to respond to the new insights arising from this and many other related studies from the sub-region.

- Advocacy targeted at MPs and the leadership role of different community role models – traditional rulers, church leaders, private sector leaders, etc. – in the HIV/AIDS response should be strengthened. The HIV/AIDS leadership role programmes already in place at Parliament and the judiciary should be strengthened, and more resources allocated and expended to other strategic institutions such as the ECZ, political parties, etc. Also, the Parliamentary Health Committee provides an opportunity for political leaders to interact with technocrats and to raise issues of HIV/AIDS at the highest level of governance. However, membership should be widened to include all stakeholders not currently part of the committee.

- This study could not capture the longitudinal impacts of HIV/AIDS-related mortalities due to the absence of specific statistics and the lack of consistent maintenance of the voters' roll by the ECZ. We therefore recommend specific interventions and legislation to be put in place to encourage/facilitate the collection of such quantitative data in all strategic institutions/workplaces as this will help paint a clearer picture of how the HIV/AIDS epidemic is affecting electoral institutions and processes. Beyond this, it is important that the ECZ collects and keeps longitudinal voters' roll profiles so that there is continuity rather than moving from one system and voters' roll to another. A system of incorporating new registrations, purging dead voters, etc. must be put in place rather than calling for fresh registration of voters every time a review is required.

- To increase participation of PLWHAs in political office, there is a need for deliberate interventions or programmes to support and encourage aspiring candidates who are known to be HIV-positive to come out and stand for political office. Deliberate programmes to prop up highly potentious PLWHA for electoral candidature should be encouraged or developed. A rights-based approach should be encouraged and CSOs in the rights arena should take up these issues and advocate for the effective participation of PLWHAs.

- Related to the above, stigma remains very high in Zambia. These interventions should therefore go hand-in-hand with programmes targeted at sensitising communities so as to reduce stigma and discrimination against PLWHA. There is a strong imperative to incorporate HIV/AIDS sensitisation in governance and electoral campaigns. This is critical if we are to create the desired political impetus for raising HIV/AIDS among priority issues. These interventions should be undertaken simultaneously with efforts to lobby for legislation providing for parliamentary positions to be reserved for PLWHAs. In all these efforts, the role of political leadership, CSOs, FBOs and traditional leaders and associated structures would be critical, particularly in the rural areas.

- While reducing stigma and discrimination would help increase the participation of PLWHAs in electoral processes, the study revealed that the structural hindrances are more effective barriers to participation than psychosocial factors, particularly as far as registering as voters and voting are concerned. As a result, taking care of the structural aspects of the whole electoral process would greatly increase the participation of PLWHAs, especially given that in Zambia the mechanism of a special vote was resisted by a significant number of participants.

- Overall, an electoral system that seeks to control the replacement costs that come with the increasing incidence of by-elections would be most suitable, and ought to be on the electoral reform agenda for the country. It is therefore the belief of this team that Zambia as a nation should consider reviewing its electoral system from FPTP to the PR model. In the current HIV/AIDS-prone environment, the costs which were intended to be saved by adopting the simpler FPTP electoral system are likely to be surpassed by the inevitable costs that come with by-elections due to increasing HIV/AIDS-related deaths among elected political leaders.

Endnote

1   Official statement from the Electoral Commission of Zambia (ECZ) signed by Acting Director Priscilla Isaacs April 18, 2007.

References

Alcantara, C.H.D. (1998), "Uses and Abuses of the Concept of Governance", *International Social Science Journal* Vol. 155, pp 104-113.

Apter, D. and C. Roseberg (1994), *Political Development and New Realism in Sub Saharan Africa*. Charlottesville: University of Michigan Press.

Barnett, T. & A. Whiteside (2002), *AIDS in the 21st Century: Disease and Globalization*, Basingstoke and New York: Palgrave Macmillan.

Chikulo, B. C. and O. B. Sichone (eds) (1996) "Democracy in Zambia: Challenges for the Third Republic". Harare: SAPES Books.

Chikulo, C. Bornwell (1989), "Elections in a One Party Participatory Democracy", in Ben Turok (ed) Development in Zambia, London: Zed Books.

Chirambo, K. (2003) "Impact of HIV/AIDS on Electoral Processes in Southern Africa", presentation at the 13th ICASA Conference, Nairobi, September.

CSO (2003), *Zambia DHS EdData Survey 2002: Education Data for Decision-Making*. Central Statistics Office (Zambia) and ORC Macro.

CSO (2000), *2000 Census Report*, Lusaka: Central Statistical Office.

De Waal, Alex (2006), "How will HIV/AIDS transform African governance?" Justice Africa: See also http://afraf.oxfordjournals.org/cgi/content/abstract/102/406/1

Diamond, Larry (1999), *Developing Democracy: Towards Consolidation*, Baltimore: John Hopkins University Press

ECZ Website (2006), See www.elections.org.zm

ERTC (2006), Report of the ERTC. Lusaka. Also see www.ertc.zm/technical_committee

FODEP (2005), See www.fodep.org.zm

Garbus, Lisa (2003), HIV/AIDS in Zambia, UCSF, March.

Grassly, N.C. *et al*, (2003), "The Economic Impact of HIV/AIDS on the Education Sector in Zambia", AIDS 17: 1039-1044.

GRZ (1991), *Constitution of the Republic of Zambia*, 24th August 1991, amended in 1996.

GRZ (2001), *Zambia Demographic Health Survey (2001 – 2002)*. Lusaka: Central Statistical Office

GRZ (2004), *Zambia Antenatal Clinic Sentinel Surveillance Report (1994 – 2004)*. Lusaka.

GRZ (2004), *Zambia Poverty Reduction Strategy Plan* (PRSP). Lusaka: Ministry of Finance and Economic Planning.

GRZ (2006), "Government Reaction to the Electoral Reform Technical Committee Report" (Unpublished).

GRZ/NAC (2004), *Joint Review of the National HIV/AIDS/STI/TB Intervention Strategic Plan (2002 – 2005) and the operations of the National AIDS Council*. Lusaka: NAC.

Hangoma, Mumba Moonga (2004), "Marriage of Convenience: State-Civil Society Partnership in the PRSP Formulation Process in Zambia". M.A. Thesis, Institute of Social Studies (ISS), The Hague, The Netherlands.

Harle, Jon (2006), "AIDS, Governance and Quality in Tanzanian Education." Justice Africa.

Hegel, G.W.F. (1953), "Philosophy of Right and Law", in Carl J. Friedrich (ed.), *The Philosophy of Hegel*, New York: Random House.

Jackson Reynolds and D. Jackson (1999), *A Comparative Introduction to Political Science*, N. J. Printice Hall.

Leys, Colin (1996), *The Rise and Fall of Development Theory*, Blooming: Indiana University Press.

MoE (2000), "Recent Developments in the fight against HIV/AIDS in the Ministry of Education in Zambia", Ministry of Education, September 2000, hivaidsclearinghouse.unesco.org

MoE (2001), "HIV/AIDS Education Strategic Plan (2001-2005)", Lusaka: MoE.

MoE (2004), *Accelerating the Education Response by Mainstreaming HIV/AIDS, Equity and Gender, Special Education Needs, School Health and Nutrition in Decentralised Planning in Zambia*: Workshop Report, 8th-13th August, Lusaka.

Mutasa, K. (2005) Paper presented at the first PEPSA Conference on Electoral Reforms held in Johannesburg on sustainable electoral systems.

NAC (2000), Strategic Framework 2001-2003, October.

NAC (2002), HIV/AIDS Care and Support Capacity and Needs in Zambia: An Assessment in Four Districts – Final Report.

NAC (2004), *The HIV/AIDS Epidemic in Zambia: Where are we now? Where are we going?* Lusaka: September.

NAC (2004), *HIV/AIDS Communication Strategy.* Lusaka – May.

NAC (2005), Joint Review of the National HIV/AIDS/STI/TB Intervention Strategic Plan (2002-2005) and Operations of the National AIDS Council, Lusaka: NAC/GRZ.

Noble Rob (2006), "HIV and AIDS in Zambia: the Epidemic and its Impact".

Pact Zambia (2005), "A-Watch Project Baseline Survey Report", Lusaka: Pact Zambia.

PANOS/UNICEF (2004) Stigma, HIV/AIDS and Prevention of Mother-to-Child Transmission: A pilot study in Zambia, Ukraine, India and Burkina Faso. London: Panos/UNICEF.

Rugalema, G. (2002), "HIV/AIDS and land issues: beyond proximate linkages," opening remarks prepared for the FAO/HSRC-SARPN Workshop on the "Impact of HIV/AIDS on Land Issues", Pretoria, 24-25 June.

Strand, P., Matlosa, K., Strode, A. & Chirombo, K. (2005), *HIV/AIDS and Democratic Governance: Illustrating the Impact on Electoral Processes.* Cape Town: Idasa.

The Namibian Newspaper Online

Times of Zambia (2004), "Let's Fight HIV/AIDS Stigma", 29th December; see http/www.allafrica.com

TIZ (2003), Government Machinery for Accountability: A Survey of Existing Laws and Institutional Framework in Zambia for Combating Corruption. Lusaka: TIZ

UNAIDS/WHO (2004), Epidemiological Fact Sheet – 2004 Update, Zambia.

UNAIDS/WHO (2006), Report on the Global AIDS Epidemic.

USAID (2002), HIV/AIDS Care and Support Capacity and Needs in Zambia: An Assessment in Four Districts, Lusaka: USAID/NAC/Cara Counselling.

Van de Walle, N. and Butler, K. (2006), "The links between HIV/AIDS and Democratic Governance in Africa", London: Justice Africa & GAIN, adapted from presentations at Justice Africa, 30 October 2003 and Oslo Governance Centre, 3 November 2003.

Weiner M. (1967), *Party building in a New Nation.* Chicago: Chicago University Press.

WHO/UNAIDS (2004), Zambia Summary Country Profile for HIV/AIDS Treatment Scale-Up, July.

ZDH (2002), ZDH Survey 2001-2002.

Interviews

1. The Executive Director, Anti-AIDS Teachers Association of Zambia, May 2006.
2. The Executive Director, Zambia AIDS Research and Advocacy Network (ZARAN), Lusaka
3. AMICAALL
4. NZP+
5. NZP+ - Mirriam Banda (National Coordinator)
6. ECZ – Mr Kunda – Human Resources Dept.
7. ECZ – Mr Dan Kalale, Director.
8. NWLG – Ms Prisca Chikwashi, Executive Director.
9. NAC – Dr Alex Simwanza – Head of Programmes
10. CBoH – Dr Ben Chirwa
11. LCC (Lusaka City Council).

Appendix: Provincial and District figures

The table indicates estimated HIV prevalence rate by province and district for 2004 (estimated by NAC, 2004).

District	Prevalence (%)	HIV+ people
Central	**14.4**	**87,435**
Chibombo	11.6	15,387
Kabwe	23.8	24,939
Kapiri-mposhi	18.5	21,063
Mkushi	11.6	7,171
Mumbwa	11.6	10,239
Serenje	11.6	8,636
Copperbelt	**18.5**	**270,525**
Chililabombwe	19.0	10,287
Chingola	26.6	35,982
Kalulushi	19.0	11,025
Kitwe	26.6	77,066
Luanshya	19.0	21,632
Lufwanyama	11.3	4,744
Masaiti	11.3	7,149
Mpongwe	11.3	4,940
Mufulira	19.0	21,367
Ndola	26.6	76,334
Northern	**8.0**	**63,812**
Chilubi	5.2	1,538
Chinsali	5.4	3,110
Isoka	5.3	2,247
Kaputa	5.2	2,029
Kasama	12.6	14,941
Luwingu	5.2	1,813
Mbala	8.9	8,487
Mpika	12.6	12,941
Mporokoso	5.2	1,765
Mpulungu	12.6	5,877
Mingwi	5.2	2,624
Nakonde	12.6	6,441
Western	**12.6**	**58,347**
Kalabo	10.0	6,172
Kaoma	10.0	9,036
Lukulu	10.0	3,881
Mongu	22.2	22,236
Senanga	10.0	5,798

District	Prevalence (%)	HIV+ people
Sesheke	16.1	7,485
Shang'ombo	10.0	3,736
Lusaka	**20.7**	**157,997**
Chongwe	19.0	13,411
Kafue	22.4	17,489
Luangwa	19.0	1,888
Lusaka	22.4	125,209
Eastern	**13.2**	**81,785**
Chadiza	9.8	2,891
Chama	9.8	2,466
Chipata	26.3	35,884
Katete	18.1	16,687
Lundazi	18.1	13,089
Mambwe	9.8	1,509
Nyimba	9.3	2,266
Petauke	9.3	6,993
Luapula	**10.6**	**49,462**
Chiengi	8.2	5,362
Kawambwa	8.2	6,707
Mansa	11.6	17,822
Milenge	8.2	1,758
Mwense	8.2	6,724
Nchelenge	9.8	8,814
Samfya	9.7	2,275
Southern	**16.2**	**120,768**
Choma	19.2	19,918
Gwembe	7.5	1,103
Itezhi-tezhi	7.5	1,415
Kalomo	18.6	17,003
Kazungula	18.6	6,713
Livingstone	30.9	19,184
Mazabuka	22.5	25,024
Monze	19.2	16,879
Namwala	7.5	2,802
Siavonga	19.2	8,044
Sinazongwe	7.5	2,684
North-Western	**8.6**	**27,587**
Chavuma	8.8	1,228
Kabompo	7.2	2,246
Kasempa	7.4	1,721
Mufumbwe	7.3	1,439
Mwinilunga	8.8	5,010
Solwezi	12.3	13,250
Zambezi	8.8	2,694

Abbreviations

AATAZ	Anti-AIDS Teachers' Association of Zambia
AIDS	Acquired Immunodeficiency Syndrome
ANC	African National Congress
APC	People's Congress Party
ART	Anti-retroviral therapy
ARVs	Anti-retroviral drugs
BCC	Behavioural Change Communication
CA	Constituent Assembly
CBoH	Central Board of Health
CBOs	Community Based Organisations
CCRC	Chona Constitutional Review Commission
CRC	Constitutional Review Commission
CSO	Central Statistical Office
CSOs	Civil Society Organisations
DATFs	District AIDS Task Forces
DHMTs	District Health Management Teams
ECZ	Electoral Commission of Zambia
ERTC	Electoral Reform Technical Committee
FBOs	Faith-Based Organisations
FDD	Forum for Democracy and Development
FGDs	Focus Group Discussions
FODEP	Foundation for Democratic Process
FPTP	First Past The Post
GAP	Governance and AIDS Programme
HIV	Human Immuno Virus
HP	Heritage Party
IDASA	Institute for Democracy in South Africa
MCRC	Mvunga Constitutional Review Commission
MMD	Movement for Multiparty Democracy
MoE	Ministry of Education
MoH	Ministry of Health
MPs	Members of Parliament
MTP 1	First Medium Term Plan
MTP 2	Second Medium Term Plan
NAC	National AIDS Council
NACP	National AIDS Prevention and Control Programme
NDF	National Democratic Focus
NGOs	Non-Governmental Organisations
NHAA	National HIV/AIDS Accounts
NPP	National Progressive Party
NZP+	Network for Zambian People Living with HIV/AIDS
OMR	Optical Mark Recognition
OVCs	Orphans and Vulnerable Children
PF	Patriotic Front
PLWHAs	People Living with HIV/AIDS
PMTCT	Prevention of Mother-to-Child Transmission
PR	Proportional Representation
PRSP	Poverty Reduction Strategy Paper
RP	Reform Party
SMM	Single Member Majority
SMP	Single Member Plurality
STIs	Sexually Transmitted Infections
STV	Single Transferable Vote
TB	Tuberculosis
UDA	United Democratic Alliance
UFP	United Federal Party
UN	United Nations
UNIP	United National Independence Party
UPND	United Party for National Development
UTH	University Teaching Hospital
VCT	Voluntary Counselling and Testing
WHO	World Health Organisation
WHO/GPA	World Health Organisation's Global Programme on HIV/AIDS
ZAMCOM	Zambia Institute of Mass Communication
ZANC	Zambia African National Congress
ZEMCC	Zambia Elections Monitoring Coordinating Committee
ZHECT	Zambian Health, Education and Communications Trust
ZINGO	Zambia Inter-Faith Network Group on HIV/AIDS
ZNAN	Zambia National AIDS Network

Senegal: Rethinking HIV/AIDS and democratic governance

Cheikh Ibrahima Niang

1. Introduction

According to socioeconomic indicators, Senegal is among the poorest countries in the world. Life expectancy is 50 for men and 52 for women, with 57% of men and 77% of women being illiterate. Though the overall rates of prevalence of HIV/AIDS in Senegal are considered to be relatively low and stable (EDS-IV, 2005; UNAIDS, 2006), higher prevalence rates are recorded among vulnerable groups, such as commercial sex workers and men who have sex with other men.

Shortly after the existence of HIV in the country was recognised, a strong political commitment to countering the epidemic led to the adoption of a multisectoral strategy, involving social dialogue, community mobilisation and the involvement of religious leaders. The government of Senegal was also among the first in Africa to budget for reducing the price of antiretroviral drugs, and, later, to issue them freely to people living with HIV/AIDS (PLWHAs).

The present case study aims to analyse:

- The profile and evolution of the HIV epidemic and the policies of response to AIDS in Senegal;

- The political aspects of vulnerability to HIV/AIDS in Senegal;

- How HIV/AIDS affects elected bodies and the electoral processes; and

- Support for HIV/AIDS and democratic governance.

A shift is needed from the prevailing biomedical paradigms and the Western concept of democracy. HIV/AIDS and health are thought of as shaped by sociohistoric perceptions of power.

Previous Senegal-based research emphasised the difficulty of measuring the impact of HIV/AIDS at a national level in their use of demographic and epidemiological data. Yet, analyses of the effects of HIV/AIDS at both family and individual level have shown that families and individuals have been ravaged by the disease, leading to the shrinking of assets and savings, and to a decline in educational standards. All such effects might also have political consequences (Niang, 2001).

Though the voters' roll and demographic/epidemiological data were quantitatively analysed, the focus is mainly on ethnographic and historical sociocultural analysis. The Senegalese strategy adopted towards the epidemic was analysed on the grounds of a literature review.

The Senegalese study highlights the difficulties of finding comparative groups and of accessing useful and exhaustive timely data, and so of reaching meaningful findings based on statistical procedures, in countries with a low prevalence. The statistical analysis is, accordingly, biased. Nevertheless, the exploratory nature of the exercise could encourage related studies.

The regions of Dakar, Kolda and Thiès were selected as representative of the HIV/AIDS epidemic, ethnic diversity and political and socioeconomic contexts, due to:

- Dakar being the administrative and economic capital of the country, as it hosts the government, Parliament and almost all state institutions, with the largest number of registered voters;

- Kolda being one of the poorest regions in Senegal, with one of the highest HIV/AIDS prevalence rates; and

- Thiès experiencing the intense external migration associated with relatively high HIV/AIDS prevalence.

The criteria for selecting participants for focus group discussions (FGDs), as well as regular and key informants, were as follows:

- The elderly (including traditional communicators), who have extensive knowledge of local history and culture;

- Political leaders and members of political parties;

- PLWHAs;

- Members of NGOs and traditional associations involved in efforts to counter HIV/AIDS;

- Members of Parliament (MPs) and of local elected bodies;

- Members of the Electoral Management Body;

- Members of the Ministry of Health and of the National AIDS Committee;

- Men who have sex with other men; and

- Commercial sex workers.

Data collection involved holding both unstructured individual and semistructured interviews (n=120) and FGDs (n=12), as well as recording case narratives (n=6). Participants in the FGDs validated previous findings, drawn from different research methods. Participants in a workshop, held to validate the research design and preliminary findings, included MPs and political leaders; PLWHAs; NGOs; traditional associations; members of the Electoral Management Body, ministries and the National AIDS

Committee; commercial sex workers; men having sex with other men; researchers; and academics.

The present work comprises six sections:

- An introductory analysis of the core elements of conceptual and theoretical frameworks used;
- An analysis of the HIV/AIDS situation in Senegal and related policy responses;
- A description of the official political institutions; and
- An analysis of the impact of HIV/AIDS on socio-politics.

2. Conceptual shifts

UNAIDS (2004) regards AIDS as "an exceptional epidemic. It requires an exceptional response that has to remain flexible, creative, energetic and vigilant."

2.1 Rethinking HIV/AIDS

According to Airhihenbuwa, African epidemiological research and interventions are still dominated by models and theories more applicable to the West (UNAIDS, 2000). Such models emphasise the centrality of individual risk[1] to intervention strategies and research designs. The first countermeasures adopted towards the HIV/AIDS pandemic focused on reducing levels of risky behaviour in the high risk groups.[2] According to Airhihenbuwa and other authors (ONUSIDA/Pennstate, 2000), such behaviour change theories and models regard individuals as totally controlling their own behaviour, ignoring the role played by context. Schoepf, an early critic of knowledge, attitudes and practices (KAP) studies, described the still-dominant linear model of relationship between knowledge, risk perception and behavioural change:

> Ignoring declining health services, gender inequality and mounting poverty, planners funded "KAP" surveys on AIDS knowledge, attitudes and sexual practices around the world. They acted as though increased information would be sufficient to change complexly determined actions and as though individuals could exercise control over the social and cultural constraints imposed on prevention. They focused on individuals in special "risk groups" and their "high risk behav-

iours" rather than on processes of economic empowerment and socio-cultural change. (Schoepf, 2004a)

According to Campbell (2003), many, despite knowing about HIV/AIDS, continue to have unprotected sex, often with multiple partners: "the forces shaping sexual behaviour and sexual health are far more complex than individual rational decisions based on simple factual knowledge about health risks, and the availability of medical services." The individualist and quantitative framework is one within which interventions and responses are designed and evaluated as isolated actions, which is often misleading in the African context.

Choice of model depends on given policies and interests. Schoepf states that the first epidemiological model was marked by the lack of political will to use the necessary funds for extended struggle efforts. By defining AIDS as an outcome of individual behaviour, political authorities at both national and international levels could deny their responsibility in this regard: In the case of AIDS in Africa, the defining power is laid in the international biomedical arena, but the definitions met with enduring disease representations and practices, especially in the most afflicted societies (Schoepf, 2004a).

Individual-focused approaches allow for violation of ethics in clinical trials, by ignoring the power relations and economic concerns influencing individual decision-making. The African concept of personhood, which largely differs from the Western, holds that "persons exist only in relation to other persons" (Niekerk et al., 2005). For example, the Senegalese Wolof use "xamal sa bop" ("know who you are") to mean "know your relationship to others" ("know your genealogy as well").

Any consideration of HIV/AIDS must include globalisation,[3] as such international social and economic restructuring causes both an unprecedented concentration of wealth and political power in the hands of a few, and an increase in the number of poor (Ziegler, 1999). Stiglitz[4] (2002) wrote: "If, in too many instances, the benefits of globalisation have been less than its advocates claim, the price paid has been greater, as the environment has been destroyed, as political processes have been corrupted, and as the rapid pace of change has not allowed countries time for cultural adaptation. The crises that have brought in their wake massive unemployment have, in turn, been followed by long-term problems of social dissolution – from urban violence [...] to ethnic conflicts [...]."

Schoepf (2004a) detected the link between HIV/

AIDS and the social devastation resulting from globalisation, claiming:

> Disease epidemics are social processes. The spread of infection is propelled by history, political economy, and culture. The destructive impact of ongoing economic crisis on the health of poor communities takes from less dramatic than violent conflict, yet which may be just as devastating. Structural and social violence has contributed decisively to the dissemination of the Human Immunodeficiency Virus (HIV) on the African continent as economic crisis spread across the continent. In the late 1970s, HIV silently spread as well. Seemingly unrelated, the two phenomena are, in fact, intimately entwined. The effects of poverty accelerated the effect of the virus in the 1980s. By the 1990s, the ravages of AIDS in turn plunged afflicted regions deeper into economic crisis.

When the first AIDS cases were reported, many African presidents remained silent or declared that the foreign press was conducting a campaign against their country. The initial denial resulted from a fear of Western stigma and racist attitudes to HIV and its potential economic, social, and political impacts (Sabatier, 1989). Schoepf (2004b) states: "Knowledge of AIDS in Africa is about power: the power to name and define; the power to know; the power to attract funds; the power to act to reduce risks of becoming infected with HIV."

O'Manique (2004) pointed out that African responses to AIDS evolved in the context of a massive debt burden, a severe economic and political crisis and a failure of states to provide basic social services. HIV/AIDS-related successes tend to have resulted from resistance across a broad front, involving the mobilisation of resources supplied both by foreign donors and by local African societies and states.

2.2 Integrating societies and cultures

The Senegalese study focuses on socially constructed identities and communities. Social capital and cohesion are central to gaining and maintaining the well-being of society, with the latter facilitating the building of health-enabling communities,[5] while the former emphasises the social networks used to access and mobilise human resources. A Wolof proverb states "*Am nit moo gen am alaP*" (having people supporting you is better than having material wealth). Social capital comprises the collective mobilisation, about which Wolofs say "*Boo woote, ñu wuyi si la*" (when you call a gathering, people come).

In many African cultures, social capital comprises a form of payback received by someone who has helped others. Having large social capital confers social prestige, with, in Wolof, "*borom daraja*" conveying both the idea of having much social capital and of benefiting from increased respect from the community.

Low-Beer *et al.* (as cited in Barnett and Whiteside, 2002) have shown that the most important behavioural changes in Uganda have been fewer youth having sex, delay of the start of sexual activity and the tendency to have fewer nonregular partners.[6]

Barnett and Whiteside (2002) point out that Ugandans developed personal behavioural strategies that significantly reduced HIV prevalence, in line with changes driven by informative communication networks. However, HIV/AIDS-related discussion among friends and family proved more effective than did mass communication channels.

Recent studies have highlighted the structural role of women in conflict resolution in various parts of Africa (UNESCO, 2003).

Bourdieu (1986) defines *habitus* as the set of durable principles embodied in rituals, symbols, practices, beliefs, taboos, rules and representations, which are transmitted from generation to generation and provide a group of individuals with a sense of collective identity, creativity and social organisation. He sees culture as a form of capital that, like social capital, can help both individuals and groups to face social trauma and enhance their position in the social and political order.[7]

Rao and Walton advocate an "institutional demand for cultural democracy" by way of basic education, free media, free electoral participation and basic civil rights (Rao and Watson, 2004). However, providing basic education in the colonial languages could lead to a loss of cultural heritage; the media can only be free if they voice the needs of the marginalised groups; and elections can be held in regimes denying civil rights to those who do not conform to prevailing cultural models.

The prevailing HIV/AIDS-related approaches tend to explain AIDS-related health problems solely as risky cultural practices. Dominant national and international policy-makers tend to be subject to

Western cultural biases and stereotypes that exclude marginalised groups from decision-making. The Senegalese case study considers how greater cultural awareness can foster PLWHAs gaining equity and improved access to health, political power and resources.

2.3 Shifts in approaching gender and sexuality

The imposition of largely Western constructs of "homosexuality" as both a sexual behaviour and a social identity has obscured the reality of male–to–male sex in Africa. So, Hardy wrote at the beginning of the HIV/AIDS pandemic: "Homosexuality is not part of traditional societies in Sub-Saharan Africa", whereas social anthropological studies have revealed socially and culturally rooted same-sex sexuality in many African countries and exposed the connection between same-sex sexuality and gender constructions (Niang *et al.*, 2004).

This study considers the historic and cultural context in which women were extremely powerful. Though many African states are described as models of both undemocratic and patriarchal systems, in some areas in Senegal only women are eligible for the highest level of leadership. Political systems of a man and woman co-ruling were known in many studies of precolonial African forms of government, with women having more power in relationships with men than has generally been common in the West (Skard, 2003). However, many women do suffer oppression and structural violence throughout Africa.

As Siplon points out, "The current patriarchal systems of African states were strongly reinforced by colonial events." Schraeder, cited by Siplon, notes that, in many regions of precolonial Africa, parallel gender-segregated systems of governance allowed women to make certain decisions. However, the colonial powers, by refusing to recognise any but male authorities, destroyed the authority and capacity of such women-controlled decision-making bodies, stifling the occasional emergence of women as national leaders. Similarly, the imposition of a patriarchal form of Christianity by missionaries meant both that men would dominate the church hierarchies and that patriarchal interpretation of the Bible would be used to justify discrimination against women. According to Siplon (2005), "The resulting legacy of patriarchal structures that directly or indirectly deny women economic resources and deci-

sion- making capacity is deadly in the age of AIDS." Reconceptualising AIDS, democracy and gender in Africa should consider African historical models of nonpatriarchal societies, as well as contemporary gender inequalities, social exclusion, violence and structural violence that increase women's vulnerability to HIV/AIDS.

2.4 Redefining democracy

In the Senegalese case study, the theoretical assumption is that any construction of political power is accompanied by diverse forms of self-affirmation and struggle for political, religious, social and economic rights. The etymological definition of democracy as rule by the people agrees with many African concepts associating the people with political power. A Wolof proverb says "*Mbolo moy doole*" (the people are the power). The Wolof concept of "*mbolo*" is associated with power-sharing (with the verb "*bolo*" meaning to gather). *Mbolo* is also used to refer to an assembly or an institution made up of several constituents. The standard opening address of an "*mboloo*" indicates the group (at macrolevel), the family and kinships (at mesolevel) and the individual's first name (at microlevel). In such terms, power is seen as a collective enterprise, to which both individuals and groups contribute and by means of which they can exercise their rights.[8]

As Mafeje (1995) points out, the central question is: Who are the people? This central question leads to the issue of who defines the people and what prevents individuals and groups from exercising their rights.

The Western concept of democracy fails to include environmental and ecological issues associated with community and societal access to natural resources, security and well-being. Though democracy and free elections might meet Western standards, they might exclude certain people on sociocultural grounds. The Western push for democracy often fails to critically analyse the reproduction of the control of the political power by "elitist" privilege and westernised minorities, even if such control is achieved though regular, multipartisan elections.

2.5 Rethinking governance

Policy is generally defined as a relatively stable, purposive course of action to be followed by an actor or a set of actors in dealing with a problem or issue of concern. A study conducted by Idasa (Strand *et al.*, 2005) states:

> Governance is deemed to be "good" when it tends toward the general progression of humankind on all fronts. Good governance should be able to widen people's choices and their well being, rendering three key elements – a healthy life, acquisition of knowledge and access to resources. This also includes ensuring that all people have an opportunity to fully participate in community decisions and enjoy human rights and economic and political freedoms.

IDASA argues for locating the HIV/AIDS policies and responses within the realm of good governance:

> This would ensure, inter alia, that the epidemic is considered as one of the national priorities, thus mainstreaming HIV/AIDS-related matters in resource mobilisation and allocation, and allowing for accountability of leadership, transparency, rule of law, participation, decentralisation of authority, decision-making and service delivery, economic justice and human rights.

The notion of good governance, mainly initiated by the World Bank and donor agencies, reflects a public management approach based on rules of efficiency and on a logic of liberal economy, overlooking the large amount of donor funding aimed at combating AIDS in Africa, but which is not spent in African countries, but instead in donor countries. Good governance is generally conceived as a multiparty system, with the staging of regular competitive elections seen as a direct form of participation in public affairs, allowing the largest number of people to choose their leaders.

The framework of good governance fails to address the control of decision-making and the determination of economically, politically and culturally limited options. Even when the prevailing definitions state that: "Good governance ensures that political, social and economic priorities are based on broad consensus in society and that the voices of the poorest and the most vulnerable are heard in decision-making over the allocation of resources" (Strand *et al.*, 2005), such consensus depends on power relations within the sociocultural framework.

After the prevailing Western cooperation paradigms, states are blamed for corruption and incompetence; so, instead of supporting local initiatives and reactions against mismanagement and in favour of state reforms, NGOs often ignore the public health institution. Historically, the notion of good governance emerged with neoliberal arguments in favour of the reduction of state expenditure on health, education and social services.

Patterson (2006) notices that, because of the decrease in state expenditure on health and education, African states rely more on Western donors and non-governmental organisations (NGOs) to provide them with basic human services. The NGOs and donors are outside the control of the state and, due to the large amount of funding that they provide for AIDS programmes, international organisations play a leading role in many state AIDS programmes and decision-making institutions throughout Africa. Moreover, HIV/AIDS-related studies are generally confined to universities or consultancies in Western countries. Such external evaluation pays scant attention to processes and to local meanings, with the donors indicating what is to be done and how and the evaluators often lacking community validation. The misuse of AIDS funding indicates not only formal rules of transparency, but also solidarity that transcends the individualistic framework.

Often, in the NGO-dominated Western-driven official discourses, community is considered a major stakeholder, with its participation regarded as an important part of strategy. However, little is known about whether communities conceive the strategies or only participate in predesigned strategies.

NGOs make up the driving force of civil society in many countries in Africa. Fowler, cited by Strand *et al.*, 2005, defines civil society as:

> an array of people's organisations, voluntary associations, self-help clubs, interest groups, religious bodies, non-governmental development organisations, foundations, and social movements that may be formal or informal in nature, that are not part of government, and that are not established to make profits.

The constituents of civil society seem to be part of a larger framework that defines the ways of, and criteria for, participation in the ensemble.

The NGOs working in the fight against AIDS often share the attitudes of those involved with cooperation aimed at development. As Gueneau, cited by Niang, 2002, says:

> When people from the administration or those working in a project come to work with them, village dwellers do not tell their needs... they wait for proposi-

tions. A project set up for buying salt or setting up a small enterprise will receive the same welcome; those people will say: let them do. All programme managers tell people what to do. People are used to that. Help from outside arrives with what they are willing to do...Donors come with big words, big questions; we, we are here. The president gazes at the secretary, the secretary gazes at the treasurer, but no one knows what to answer, since the questions they ask are their own questions.

Botes and Van Rensburg (cited by Niang, 2002) record an Indian village dweller saying: "They (developers) arrived already knowing everything. They look around, but they see only what is not here."

Farmer (2007) questioned:

There are now more than 60 000 AIDS alone related NGOs. Yet by 2006, after a global campaign to bring HIV/AIDS care to Africa, less than 25% of the Africans who needed antiretrovirals to survive were receiving them, with the fraction dwindling to less than 5% in rural areas. Worse, new infections continue apace. So what on earth, one might ask, are all these AIDS focused NGOs doing?

Many NGOs in Africa have refocused on dealing with the HIV/AIDS pandemic. HIV/AIDS appears increasingly as an international industry, with financial influx completely out of the control of people and societies that are the worst affected by the pandemic.

Farmer (2007) states, "When programmes are properly designed to reflect the patient's needs rather than the wishes of donors, AIDS funding can strengthen primary care". With examples taken from Haiti, Rwanda and Malawi, he points out the importance of working under the aegis of the Ministries of Health to promote health as a human right and, in some cases, of rebuilding the public infrastructures damaged by war, neglect, or the misguided advice of outside experts.

2.6 Rethinking health and democracy

The link between democracy and better health is based upon unverifiable assumptions:

- that democracy protects the well-being of citizens; and

- that democratically elected leaders are more likely to invest in the public good and to use state resources for the benefit of small groups, as well as to address major societal problems, as they are watched by free media, opposition parties, and civil society organisations (Paterson, 2005).

Democracies are also considered as meeting the conditions that favour the perception of risk of being infected by the virus, which, in the classical Western behavioural models, is an important step towards behavioural change. Paterson cites the case of Senegal: "Among all African women, those in Senegal are the most likely to report feeling this risk". However, according to a study conducted in Senegal, only 12% of female students in Dakar and 10% in other regions felt that they were at risk of infection due to their previous behaviour. Only 1% of female students in Senegal, 0.20% of the saleswomen in Dakar and 5% of the female population in the other regions surveyed said that they felt that their current behaviour was high risk. The commercial sex workers who thought that they had previously risked being infected represented 27% of those registered in Dakar. 84% of the traders in Dakar felt that they had taken no risk (FHI-BSS, 2001). Douglas's cultural theory shows, in this regard, the fundamental bias of statistically grounded individualistic perspectives (Douglas, 1992).

Risk is culturally constructed, being associated with self-image, philosophy of life and death. Those from rural areas, when asked whether they felt at risk of contracting HIV, closed their ears in a way that expressed strong negation; they did not even want to hear about such a possibility, rather emphasising their positive behaviour and optimism.

Another assumption is that health benefits result from larger government health budgets that derive from democracies (Ghobarah et al., 2004, cited by Patterson, 2006). To assess the link between democracy and health expenditure, Paterson used the percentage of the budget spent on health, as in the analytical framework and criteria defined by Freedom House. She concluded that Africa has become more democratic since 1980, with health expenditures having generally increased in most free countries, where she discovered a correlation between health expenditures and democracy: "The highest correlation is between democracy and health spending in 1980, showing that those countries that were free in 1980 were more likely to spend on health" (Patterson, 2006). However, such correlation appears to occur between a limited number of variables, disconnected from their historic and global contexts.

Her analysis, which includes a comparison of health budgets, seems to completely ignore the drastic reduction of those same health budgets through the policies of structural adjustment worked out within Western paradigms and economic models. In most African countries, most public health progress was achieved within the post-independence decade.

In Senegal, from 1960 to 1970, the share of the Ministry of Health in public spending kept growing, reaching 9% of the state budget from 1970 to 1972 (Wone et al., 1984). From 1972 onwards, the percentage has declined, reaching its lowest point of 4.16% in the mid-1990s at the peak of its Western-style democracy, while the health budget started increasing again in 1995, reaching 7% in the late 1990s, but not again attaining the level at which it stood immediately after independence.

As soon as independence was declared, many African governments made big investments in expanding the health care services in their country in an effort to make them efficient and available to all citizens. Such health policies were in the line with the Alma-Ata Declaration that called for a collective response to achieve "Health for all by the year 2000", by means of state-organised comprehensive primary health care programmes involving all communities.

The international financial institutions, which create a neoliberal framework for global health care within a global market economy and Western democracy, challenged the concept of "health for all". Within the framework, full-scale privatisation of health took place, with the quasidismantling of state public health services.

Farmer (2007) urges for enlarging the analysis of AIDS fund flows by including consideration of Western policies, blaming corrupt governments for diverting many resources to the relatively wealthy. Garret cites a 2006 World Bank report as indicating that "about half of all funds donated for health efforts in Sub-Saharan Africa never reach the clinics and hospitals at the end of the line".

The international financial institutions that issue such reports also worsen the situation, having long suggested "capping" social expenditures on health and education and having even made restructuring of national budgets a precondition for access to the financial help on which poor governments depend for survival.

When the HIV/AIDS pandemic started, Senegal was experiencing a health and social services collapse, worsened by a severe economic crisis and the devaluation of its currency under the World Bank's and the International Monetary Fund's economic adjustment programmes. The ratio of inhabitants to health personnel most markedly decreased from 1965 to 1974, while increasing from 1974 to the present with regard to all indicators. The ratio in 1999, during the multiparty regime, was much higher than that between 1965 and 1969, during the single-party era (see Table 2.1).

The ratio of medical personnel to population relates to the government's macroeconomic policies. At the end of the 1970s, Senegal adopted structural adjustment programmes that caused the government to freeze the recruitment of public health staff. As a consequence, there was a decline in the renewal of public health personnel posts, which resulted in a sharp drop in their number, which was also fuelled by deaths, resignations and retirements. Hence, the number of health experts plummeted from 5 904 in 1989 to 4 886 in 1995 (Ministère de la Santé Publique et de l'action sociale, 1995).

Globalisation and pressures for a Western-style democracy coincided with many health professionals leaving African countries to go to mainly Western industrialised countries (IOM, 2001). The World Health Organisation estimates that 7 281 health professionals left 16 African countries from 1993 to 2002 (WHO, 2006). Many Western-style democracies have the highest number of PLWHAs and the highest HIV prevalence rates, while regions of countries labelled "nondemocratic" or that are the least subject to such influences, such as southern Senegal, are among those with the lowest HIV prevalence rate (Lagarde et al., 1992).

Table 2.1: Number of inhabitants in relation to health personnel

No. inhabitants by health personnel	1960-64	1965-69	1970-74	1974-79	1999
No. inhabitants to each physician	18 200	14 200	14 600	14 700	17 000
No. women in age of reproduction to each midwife	5 137	4 178	3 290	8 201	4 600
No. inhabitants to each nurse	3 000	2 400	1 900	2 200	8 700
Source: Ministère de l'Economie et des Finances (1999).					

2.7 Rethinking social cohesion: The precolonial heritage

The assumption underlying the cultural and historical analysis is that the current fight for political, economic and social rights in Africa is rooted in history and culture resistant to the Western colonial invasion. The upsurge of multiparty elections led to the undermining of state by personal, ethnic, clan-based and religious interests.

2.8 Rethinking pluralism and political equilibrium

The Mali Empire of the 13th to 15th centuries, a confederation of political systems led by one sovereign ruler, managed a diversity of ethnic, religious and territorial communities, which maintained specific forms of government, as well as much cultural and economic autonomy (Cissoko, 1975; Diagne, 1981; Diop, 1981; and Niane, 1975). At a local level, diverse organisations and networks (consisting of age groups, lineages, self-help associations and ritual groups) administered decision-making.

Certain precolonial kingdoms, such as the Wolof, Mandinka and Fulani kingdoms and the Diola political systems, withdrew from the great empires. The Waalo kingdom of the 12th to 18th centuries was the first Wolof kingdom that can be considered the prototype of the later Wolof kingdoms that preceded the setting up of present-day Senegal. The Waalo kingdom lacked a homogenous ethnic composition, consisting of several complicated power-regulating organs (Barry, 1972).

In the Wolof kingdoms, women bearing the title of *lingeer* (the king's mother or sister) and *awo* (the king's wife) participated in decision-making at the highest level, holding pre-eminent roles in the structure and functioning of the central power (Battûta, 1997). Women also had freedom of expression and engaged in protests to challenge unpopular decisions (Diop, 1967). Protest by women networks also characterised the colonial era (Banda, 1985).

Present-day women's self-support networks (*natt, mbotaay, tuur, Dimbatulon, Kanyaleen*), whose existence dates back to the precolonial period, constitute entrenched social forms that ensure pre-eminent roles in the dissemination of information and the organisation of collective responses concerning issues related to sexuality and the health of woman and child.

2.9 Elections and civic participation

In precolonial Waalo, the sovereign (the *brak*) was elected by an honourable electoral college called *seb ak baor*, which was the authority designed to settle, through peaceful means, the rivalries between matriarchal descents that were struggling for power. However, the *brak* could not designate a successor and neither other members of his family nor his descendents took part in the electoral college. In return, those who had the power to elect the sovereign could not contest this position.

According to Barry (1972), in the case of the Senegalese kingdom of Waalo, the *seb ak baor* comprised representatives of the most diverse statutory groups. Its members were, among others, the recognised descendants of the first settlers; the *jogomay* lineage (masters of the waters); the *jawdin* lineage (masters of the land); the *maalo* descent (in charge of the Exchequer); the lineages in charge of the expenses; representatives of the king's slaves; and representatives of all the social statuses, all the casts and ethnic groups living in the kingdom. The aim was to have an inclusive body whose diversity could reflect society in its entirety. Within this framework, policies imply flexibility, an array of arrangements, and sensitivity and adaptation to particular aspects.

As had other kingdoms of the time, precolonial Waalo had very advanced forms of recognition of civil society. In Wolof society, the *jambuur* comprised a social category (an order) independent of established powers (Diop, 1985). In contemporary language, the term *jambuur* refers to a person who respects the intimacy or the rights of the others, keeps his distance from partisan quarrels and manifests an attachment to peace in society. This attachment to societal peace is why this person is attributed a spiritual dimension, as seen in the expression "*jmbuuru yalla*".

A Wolof proverb goes: "*Temeeri nak, benn bant a len di samm, temeeri nit, temeeri bant a len di samm*" (to herd along 100 cows, one stick suffices; to guide 100 people, you need 100 sticks).

Peace is seen as an essential condition for social life and individual or collective accomplishment "*Jamm ci la lep xec*" (only in the context of peace can a project take place). In Wolof, the word *jamm* refers both to peace and health. The expression more precisely used to designate individual health is *jammu yaram*, literally meaning peace of body, with the mind being regarded as part of the body. *Jamm* is a holistic concept, which refers to the harmony within different levels of social organisation (the family, kinship and community) and within the whole cosmological system (meaning harmony with nature). The societies were anchored by underlying values, facilitating the granting of networking, support and compassion to the disadvantaged. PLWHAs are entertained by high-ranking government officials in Senegal as an expression of this.

The predominant concept of civil society refers mainly to Western models, lacking an ethical and spiritual perspective and an African historical perspective, so that civil society is represented by mostly urban-based Western types of NGOs, whose members are highly educated. Many civil society members use civil society as a means to attain government positions. Reconceptualising civil society from an African perspective would help to promote political autonomy and critical thinking about political institutions.

Consultation as a way of using cultural modes and socially constructed networks is still missing from official HIV/AIDS policies, programmes and interventions. Usually questions are raised only about how to implement externally produced solutions (mainly preventive devices and methods), instead of how social groups, networks and various identities might conceive their own solutions.

3. HIV/AIDS in Senegal: Evolution, responses

Senegal has a low, stable prevalence of HIV/AIDS, of which two types (HIVI and HIVII) are present (Mboup *et al.*, 1998). The dominant modes of transmission are believed to be the heterosexual mode and mother–to–child transmission, though recent studies suggest relatively high transmission among men having sex with other men.

The low HIV prevalence rate has led to research into the existence of biological factors likely to limit the spread of the HIV. Mboup has suggested that the presence of HIVII might, to a certain extent, prevent additional infection by HIVI (Mboup, 1998). However, considering the high prevalence of HIVII in some African countries in which HIVI has

also reached pandemic proportions, the biological hypotheses do not seem fully to account for the Senegalese situation.

The literature review reveals that sociocultural factors have been analysed to see how they influence the situation. Diverse societal factors, religious factors and social cohesion have been examined.

3.1 Epidemiological profile

The population of Senegal is estimated at 11 658 000 inhabitants (UNAIDS, 2006). The current estimates of HIV/AIDS prevalence among the general population vary between 0.7% and 9% (EDS-IV, 2005; UNAIDS, 2006). These rates, considered as relatively low in the Sub-Saharan African context, nevertheless hide large disparities between the various regions of the country, ranging from 0.1 in Diourbel to 2.2 in Ziguinchor. Prevalence rates among women and the difference between the rates of men and women also vary between regions. The ratio of women to men is highest in Ziguinchor (4.25), which also has the highest rate of HIV infection among women (3.4%).

Table 3.1 is drawn from the latest Demographic and Health Survey (EDS IV, 2005), which did not record HIV/AIDS cases in regions where samples were too small or the prevalence of HIV was probably too low, so that the ratio of women to men cannot be estimated in those regions, given the available data.

Regions	Women	Men	Ratio of women to men	Global prevalence
Dakar	0.7	0.5	1.4	0.6
Diourbel	0.1	0.0		0.1
Fatick	0.9	0.9	1	0.9
Kaolack	1	0.2	1.11	0.7
Kolda	2.7	1.1	2.45	2.0
Louga	0.7	0.0		0.5
Matam	0.5	0.8	0.62	0.6
St Louis	0.9	0.0		0.5
Tambacounda	0.3	0.5	0.6	0.4
Thiès	0.4	0.3	0.7	0.4
Ziguinchor	3.4	0.8	4.25	2.2
Total	0.9	0.4	2.25	0.7

Table 3.1: HIV prevalence for age group 15-49 years by region, gender

Source: EDS–IV, 2005.

The region of Ziguinchor, which has the highest prevalence rate among women and the highest ratio of women to men, is also the most affected by the internal conflict in Casamance. Studies should be carried out to assess possible links between HIV/AIDS and particular aspects of internal conflicts. Moreover, the sites situated in Dakar region (the capital of the country) and the central and north-west regions of the country (Diourbel, Saint Louis and Louga), with the exception of Kaolack region (which has a rate of 2%), rates lower, or equal to, the national average.

Due to their demographic weight and the concentration in them of the principal political, economic, social and health infrastructures of the country, the Dakar region and the central region of the country host the biggest number of individuals living with HIV. In 2003, sampling carried out in the sentinel surveillance sites of the regions in the south, southeast and extreme north indicated prevalence rates at least twice higher than the national average (2.2% for Ziguinchor; 2.8% for Kolda; 2.6% for Tambacounda; and 2.2% for Matam).

However, much higher prevalence rates are recorded in some of the poorest areas and in some of the regions subject to much emigration. Thus, in the extreme north of Senegal, high rates of up to 27% of adults have been recorded from the early stages of the epidemic and have also been strongly correlated to past migration history (Decossas et al., 1995). Likewise, Kolda and Tambacounda, which have the highest prevalence rate, are part of the poorest and most remote regions of the country.

Generally, Senegal recorded a higher number of women infected with HIV than men. In 2003, the number of PLWHAs was estimated at 74 890, 34 300 of whom were men and 40 590 women. For the same year, the number of new HIV infections was estimated at 12 700 adults, of whom 6 630 were women and 6 070 men (Bulletin Epidémiologique, 2004). The demographic and health inquiry data also emphasise the much higher female HIV prevalence of 0.9% among women, as opposed to 0.4% among men (EDS-IV, 2005). The gap between the rates of men and women seems to be widening in regions where the prevalence is higher. In Ziguinchor region, the male to female ratio is 4.25. Even in the regions with the lowest prevalence, the female rate is higher than the male rate (EDS-V, 2005).

The data analysis revealed major age differences. According to estimates made in 2000 from data recorded at the sentinel sites, more than 90% of cases (77 000 out of 80 000 PLWHAs) are aged between 15 and 49 years (Bulletin Epidémiologique, 2000). Likewise, age analysis reveals a higher female HIV prevalence in people under 25 years of age, up to a ratio of four females for every one male living with HIV.

Table 3.2: HIV prevalence by age group and gender, 2005				
Age group	Women	Men	Ratio of women to men	Global prevalence
15–19	0.2	0.0		0.1
20–24	0.8	0.2	4	0.5
25–29	1.5	0.0		0.9
30–34	0.9	1.2	0.75	1
35–39	0.6	0.8	0.75	0.7
40–44	1.7	1.6	1.06	1.7
45–49	1.9	0.6	3.16	1.3
Source: EDS IV, 2005.				

The highest prevalence rate among women is observed in the 45–49 age group and among men in the 40–49 age group. The largest imbalance rate is noted in the 20–24 age group, in which group one man to more than four women lives with HIV and in the 45–49 age group, in which group three women to every man lives with HIV (EDS-IV, 2005). In the late 1990s, a study carried out in the Principal Hospital infectious diseases clinic (Sow, 1997) indicated that 25% of infected women were between 20 and 30 years of age and 72% between 30 and 40 years.

Moreover, large disparities are noted between the social groups in which serological samplings have been taken. Thus, early after the advent of the epidemic, the highest prevalence was recorded among commercial sex workers, with a 1989 study recording a rate of 44.8% among Ziguinchor commercial sex workers, while rates higher than 30% were also recorded in Kaolack (Sankalé et al., 1989). Recent data show a prevalence of 20% among Dakar commercial sex workers. High prevalence rates of 27% have also been found among men with experience of migration. Recent studies found 21% of PLWHAs among men having sex with other men (IDA, 2005).

HIV prevalence data rely heavily on estimates from the limited samples available. VCT is still very limited and in Senegal as well as in most African countries, most of PLWHAs (an estimation of 90%) do not know their sero status.

The issue of voluntary counselling and testing

(VCT) raises issues of confidentiality and access to care and treatment, according to which political institutions can regulate and build responses. Official institutions, including health services, are often plagued by distrust and lack of confidence, being perceived as hostile, or at least disrespectful, to marginalised groups and those who do not speak Western languages. They are often regarded as conveying colonial or postcolonial state violence and power, resulting in an attitude of "You only go to these when you really do not have any other choice."

Regarding the underutilisation of VCT, a key issue is how to make, socially, culturally and politically, such services more accessible. In 2000, the estimated total number of AIDS-related deaths for the whole of Senegal was 30 000, with the number of deaths for 2000 alone estimated at 5 000. In 2000, Dakar region recorded the largest number (21%) of AIDS-related deaths for the year, while the Kaolack region recorded the highest number of cumulative deaths. Probably, due to disparities in demography and medical infrastructures, the regions with the highest HIV prevalence rates (Ziguinchor, Tambacounda and Kolda) have the lowest number of deaths.

Table 3.3: Number of HIV/AIDS-related deaths by region, 2000

Region	Deaths in 2000		Cumulative deaths	
	Numbers	%	Numbers	%
Dakar	1 050	21	5 300	18
Thiès	500	10	3 200	11
Kaolack	1 000	20	6 600	22
Saint-Louis	300	6	1 900	6
Kolda	300	6	1 300	4
Louga	400	8	3 800	13
Diourbel	500	10	2 900	10
Fatick	500	10	3 000	10
Tambacounda	250	5	950	3
Ziguinchor	200	4	1 050	3
Senegal	5 000		30 000	

Source: Bulletin Epidémiologique, 2000.

UNAIDS estimates for 2005 indicated 5 200 cumulative AIDS-related deaths in Senegal. The figures were not broken down by geographic area, sex, age or other social characteristics that might otherwise have allowed the development of an analysis of the socioeconomic impacts of AIDS mortality at regional level.

3.2 Evolution of the epidemic and projections

According to official statistics, the evolution of the epidemic in Senegal appears to be relatively stable, including groups where prevalence is relatively high. According to Méda, even in groups where prevalence increased substantially toward the end of the 1980s, the rates appeared more stable during the 1990s. According to the compilations of Méda *et al.* (1998), HIV-II prevalence has also only slightly fluctuated about 1% among pregnant women.

According to the sentinel surveillance site data, the overall prevalence appears to have been relatively stable over the years, though the rates clearly increased from 1994 to 2003 in the South (*Bulletin Epidémiologique*, 2004).

In the regions where the HIV sero-prevalence surveillance sites were only relatively recently constructed, large increases have been noted. Such appears to be the case in Tambacounda region, where HIV prevalence has increased from 0.8% in 2002 to 2.6% in 2003.

Moreover, the overall stability hides an escalation of the epidemic among women, with, for every man living with HIV, there are two women; whereas, in 1987, the ration was one woman to nine men, and, in 1992, the ratio was three women to every seven men. The prevalence rate among pregnant women has also increased from 1.2% in 2002 to 1.5% in 2003 (*Bulletin Epidémiologique*, 2004).

The increased rate of HIV among pregnant women emphasises cultural misconceptions of pregnancy. For example, in Wolof culture, pregnancy is considered as one of the most vulnerable periods, resulting in the collective mobilisation of family and community members for protection. The Wolof say: "if you are pregnant, your husband is pregnant; your mother is pregnant; your mother-in-law is pregnant". Yet, in current HIV prevention discourses, community mobilisation to protect pregnant women from AIDS is rare.

Predictions foresee a continuation of HIV prevalence rate stability among those aged 15 to 49 years that globally should remain lower than 1% until 2010. Such rates might decrease slightly, being lower than 0.7% from 2007. Yet, the prevalence rates foreseen are still likely to be higher among women than among men (*Bulletin Epidémiologique*, 2004).

Table 3.4: Evolution of HIV/AIDS prevalence for the age group 15 to 49 years by region, 1994–2003

Region	1994	1995	1996	1997	1998	1999	2000	2001	2002	2003
Dakar	0.5	1.3	0.4	0.4	2.1	1.7	1.2	0.7	1.2	1.7
Kaolack	1.4	0.9	0.4	1.3	1.2	2.2	1.2	1.1	1.2	2
Ziguinchor	1.6	1.2	0.8	2.4	1.8	1.2	1.8	3	1.8	2.2
Thiès	0.5	1	0.6	0.3	0.5	0.9	1.5	1	0.5	0.7
Saint Louis					0.2	0.3	0.4	0.2	0.2	0.5
Fatick					1.4	1.9	1.3	1.5	1.5	1.2
Louga					0.4	0.7	0.9	1.1	1.1	0.8

Source: Bulletin Epidémiologique, 2004.

Table 3.5: HIV prevalence projection by gender for age group 15-49 years, 2006-2010

Year	Men (15-49 yrs)	Women (15-49 yrs)	Total no. adults (15-49)
2006	0.61	0.79	0.7
2007	0.6	0.78	0.69
2008	0.6	0.78	0.69
2009	0.59	0.77	0.68
2010	0.59	0.77	0.68

Source: Bulletin Epidémiologique, 2004.

As shown in Table 3.5, estimates project that HIV prevalence will remain relatively stable from 2006 to 2010. The HIV/AIDS prevalence rate is expected to drop to less than 0.6% in 2009 among men, while, for women, it is expected to stay close to 0.8%, up to 2010. However, little is known about the social characteristics of those women who put themselves at risk of contracting HIV/AIDS.

Projections of HIV prevalence among children are alarming, given that they show an exponential evolution curve, as indicated in Figure 3.1. The estimated number of children living with HIV/AIDS doubled triennially between 1981 and 1990, with, up to the mid-90s, the estimated progression being about the same. The figure of 2 000 is, however, estimated to double in 2010.

The seriousness of the HIV/AIDS situation among children is highlighted by the poor results of prevention of mother–to–child transmission programmes, with only 1.4% of women accessing the programmes. Without data according to region and age group, and the social status and sex of the parents of such children, the HIV/AIDS situation among children could be much worse in specific vulnerable situations.

Anecdotal accounts reveal that the births of chil-

Figure 3.1: Estimates and projections of number of new HIV infections among children, 1980-2010

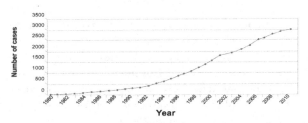

Source: Bulletin Epidémiologique, 2004.

dren of commercial sex workers living with HIV/AIDS are often not registered, either because they are not recognised by their biological father, or because they are not taken care of by the latter, or for both reasons. Such lack of registration is likely later to make it difficult for them to get the necessary documents to enable them to register to vote. The lack of recognition by the father in an increasingly patrilineal society leads to social exclusion, resulting in the denial of political and human rights.

Table 3.6: Projections of the number of HIV-related deaths and orphans

Year	Adult males	Adult females	Children
2006	2700	2850	1640
2007	3030	3220	1780
2008	3380	3600	1920
2009	3740	4000	2060
2010	4100	4420	2190

Source: Bulletin Epidémiologique, 2004.

The 2004 estimates project that the number of deaths among women will have doubled by 2010, with many more deaths among children as well. Projections foresee an increase in the number of orphans due to AIDS, which would double in less than 10 years, rising from 18 600 cases in 2003 to 40 260 in 2010 (*Bulletin Epidémiologique*, 2004).

Figure 3.2: Estimates and projections of number of orphans from AIDS-related deaths, 1980-2010

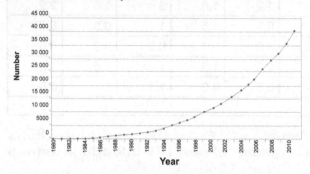

Source: Bulletin Epidémiologique, 2004.

The number of infant orphans, as shown in the graph above, risks increasing exponentially, which is likely to complicate the socialisation of such children into a democratic environment. Studies in other African countries have already emphasised social exclusion phenomena suffered by HIV-affected children (Gow and Desmond, 2002).

3.3 National strategic responses to HIV/AIDS

The national response to HIV/AIDS seems to have benefited from the successes with social and health policies enforced before the outbreak of the HIV/AIDS epidemic. Previously, Senegal had set up a number of political, legal and social arrangements aimed at: disease control and the improvement of sanitation; sex work regulation; blood transfusion safety policies; sexually transmitted disease management; health system reform; women and youth support networks and public health (UNAIDS, 1999).

Since 2001, the National Agency of the Coordination of the Fight against AIDS has resided under the authority of the prime minister, with its focus on: devolution; decentralisation; multisectoral planning; respect for equity and the rights of PLWHAs; and continuous evaluation, according to UNAIDS guidelines. The Senegalese government was also considered a driving force behind the 1992 Africa Heads of State Declaration on AIDS, which emphasised the need for political, religious and community leadership in the struggle against the HIV/AIDS epidemic.

Studies carried out by the Senegalese scientific

community and international partners generated credible, contextualised data that helped develop an indigenous, independent perspective and gain more political support.

During the early phases of the epidemic, the government played a leading role in providing HIV/AIDS-related education to parliamentarians, researchers, religious leaders and the media, investing about US$20 million in AIDS prevention programmes between 1992 and 1996 (UNAIDS, 1999).

The political leadership laid the groundwork for productive dialogue between many different stakeholders, including religious and community leaders, enabling consensus building between various political and religious actors in setting up a national policy response. Religious leaders played a positive role in the struggle against the epidemic from the start, with both Muslim and Christian religious leaders promoting sexuality only within marriage to reduce HIV infection risk. HIV/AIDS prevention messages were often integrated into homilies, sermons and public addresses made by the religious leaders. Such interventions agreed with wider sociocultural construction of sexual norms.

At the start of the epidemic, the government supported a survey directed at Muslim and Christian leaders, which showed that, though they were poorly informed about HIV/AIDS, they wanted to participate in the response by guiding their followers. In response, they were given the needed educational materials. A 1995 conference on AIDS was organised with 260 senior Islamic leaders, who vowed support of universal access to full and accurate information about HIV/AIDS, as well as of respect for PLWHAs. In 1996, all Christian religious leaders attended a conference on AIDS and religion. Led by a Catholic NGO, SIDA Service, the churches developed a comprehensive programme of prevention, free and confidential counselling and testing, as well as access to treatment (UNAIDS, 1999). As many social activities are organised around religious associations, the involvement of religious leaders helped create a dynamic social response, allowing activists and health officials to work productively at providing access to prevention, care and treatment.

The official policy continued the strategies previously developed, towards the end of the 1960s, in response to sexually transmitted epidemic diseases. Commercial sex work was legalised in 1969, after which registered sex workers were required to undergo regular medical checks and be treated for curable STDs. A national STD control programme was also integrated into regular primary health services (UNAIDS, 1999).

In 1998, Senegal was the first country in Sub-Saharan Africa to develop a government-driven antiretroviral treatment programme for the general public, the Senegalese Initiative of Access to Antiretrovirals (Initiative Senegalaise d'Accès aux Antiretroviraux [ISAARV]) (Ndoye *et al.*, 2002). ISAARV faced a situation marked by limited state resources, with the cost of treatment being extremely high. International consensus, therefore, influenced by the Donors Community, recommended prevention rather than treatment for Africa, with no international institution accepting the liability of financing access to treatment in sub-Saharan Africa. However, ISAARV implemented a programme aimed at lobbying the pharmaceutical industries, which accepted, upon massive coordinated purchases, to apply preferential prices, thanks to CFA 250 million (US$500 000) government credit (Ndoye *et al.*, 2002).

ISAARV led to the adoption of free AIDS medication in 2000, with VCT being integrated into the overall prevention strategy. Senegal had the required competences to correctly administer treatments, succeeding in reducing the cost of antiretroviral drugs by 10% through appropriate purchasing strategies.

Only 47% of PLWHAs benefit from taking antiretrovirals, showing that universal access is still far from being achieved. Despite the will to decentralise being contained in the latest strategic plans of the National Commission of the Struggle against AIDS, services are still largely centralised in Dakar, bioclinical tests are not free, transport is expensive, and there is fear of stigmatisation. Commercial sex workers and men having sex with other men also seem unwilling to access treatment, because they fear a double stigmatisation, both as PLWHAs and as members of a social group that was already stigmatised before the advent of AIDS.

3.4 Private sector and workplace responses

The Senegalese response, in agreement with ILO principles, embraces:

- Recognising HIV/AIDS as a key issue in the workplace, requiring a healthy work environment and a continuum of prevention and access to treatment and care;
- Rejecting all forms of exclusion and discrimination towards the PLWHAs, respecting the confidentiality of serologic data and rejecting imposed testing and the use of test results aiming at excluding or discriminating against employees; and
- Applying gender equality and respect for women's rights, to reduce their vulnerability to HIV and to eliminate gender-biased access to treatment.

Senegal set up tripartite state, employer and trade union commissions for coordinating responses in the workplace. The workplace is always represented in national response strategic planning. Partnership between the private and public sector might enhance prevention and access to care, not only for workers and their families, but also for vulnerable groups. Some companies, like those in the chemical and the mining industry, have pioneered initiatives to provide workers and their families with antiretroviral medicines, as well as invested in prevention in the workplace. In 2002, Senegal helped the International Conference of African Trade Unions (ICATU) devise instruments for promoting advocacy, training and concerted reaction to HIV/AIDS in companies.

Company coalitions formed against HIV/AIDS aimed to reduce the risk of infection, to protect the rights and dignity of PLWHAs, as well as to supply treatment and care. Advocacy programmes have also been undertaken in several companies, with a charter, "Companies against AIDS", created in 2003, and already signed by more than 80 companies, aimed at reversing HIV trends by practically implementing the *ILO Code of Practice on HIV/AIDS and the World of Work.* An interministerial Committee of Struggle against HIV/AIDS has been set up under the leadership of the Ministry of Labour to strengthen the capacity reinforcement programme and sensitise ministries.

However, studies dealing with HIV/AIDS-related policies and responses in the workplace are relatively rare, often being uninformed of the HIV situation in the work environment. Such knowledge would allow better adaptation of responses and measurement of their impact through relevant indicators of risk behaviours and HIV incidence.

Knowledge of the socioeconomic impact of HIV/AIDS in companies is also still very limited, resulting in inadequate efforts to reduce the effects of the epidemic on companies, workers, their families and communities, as well as in national and subregional development. Studies of stigmatisation and discrimination are also lacking, which constitutes a major obstacle to prevention and access to care and treatment. Neither legal responses nor actions are systematically evaluated, so that few benchmark practices exist.

3.5 Community and societal responses

Senegalese society has a tradition of active community involvement in health issues. From many local cultural perspectives, health is considered as the primary asset of communities and individuals. When AIDS appeared as a threat to communities, women's and youth networks reacted quickly. By 1995, 200 NGOs were already active in the fight against AIDS. Thousands of women's groups, with a total of half a million members, also are estimated to have supported AIDS-related activities at the time (UNAIDS, 1996).

The community-based responses supportive of marginalised and vulnerable groups were informed by many social science studies, which suggested complementary public health, human rights and culture-based approaches to strategising.

The public health approach views HIV/AIDS as a major threat to the health of individuals, as well as to society, focusing on the development of immediate widespread responses. The approach aimed for a political compromise acceptable to the partners, the official agencies, the religious leaders and to groups beset by conflicting moral values.

The human rights approach questioned the discrimination and violence that prevented marginalised and vulnerable groups from accessing prevention and treatment in accordance with their human rights. Vulnerable groups had their constitutional rights affirmed by way of international conventions[9] ratified by the Republic of Senegal.

The cultural approach draws on local cultures to develop responses and strategies in which local communities can find historic and cultural continuity. Dimba is a solidarity group in southern Senegal consisting of women who have experienced problems with childbirth and children. As well as helping one another socially, financially and with farming, members hold community rituals and ceremonies and advise women and couples. Laobe women sell various sex enhancement products (Niang, 1995). Both groups have proved themselves as credible communication and community mobilisation channels for HIV/AIDS prevention (Niang, 1995).

3.6 The legislative response

Senegal has ratified all international texts considered key in the fight against the epidemic:

1. Senegal has signed the *UNGASS Declaration* compiled during the twentieth Special Session of the United Nations General Assembly on HIV/AIDS, held in New York from 25 to 27 June 2001, which exhorts states to promulgate, reinforce and enforce laws, regulations and other measures aimed at eliminating all forms of discrimination against PLWHAs and members of vulnerable groups, ensuring that they enjoy all their rights and fundamental freedoms to the full.

2. Senegal also signed the Abuja Declaration during the African Summit on HIV/AIDS, Tuberculosis and Other Related Infectious Diseases, held from 24 to 27 April 2001, which recognises that the urgency of the HIV situation in Africa demands them "to mobilise all necessary human, material and financial resources to provide care and support to the HIV infected populations". The declaration exhorted African countries to allocate at least 15% of their annual budget to the health sector, though such an aim is far from being reached in many countries, including Senegal.

3. The Senegalese Parliament also ratified the United Nations Convention on the Elimination of All Forms of Discrimination against Women, the Convention related to the rights of the child contained in the 1989 African Charter on the Rights and Welfare of the Child, as adopted by the 26th Conference of Heads of State and Government of the Organisation of African Unity.

4. The International Convention on the Protection of the Rights of All Migrants and Members of Their Families, adopted by the General Assembly in 1990, was also ratified by Parliament.

MPs and several other elected officials are involved in associative movements. All the parliamentarians interviewed for this study declared that they had taken individual initiatives in the fight against HIV, consisting especially of sensitisation actions and involvement in prevention campaigns at a local level. The network Population and Development in the National Assembly carries out *ad hoc* sensitisation and holds HIV/AIDS-related information workshops for parliamentarians and parliamentary employees.

However, the political institutions appear not to have developed internal HIV prevention action plans aimed at accessing care and treatment for those of their members who are PLWHAs. Similarly, stigmatisation and discrimination countermeasures do not seem to have been taken.

Many FGD participants criticised Parliament for not distinguishing itself in HIV-related media debates, in which few parliamentarians participated. One MP remarked that AIDS does not constitute a major priority for Senegal, which has one of the lowest prevalence rates in Africa: "At this moment, it must all the same be recognised that sectors like education, agriculture and the fight against poverty have priority over the other ones…"

Many PLWHAs think that the fight against HIV is the responsibility of the executive, communities and society and that the legislative body seems to have contributed little to the response. No law as yet protects PLWHAs from discrimination, regulates HIV/AIDS testing or guarantees the rights of women and children infected or affected by HIV/AIDS. Though a draft Bill is in circulation in Parliament, MPs have generally disregarded the urgent need for such a law.

Parliament ought to play a major role in recognising the human rights of members of the vulnerable groups. No strong political will exists to protect such vulnerable groups as live in situations of violence and social exclusion that add to their vulnerability to HIV/AIDS.

4. HIV/AIDS and the political system

The official elected bodies of the Senegalese political regime comprise the president of the Republic, the Parliament, the High Council for Economic and Social Affairs and the decentralised elected bodies in the local communities. The qualitative analysis performed for this section was based on quantitative data collected during the study and on the work carried out by Tamba (2006).

4.1 The Executive

The president of the Republic is elected for a period of five years, renewable once, through direct universal suffrage polling on a majority basis, though two-round voting is envisaged for such election. Before its suppression on 3 November 2006, article 33 of the Constitution of the Republic of Senegal specified that no candidate could be elected in the first round without an absolute majority of the votes cast, representing at least a quarter of the registered voters. If no candidate gets such an absolute majority, a

second round of voting is held to elect the candidate with the highest number of votes.

In cases of resignation, incapacitation or death, the president of the Republic is replaced by the president of Parliament, and elections are held within an interval of 60 to 90 days. Thus, for the president of the Republic, contrary to other elective functions, in which the substitute completes the mandate of his/her predecessor, elections are organised where a vacancy opens up, resulting in great expense.

The Constitution in force at the end of the 1970s provided for the prime minister to complete the mandate of the president of the Republic, where a vacancy fell open. The president of the Republic had the power to designate his own successor and the latter, once installed, would use the state apparatus to secure his power, notably through manoeuvred elections. This provision was removed at the beginning of the 1980s.

In principle, the president of the Republic, who chairs the council of ministers and presidential meetings, determines the national policy that is to be enforced by the government under the guidance of the prime minister. The president signs orders and decrees, and nominates civil servants and military functionaries. The head of state is the commander-in-chief of the armed forces and has the armed forces at his disposal. He may dissolve Parliament (the National Assembly), when the latter has voted a motion of censure. The president of the Republic appoints the prime minister and the members of government, as well as putting an end to their functions. The powers of the executive body are formally limited by the legislative and the judiciary organs. However, as in a number of cases in Western democracies, the executive has many different ways in which to exert pressure on and influence the legislative and the judiciary organs.

In Senegal, the president of the Republic is less limited by the legislative and the judicial powers than by "unofficial influences", represented by historically and culturally constructed forces, such as religious leaders, traditional leaders and community networks. For example, the first president of the Republic was a Catholic, despite most of the population being Muslims; however, he built strong political ties with the Muslim religious supreme leaders (the Khalifs), ruling in close consultation with them. His example was followed by all his successors, leading to stability resulting from subtle power sharing between the state, the politicians and the religious networks (O'Brien, 1975).

As well as a delicate balance between religious

identities, provinces and precolonial political entities, there is also continuing change in the style of communication, with the president of the Republic increasingly communicating in national languages, though French is still the only official language.

4.2   The Parliament

Parliament is a single chamber, after having been bicameral for a short period during the 1990s. At the time, a senate was instituted alongside a lower house, which was expected to be instituted again following the June 2007 legislative elections. However, at the time of writing, Parliament was made up of the National Assembly, which includes all the MPs.

The National Assembly, on 20 August 1960, is the institution to which the people delegate their sovereign legislative power, with MPs being considered the representatives of the people. The mission of the National Assembly is to exercise legislative power by voting in laws and controlling government activities. The president of the Republic initiates Bills, while the MPs initiate legislative proposals. Bills or legislative proposals are submitted to the president of the Republic for promulgation, with the MPs being empowered to ask the ministers written or oral questions. The National Assembly can constitute commissions of inquiry and force the government to resign after voting a motion of censure.

The National Assembly is headed by a president; a bureau, renewed every year at the first ordinary session; and a conference of chairpersons of commissions. The president of the National Assembly is elected for the duration of the legislature. The national languages and French are commonly used during Assembly sessions. The statutory texts of the National Assembly stipulate that MPs can organise themselves according to political affinities in groups of at least ten members called parliamentary groups, comprising a chairperson and a deputy chairperson. In case of absence or an inability to attend, chairpersons of parliamentary groups are replaced by their deputy chairpersons. The 10th National Assembly legislature comprises three parliamentary groups and two independent MPs.

MPs are elected by means of direct universal suffrage, with the duration of their mandate being five years, which can only be cut short by the dissolution of the National Assembly. The mode of election provides for the election of 65 representatives of government departments, after one-round majority voting and, on the basis of national registers presented by the competing parties, of 55 other members, using

the system of proportional representation (PR). PR was introduced in the 1980s to bring about more diversity in the Parliament, as the initial first-past-the-post (FPTP) mode was considered to favour the ruling party, which usually controlled the electoral districts.

The lists presented for the FPTP and the proportional votes were considered to bring stability and the continuous representation of constituencies, in case of death or a vacancy of the elected MP. Voters have to choose between lists already made up by the parties or their leadership. Increasingly, it seems that MPs show more loyalty to the leader of their party than to their constituencies.

Senegal has had ten legislatures from 1957 to 2005: in the first, there were 80 MPs in the National Assembly, increasing to 120 from 1993 to 1998, and then to 140 during the 1998 to 2001 legislature. After the reforms resulting from the 2001 Constitutional changes, the number of MPs is once more 120, while the next legislature, starting in June 2007, is expected to comprise 150 MPs, with 90 elected from the lists of the FPTP mode of election and 60 elected from the lists of the proportional vote, which suggests a mixed member proportional electoral system (Reynolds et al, 2005).

Since the first legislature in 1957, the poorest social and professional categories, who represent most of the population, have been overlooked in representation in Parliament, in favour of senior public servants and the managers of private companies, who have made up to more than half the number of MPs in some legislatures. Farmers, stockbreeders and fishers, despite representing at least two-thirds of the general population, have consistently had almost no parliamentary representative. The figure below presents the socioprofessional statuses represented in Parliament from 1957 to 2001.

Figure 4.1: Distribution of MPs by profession, 1957-2001

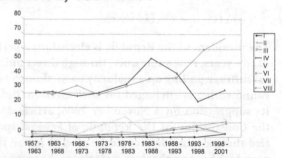

Key: I = farmers, stockbreeders and fishers; II = craftspeople, salespeople, industrialists, and heads of companies; III = managers and academics; IV = middle management; V = employees; VI = factory workers; VII = retired persons; VIII = the unemployed; IX = not identified. Source: Tamba, 2006.

In the 2001 to 2007 legislature, the socioprofessional profiles do not appear to have changed to bridge the gap between the socioeconomic categories that represent most of the general population and those that are represented in Parliament. As shown in the figure below, professions that require a Western type of education (such as managers, administrators and highly qualified professionals) are overrepresented. Only 5% of MPs are farmers and stockbreeders, whereas they constitute over 60% of the general population. Despite many youth being unemployed, they are also not represented.

Figure 4.2: Distribution of MPs by profession, 2001-2007

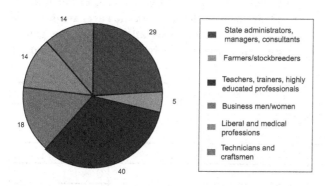

Commercial sex workers, men who have sex with other men, migrants and informal sector workers are not present in Parliament. However, during one past legislature, a female former bar manager was elected MP.

More than half of the MPs have completed higher education studies, whereas they represent less than 1% of the general population; official estimates indicate 470 students (university, college or higher education) for 100 000 inhabitants. Those who have not attended school represent one-tenth of the total number of MPs, whereas, in the general population, they represent about 70%.

Table 4.1: Distribution of Members of Parliament in the Legislature by level of education, 2001–07

Level of education	Number	(%)
None	14	11.7
Primary school	7	5.8
Secondary intermediate studies	26	21.7
Secondary studies	11	9.2
Higher education	62	51.7

Moreover, the underrepresentation of particular socioprofessional categories coincides with the underrepresentation of the poor and those of lower economic status. Hidden mechanisms of social exclusion reproduce the political exclusion of most of the population.

Though HIV/AIDS affects all socioprofessional categories, some of their working and living conditions render their members more vulnerable.

Parliament uses French as the only official and major working language, thereby excluding most citizens from participation. By excluding those who do not read and speak French, not only are local languages excluded, but also specific non-Western world visions and cultural concepts, especially social relations and dynamics. The data on the legislature from 2001 to 2007 agrees with those on previous legislatures (1957–2001) as they appear in Tamba's (2006) work.

Table 4.2: Distribution of MPs by Legislature, level of education, 1957–2006

Legislature	Not taught in French	Primary level	Secondary level	Higher education level	Unidentified	Total
1957–1963	05	07	39	24	05	80
1963–68	07	04	46	20	03	80
1968–73	09	01	34	25	11	80
1973–78	10	02	38	20	10	80
1978–83	16	05	50	29	0	100
1983–88	16	05	61	38	0	120
1988–93	19	15	46	40	0	120
1993–98	15	21	37	47	0	120
1998–2001	23	09	40	68	0	140
Source: Tamba, 2006.						

Those with a secondary level of education or with no education have a higher HIV/AIDS prevalence, with those with the lowest education level, who are among the more vulnerable, being the least present in Parliament.

One of the most prominent gaps between Parliament and the general population is that related to the age of MPs, with the average age of members of the current legislature being 55.64 years (50.73 for female MPs and 56.74 for male MPs). When distributed by age groups, younger generations appear largely underrepresented, considering that about half the general population is under 25 years old.

The data presented by Tamba for the previous legislatures (1957–2001) show the same pattern of exclusion of the youngest age groups. From 1957 to 1973 and from 1988 to 1993, no legislature had a representative in the 20 to 29 age group, while, in the 1973 to 1978 legislature, only one MP belonged

to the age group, which, at no point, had more than four representatives. By contrast, the age group older than 59 years has always been represented, with one-third of MPs being 60 years of age or older in the legislatures between 1988 and 2000. The legislatures also socially excluded the age groups that, for the same periods, made up most of the general population, with the censuses showing that about 65% of the general population of the country were under 30 years old, while about only 6% were 60 years of age or older.

At the end of the 1960s, the state faced strong challenges, antiauthoritarianism and unrest among the youth, to which it responded mainly by coercion and by the adoption of repressive laws, while no one under the age of 30 was sitting in Parliament. Contrary to what happens in the rural areas, where many social mechanisms allow filling the generation gap between the institutions controlled by

Table 4.3: Distribution of Members of Parliament by age and gender

Age groups	Total Members of Parliament		Female MPs		Male MPs	
	Number	(%)	Number	%	Number	%
Under 30	0	0	0	0	0	0
30–34	3	2.5	1	4.54	2	2.04
35–39	6	5.0	2	9.09	4	4.08
40–44	4	3.3	1	4.54	3	3.06
45–49	16	13.3	5	22.72	11	11.22
50–54	28	23.3	4	18.18	24	24.48
55–59	22	18.3	7	31.81	15	15.30
60–64	19	15.8	2	9.09	17	17.34
65+	22	18.3	0	0	22	22.44
Total	120	100	22	100	98	100

Table 4.4: Distribution of MPs by Legislature and age group, 1957–2001

Legislature	20-29 yrs	30-39 yrs	40-49 yrs	50-59 yrs	60 & more	Unidentified	Total
1957–63	00	20	35	16	04	05	80
1963–68	00	23	33	17	04	03	80
1968–73	00	12	35	18	04	11	80
1973–78	01	10	33	22	06	08	80
1978–83	04	15	32	36	13	00	100
1983–88	02	12	40	49	17	00	120
1988–93	00	10	34	43	33	00	120
1993–98	00	05	28	32	29	16	120
1998–2001	01	09	54	45	28	03	140

Source: Tamba, 2006.

seniors and the younger age classes, the elected bodies inspired by the Western conceptions of democracy were not providing bridges to facilitate inter-generational dialogue.

The age gap between Parliament and the general population might have implications to be taken into account in epidemiological analysis, with the age groups most affected by HIV/AIDS being less represented.

Historical analysis suggests the social exclusion of women from the legislative body. Since the creation of Parliament in 1957, women remain underrepresented and misrepresented in this institution, with their presence evolving only very slowly in the course of the history of independent Senegal.

As shown in Table 4.5, in the course of the first legislature, there was no woman in the National Assembly. The total number of women over the past 10 legislatures represents only 10% of the total number of MPs. Hidden mechanisms of social exclusion might prevent women from benefiting from their recognised political and individual rights.

The first woman MP was elected in 1963, and the second in 1968. The proportion of women among the parliamentarians then increased progressively, except in 1993, with renewals of Parliament. However, progression was very slow, with it taking 20 years before women (who represent 51% of the population) making up little over 10% of parliamentarians and 20 more years (or 40 years after the election of the first female parliamentarian) before they could account for slightly more than 20% of the MPs. Women hold very few key positions in the National

Assembly, with no woman having yet been either president of the National Assembly or chairperson of a parliamentary group.

Older people, predominantly men, sit together for sessions, where women are in the minority, Parliament offers no culturally sensitive space for discussion of sexuality. The culture of Senegalese Parliament clashes with that of local culture, with regard to the models of communication traditionally used in Senegalese society. When participants belong to different sex and age groups, public discussion of sexuality tend to be mostly allusive, using inappropriate metaphors and symbols. Moreover, those political parties whose members compete to be elected to Parliament reproduce the same gaps, reverting to the colonial period, during which old men were the chief administrators.

The fact that the same gaps exist throughout all the legislatures suggests the existence of selection bias. Unofficial mechanisms, conflicting with the proclaimed conditions for eligibility, reproduce the marginalisation of groups and social categories that, paradoxically, represent most of the population.

Since the marginalised groups lack a voice in Parliament, the political system reinforces the conditions of their marginalisation and its consequences for their health.

Statistical analysis did not reveal any HIV/AIDS impact on the mortality rate among MPs. In the course of the current legislature (2001–2007), there have been three deaths among MPs. Such a figure does not indicate any increase in the number of deaths compared with the previous legislatures, notably

Table 4.5: Distribution of MPs by Legislature and gender, 1957–2006

Legislature	Women		Men		Total	
	Number	%	Number	%	Number	%
1957–63	0	0	80	100	80	100
1963–68	1	1.2	79	98.8	80	100
1968–73	2	2.5	78	97.5	80	100
1973–78	4	5	76	95	80	100
1978–83	8	8	92	92	100	100
1983–88	13	11	107	89	120	100
1988–93	18	15	102	85	120	100
1993–98	14	11,5	106	88.5	120	100
1998–2001	21	15	119	85	140	100
2001–2006	24	20	96	80	120	100
Total	104	10	936	90	1 040	100

Source: Tamba, 2006.

those preceding the advent of AIDS. Whether there are more deaths in the decentralised elected body also cannot be established. Official reports of causes of death among parliamentarians and members of decentralised elected bodies do not refer to AIDS, so that it would be highly speculative and methodologically invalid to blame them on the epidemic.

The present system provides for the automatic replacement of a deceased office-bearer by the person who follows him/her on the list presented to the electoral body by his/her party before the elections. Thus, a higher mortality rate due to AIDS certainly has no impact on the frequency of legislative or municipal elections.

Before the high prevalence of AIDS, many Senegalese complained about absenteeism in the National Assembly and local elected bodies. Therefore, neither can the absenteeism noted in the media be related to AIDS, nor is there any record of expenses related to medical treatment or funerals. Any statistical analysis of the direct financial or economic impact of HIV/AIDS on the elected bodies and the political system would, therefore, be highly speculative and, to some extent, groundless.

4.3 High Council for Economic and Social Affairs and local communities

The National Council for Economic and Social Affairs was set up on 19 June 2003 (Act No. 15 of 2003) on the occasion of the Constitutional reform. The Council is a consultative assembly, whose explicit mission is to "rationalise the institutional space of the country" and to "to move forward in the democratic process and local governance through the consultation of the citizens and their participation in the harmonious development of the country". All aspects of national life are of interest to the Council of the Republic, with issues being referred to it or its accepting responsibility for handling all matters of national importance. However, their opinion does not place a binding obligation on the recipients to abide by what they say.

The National Council for Economic and Social Affairs reproduces the same gaps as Parliament. The Council comprises 100 members (the counsellors of the Republic), who are at least 35 years old. Their mandate lasts 5 years. with 25 of them appointed directly by the president, 25 designated by socio-

professional organisations and 50 locally elected by their peers. The Council is headed by a chairperson and a bureau comprising three deputy chairpersons and four elected secretaries. 25 of the counsellors are women.

For many leaders of associations of PLWHAs, the High Council of the Republic for Economic and Social Affairs does not include HIV/AIDS in its core thinking, though the issue is raised from time to time by the ministers concerned. Potentially, the High Council of the Republic could strategically reflect on the relationship between HIV/AIDS and development issues within a multisectoral perspective affecting all health sectors. The Social and Economic Council could then set up a strategic think-tank capable of informing decision-makers at all levels of the actions to be taken to curb socioeconomic vulnerability.

Concerning the elected decentralised bodies soon after independence, the government formally committed itself to promoting democracy at grassroots level through a series of administrative and territorial reforms. In 1960, 30 existing communes had been erected into fully functioning entities. A law was passed on 19 April 1972, increasing the number of communes to 37 and creating rural communities. In February 1983, the Dakar urban community was created. In 1992, the law granted the communes and rural communities financial autonomy and the status of moral personality.

In 1992, the regions and departments were transformed into territorial collectivities with enlarged responsibilities. The state representatives at local level, consisting of the governor, the prefect and sub-prefect, are in charge of each level of the territorial administration.

In the 1996 local elections, the ruling party won 300 rural communities out of 320, 56 city hall municipal councils out of 60, all of the ten regions, and 38 decentralised municipal councils out of 43 in the Dakar urban community, which, as a result, came to be headed by a socialist mayor. In 2002, the ruling coalition that won the 2001 presidential elections also won the local elections.

Local communities are considered as affirming local cultural identities because of the emergence of political spheres and the empowerment of local actors. The 2001 Constitution provides that "the region, the commune and the rural community have moral personality and financial autonomy. They are freely administered by councillors elected through universal suffrage."

The laws on decentralisation transferred to the decentralised elected bodies education, health, management of natural resources and development planning competences that were, until then, the domain of the central government. However, often, the essential problem is the lack of financial, material and human resources for the effective exercise of such transferred competences.

The region, which is the main administrative subdivision of the national territory, is administered by a regional council, which brings together regional councillors elected through direct universal suffrage for a five-year mandate. The regional council is headed by a chairperson and a bureau, elected by regional councillors for a five-year mandate. The regional council relies on a technical tool called the regional development agency and consultative organs, like the Economic and Social Committee, whose intent is to implement its development programmes.

In the urban areas, the main local community unit is the commune, which is headed by the mayor and municipal council. The political parties present their list of would-be members of the municipal council at the municipal elections, with the first person on the list becoming mayor, while the two runners up assume the positions of deputy. According to the code of local collectivities, the municipal council conducts the businesses of the commune through its deliberations. The council is responsible for local planning and development, and has to give its opinion on all issues related to the commune's affairs. The municipal councillors are elected for a five-year mandate.

The rural community is defined as constituted by a certain number of villages "belonging to the same territory, united by a neighbourhood solidarity, with the same common interests and capable of finding the necessary resources for their development". The 1990 law transferred to the chairperson of the rural council the management of the budget and the disbursements, which, until then, were exercised by a representative of the executive power (the sub-prefect). Rural councillors are elected through one-round elections on a majority basis and the other half on a proportional basis, with the application of the rural quotient.

In 2004, Senegal had 11 regional councils, the same number of city hall councils, 110 decentralised communes, 320 rural communities and a total of 13 830 councillors elected at the various levels (République du Sénégal, 2003).

In 2004, the rural communities had the largest number of elected councillors, as they were regrouping 40% of all the elected officials local collectivities. Kolda and Kaolack regions have the largest number of rural councillors. The political exclusion of women can be seen in their very poor representation in all the local communities. such as in 2000, when they represented only 8%.

The poor representation of women limits their capacity to mobilise more resources in the local communities. The underrepresentation of women appears still more clearly in an analysis of the positions that they occupy in the local communities. They also represent only a minute proportion of people elected to head such structures.

The inadequate representation of women is all

Table 4.6: Number of elected councillors by region and local communities					
Regions	Regional councillors	Communes	Decentralised communes	Rural communities	Total
Dakar	62	442	1 916	64	2 464
Diourbel	52	158	–	964	1 174
Fatick	42	238	–	960	1 240
Kaolack	52	260	–	1 276	1 588
Kolda	52	188	–	1 284	1 524
Louga	42	164	–	1 156	1 362
Matam	42	206	–	408	656
St. Louis	42	302	–	484	828
Tambacounda	42	152	–	1 130	1 130
Thies	52	462	–	976	1 490
Ziguinchor	42	166	–	688	896
Total	522	2 718	1 916	9 196	13 830

Table 4.7: Women in rural communities elected as local councillors, 2000

Local elected councillors	Total no. elected councillors	No. elected women	% elected women
Rural councillors	9 092	694	8
Municipal councillors	2 442	158	6
Regional councillors	470	61	13
Total	12 004	913	8

Table 4.8: Female leaders of local administrations, 2000

Post	Total no. elected councillors	No. elected women	% elected women
Chairpersons of rural councils	320	2	0.62
Mayors of towns	60	2	3.33
Chairpersons of regional councils	10	1	10
Mayors of decentralised communes	43	4	9.30
Total	433	9	2.07

the more paradoxical because, generally, they are the ones who are the most directly confronted affected by mismanagement of problems related to the transfer of competences to local communities. For example, in health matters, they are the ones who give priority attention to health care at home and take care of the deceased. In environmental management, they are also the first concerned with refuse disposal, water supply or domestic energy.

HIV/AIDS interventions and projects form a patchwork of projects, interventions and programmes or activities without overall coherence. NGOs in the regions are often controlled by foreign donors who come with their own indicators and approaches that often are not the most reliable and applicable. So, the regional council could serve as a coordination and evaluation unit of all these initiatives.

The city hall councils, the decentralised communes and the rural communities are not much involved in the fight against HIV/AIDS, though public health is part of their prerogative. The councils manage infrastructure building budgets or the recruitment of health personnel, monitoring and evaluating the actions and not feeling it mandatory to provide feedback on completed projects. According to some of them, the communes and the rural communities could further involve health committees in the HIV/AIDS battle.

The health committees representing the rural communities in public health structures have their members elected during deliberative assemblies. The committees are in charge of the organisation and supervision of rural community participation in health service provision efforts. They are also in

charge of the evaluation and monitoring of the performance of medical structures. However, they do not seem much involved in community mobilisation around crucial issues related to AIDS, such as prevention, the overcoming of stigmatisation, reduction of the socioeconomic impacts of HIV on children, orphans or affected people and access to HIV/AIDS care and treatment.

4.4 Political parties

At the end of about ten years of one-party rule, Senegal resumed a multiparty system in the mid-1970s. In 2000, the officially recognised parties numbered 57. In 2004, the number of political parties rose to 78, of which several had regrouped in coalitions. The Sopi coalition, supportive of the president of the Republic, won 89 seats in the 2001 legislative elections, while the Alliance des Forces Patriotiques (AFP) won 11 seats, Parti Socialiste (PS) 10 seats, and five other parties won one seat each.

Moreover, an analysis of the programmes and structures of the parties revealed poor interest by political parties in embracing AIDS-related issues. During the 2007 presidential campaign, only one candidate mentioned AIDS in a public declaration.

Political parties seem to marginalise women on the outskirts of contemporary political power. All the parties represented in Parliament have fewer female MPs than male.

Table 4.9: Number of women and men representing political parties in Parliament

Political parties	Female MPs	Male MPs
PDS	15	68
PS	3	8
AFP	2	10
URD	0	4
AJ/PADS	1	1
LD/MPT	1	4
PIT	0	1
Jef-Jel	0	1
PLS	0	1

Kassé showed how the multiparty approach enabled women to garner political gains. In 1994, a group of women belonging to political parties, trade unions and women's organisations decided to create a unified structure for the promotion of women's initiatives, especially in the political domain, the Council of Senegalese Women (COSW).

The first meetings between COSW delegates from several political parties and the leading national structures of political parties were held in 1996, on the eve of municipal and rural elections. In 1997, efforts were made to consolidate COSW structures at grassroots level, to set up training programmes for women and to raise the level of gender awareness of those who stood to be elected about gender issues. The 1998 legislative elections were preceded by a strong campaign that harmonised actions directed at the parties, the media and the general public. The campaign included a press conference, campaign posters, national press releases and the production and distribution of a cassette. Under such pressure, some parties instituted a system of quotas of women representatives within a range varying between 25% and 40%. In 2007, the government introduced a Bill that was approved by Parliament, providing that women represent half of the candidates on the national list to be presented by political parties in the legislative elections. However, the Bill was declared unconstitutional by the judiciary power. In several domains, the Constitution continues to reproduce latent social exclusion of women, in keeping with the French institutional tradition.

However, the presence of women on the lists of candidates started to increase from the end of the 1990s. Out of 20 national lists, two listed a woman second, just after the party leader. In three parties,

the first woman occupied the third position and, in two others, the first woman came fourth. In 23 out of the 34 departments that constitute Senegal, 12 parties registered women in first place on the departmental lists, with the percentage of women being between 1% and 20%, while, on the national list, they were between 13% and 50% (Kassé, 2003).

By spreading more rapidly among women and the youth, HIV might affect the mobilisation capacity of political parties, in so far as it was especially linked to the presence and action of youth and women. However, such an assumption requires confirmation by other types of research designs.

In conclusion, analyses using quantitative data and statistical procedures do not show an impact of HIV/AIDS on political institutions, though they emphasise the underrepresentation of the most vulnerable groups. The political impact of HIV can, however, be analysed at the microlevel of the family and the individual.

The impact of HIV/AIDS on political parties and elected bodies is difficult to measure. None of the political institutions has, up till now, undertaken a situational analysis of the prevalence of HIV/AIDS, of access to treatment and care, or of the protection of PLWHAs from discrimination or stigma. No data exists on the number of elected MPs or councillors, nor of members of political parties living with HIV, nor of those who have died due to AIDS.

5. HIV/AIDS and the electoral system

This section describes the legal and institutional framework of the elections and develops statistical procedures to assess whether HIV/AIDS affects the elections. Regarding the registration of voters, no comparison was possible of different historical periods (such as before the epidemic began and after its onset), because the voters' roll was unavailable, due to Senegal revising its register of voters. The 2000 voter registration figures on the Internet site of the Ministry of Interior, on which Dé-Diop's wide-ranging, detailed study is also based. were, nevertheless, utilised during the research. As well as a secondary analysis of Dé-Diop's data, extra analyses were carried out on the published data related to the 2007 presidential elections.

5.1 Legal framework of electoral process

The electoral code used during the 2000 presidential elections was the object of broad discussion and consensus between the political parties, which set the provisions needed in the presidential, parliamentary and local administration elections. The code defined the roles and responsibilities of the different parties in the electoral process, as well as the nature and implementation conditions of the various stages of the electoral process: the voters' roll registration; the submission of candidatures; the electoral campaign; the organisation and counting of votes; the announcement of the results; and the management of disputes.

5.1.1 The electoral process

The Ministry of the Interior is in charge at both local and national level of the material organisation of the elections, particularly of all the registration procedures on the register of voters; the submission of candidatures; electoral file design; the setting up of the different committees in charge of the management of the electoral files; the processing of voter cards; the publication of the register of voters; the design and installation of polling stations and their equipment; the conveyance of booths; the security of candidates; and the electoral process itself.

The Ministry of the Interior should work closely with the representatives of the different political parties and the independent bodies in charge of monitoring elections. Local administrations also support various procedures, such as the registration on the voters' roll, the withdrawal of the voter cards, and the setting up of the voting polls

The national committee in charge of the counting of the votes is chaired by the president of the Court of Appeal of Dakar and includes the representatives of the candidates or of the competing parties. The committee is responsible for checking and correcting the district committee minutes, as well as for compiling the results and announcing the provisional election results.

The Court of Appeal is represented by the delegates, appointed by decree, who visit the polling stations to inquire about the correct unfolding of the voting procedures, the transparent counting of the votes and the respect to be granted voter and candidate rights. The Constitutional Court is responsible for resolving the disputes submitted to its attention, as well as for announcing the final election results.

5.1.2 Election monitoring and supervision

Until 1992, the whole electoral process was managed by the Ministry of the Interior. From 1993, an independent body for the monitoring of the elections, the *Observatoire National des Elections* (the National Observatory of the Elections) (ONEL), was created. The members of ONEL were selected from among the independent authorities and known for their moral integrity, intellectual honesty, neutrality and impartiality. Nominated by decree after consultation with civil society, ONEL was limited in its mandate, because it lacked coercive power and had no permanent legal status.

In 2005, a law creating the *Commission Electorale Nationale Autonome* (the Autonomous National Electoral Commission) (CENA) was passed. The CENA is a permanent structure, with a permanent legal status, including some financial autonomy. The commission is responsible for ensuring that legislation is complied with and that voting is transparent and sincere, by guaranteeing the free expression of the rights of both voters and candidates. The CENA is empowered to submit a case to competent courts, and to punish or correct in cases of the electoral law being violated. In the exercise of their duties, the members of CENA must not receive instructions or orders from any private or public authority.

The law defines, the mandates of the CENA in such fields as the control and the monitoring of the electoral process, particularly in:

1. The Constitution and management of the registration of voters: The CENA has the right of access to:

- any relevant documentation;
- the physical layout of equipment, including computers;
- the programming and processing of court submissions; and
- the updating, processing and restoring of data.

   The CENA is responsible for:

- controlling the design and revision of the voters' registers;
- printing and distributing voter cards, including tender offers or takeover bids for the supplying such cards;
- counting cards that have not been withdrawn;

- publishing the voters' roll; and
- correcting procedures.

2. The vote: The CENA is responsible for:

- controlling the ordering and printing of ballot papers;
- publishing polling stations lists;
- installing both the equipment and the electoral documents;
- installing the members of the polling stations appointed by the administration;
- selecting inspectors to be sent to all the polling stations;
- participating in the accrediting of national and international observers; and
- keeping the list of representatives of candidates or parties.

3. The counting of votes: The CENA monitors the collection and transfer of the minutes from the polling stations to the places of counting and centralisation of the results.

4. The CENA participates in the work of the regional, departmental and national commissions in respect of the counting of the vote and the keeping of copies of all electoral documents.

The CENA, which comprises twelve members, is managed by a president, who is helped by a vice-president and general secretary. Its members are selected from among independent authorities reputed for their moral integrity, intellectual honesty and impartiality, after consultation with institutions that are relatively independent from the political scene. In the regions, departments, embassies and consulates, the CENA has to set up reporting structures that can help them fulfil their mandate. By the 2000 elections, the ONEL (which has been replaced by the CENA) created 10 regional, and 40 departmental, bodies, as well as nominating 9 000 delegates, to represent them in each polling station.

The members of the support team to the electoral management body are often recruited from among teachers and middle public executives, which do not appear to be particularly vulnerable to HIV/AIDS, compared with the migrants, the commercial sex workers and other social categories studied in the epidemiological and behavioural surveys. Few know their HIV sero status, so any estimate of the impact of HIV/AIDS on the electoral management body would be highly speculative.

A High Council of the Audiovisual Press was also created to ensure equal treatment to all candidates, in compliance with the institutions of the Republic. The High Council for the Audiovisual Press rules on the production and broadcasting of the announcements and debates of candidates during electoral campaigns.

The officially recognised civil society members (gathered within a group of ten NGOs and civil associations) were involved in the electoral process that led to the change of government in 2000. Generally, civil society members focused on:

- Boosting public confidence and participation in the electoral process (the previous elections experienced low voter turnout due to their being undervalued);
- Discouraging fraud, irregularities, intimidation and violence associated with the electoral process;
- Ensuring that the administration was impartial;
- Helping to check results and to ensure that the electoral process was transparent; and
- Mediating between the candidates to avoid potential conflict.

The privately run radio stations and the private press are also part of the electoral process, in that they guarantee that the elections are transparent. Some analysts said that, in 2000, the wide coverage of the elections helped to reduce electoral defrauding of which the party in power and the state representatives were traditionally accused.

No anecdotal records and no statistical confirmation exist that HIV/AIDS has significantly affected the members of civil society (and the private radio stations), who were involved in the 2000 and the 2007 electoral processes.

5.2 2000 voters' roll

Until 2000, continuous registration took place, which did not fully account for deceased voters or changes to voters' personal details. For the 2000 elections, however, a law was passed in 1999 (Act No. 75 of 1999), which allowed for auditing by opposition parties and the posting on the Internet of the voters' register by the Ministry of the Interior. Most of the analysis relating to the registration of voters is based on the electoral files of 2000.

For the elections of 2007, the Ministry of the Interior compiled a totally new register of voters. Each Senegalese citizen who meets the legal requirements has to register and get a voter's card and the national identity card. No cases of exclusion of PLWHAs from registration were documented. PLWHAs also did not seem to be disinclined to register for the 2007 elections.

5.2.1 Demographic characteristics of the register of voters for 2000

A comparison of the data from the sociodemographic survey with those got from the register of voters points out that more than half (55%) of the Senegalese, who had reached the age (18 years or older) to vote registered for the 2000 elections. The number of registered voters was 2 619 808, with the number of people who had reached the age to vote being estimated at 4 789 419. However, the rate of

registration differs between regions, as shown in Table 5.1.

The highest rate of registration (higher than 55%) was recorded in Louga region, with the highest rate in the country (77%), followed by Saint Louis (64%), Tambacounda (61%), Dakar and Fatick (57%). Kolda, Thies and Kaolack have an average rate of registration, while Diourbel (39%) and Ziguinchor (46%) recorded the lowest rates. In Ziguinchor, the low number of registrations is probably due to the climate of insecurity resulting from the armed conflict that has been going on since early 1980. In Diourbel, the high level of male emigration and a lack of interest in politics resulting from religious concerns seem to explain the low rate of registration.

In the 2000 registration of voters, women accounted for 51% of the registered voters (1 328, 829), while

Table 5.1: Population and registration by region

Regions	Total population	Voting age population	No. registered voters	% registered voters
Dakar	2 050 000	1 165 954	684 831	59
Thiès	1 210 000	760 147	385 236	51
Kaolack	1 120 000	612 299	310 502	51
Saint-Louis	840 000	384 529	244 930	64
Kolda	740 000	364 919	201 441	55
Louga	650 000	253 821	194 388	77
Diourbel	820 000	438 782	172 738	39
Fatick	650 000	288 356	163 099	57
Tambacounda	560 000	236 846	145 593	61
Ziguinchor	560 000	253 766	117 050	46
Total	9 200 000	4 759 419	2 619 808	55

Sources: Diop, 2000; Direction de la Prévision et de la Statistique, 2006.

Table 5.2: Distribution of registration by gender and region, 2000

Region	No. registered women	No. registered men	% total registered voters
Dakar	299 857	384 974	44
Thies	201 348	183 888	52
Kaolack	163 427	147 075	53
Saint-Louis	133 944	110 986	55
Kolda	103 791	97 650	52
Louga	105 215	89 173	54
Diourbel	99 961	72 777	58
Fatick	88 754	74 345	54
Tambacounda	73 360	72 233	50
Ziguinchor	59 172	57 878	51

Sources: Diop, 2000; Ministére de l'Economie et des Finances, 2006

men accounted for 1 290 979, representing a percentage of 49%. The meta-analysis prevented conclusions from being drawn as to the age of people registered to vote. Overall, mostly the young register, with 60% of women voters being between 18 and 35 years old (Diop, 2000).

In all the regions, apart from Dakar, more women registered than did men. Women especially predominate on the voters' roll in the Diourbel region, where they account for 58% of registered voters and for 53% of the total population. In Dakar, the capital, fewer women are registered than men, though the 2002 demographic statistics indicate that there are more women than men in the capital. The imbalance might be due to women's time-consuming domestic responsibilities.

The most populated regions are generally those with the higher number of registered voters, who, therefore, exert more electoral leverage. However, if the same situation prevails in almost all the regions, demographic weight might not correspond with electoral weight. Such was clearly the case in the Diourbel

region, which is more populated than the Louga and Kolda regions, but has a lower number of registered voters. The situation is similar in Ziguinchor, which has the same population as Tambacounda, but where fewer people registered.

A gender analysis of the statistics indicates that demographic weight does not necessarily translate into electoral weight or higher registration of a predominant sex.

In rural areas, more women appear on the 2000 voter register. According to a study conducted by Diop, the Kaolack region has the highest number of women registered from among the rural areas, followed by Kolda and Thies. In the decentralised communes of Dakar, women are less represented on the voters' register, as shown in Table 5.4.

Women constitute 54% of the total number of voters in rural communities and 52% in communes. According to a study conducted by Diop (2000), more women are registered in 46 communes out of the 56 in existence.

Table 5.3: Electoral weight by region and gender

Region	Total		Women		Men	
	No. registered voters	% registered voters	No. registered voters	% registered voters	No. registered voters	% registered voters
Dakar	684 831	26	299 857	11	384 974	15
Thiès	385 236	15	201 348	8	183 888	7
Kaolack	310 502	12	163 427	6	147 075	6
Saint Louis	244 930	9	133 944	5	110 986	4
Kolda	201 441	8	103 791	4	97 650	4
Louga	194 388	7	105 215	4	89 173	3
Diourbel	172 738	7	99 961	4	72 777	3
Fatick	163 099	6	88 754	3	74 345	3
Tamba	145 593	6	73 360	3	7 233	3
Ziguinchor	117 050	4	59 172	2	57 878	2

Sources: Diop, 2000; Ministére de l'Economie et des Finances, 2006.

Table 5.4: Registration in communes and rural communities, 2000

Local subdivisions	Total registered voters		No. registered women	No. registered men	% women
	Total population	% on voters' roll			
Communes	571,503	22	296,341	275,162	52
Decentralised communes (Dakar)	644,213	25	279,116	365,097	43
Rural communities	1,404,092	54	753,372	650,720	54

Source: Diop, 2000.

Table 5.5: Registered voters, number of people with HIV/AIDS by region, 2000

Region	% registered voters	No. living with HIV/AIDS	No. registered voters among PLWHAs	% PLWHAs among registered voters
Dakar	59	19 400	11 395	2
Thies	51	8 500	4 308	1
Kaolack	51	13 600	6 897	2
Saint Louis	64	5 500	3 503	1
Kolda	55	4 300	2 374	1
Louga	77	5 200	3 982	2
Diourbel	39	7 000	2 756	2
Fatick	57	7 400	4 186	3
Tamba	61	2 800	1 721	2
Ziguinchor	46	3 300	1 522	1
Total	55	77 000	42 384	2

Sources: Diop, 2000; Bulletin Epidémiologique, 2000.

A comparative analysis was undertaken between the number of registered voters and the estimated number of PLWHAs in the different regions of Senegal. The data, analysed by Diop, were extracted from the 2000 voters' registers and from the Senegalese *Bulletin Epidémiologique*, 2000.

By applying the ratio of registered voters/population who have reached the age to vote to the PLWHAs in each region, we have 1% to 3% of PLWHAs in the registered population. Envisaging a scenario in which all PLWHAs are registered in the 2000 reg-

ister of electors (a universal registration scenario) allowed us to estimate the weight that they would have represented in the register of voters according to that particular scenario.

The rate of PLWHAs is higher in the population of registered males than in the population of registered females in all regions, excepting Dakar. By applying the parametric comparative test of the two ratios, we can compare the rates of PLWHAs among both women and men. The results show that the ratios are proportionally different for men and women, except

Table 5.6: Electoral weight of people living with HIV/AIDS by gender in the universal registration scenario

Region	Women			Men			Difference in % men and women
	No. registered voters	No. of PLWHAs	% of PLWHAs	No. registered voters	No. of PLWHAs	% of PLWHAs	
Dakar	299 857	9 000	3.0	384 974	10 400	2.7	+1.7
Thies	201 348	4 000	2.0	183 888	4 500	2.4	-0.4
Kaolack	163 427	6 000	3.7	147 075	7 600	5.2	-1.5
St Louis	133 944	2 600	1.9	110 986	2 900	2.6	-0.7
Kolda	131 791	2 000	1.5	97 650	2 300	2.4	-0.9
Louga	105 215	2 400	2.3	89 173	2 800	3.1	-0.7
Diourbel	99 961	3 100	3.1	72 777	3 900	5.4	-2.3
Fatick	88 754	3 000	3.4	74 345	4 400	5.9	-2.5
Tamba	73 360	1 400	1.9	72 233	1 400	1.9	0
Ziguinchor	59 172	1 500	2.5	57 878	1 800	3.1	-0.6
Total	1 356 829	35 000	2.6	1 290 979	42 000	3.3	-0.7

Sources: Direction de la Prévision et de la Statistique, 2006; Bulletin Epidémiologique, 2000.

for in the Tambacounda region. However, this is only a hypothetical situation: all PLWHAs aged 18 and above were assumed to be on the 2000 voters' register, as the percentage of PLWHAs who registered for the 2000 elections is unknown.

5.2.2 Estimated impact and projections based on the 2000 register of voters

The study was undertaken in terms of a universal registration scenario, according to which all those who died from AIDS were previously registered. Table 5.7 indicates the impact that AIDS deaths could have on the voters' register in that scenario; in the scope and design of the study, we have no means of finding out how many voters, whose names were on the 2000 voters' register, died from AIDS-related causes.

Even if the extreme case was assumed where all those who died from AIDS were registered, the impact on the voters' register would still be insignificant, since the calculated rate of registrations, after withdrawal of those who died from AIDS, does not then vary, probably because of the relatively insignificant number of deaths from AIDS.

Moreover, if all the people who died from AIDS-related causes were previously registered, the proportion of deaths from AIDS among registered voters would be less than 0.3% in all the regions. On the basis of such estimates, we can state that deaths from AIDS have only an insignificant impact on the voters' register, both at national and regional levels.

For the projections regarding the lag of time between 2005 and 2010, we have used the demographic projections of the Ministry of Interior and those made by the National Committee for AIDS Control.

On this basis, the following assumptions were made:

1. Between 2005 and 2010, the percentage of registered voters who will reach voting age will remain at the same level as in 2000.

2. Between 2005 and 2010 the proportion, in the general population, of people who will reach voting age will also remain the same as in 2000.

The (a) and (b) scenarios, correspond respectively to the assumption that all the PLWHAs would be registered and to the assumption that only half of the PLWHAs would be registered. Further, the two scenarios predict that the proportion of PLWHAs on the voters' roll could reach 2.5% (for scenario b) and 4.11% (for scenario a) in 2010 respectively.

Table 5.7: Estimated number of adult deaths and percentage of registered voters by region, 2000

Region	No. of registered voters	% registered voters compared with population of age to vote	No. of adult deaths	No. remaining registered voters*	% deaths from AIDS among registered voters	% registered voters compared with population of age to vote, minus AIDS deaths
Dakar	684 831	59	771	684 060	0.11	59
Thies	385 236	51	367	384 869	0.10	51
Kaolack	310 502	51	734	309 768	0.24	51
Saint Louis	244 930	64	220	244 710	0.09	64
Kolda	201 441	55	220	201 221	0.11	55
Louga	194 388	77	294	194 094	0.15	76
Diourbel	172 738	39	367	172 371	0.21	39
Fatick	163 099	57	367	162 732	0.23	56
Tamba	145 593	61	184	145 409	0.13	61
Ziguinchor	117 050	46	147	116 903	0.13	46
Total	2 619 808	55	3672	2 616 136	0.14	55

* If all those who died from AIDS were previously registered in the region.
Sources: Direction de la Prévision et de la Statistique, 2006; Bulletin Epidémiologique, 2000.

Table 5.8: Proportion of people living with HIV/AIDS among registered voters, according to universal and 50% registration assumptions

Year	Population of Senegal	No. of people of an age to vote	Estimated no. of registered voters	Estimates of no. PLWHAs	% PLWHAs among registered voters[a]	% PLWHAs among registered voters[b]
2005	10 817 844	5 376 468	2 957 058	92 340	3.12	1.56
2006	11 077 484	5 505 510	3 028 030	101 320	3.35	1.67
2007	11 343 328	5 637 634	3 100 699	110 400	3.56	1.78
2008	11 615 586	5 772 946	3 175 120	119 330	3.76	1.88
2009	11 894 343	5 911 488	3 251 319	128 120	3.94	1.97
2010	12 179 368	6 053 146	3 329 230	136 670	4.11	2.05

Sources: Direction de la Prévision et de la Statistique, 2006; Bulletin Epidémiologique, 2000.

Considering that, in the 2001 legislative elections, political parties that got 4.05% or 1% of the total votes cast were able to secure a similar proportion of seats in Parliament, and also, taking the PR system into account, every vote counts, with the number of PLWHAs on the register forming a significant electoral leverage. Moreover, the projections related to the weight of the deaths from AIDS on the voters' register were carried out on the basis of the same projections of the number of registered voters, as well as on the basis of the assumption that all the deceased people were previously registered.

On the basis of the envisaged scenario, the percentage represented by the deceased on the voters' register would certainly tend to increase, but would remain relatively insignificant, with an expected rate of only 0.26% in 2010.

5.2.3 Updated analysis using 2007 voters' roll

The published data drawn from the 2007 register show only the number of registered voters in each region, as no other recent data were made available. For 2007, the available data on the Senegalese population give no information as to either the total number of people in each region in 2006 or the total number of voting age population in 2006. Such published data for 2004 and generated estimates for 2006.

The estimates of the voting age is made using both the population natural growth rate in each region and the projections made by the Department of Planning and Statistics for 2004. Those estimates will be used to carry out the analysis.

The comparison of the demographic estimates data with those of the voters' register shows that 85% of the Senegalese who had reached voting age. That important increase in the number of the registered voters comparatively to 2000 could be explained by the total reconstruction of the voter registers by the Ministry of Interior. Indeed, any citizens who meet the legal requirements have to register to get not only their voters' cards, but especially their digitised national identity cards, which offer extra motivation for registering.

In Dakar, the number of newly registered voters was found to exceed that of those who had reached the age to vote. Apart from the reasons cited earlier

Table 5.9: Estimated proportion of deaths in universal registration scenario

Year	Estimated no. registered voters	Estimated no. deaths	Proportion of no. deaths/ registered voters (%)
2005	2 957 058	4 900	0.17
2006	3 028 030	5 550	0.18
2007	3 100 699	6 250	0.20
2008	3 175 120	6 980	0.22
2009	3 251 319	7 740	0.24
2010	3 329 230	8 520	0.26

Sources: Direction de la Prévision et de la Statistique, 2006; Bulletin Epidémiologique, 2000.

Table 5.10: Estimated population having reached voting age by 2006

Region	Total population in 2004	Voting age population in 2004	Proportion of population of age to vote in 2004	Population growth rate	Estimated population in 2006	Estimated population of age to vote in 2006
Dakar	2 399 451	1 343 693	0.56	2.79	2 535 208	1 419 717
Diourbel	1 144,009	547 980	0.48	2.17	1 194 198	572 020
Fatick	643 505	301 160	0.47	1.87	667 797	312 529
Kaolack	1 114 292	638 489	0.57	0.41	1 123 448	643 735
Kolda	893 867	412 967	0.46	2.51	939 302	433 958
Louga	714 732	345 216	0.48	2.24	747 111	360 855
Matam	461 836	217 571	0.47	3.67	496 357	233 834
Saint Louis	738 724	342 029	0.46	1.39	759 403	351 603
Tambacounda	650 399	295 281	0.45	3.26	693 496	314 847
Thies	1 358 658	760 577	056	0.73	1 378 567	771 722
Ziguinchor		220 636	0.50	2.55	467 806	232 032
Total	10 564 303	5 425 599	0.51		11 002 692	5 646 853

Source: Projections about the Senegalese population on the basis of the 2002 population general census, Department of Planning and Statistics.

Table 5.11: Electoral weight by region

Region	No. registered voters	% registered voters in 2006 by region	Electoral weight of region (%)
Dakar	1 518 044	107	31.5
Thies	629 502	82	13.0
Kaolack	455 724	71	9.4
Saint Louis	349 015	99	7.2
Kolda	321 307	74	6.7
Louga	294 915	82	6.1
Diourbel	410 412	72	8.5
Fatick	249 726	80	5.2
Tamba	221 420	70	4.6
Ziguinchor	211 559	91	4.4
Matam	164 281	70	3.4
Total	4 825 905	85	100

Source: The national daily newspaper, *Le Soleil*, 2 March 2007

in this section, this fact could also be explained by the liberalised voting procedures introduced by the Home Ministry, allowing citizens to register anywhere and also to vote in a station of their choice. Consequently, the citizens living in Dakar and originating from the other regions of Senegal had the opportunity to register in Dakar and vote in their regions of origin.

Table 5.12 applies the universal registration scenario to PLWHAs on the 2006 voters' register to measure the weight they could represent in each situation. Case 1 of the exercise estimates the number of PLWHAs based on the 2005 sociodemographic rate

If all PLWHAs were registered on the 2006 voters' register, they would remain below 2% of the total numbers of voters in all the regions, except in Kolda and Matam where the prevalence would respectively reach 27% and 3.13%. Consequently, we have noticed that the prevalence rate remains low and is in line with the results got with the same scenario used for 2000.

Table 5.12: Registrations and number of people living with HIV by region

Region	No. registered voters in 2006	No. adults (18 or older) in 2006	HIV prevalence from 2005 socio-demographic survey	Estimated no. PLWHAs	% PLWHAs out of total no. registered voters
Dakar	1 518 044	1 419 717	0.6	8 518	0.56
Thies	629 502	771 722	0.1	772	0.12
Kaolack	455 724	643 735	0.9	5 794	1.27
Saint Louis	349 015	351 603	0.7	2 461	0.71
Kolda	321 307	433 958	2.0	8 679	2.70
Louga	294 915	360 855	0.5	1 804	0.61
Diourbel	410 412	572 020	0.6	3 432	0.84
Fatick	249 726	312 529	0.5	1 563	0.63
Tamba	221 420	314 847	0.4	1 259	0.57
Ziguinchor	211 559	232 032	0.4	928	0.44
Matam	164 281	233 834	2.2	5 144	3.13
Total	4 825 905	5 646 853		40 355	0.82

Source: The 2005 Sociodemographic survey, projections about the Senegalese population from 2002 national general census conducted by the Department of Planning and Statistics.

Case 2 of our exercise estimates the number of PLWHAs using the prevalence rate estimated at 1% among adults by UNAIDS in 2006 and on the basis of the proportional distribution that appears in the 2005 sociodemographic survey.

Based on the estimated prevalence rate of 1% among adults, the number of PLWHAs would be 56 468 in 2006. Though the regional distribution of PLWHAs would differ from that got on the basis of 2005 sociodemographic survey rates, the proportion of PLWHAs among the registered voters would still be low compared with the universal registration scenario, except in Kolda and Matam.

We then notice that, in both situations, the rate of the PLWHAs on the voters' register remains low (about 1.17% in a universal registration scenario).

Table 5.13: Registrations, number of people with HIV/AIDS by region (cont.)

Region	No. of registered voters in 2006	Adults older than 18 in 2006	Prevalence of HIV/AIDS (from 2005 socio-demographic survey)	No. PLWHAs (2005 socio-demographic survey)	No. adults with HIV/AIDS, (UNAIDS, 2006, 2005 sociodemographic survey)	% PLWHAs, out of total no. registered voters
Dakar	1 518 044	1 419 717	0.6	8 518	11 920	0.79
Thies	629 502	771 722	0.1	772	1 080	0.17
Kaolack	455 724	643 735	0.9	5 794	8 107	1.78
Saint Louis	349 015	351 603	0.7	2 461	3 444	0.99
Kolda	321 307	433 958	2	8 679	12 145	3.78
Louga	294 915	360 855	0.5	1 804	2 525	0.86
Diourbel	410 412	572 020	0.6	3 432	4 803	1.17
Fatick	249 726	312 529	0.5	1 563	2 187	0.88
Tamba	221 420	314 847	0.4	1 259	1 762	0.80
Ziguinchor	211 559	232 032	0.4	928	1 299	0.61
Matam	164 281	233 834	2.2	5 144	7 198	4.38
Total	4 825 905	5 646 853	0.7	40 355	56 468	1.17

But using the projection provided by the Senegalese *HIV Epidemiological Bulletin*, we can foresee a probable increase of that percentage in the years to come (up to 2010) as shown in Table 5.14 (in the perspective of the hypothetical situation where (scenario a) all PLWHAs would be registered and (scenario b) in the perspective of the situation in which only half of them would be registered).

The data shown in Table 5.14 could lead us to think that in the elections based on the PR system, the weight of PLWHAs could be important in the years to come and radically influence vote outcomes. On the other hand, we used the 2007 voters' register to estimate the impact of AIDS deaths, based on the scenario in which all people who died from AIDS-related causes were registered. The statistics on the distribution of adults' deaths from AIDS-related causes in 2006 in each region are not yet available.

The exercise shows that the impact of AIDS on the voters' register remains insignificant (below 0.02%) and is even lower than in 2000. The overall low and stable HIV prevalence rates in Senegal added to a high increase of the registration rate in 2006 explain the less noticeable impact of HIV/AIDS on the voters' register, compared with 2000.

6. HIV/AIDS: Political vulnerability, impact on society

Both social cohesion and social capital result from the social infrastructure, shared emotional intelligence[10] and social control.

6.1 Social cohesion, sexual control and vulnerability

Vulnerability to HIV is increased by constant displacements, the separation of spouses and gender

Table 5.14: Proportion of PLWHAs among registered voters, based on (a) universal registration assumptions, or (b) registration of 50% of such people						
Year	Population of Senegal	Voting age population in 2006	No. registered voters	Estimated no. PLWHAs	% PLWHAs among registered voters[a]	% PLWHAs among registered voters[b]
2006	11 077 484	5 505 510	4 825 905	101 320	2.10	1.05
2007	11 343 328	5 637 634	4 791 989	110 400	2.30	1.15
2008	11 615 586	5 772 946	4 907 004	119 330	2.43	1.22
2009	11 894 343	5 911 488	5 024 765	128 120	2.55	1.27
2010	12 179 368	6 053 146	5 145 174	136 670	2.66	1.33
Source: Author's calculations.						

Table 5.15: Estimated number of adult deaths in each region				
Region	No. registered voters in 2006	No. adult deaths in 2000	Estimated adult deaths in 2006	No. remaining registered voters	% deaths from AIDS among registered voters
Dakar	1 518 044	771	634	1 517 410	0.04
Thies	629 502	367	302	629 200	0.05
Kaolack	455 724	734	604	455 120	0.13
Saint Louis	349 015	220	181.2	348 833.8	0.05
Kolda	321 307	220	181.2	321 125.8	0.06
Louga	294 915	294	241.6	294 673.4	0.08
Diourbel	410 412	367	302	410 110	0.07
Fatick	249 726	367	302	249 424	0.12
Tamba	221 420	184	151	221 269	0.07
Ziguinchor	211 559	147	120.8	211 438.2	0.06
Source: Author's calculations.				

inequities in negotiating sex, associated with institutional political power. Though political leaders might experience increased vulnerability to HIV/AIDS due to their intensive travelling, during which they are often separated from their spouses, and their political and financial power, their fear of loss of social prestige could dissuade them from risky behaviour.

Elected politicians are subject to locally developed sexual norms, such as how many partners a man might have. Though polygamy is common in Senegal, a man having multiple extramarital sexual partners or having sex with girls is called *ñak fayda* (lacking values that promote a positive image) and could be considered unfit to be in a position of leadership.

Much stricter sexual norms apply to women, with female politicians avoiding extramarital affairs for fear of damaging their moral leadership status. Often, they are respected and extend their social obligations to their husband's extended family, who control their sexual behaviour. Women younger than 40 are under intense social pressure to avoid much travel, so that their capacity to run for political office is undermined.

Diourbel has the lowest HIV regional prevalence and the lowest prevalence among women, though it is one of the regions with the highest rate of external migration and the highest number of people living below the poverty line. Diourbel is largely inhabited by the anticolonialist Islamic Murids, who are marked by strong social cohesion.

Similarly, Mlomp, a rural enclave in southern Senegal, is marked by strong social cohesion, animated by rituals and institutions derived from African traditional religions. As Emmanuel Lagarde *et al.* pointed out, the sociodemographic and epidemiological data collected in Mlomp show that a large part of the adult population, (80% of women between 15 and 24 years of age and 82% of men aged 20 to 40 years old), migrate seasonally to the Senegalese or Gambian metropoli. However, in October 1990, an exhaustive seroprevalence survey (Lagarde *et al.*, 1992) of those aged 20 years or older, during which 3 230 people were tested) showed that 0.8% was HIVII, and 0.1% HIVI, seropositive. Social cohesion cuts vulnerability beyond the immediate community.

6.2   Society, politics

Voters might reject candidates who declare that they are living with HIV/AIDS. An MP declared:

I think that in Senegal, it will be difficult at this moment for a political leader to say that he/she is living with HIV/AIDS, because of the stigmatisation associated with AIDS. Even if they could be in that situation, political leaders (in particular the Members of Parliament) will carefully avoid saying publicly that they are living with HIV/AIDS. It would be like a political suicide.

Besides the stigmatisation, disclosure might lead to attempts to prevent PLWHAs from assuming political office.

Medical records suggesting the coming death of the president tend to be treated as state secrets in many contemporary industrialised nations in the West, as they were in the former Soviet Union; in Africa, ethnographic and historical research reveals kings being killed or being forced to kill themselves at the least sign of disease or weakness. The reversal of the social exclusion of PLWHAs and its political implications should be analysed to find out how to dissociate AIDS from death. Such an analysis would involve clarifying access to antiretroviral treatment and reconstructing how to represent the social aspects of the disease.

Many PLWHAs fear that their political opponents might use their HIV positive status against them. Revealing an HIV-positive status can lead to social disaster. Women living with HIV fear that, by becoming involved in politics, they risk exposing their private lives, families and children to stigmatisation and discrimination. PLWHAs are less likely to experience social solidarity.

An HIV-positive status can also hamper involvement in political contests, by reducing the material and financial resources needed for such involvement. Rural PLWHAs who sell their livestock are often thought to be doing so to pay for their care. By reducing the outward signs of wealth, which are a mark of social prestige, the sellers limit their participation in politics. PLWHAs, especially women, say that having AIDS has negatively affected their lifestyle and plans for the future, as well as their priorities and financial prospects. Those without a stable source of income have little chance of participating in politics.

As heightened AIDS prevalence results in more deaths, families of whom one or more members are living with AIDS have to pay for expensive funerals, which might impoverish them. Catering for large gatherings at funerals is regarded as a way of ensuring that the deceased person has a favourable afterlife. Funerals allow for the reaffirmation of social ties, by enabling the family of the deceased person to display their power within the community. Large gatherings during funerals can add the political weight of the families responsible for their organisation.

Political capital is the sum of people and social networks that one can mobilise in support of one's political positions and actions. In traditionalist families, many people share the same meals, even if they don't live in the same compound. Such community sharing is sometimes seen as a sign of wealth or social prestige. However, when families suffer financially because of illness, the number of people who eat together might decrease (SAHARA, unpublished data). When exacerbated by stigmatisation, families with an HIV-infected member become relatively isolated.

HIV/AIDS affects family size and composition. The families of PLWHAs (especially if the person with the disease is the head of this family) tend to have fewer children staying with them than other families do. Families with no HIV-positive member tend to live with people other than the nuclear family unit, such as brothers, sisters, nephews, nieces, parents-in-law, and orphans, who all live in the compound of the head of the family (Niang, 2001; SAHARA, unpublished data). Large families, due to their accounting for many votes, can influence the decision-making process.

Divorcees and widows tend more often to be PLWHAs, with remarriage being unlikely when a woman is known to be HIV-positive. The widows of emigrants seldom remarry, because their deceased husbands are suspected of having died of AIDS-related illness. With marriage being considered necessary for social integration, which is key to being a leader, unmarried people (especially women) have less chance of being elected to a political position.

Social exclusion and political marginalisation are related to difficulties with communication, trust and confidence. Many representatives of associations of PLWHAs say that they are exploited by politicians, whose sincerity they doubt, stating: "When you are with them [politicians], they give the impression of showing solidarity, whereas indeed, they stay with you just because they want to protect their own interests." Another goes further: "My uncle is a Member of Parliament, he reacted very badly when I informed him that I was living with HIV/AIDS. I was living in his house at that time; but he did not hesitate to turn me out from the house, when I informed him." For many PLWHAs, political leaders typify the stigmatisation that they have perpetrated against them.

Many leaders of associations of PLWHAs state that they suspect that they are exploited for the vote or to sway the balance of power between competing groups within the same political party. A 33-year-old woman stated:

Politicians use us in order to progress. Some of them come to visit us, make promises and then leave, such as on the occasion of the Women's Rights Day two weeks ago, a female politician told us if we supported her she would help us cope with our needs in medicines and medical costs, and at the outset she offered us some but after nothing else came.

Politicians were described by participants in the FGDs as people who intervene only when they seek to mobilise votes.

A 44-year-old man said:

Six months ago, some members of our association made some testimonies for some politicians and they made us believe that they wanted to build programmes to take care of us. They seemed very motivated, but six months after we are still running after them in order to meet them, they have forgotten us...all of them are liars.

Moreover, many PLWHAs think that politicians only discuss AIDS on specific occasions, such as on 1 December (AIDS Day), while the political party programme has no reference to the disease. One 46-year-old said: "I am involved in the political sector, but I have not yet heard a politician who once took AIDS as a topic in his programme. They put everything in the health sector and do not talk about it any more. In Senegal, people still avoid talking about AIDS."

According to a 45-year-old association leader: "Politicians consider us as simple beneficiaries and not as stakeholders; they have to involve us in the combat against AIDS and take into account our experiences." Another association leader stated more precisely: "People living with HIV/AIDS should be invited to join the parliamentary committees in order to make these committees more useful to the responses against AIDS."

However, for many PLWHAs, AIDS is a lucrative topic for NGOs and politicians who interact with international cooperation agencies. Therefore politicians are more easily influenced by donors than by beneficiaries or constituencies, given that their motive is primarily financial.

The ability to lead a community strongly relates

to one's ability to be sensitive to both individual and family personal basic needs, so that the capacity to redistribute resources is an important criterion for selection. Accordingly, those in power provide extensive funding to their leaders elected at local level.

The voter education campaigns are associated with intense competition between candidates and a migrational population, symbolic chaos, verbal and physical violence and the slackening of social control over sexuality, all of which could make people more vulnerable to HIV/AIDS. Before the voter education campaign, the political parties nominated their candidate, with the nomination depending on the renewal of the authorities and/or of the decisions taken by their executive structure. Due to the stigmatisation, PLWHAs who make their status public would probably be eliminated from the competitions existing within the political parties for the nomination of candidates. African cultural perspectives still need to be fully explored in relation both to the HIV pandemic and to political transformation.

7. Conclusion

The conceptual framework highlights shifts from the prevailing biomedical paradigms, from the Western conception of democracy and from the statistical analysis stating the link between health and indicators derived from the Western conception of democracy. The main assumption is that HIV/AIDS and health are shaped by various factors related to societal contexts, historical circumstances, predominant paradigms, and internal and external power relations, and not only by adherence to the prevailing models of democracy.

The statistical analysis has shown no effect of HIV/AIDS on political institutions, the voters' register and on the overall electoral process. The institutional analysis focused on the social exclusion of youth, women, the illiterate and social categories representing most of the locals. The social analysis highlighted social capital and social cohesion as key concepts in understanding vulnerability to the HIV/AIDS political impact. The study suggests, also, that fear of stigma could have an impact on the political rights and on the participation of PLWHAs in political institutions and processes.

The success of Senegal in its fight against AIDS could be linked with the capital of social cohesion inherited from the precolonial political systems and from political, cultural and social resistance to the colonial system.

The Senegalese response requires government commitment to the fight against AIDS. Political power must be shared with women and the most vulnerable groups, relying on the emergence of paradigms that recognise the historic legacy of African societies.

7.1 Recommendations

As Senegal maintains a low prevalence rate of HIV/AIDS infection, more studies need to be carried out to learn from its experience, enabling it to face the increasing number of pregnant women and children living with HIV/AIDS and the high prevalence of HIV/AIDS among marginalised groups.

The political commitment that shaped the early response to the epidemic should be affirmed in legislation, as well as in policy, entrenching the universal right to health, including access to HIV/AIDS care and treatment.

The impact of HIV/AIDS on elected representatives and on the electoral processes, as well as on the context of vulnerability and responses to HIV/AIDS, should be analysed within larger conceptual and methodological frameworks that include cultural and social in-depth analysis. The political analysis and intervention should include consideration of cultural aspects.

Though Senegal has expended much effort on providing access to antiretroviral treatment, the fear of stigma still limits the outcomes of such efforts. A holistic approach is needed to identify the cultural, economic and social factors associated with the stigma, to enable designing of more appropriate responses, including the legislative and political measures adopted to counter both stigma and discrimination in relation to PLWHAs.

Such measures should be informed by scientific research aimed at implementing alternative preventive methods. Often politicians are unaware of advances made in the biomedical and social sciences, while researchers in these fields are unaware of the need for, as well as the opportunities granted by, political organs, resulting in a need for institutionalised dialogue. Decentralised political bodies could also be informed to play a key role in the coordination and evaluation and escalation of community-based interventions.

As regional intervention often comprises uncoordinated projects, programmes and activities, regional, decentralised elected bodies should be capacitated to exercise input, control, coordination, supervision and evaluation of countermeasures to HIV/AIDS.

Though the electoral process is a strong indicator of democratic governance, it is often biased in the projections of Western cultural models, which tend to ignore issues related to hidden social, economic and cultural exclusion; to the participation of various communities and identities in conceptualisation; and to collective participation in the conception and evaluation of political decision-making. The electoral processes could be inspired by experiences relating to the dynamics of the transfer of power within the framework of various African political cultures.

Political institutions seem to exclude the most vulnerable groups, failing to reflect their basic social, cultural and demographic characteristics, which should be considered in the transformation of political institutions. The representation of multiple identities, women and various age and social categories in legislative and elected bodies should be furthered, while civil society should be informed by African social and cultural models to consolidate all efforts made in the fight against HIV/AIDS.

Looking beyond the paradigms dominated by the biomedical approach and narrow Western political models is important not only for researchers but also for the elected members of political institutions. Instead, the emphasis should be on the wider community, societal debates (using local languages, social networks and cultures) on HIV/AIDS and democratic rights. A Wolof proverb teaches: "*réroo amul, ñak waxtam na am*" (Misunderstanding doesn't exist, it's the absence of social dialogue that exists). Such debates should animate consensus building beyond the recognition of cultural diversities.

Endnotes

1. Risk is defined as the probability that a person might be infected by a disease, with some individual behaviours considered likely to increase the probability.

2. Members of high-risk groups are individuals considered to engage in frequent individual high risk behaviour.

3. Globalisation refers to the complex international social and economic restructuring that accelerated at about the same time as the global HIV pandemic began, in the late twentieth century (Parker, 2002).

4. A former senior officer of the World Bank and winner of the 2001 Nobel Prize in economics.

5. As defined by Campbel (2003), "a 'health-enabling community"

refers to "a social and community context that enables or supports the renegotiation of social identities and the development of empowerment and critical consciousness, which are important preconditions for health-enhancing behaviour change".

6. Condom use did not appear to be significantly associated with the reduction of HIV incidence.

7. Cultural capital is also defined by Bourdieu as "cultivated dispositions that are internalized by the individual through socialization and that constitute schemes of appreciation and understanding" (Bourdieu, 1986).

8. The Wolof word for parts ("cër") also means rights.

9. Such as the Universal Declaration of Human Rights; the International Covenant on Civil and Political Rights; the International Covenant on Economic, Social and Cultural Rights; the Convention on the Elimination of All Forms of Discrimination against Women; the Convention against Torture and other Cruel, Inhuman or Degrading Treatment or Punishment; the Convention on the Rights of the Child; the African Charter of Human Rights and People's Rights; The Declaration of the UN Conference on Population and Development, Cairo, 1994; and the Declaration of the UN Conference on Women's Rights, Beijing, 1995.

10. Emotional intelligence facilitates tension release and peace-building.

References

Allemand, S., 2002. "Gouvernance, le Pouvoir Partagé", in *Le Pouvoir*, Editions Sciences Humaines, pp. 109–119.

Arnfred, S., 2004. *Re-thinking Sexualities in Africa*.

Augé, M., 1977. *Pouvoirs de Vie, Pouvoir de Morts*, Flammarion.

Banda, K., 1985. *Réflexion sur la Situation des Femmes Africaines*, Pro Mundi Vita, Dossiers, 2.

Barnett, T. et al., 2002. *AIDS in the Twenty-First Century: Disease and Globalization*.

Barnett, T. and Blaikies, P., 1992. *AIDS in Africa – Its Present and Future Impact*.

Barry, B., 1972. *Le Royaume du Waalo: Le Sénégal Avant la Conquête*. Maspéro.

Battûta, I., 1997. Voyage, III. *Indes Estrème-Orient, Espagne et Soudan*.

Beck, L.J., 2002. "Le Clientélisme au Sénégal, Un Adieu Sans Regrets?", in Diop, M.C. (ed.), *Le Sénégal Contemporain*, Karthala, pp. 529–547.

Bourdieu, P., 1986. "Three Forms of Capital", in *The Handbook of Theory and Research for the Sociology of Education*.

Bulletin Epidémiologique HIV, 2000, (8), December, CNLS, Senegal.

Bulletin Epidémiologique HIV, 2004, (11), September, CNLS, Senegal

Campbell, C., 2003. *African Issues: Letting Them Die – Why HIV/AIDS Prevention Programmes Fail.*

Chilungu, S.W., 1989. "Introduction to African Continuities", in Chilungu, S. W. and Niang, S. (eds), *African Continuities.*

Chomsky, N., 1989. *Necessary Illusions: Thought Control in Democratic Societies*, Boston, Mass.: South End Press.

Chua, A., 2003. *World on Fire: How Exporting Free Market Democracy Breeds Ethnic Hatred and Global Instability.*

Cissoko, S.M., 1975. *Tombouctou et l'Empire Songhay.* Nouvelles Editions Africaines.

Collins, O.A., 1995. *Health and Culture: Beyond the Western Paradigm.*

Dahl, R.A., 1989. *Democracy and Its Critics.* New Haven: Yale University Press.

Dawkins, R., 1989. *The Selfish Gene.*

Decossas, J.; Kare, F.; Anarpi, J.K.; Sodji, K.D.R.; Wagner, H.U., 1995. "Migration and AIDS," Lancet, Vol 346, No 8978: 826-828, September.

Diagne, P., 1981. "Le Pouvoir en Afrique", in UNESCO (ed.), *Le Concept de Pouvoir en Afrique*, Presses de l'UNESCO, pp. 28–55.

Diop, A.B., 1985. *La Société Wolof*, Paris: Karthala.

Diop, C.A., 1981. *Civilisation ou Barbarie.* Présence Africaine.

Diop, C.A.D. 1967. *L'Unité Culturelle de l'Afrique Noire.* Présence Africaine.

Diop, C.A.D., 1987. *L'Afrique Noire Pré-coloniale.* Présence Africaine.

Diop, D.A., 2000. *Femmes, Enjeu électorale: Des Chiffres Qui Parlent*, Institut Africain Pour la Démocratie, Edition Démocratie Africaine.

Diouf, M., 2001. *Histoire du Sénégal*, Maisonneuve & Larose.

Direction de la Prévision et de la Statistique, 2006. *Estimation de la Population du Sénégal de 2005 à 2015.*

Direction de la Prévision et de la Statistique, 2004. *Projections de Population du Sénégal issues du Recensement de 2002.*

Direction de la Prévision et de la Statistique, 1997. "Enquête Sénégalaise Auprès des Ménages", Rapport de Synthèse Direction de la Prévision et de la Statistique.

Direction de la Prévision et de la Statistique, 2001. "Enquête Sénégalaise Auprès des Ménages", Rapport de Synthèse Direction de la Prévision et de la Statistique.

Douglas, M., 1992. *Risk and Blame: Essays in Cultural Theory.*

Echenberg, M., 2002. *Black Death, White Medicine: Social History of Africa.* Cape Town: David Philip.

EDS-III, 1997. *Enquête Démographique et de Santé*, Senegal.

EDS-IV, 2005. *Enquête Démographique et de Santé*, Senegal.

Evans Pritchard, E.E., 1968. *Les Nuers*, Editions Gallimard NRF.

Farmer, P., 2007. "From 'Marvelous Momentum' to Health Care for All: Success Is Possible With the Right Programs", in Wars, G. (ed.), Foreign Affairs.

Fassin, D., 2004. *Afflictions – L'Afrique du Sud, de l'Apartheid au SIDA.*

FHI – BSS, 2001. *Sénégal.* Round 3.

French, M. *et al.*, 1992. *La Guerre Contre les Femmes.*

Gellar, S., 2002. "Pluralisme ou Jacobisme : Quelle Démocratie pour le Sénégal?", in Diop, M.C. (ed.), *Le Sénégal Contemporain*, Karthala, pp. 507–528.

Gluckman, M., 1965. *Law and Ritual in Tribal Society*, Oxford.

Goerg, O., 1997. "Femmes Africaines et Politique: Les Colonisées au Féminin en Afrique Occidentale", in *Femme d'Afrique*, Clio, Presses Universitaires du Murail.

Gow, J. and Desmond, 2002. *Impacts and Interventions: The HIV/AIDS Epidemic and the Children of South Africa.*

Habermas, J., 1994. "Struggles for Recognition in Democratic Constitutional State", in Gutmann, A. (ed.), *Multiculturalism: Examining the Politics of Recognition*, Princeton University Press.

Harrison, L. *et al.*, 2000. *Culture Matters: How Values Shape Human Progress.*

Huntington, S.P. 2000. "Foreword: Cultures Count", in Harrison, L. D. and Huntington, S. P. (eds), *Culture Matters: How Values Shape Human Progress.*

Ibn Battûta, 1997. *Voyage III, Inde: Extrême-Orient, Espagne et Soudan*, La Découverte/Poche.

IDA, 2005. *Rapport Mission, Revue Mi Parcours.*

Jeffrey, D. *et al.*, 2001. *Macroeconomics and Health: Investing in Health for Economic Development.*

Kaarsholm, P., 2006. *Violence, Political Culture and Development in Africa.*

Kalipeni, E. *et al.*, 2004. *HIV and AIDS in Africa: Beyond Epidemiology.*

Kassé, A.F., 2003. "Women in Politics in Senegal", IDEA/EISA/SADC Parliamentary Forum Conference, Pretoria, South Africa, 11–12 November.

Kent, S., 1998. *Gender in African Prehistory.*

Kim, J.Y., Millen, J.V., Irwin, A. and Gershman, J., 2000. *Dying for Growth: Global Inequality and the Health of the Poor.*

Lacroix, J.B. and Mbaye, S., 1976. "Le Vote des Femmes au Sénégal", *Revue Ethiopique*, (6), pp. 26–43.

Lagarde, E., Pison, G., Le Gueno, B., Enel, C. and Seck, C. 1992, "Les Facteurs de Riques de l'Infection à VIH2 Dans Une Région Rurale au Senegal", *Dossiers et Recherches*, (37), October,

Mafeje, A., 1995. "Théories de la Démocratie et Discours Africain: 'Cassons la Croûte, Mes Compagnons de Voyages!'", in Chole, E. and Ibrahim, J. (eds), *Processus de Démocratisation en Afrique: Problème et Perspectives*, pp. 1–3.

Mboup, S., Ndoye, I., Samb, D., 1988. HIV and Later Viruses in Senegal, IV International Conference on AIDS, Stockholm, Poster 5024.

Meda, N., Ndoye, I., Mboup, S., Wade, A., Ndiaye, S. and Niang, C., 1999. "Low and Stable HIV Infection Rates in Senegal: Nature Course for the Epidemic or Evidence for Success of Prevention?", *AIDS*, (13), pp. 1397–1405.

Ministère de la Santé Publique et de l'action Sociale. Division des Statistiques: Statistiques Sanitaires et Démographiques. 1994-1995, Dakar, Juillet 1996.

Ministère de la Santé Publique et de l'action Sociale. 1999.

Nadel, S.F., 1971. *Byzance Noire, le Royaume des Nupe du Nigeria*, François Maspero.

Ndiaye, S., 2001. *Femmes et Politique au Sénégal: Contribution à la Réflexion sur la Participation des Femmes Sénégalaises à la Vie Politique de 1945 à 2001.*

Mémoire de DEA, Université de Paris I, Panthéon, Sorbonne.

Ndoye, I., Taverne, B., Desclaux, A., Lanièce, I., Egrot, M., Delaportte, E., Sow, P.S., Mboup, S., Sylla, O. and Ciss M., 2002. *Présentation de l'Initiative Sénégalaise d'Accès aux Antirétroviraux in Agence Nationale de Recherches sur le SIDA (ANRS)*, Collection Sciences Sociales et SIDA: L'Initiative Sénégalaise d'Accès aux Antirétroviraux.

Nelson, S.M., 1998. "Reflections on Gender Studies in African and Asian Archaeology", in Kent, S. (ed.), *Gender in African Prehistory.*

Niane, D.T., 1975. *Le Soudan Occidental au teMembers of Parliament des Grands Empires XI–XVIè Siècle.* Présence Africaine.

Niang, C.I., 1988. "La Question de l'Unité Culturelle de l'Afrique Dans l'Oeuvre de Cheikh Anta Diop" in Diop, C.A. (ed.), *Panafrica: Revue Panafricaine de Recherches Scientifiques et d'Etudes Politiques*, (1), pp. 9–27.

Niang, C.I., 1995. "Integrating Laobe Women into AIDS Prevention Strategies in Kolda, Senegal" in Zeidenstein, S. and Moore, K. (eds), *Learning about Sexuality: A Practical Beginning*, New York: Population Council International Women's Health Coalition.

Niang, C.I., 2001. *The Socioeconomic Impacts of HIV/AIDS on Children: The Case of Senegal.*

Niang, C.I., 2002. *Réformer la Cooperation Technique Pour le Développement des Capacités. Etudes Focalisées: Le Cas des Pays en Développement.*

Niang, C.I., 2004. *It Is Raining Stones: Stigma, Violence and HIV Vulnerability among Men Who Have Sex with Men in Dakar, Senegal.*

Niekerk, A. *et al.*, 2005. *Ethics and AIDS in Africa: The Challenge to Our Thinking.*

O'Brien, D.B., 1975. *Saints and Politicians: Essays in the Organisation of a Senegalese Peasant Society.* Cambridge University Press.

O'Brien, R.C., 1972. *White Society in Black Africa: The French of Senegal.*

O'Manique, 2004. *Neoliberalism and AIDS Crisis in Sub-Saharan Africa: Globalization's Pandemic.*

ONUSIDA/Banque Mondiale, 2001. *SIDA: Lutte Contre la Pauvreté et Allégement de la Dette*, Geneva: ONUSIDA/Banque Mondiale Genève.

ONUSIDA/Pennstate, 2000. *Cadre de Communication sur le VIH/SIDA: Théories et Modèles Utilisés pour la Prévention du VIH/SIDA*, pp. 19–28.

ONUSIDA, 2000. "Iniative Quest Africaine pour une réponse á l'épidémie du VIH/SIDA," Résultats de recherche action projet migration et SIDA.

Organisation Mondiale de la Santé (OMS) Afrique, 2006. *La Santé des Populations: Rapport sur la Santé Dans la Région Africaine.*

Oyèwùmi, O., 1997. *The Invention of Women: Making An African Sense Of Western Gender Discourses.*

Parker, R.G., 2002. "The Global HIV/AIDS Pandemic, Structural Inequalities, and the Politics of International Health", *American Journal of Public Health*, 922(3), pp. 343–346.

Patterson, A., 2005. *The African State and the AIDS Crisis: Global Health.*

Patterson, A.S., 2006. *The Politics of AIDS in Africa.*

Rao, V. and Walton, M., 2004. *Culture and Public Action.*

République du Sénégal, 2003. *Annuaire des Collectivités Locales.*

Reynolds, A.; Reilly, B; Ellis, A. (eds). 2005. *Electoral Systems Design. The International IDEA Handbook.* IDEA, Stockholm.

Robinson, D. 2004. *Société Musulmanes et Pouvoir Colonial Français au Sénégal et en Mauritanie, 1880–1920,* Parcours d'Accommodation.

Sabatier, R. 1989. *SIDA l'épidémie Raciste.*

Sankal, J.L. S. Mboup, C.S. and Boye et al., 1989. Expérience de l'Utilisation de Tests Rapides Dans Une Enquête épidémiologique au Sénégal. Vth International Conference on AIDS and Associated Cancers, Marseille, Abstract 132.

Schoepf, B., 2004a. "AIDS, History and Struggles over Meaning in HIV and AIDS", in Kalipeni, E., Craddock, S., Oppong, J.R., (eds), *Africa: Beyond Epidemiology*, pp. 15–28.

Schoepf, B. 2004b. "AIDS in Africa: Structure, Agency, and Risk", in Kalipeni, E., Craddock, S., Oppong, J.R. and Ghosh, J. (eds), *Africa: Beyond Epidemiology.* pp. 121–132.

Siplon P., 2005. "AIDS and Patriarchy: Ideological Obstacles to Effective Policy Making", in Patterson A. S. (ed.), *The African State and the AIDS Crisis.*

Skard T., 2003. *Continent of Mothers: Understanding and Promoting Development in Africa Today, Continent of Hope.*

Slayter B., 2003. *Southern Exposure: International Development and the Global South in the Twenty-First Century.*

Sow, P. et al., 1997. Aspects épidémiologiques de l'Infection Rétro Virale à VIH à Partir d'Une Population Malade de Dakar, VIIIé Conférence Internationale sur le SIDA en Afrique, MOP54.

Stiglitz J., 2002. *Globalization and its Discontents.*

Strand. P., Mathosa, A., Strode, K. and Chirambo, 2005. "HIV/AIDS and Democratic Governance", in Strand, P. and Chirambo, K. (eds), *South Africa: Illustrating the Impact on Electoral Processes.*

Tamba, M., 2006. Approche Sociologique de l'Assemblée Nationale du Sénégal de 1960 à 2001, *Annales de la FLSH Société en Devenir: Mélanges Offerts à Boubakar LY.* Dakar: PUD.

Tyldesley, J., 1994. *Daughters of Isis: Women of Ancient Egypt.*

UNAIDS, 1999. *Acting Early to Prevent AIDS: The Case of Senegal,* 4th ed., UNAIDS.

UNAIDS, 2000. *Report on the Global AIDS Epidemic.*

UNAIDS, 2004. *Report on the Global AIDS Epidemic.*

UNAIDS, 2006. *Report on the Global AIDS Epidemic.*

UNESCO, 2003. *Women and Peace in Africa: Case Studies on Traditional Conflict Resolution Practices.*

UNESCO/BREDA, 2005. *Statistiques et Analyses Sous-régionales: Education Pour Tous en Afrique 2006,* Rapport Dakar 6.

Wars, G., 2007. *Foreign Affairs,* March/April.

Wone, I., Barondra-Haaby, E., Lallement, A.M., Sinankwa, and De Lauture, H., 1984. *Première Analyse d'Indicateurs de Santé à Partir des Statistiques Officielles du Ministère de la Santé Publique du Sénégal de 1960 à 1979.*

Ziegler J., 1999. *Les Nouveaux Maîtres du Monde et Ceux Qui Leur Résistent.* Fayard.

Abbreviations

AFP	Alliance des Forces Patriotiques
CENA	Commission Electorale Nationale Autonome
COSW	Council of Senegalese Women
FGD	focus group discussion
FPTP	first-past-the-post
ICATU	International Conference of African Trade Unions
ISAARV	Initiative Senegalaise d'Accès aux Antiretroviraux
KAP	knowledge, attitudes and practices
MMP	mixed member proportional
MP	Member of Parliament
ONEL	Observatoire National des Elections
PLWHA	people living with HIV/AIDS
PR	proportional representation
PS	Parti Socialiste
VCT	voluntary counselling and testing

Participating research institutions

Gisa's Governance and AIDS Programme (GAP)

GAP's mission is centred on promoting knowledgeable governance and developing visionary leadership and citizen agency to deal effectively with the pandemic. The approach emphasises the strong interaction between empirical research and policy actions based on communicative and collaborative citizen-state relationships. GAP's vision is to build AIDS-resilient democratic societies in Africa. The idea of resilience conveys not only improved management of the pandemic by state institutions, but the existence of thriving democratic communities, able to confront the epidemic and its consequences with confidence, looking towards a more hopeful future.

Contact: 357 Visagie St, Pretoria, South Africa 0001
Tel: (27 12) 392 0500

The Centre for Social Research (CSR)

The CSR was established at the University of Malawi in 1971. It provides research-based information to scholars, decision-makers and planners to stimulate high quality academic debate and to contribute towards the formulation of sound policies. The CSR is an organ of the University of Malawi that conducts and promotes excellence in academic and applied social science research in partnership with the public and private sector to inform policy and offer training for capacity building.

Contact: P.O. Box 278, Zomba, Malawi.
Tel: (265) 1 524 916/800; 1 525 194.
Email: csrbasis@malawi.net; csr@malawi.net

The Foundation for Democratic Process (FODEP)

FODEP is a non-partisan, voluntary and non profit civic organisation working for the promotion and protection of good governance and the democratisation process in Zambia. The foundation was formed in 1992 as a successor to the Zambia Election Monitoring and Coordinating Committee (ZEMCC).

FODEP's mission is "to promote and strengthen democracy, human rights, good governance and development in Zambia through election monitoring, lobbying and advocacy, civic education, training, information dissemination and conflict resolution".

Contact: www.fodep.org.zm

The Namibia Institute for Democracy (NID)

NID was founded in 1991 with the aim of educating Namibians about democracy. The founders of the NID have declared their commitment to a multi-party democracy which they consider to be the only viable form of governance for the Republic of Namibia. Registered as an Association not for Gain in accordance with Article 21 of the Companies Act, No. 61 of 1973, NID is a non-political institution which guards its political neutrality and objectivity. The operations of NID are structured into four divisions: The Civic Education Program, the Public Dialogue Centre, the Civil Society Support Program and the AIDS and Governance Program.

Contact: 29 Feld St, Central Windhoek PO Box 11956, Klein Windhoek

Tel (264 61) 229117/8
Fax (264 61) 229119

Economic and Social Research Foundation (ESRF)

ESRF was established in 1993 as an independent not-for-profit non-governmental research institute for capacity building in economic and social policy analysis. The Foundation started its operations in April 1994. The main objective of ESRF is to build and strengthen human and institutional capabilities in economic and social policy analysis and decision-making and to enhance the understanding of policy options within the government, public sector, donor community and in the growing national non-governmental sector, mainly, but not only, in Tanzania.

Contact: 51 Uporoto street, Ursino estates
PO Box 31226 Dar es Salaam
Tel (255 22) 2760260 or 2760751.
Fax (255 713) 3245078

Institut des Sciences de l'Environnement/Institute for Environmental Studies, Cheikh Anta Diop University

The Institut des Sciences de l'Environnment (ISE) is a doctored level institute affiliated to the Faculte des Sciences et Techniques of the University Cheikh Anta Diop-Dakar, Senegal. The training supplied is based on teaching and research on environmental issues. It was created in June 1979 and started with technical and financial support from the Belgium government.

Contact: Universite Cheick Anta Diop
PO Box 5005 Dakar-Fann, Senegal.
Tel +(221 869) 2766.
Fax : (221 825) 28 83
Email: rectorat@ucad.sn

ppendix: Maps

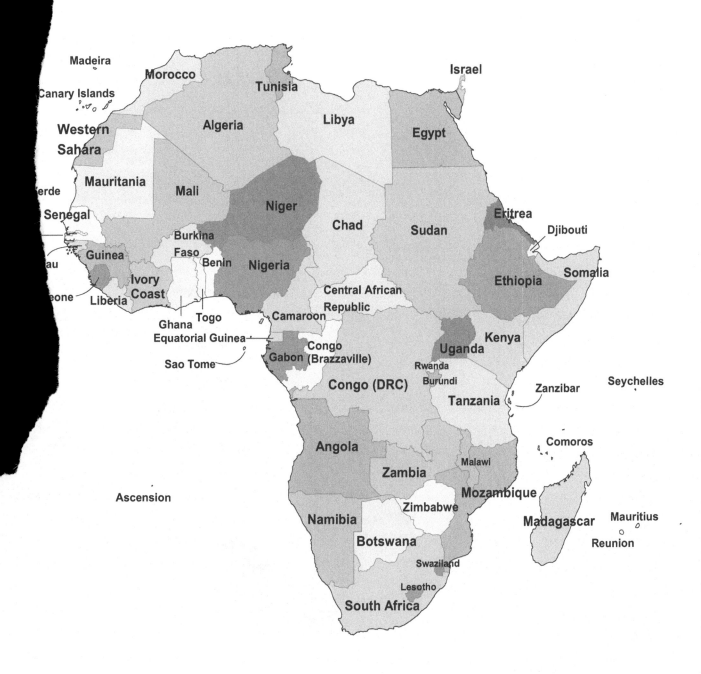

Population (2005)

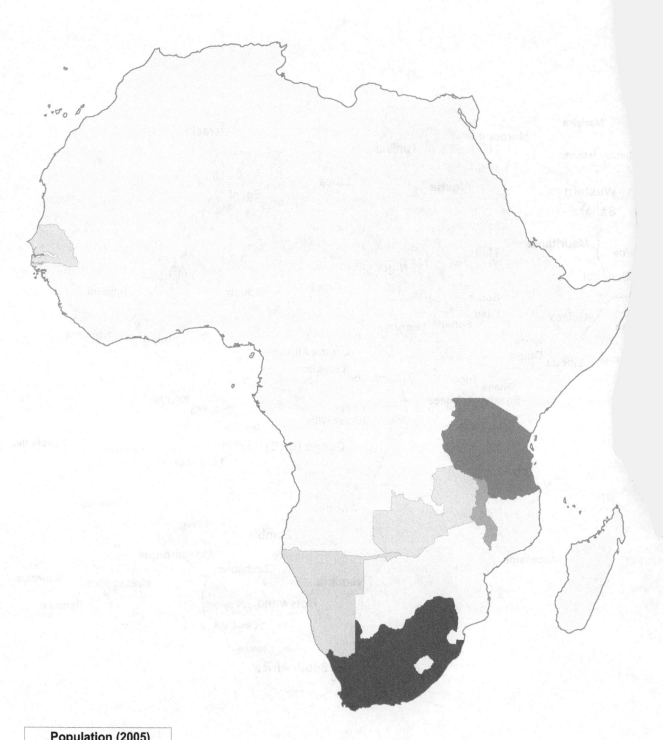

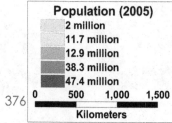

Population (2005)
- 2 million
- 11.7 million
- 12.9 million
- 38.3 million
- 47.4 million

0   500   1,000   1,500
Kilometers

der Disaggregated Population Data (2005)

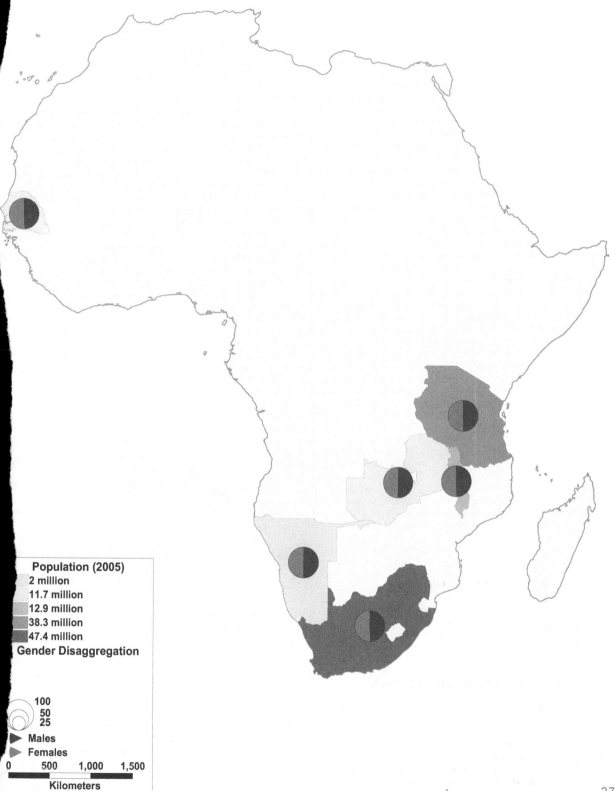

Population (2005)
- 2 million
- 11.7 million
- 12.9 million
- 38.3 million
- 47.4 million

Gender Disaggregation

100
50
25

▶ Males
▶ Females

0   500   1,000   1,500
Kilometers

Gender Disaggregated Adult Mortality per 1000 (2004)

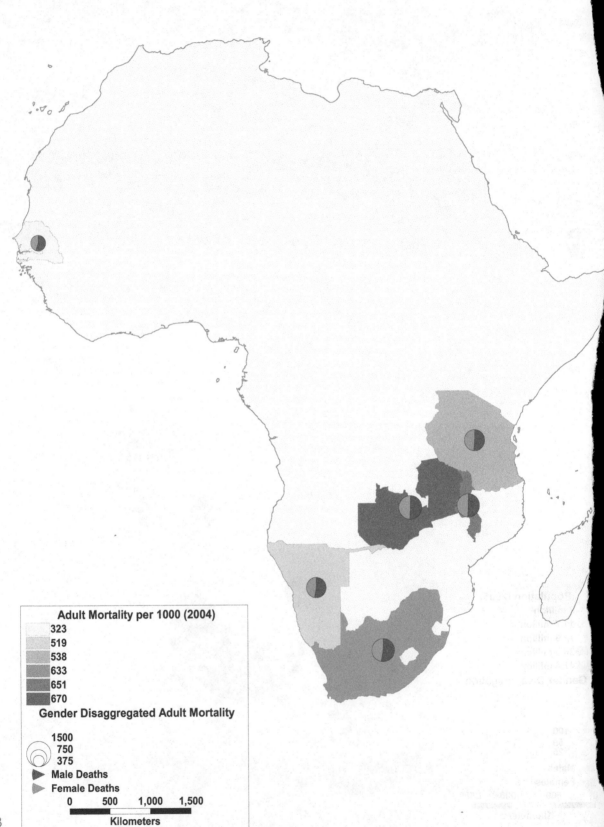

Adult Mortality per 1000 (2004)

- 323
- 519
- 538
- 633
- 651
- 670

Gender Disaggregated Adult Mortality

- 1500
- 750
- 375

▶ Male Deaths
▶ Female Deaths

0   500   1,000   1,500
Kilometers

49 Age Group HIV/AIDS Prevalence (2005)

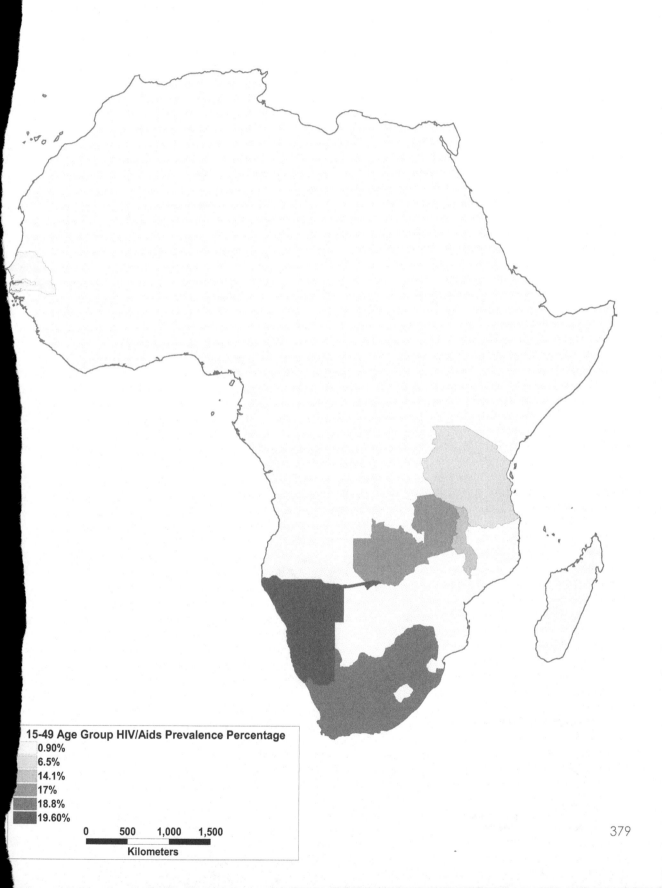

15-49 Age Group HIV/Aids Prevalence Percentage
- 0.90%
- 6.5%
- 14.1%
- 17%
- 18.8%
- 19.60%

0   500   1,000   1,500
Kilometers

Average Life Expectancy (2004)

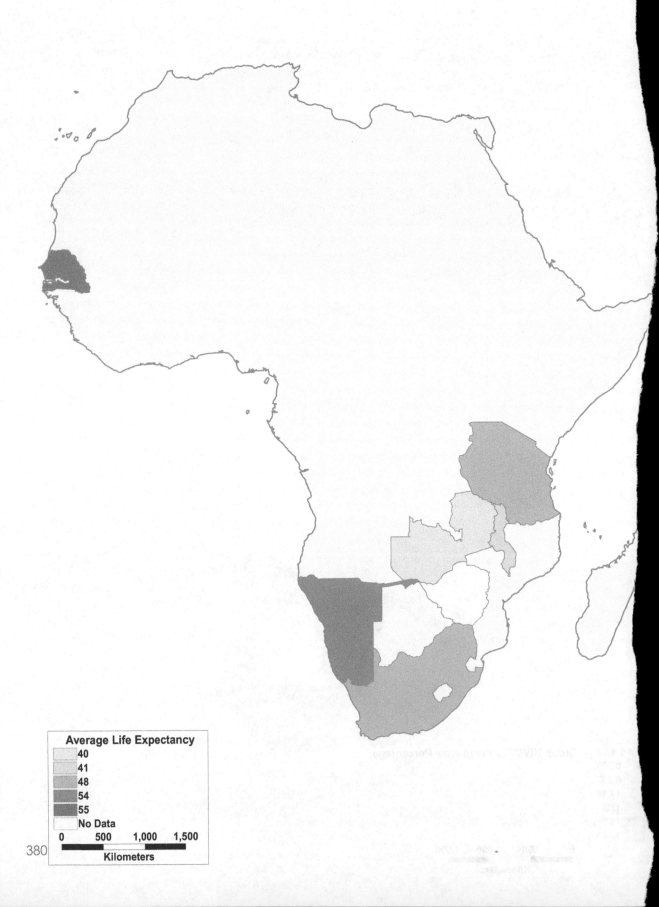

Average Life Expectancy

	40
	41
	48
	54
	55
	No Data

0   500   1,000   1,500
Kilometers

rage Male Life Expectancy (2004)

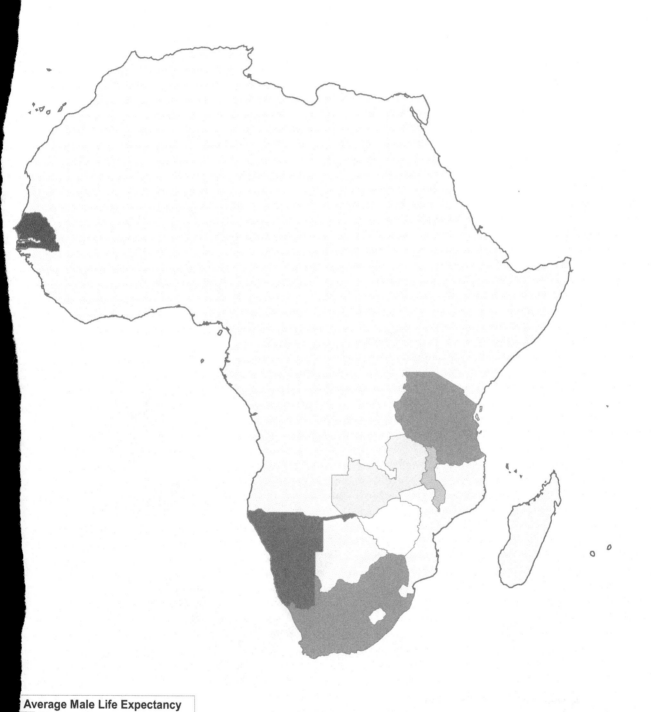

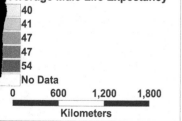

Average Male Life Expectancy

40
41
47
47
54
No Data

0   600   1,200   1,800
Kilometers

Average Female Life Expectancy (2004)

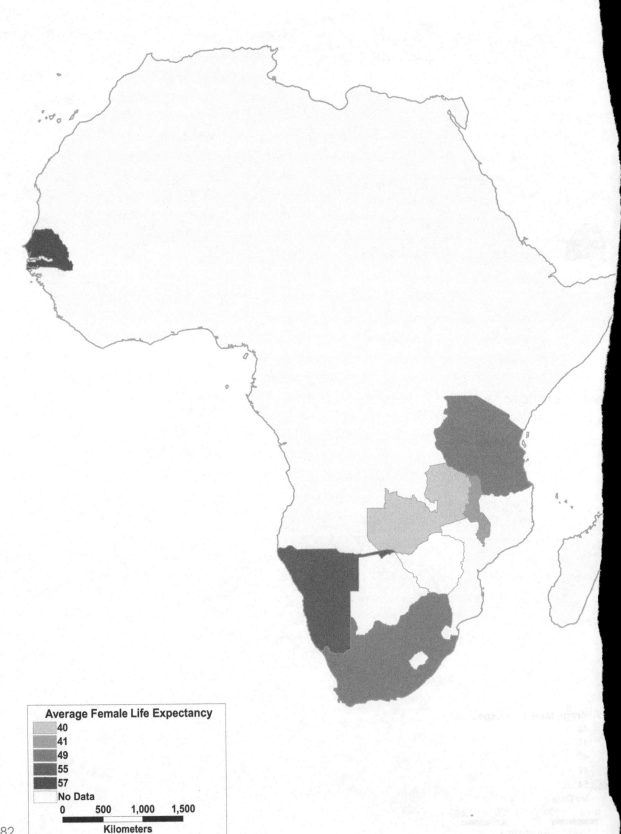

Average Female Life Expectancy
- 40
- 41
- 49
- 55
- 57
- No Data

0   500   1,000   1,500
Kilometers

S Deaths as a Percentage of All Deaths (2002)

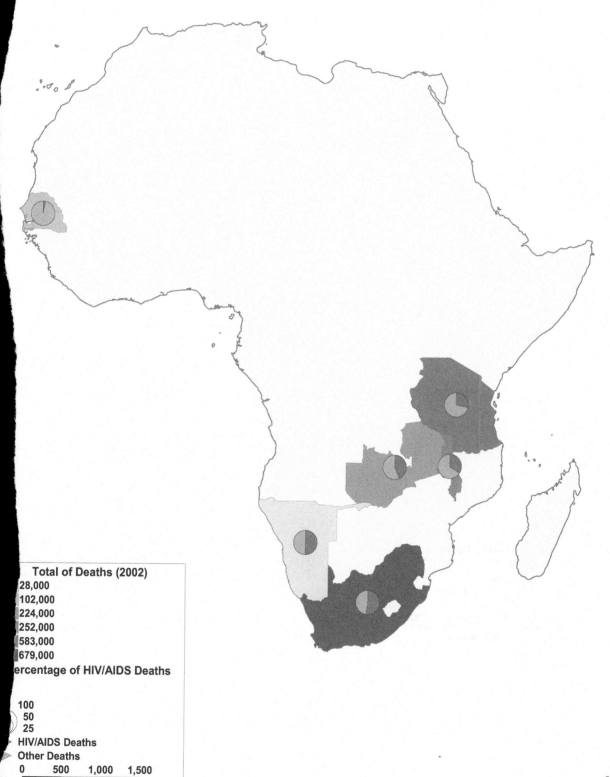

Total of Deaths (2002)
28,000
102,000
224,000
252,000
583,000
679,000

ercentage of HIV/AIDS Deaths

100
50
25

HIV/AIDS Deaths
Other Deaths

0   500   1,000   1,500

Kilometers

Types of Electoral Systems used in Countries

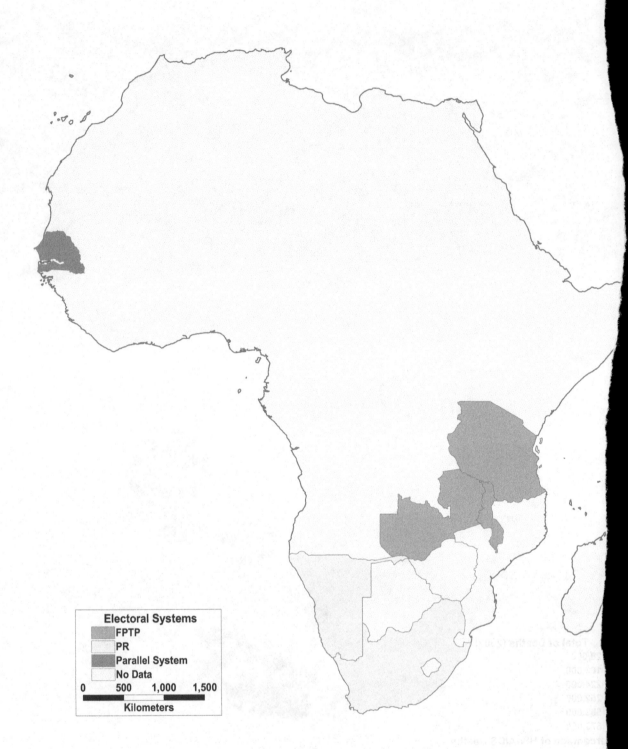

Electoral Systems
- FPTP
- PR
- Parallel System
- No Data

0   500   1,000   1,500
Kilometers

rage Cost of By-elections in FPTP and MMP Countries

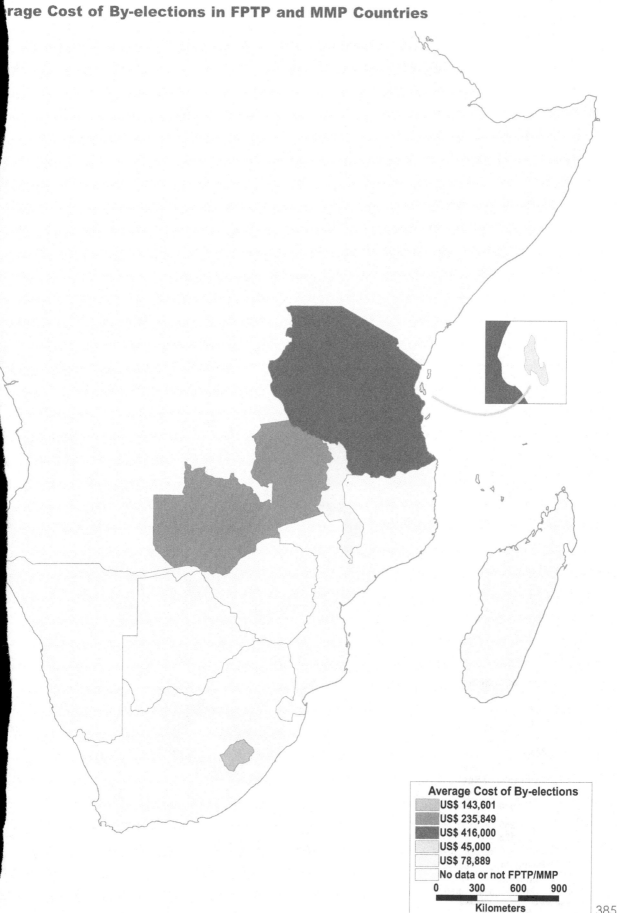

Average Cost of By-elections

	US$ 143,601
	US$ 235,849
	US$ 416,000
	US$ 45,000
	US$ 78,889
	No data or not FPTP/MMP

0	300	600	900

Kilometers

Distribution of Seats in Parliament per Country

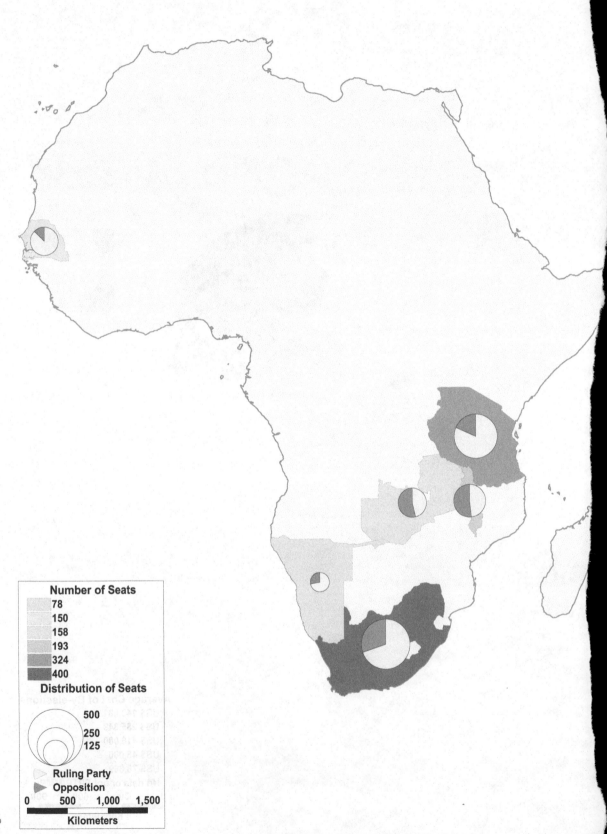

Number of Seats
- 78
- 150
- 158
- 193
- 324
- 400

Distribution of Seats

- 500
- 250
- 125

Ruling Party
Opposition

0   500   1,000   1,500
Kilometers

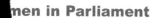

men in Parliament

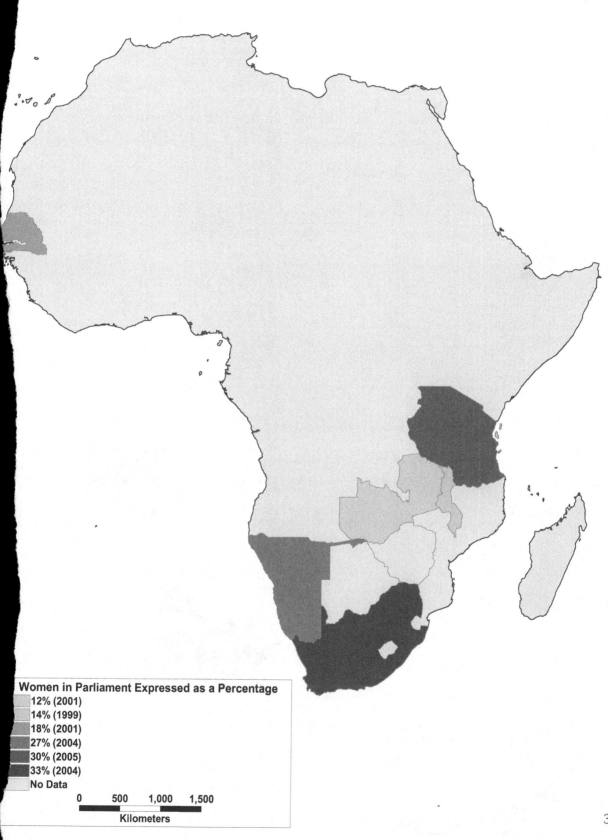

Women in Parliament Expressed as a Percentage
- 12% (2001)
- 14% (1999)
- 18% (2001)
- 27% (2004)
- 30% (2005)
- 33% (2004)
- No Data

0   500   1,000   1,500
Kilometers

Average Age of Parliamentarians

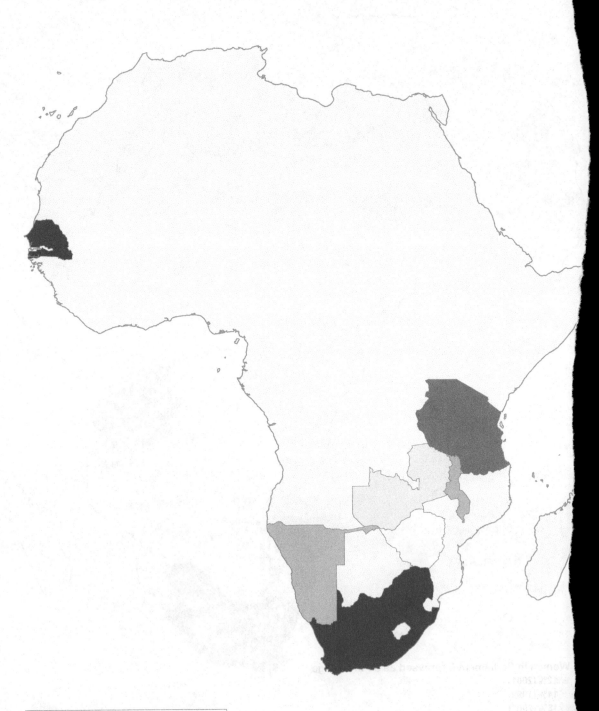

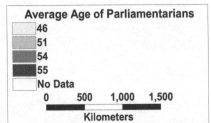

Average Age of Parliamentarians
- 46
- 51
- 54
- 55
- No Data

0   500   1,000   1,500
Kilometers

ing Age Population (2004-2006)

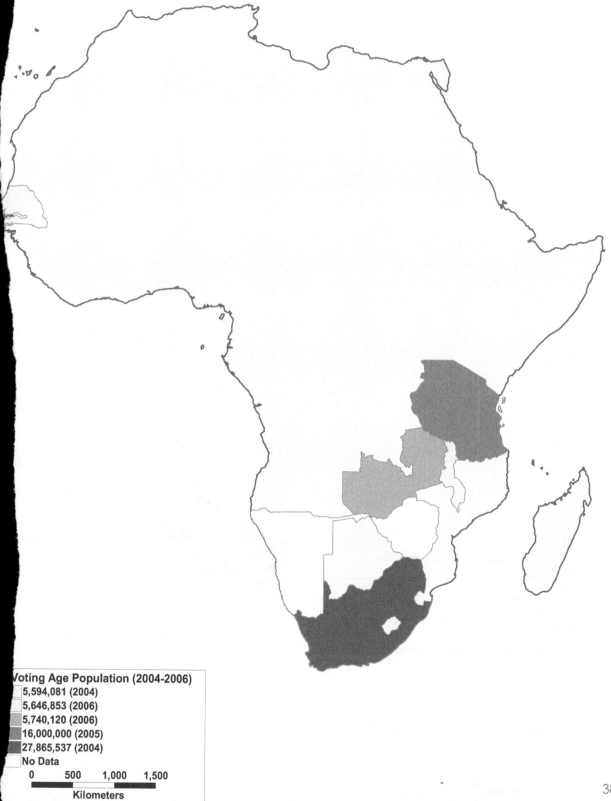

Voting Age Population (2004-2006)
- 5,594,081 (2004)
- 5,646,853 (2006)
- 5,740,120 (2006)
- 16,000,000 (2005)
- 27,865,537 (2004)
- No Data

0   500   1,000   1,500
Kilometers

Voter Turnout as a Percentage of Voting Age Population (2004-2006)

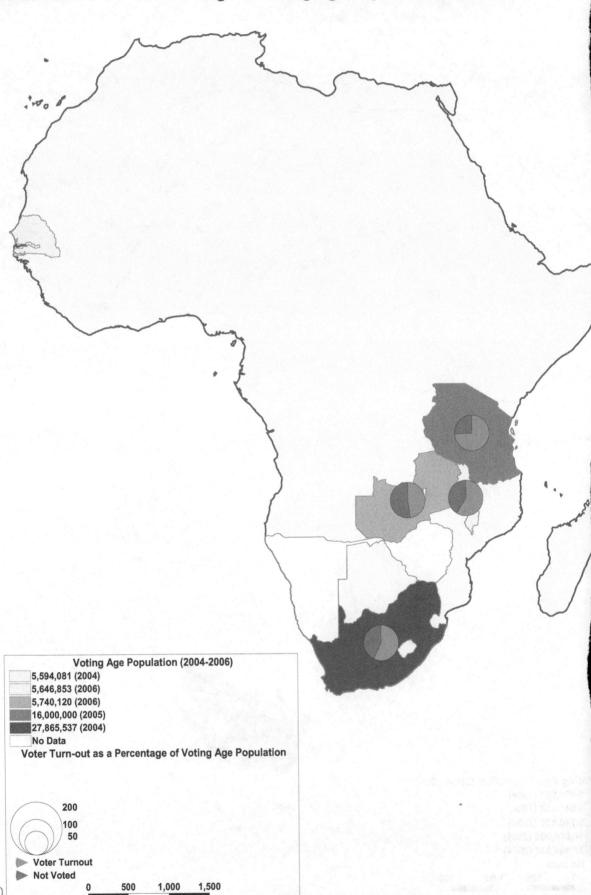

Voting Age Population (2004-2006)
- 5,594,081 (2004)
- 5,646,853 (2006)
- 5,740,120 (2006)
- 16,000,000 (2005)
- 27,865,537 (2004)
- No Data

Voter Turn-out as a Percentage of Voting Age Population

200
100
50

Voter Turnout
Not Voted

0   500   1,000   1,500
Kilometers